MYOCARDIAL HEART DISEASE
(Excluding Hypertrophic Cardiomyopathy)

Collected Reprints
(1969-2020)

By

William C. Roberts, MD

and

Colleagues

ISBN: 979-8-88862-141-7
Printed in the United States of America on acid-free paper.

Table of Contents

86.* **Endomyocardial disease and eosinophilia. A clinical and pathologic spectrum** 1
Roberts WC, Liegler DG, Carbone PP. *Am J Med.* 1969;46(1):28-42.

90. **Papillary muscle fibrosis in primary myocardial disease** 16
Marcus FI, Gomez L, Glancy DL, Ewy GA, Roberts WC. *Am Heart J.* 1969;77(5):681-685.

119. **Löffler's fibroplastic parietal endocarditis, eosinophilic leukemia, and Davies' endomyocardial fibrosis: the same disease at different stages?** 21
Roberts WC, Buja LM, Ferrans VJ. *Pathol Microbiol (Basel).* 1970;35(1):90-95.

131. **Iron in the heart. Etiology and clinical significance** 27
Buja LM, Roberts WC. *Am J Med.* 1971;51(2):209-221.

211. **Pathologic anatomy of the cardiomyopathies. Idiopathic dilated and hypertrophic types, infiltrative types, and endomyocardial disease with and without eosinophilia** 40
Roberts WC, Ferrans VJ. *Hum Pathol.* 1975;6(3):287-342.

225. **Massive myocardial hemosiderosis: a structure-function conference at the National Heart and Lung Institute** 96
Arnett EN, Nienhuis AW, Henry WL, Ferrans VJ, Redwood DR, Roberts WC. *Am Heart J.* 1975;90(6):777-787.

273. **Sarcoidosis of the heart. A clinicopathologic study of 35 necropsy patients (group 1) and review of 78 previously described necropsy patients (group 11)** 107
Roberts WC, McAllister HA Jr, Ferrans VJ. *Am J Med.* 1977;63(1):86-108.

297. **Cardiomyopathy and myocarditis: morphologic features** 130
Roberts WC. *Adv Cardiol.* 1978;(22):184-198.

309. **Myocardial biopsy: a useful diagnostic procedure or only a research tool?** 145
Ferrans VJ, Roberts WC. *Am J Cardiol.* 1978;41(5):965-967.

363. **Clinical pathologic conference. Left and right ventricular myocardial infarction in idiopathic dilated cardiomyopathy** 148
Isner JM, Virmani R, Itscoitz SB, Roberts WC. *Am Heart J.* 1980;99(2):235-242.

365. **Cardiac sarcoidosis: a major cause of sudden death in young individuals** 156
Virmani R, Bures JC, Roberts WC. *Chest.* 1980;77(3):423-428.

397. **Congenital hypoplasia of portions of both right and left ventricular myocardial walls. Clinical and necropsy observations in two patients with parchment heart syndrome** 162
Waller BF, Smith ER, Blackbourne BD, Arce FP, Sarkar NN, Roberts WC. *Am J Cardiol.* 1980;46(5):885-891.

401. **Hemochromatosis heart disease: an unemphasized cause of potentially reversible restrictive cardiomyopathy** 169
Cutler DJ, Isner JM, Bracey AW, Hufnagel CA, Conrad PW, Roberts WC, Kerwin DM, Weintraub AM. *Am J Med.* 1980;69(6):923-928.

432. **Hemodynamic cardiac constriction without anatomic myocardial restriction or pericardial constriction** 175
McManus BM, Bren GB, Robertson EA, Katz RJ, Ross AM, Roberts WC. *Am Heart J.* 1981;102(1):134-136.

483. **Atrioventricular valve replacement in the idiopathic hypereosinophilic syndrome** 178
Harley JB, McIntosh CL, Kirklin JJ, Maron BJ, Gottdiener J, Roberts WC, Fauci AS. *Am J Med.* 1982;73(1):77-81.

485. **NIH conference. The idiopathic hypereosinophilic syndrome. Clinical, pathophysiologic, and therapeutic considerations** 183
Fauci AS, Harley JB, Roberts WC, Ferrans VJ, Gralnick HR, Bjornson BH. *Ann Intern Med.* 1982;97(1):78-92.

520. **Two-dimensional echocardiographic assessment of the idiopathic hypereosinophilic syndrome. Anatomic basis of mitral regurgitation and peripheral embolization** 198
Gottdiener JS, Maron BJ, Schooley RT, Harley JB, Roberts WC, Fauci AS. *Circulation.* 1983;67(3):572-578.

529. **Clinical and morphologic cardiac findings after anthracycline chemotherapy. Analysis of 64 patients studied at necropsy** 205
Isner JM, Ferrans VJ, Cohen SR, Witkind BG, Virmani R, Gottdiener JS, Beck JR, Roberts WC. *Am J Cardiol.* 1983;51(7):1167-1174.

530. **Amyloidosis limited to small arteries causing angina pectoris and sudden death** 213
Saffitz JE, Sazama K, Roberts WC. *Am J Cardiol.* 1983;51(7):1234-1235.

540. **Cardiac amyloidosis causing cardiac dysfunction: analysis of 54 necropsy patients** 215
Roberts WC, Waller BF. *Am J Cardiol.* 1983;52(1):137-146.

581. **Cardiac involvement by Kaposi's sarcoma in acquired immune deficiency syndrome (AIDS)** 225
Silver MA. Macher AM, Reichert CM, Levens DL, Parrillo JE, Longo DL, Roberts WC. *Am J Cardiol.* 1984; 53(7):983-985.

767. **Idiopathic dilated cardiomyopathy: analysis of 152 necropsy patients** 228
Roberts WC, Siegel RJ, McManus BM. *Am J Cardiol.* 1987;60(16):1340-1355.

787. **Sudden death in hemochromatosis after closed-chest catheter ablation of the atrioventricular junction** 244
Lemery R, Brugada P, Havenith M, Barbour D, Roberts WC, Wellens HJ. *Am J Cardiol.* 1988;61(11):941-943.

800. **Serial electrocardiographic changes in idiopathic dilated cardiomyopathy confirmed at necropsy** 247
Wilensky RL, Yudelman P, Cohen AI, Fletcher RD, Atkinson J, Virmani R, Roberts WC. *Am J Cardiol.* 1988;62(4):276-283.

808. **Frequency of myocarditis, left ventricular dysfunction and ventricular tachycardia in the acquired immune deficiency syndrome** 255
Reilly JM, Cunnion RE, Anderson DW, O'Leary TJ, Simmons JT, Lane HC, Fauci AS, Roberts WC, Virmani R, Parrillo JE. *Am J Cardiol.* 1988;62(10 Pt 1):789-793.

814. **Frequency of acute and healed myocardial infarcts in fatal cardiac amyloidosis** 260
Barbour DJ, Roberts WC. *Am J Cardiol.* 1988;62(16):1134-1135.

832. **Defining idiopathic dilated cardiomyopathy: a courtroom discussion** 262
Roberts WC. *Am J Cardiol.* 1989;63(12):893-896.

880. **Pathologic findings associated with interleukin-2-based immunotherapy for cancer: a postmortem study of 19 patients** ... 266
Kragel AH, Travis WD, Feinberg L, Pittaluga S, Striker LM, Roberts WC, Lotze MT, Yang JJ, Rosenberg SA. *Hum Pathol.* 1990;21(5):493-502.

887. **Myocarditis or acute myocardial infarction associated with interleukin-2 therapy for cancer** ... 276
Kragel AH, Travis WD, Steis RG, Rosenberg SA, Roberts WC. *Cancer.* 1990;66(7):1513-1516.

998. **Gross and semiquantitative histologic findings in mononuclear cell myocarditis causing sudden death, and implications for endomyocardial biopsy** ... 280
Shirani J, Freant LJ, Roberts WC. *Am J Cardiol.* 1993;72(12):952-957.

1075. **Effectiveness of cardiac transplantation for primary (AL) cardiac amyloidosis** ... 286
Pelosi F Jr, Capehart J, Roberts WC. *Am J Cardiol.* 1997;79(4):532-535.

1215. **Acute myocarditis (predominately lymphocytic) causing sudden death without heart failure** ... 290
Theleman KP, Kuiper JJ, Roberts WC. *Am J Cardiol.* 2001;88(9):1078-1083.

1365. **Lymphocytic myocarditis as a cause of fulminant fatal heart failure** ... 296
Garner WL, Starling C, Kuiper JJ, Roberts WC. *Proc (Bayl Univ Med Cent).* 2006;19(2):122-123.

1472. **Cardiac transplantation for cardiac sarcoidosis with initial diagnosis by examination of the left ventricular apical "core" excised for insertion of a left ventricular assist device for severe chronic heart failure** ... 298
Roberts WC, Vowels TJ, Ko JM, Capehart JE, Hall SA. *Am J Cardiol.* 2009;103(1):110-114.

1488. **Diagnosing cardiac sarcoidosis clinically without tissue confirmation** ... 303
Sharma PS, Lubahn JG, Donsky AS, Yoon AD, Carry MM, Grayburn PA, Wood PB, Ko JM, Burton EC, Roberts WC. *Proc (Bayl Univ Med Cent).* 2009;22(3):236-238.

1510. **Alcohol ablation or ventricular septal myotomy/myectomy for severe obstructive hypertrophic cardiomyopathy?** ... 306
Roberts WC, Dearani J, Maron B. *Med Roundtable Cardiovasc Ed.* 2010;1:128-133.

1517. **Some previously neglected examples of arrhythmogenic right ventricular dysplasia/cardiomyopathy and frequency of its various reported manifestations** ... 312
Roberts WC, Ko JM, Kuiper JJ, Hall SA, Meyer DM. *Am J Cardiol.* 2010;106(2):268-274.

1546. **Examination of isolated ventricular noncompaction (hypertrabeculation) as a distinct entity in adults** ... 319
Roberts WC, Karia SJ, Ko JM, Grayburn PA, George BA, Hall SA, Kuiper JJ, Meyer DM. *Am J Cardiol.* 2011;108(5):747-752.

1606. **Isolated atrial amyloidosis and the importance of molecular classification** ... 325
Podduturi V, Armstrong DR, Hitchcock MA, Roberts WC, Guileyardo JM. *Proc (Bayl Univ Med Cent).* 2013;26(4):387-389.

1615. **Morphologic features of cardiac sarcoidosis in native hearts of patients having cardiac transplantation** ... 328
Roberts WC, Chung MS, Ko JM, Capehart JE, Hall SA. *Am J Cardiol.* 2014;113(4):706-712.

1618. **Cardiac restriction secondary to massive calcific deposits in the left ventricular cavity** 335
Roberts WC, Rosenblatt RL, Ko JM, Grayburn PA, Kuiper JJ, Guileyardo JM. *Am J Cardiol.* 2014;113(8):1442-1446.

1627. **Morphologic features of the recipient heart in patients having cardiac transplantation and analysis of the congruence or incongruence between the clinical and morphologic diagnoses** 340
Roberts WC, Roberts CC, Ko JM, Filardo G, Capehart JE, Hall SA. *Medicine (Baltimore).* 2014;93(5):211-235.

1639. **The two extremes of cardiac sarcoidosis and the effect of prednisone therapy** 365
Armstrong D, Gonzalez-Stawinski GV, Ko JM, Hall SA, Roberts WC. *Am J Cardiol.* 2015;115(1):150-153.

1663. **Frequency of massive cardiac adiposity (floating heart) at necropsy and comparison of clinical and morphologic variables with cases with nonmassive cardiac adiposity at a single Texas hospital, 2013 to 2014** 369
Roberts WC, Won VS, Vasudevan A, Ko JM, Guileyardo JM. *Am J Cardiol.* 2016;117(6):1006-1013.

1679. **Characteristics of hearts at necropsy in patients treated chronically with prednisone (the corticosteroid heart)** 377
Roberts WC, Won VS, Vasudevan A, Guileyardo JM. *Am J Cardiol.* 2016;118(12):1935-1940.

1702. **Usefulness of total 12-lead QRS voltage as a clue to diagnosis of patients with cardiac sarcoidosis severe enough to warrant orthotopic heart transplant** 383
Roberts WC, Becker TM, Hall SA. *JAMA Cardiol.* 2018;3(1):64-68.

1715. **Usefulness of total 12-lead QRS voltage for diagnosis of arrhythmogenic right ventricular cardiomyopathy in patients with heart failure severe enough to warrant orthotopic heart transplantation and morphologic illustration of its cardiac diversity** 388
Roberts WC, Kondapalli N, Hall SA. *Am J Cardiol.* 2018;122(6):1051-1061.

1720. **Total 12-lead QRS voltage in patients having orthotopic heart transplantation for heart failure caused by adriamycin-induced cardiomyopathy** 399
Roberts WC, Haque S, Hall SA. *Cardiology.* 2018;141(3):172-175.

1736. **Comparison of clinical and morphologic findings in patients with cardiac sarcoidosis severe enough to warrant heart transplantation in those with -vs- those without non-caseating granulomas in the explanted heart (burnt-out sarcoid)** 403
Fathima S, Roberts WC. *Am J Cardiol.* 2019;124(4):599-603.

1742. **Severe eosinophilic myocarditis in the portion of left ventricular wall excised to insert a left ventricular assist device for severe heart failure** 408
Roberts WC, Kietzman AT. *Am J Cardiol.* 2020;125(2):264-269.

1743. **Massive cardiomegaly (>1000 g heart) and obesity** 414
Roberts WC, Khan OS. *Am J Cardiol.* 2020;125(2):277-281.

*Articles are numbered based on WCR's CV.

Endomyocardial Disease and Eosinophilia*

A Clinical and Pathologic Spectrum

WILLIAM C. ROBERTS, M.D., DONALD G. LIEGLER, M.D. *and* PAUL P. CARBONE, M.D.
Bethesda, Maryland

Three patients with cardiomegaly, congestive cardiac failure and blood eosinophilia are described. Necropsy in two disclosed severe mural endocardial fibrosis with superimposed fibrin-platelet thrombi, myocardial scarring, eosinophilic hyperplasia of the bone marrow and spleen without abnormal or leukemic myeloblasts, and occasionally thrombosed small arteries in the heart, spleen, kidneys and lungs. These features are similar to those described in patients with Löffler's fibroplastic parietal endocarditis and in "eosinophilic leukemia" without abnormal myelopoiesis. It is suggested that these two conditions are the same disease. It is also suggested that the predominantly African condition, endomyocardial fibrosis without eosinophilia, may be a late or inactive stage of either Löffler's endocarditis or of "eosinophilic leukemia" without abnormal myelopoiesis.

SINCE 1953 three patients have been referred to the National Cancer Institute because of "eosinophilic leukemia." Each had large numbers of mature eosinophils in the blood and severe, ultimately fatal, congestive cardiac failure. Necropsy in two of the three patients disclosed extensive endomyocardial fibrosis with superimposed thrombi, similar to that described in Löffler's fibroplastic parietal endocarditis. In addition, small arterial and arteriolar lesions were found in several organs, an observation in accord with the thesis that "eosinophilic leukemia" and Löffler's syndrome" may be "collagen disease" [*1,2*]. Observations in these three patients are described with a discussion of their meaning.

CASE REPORTS

CASE 1. A twenty-five year old soldier (L.E., 01-95-95), who died on October 18, 1958, had been well until January 1957 when a nonproductive cough developed. In March 1957 fever (with temperatures up to 100.5°F.), pedal edema and exertional dyspnea appeared and he was hospitalized. An examination in October 1956 had disclosed no abnormalities. Examination now, however, showed distended neck veins, cardiomegaly, increased pulmonic second sound, ventricular gallop and grade 3/6 blowing apical pansystolic and grade 3/6 diastolic apical murmurs. The liver and spleen were enlarged, and the feet were edematous. The peripheral white blood cell count was 24,000 per cu. mm. with 51 per cent eosinophils, 26 per cent neutrophils and 23 per cent lymphocytes. The hematocrit was 31 per cent and the erythrocyte sedimentation rate in one hour was 37 mm. Aspirated bone marrow showed marked myeloid hyperplasia, but no other abnormalities.† Urinalysis revealed an occasional erythrocyte in the sediment. The serum urea nitrogen was 12 mg. per 100 ml. and serum protein 7.3 gm. per 100 ml. with a normal electrophoretic pattern. Blood cultures were negative. The lungs and heart appeared normal on the initial chest roentgenogram, but subsequent ones disclosed progressive cardiomegaly (Fig. 1).

A regimen consisting of bed rest, digitalis, diuretics and a low salt diet failed to alter the signs and symptoms of cardiac failure. Cortisone (380 mg. per day) then was given for four weeks, when the dosage was tapered. The white blood cell count rose (to 108,000 per cu. mm. with 50 per cent eosinophils) and the erythrocyte sedimentation rate and blood hemoglobin levels became normal. Fol-

† Tests for trichinosis, lupus erythematosus preparations, antistreptolysin titer, and examinations of feces for ova, parasites and blood in each of the three patients were negative or normal.

* From the Section of Pathology, National Heart Institute, and the Solid Tumor Service, Medicine Branch, National Cancer Institute, National Institutes of Health, Bethesda, Maryland 20014. Requests for reprints should be addressed to William C. Roberts, M.D., Section of Pathology, National Heart Institute, National Institutes of Health, Bethesda, Maryland 20014. Manuscript received January 17, 1968.

lowing discontinuance of the cortisone, the erythrocyte sedimentation rate rose to 58 mm. per hour, the hematocrit dropped to 30 per cent and the white blood cell count dropped to 4,000 per cu. mm. with 30 per cent eosinophils. In May 1957 the spleen was noted to be large and tender, and the patient was given radiation to the left upper quadrant. In addition, Myleran® (4 mg. per day) was given for several weeks, and during this time the eosinophil count decreased. On October 23, 1957, the patient was transferred to the Clinical Center. At the time of admission his only medication was digitalis.

On examination, the findings were similar to those observed seven months earlier. The temperature was 98°F. and the blood pressure, 120/70 mm. Hg. The neck veins were distended, the heart was enlarged with recordable murmurs and a ventricular gallop, and the liver and spleen were enlarged. Direct measurement of pressure in an antecubital vein was equivalent to 18 cm. of water. The peripheral white blood cell count was 29,000 per cu. mm. with 46 per cent eosinophils, 48 per cent mature and nonfilamented neutrophils, 4 per cent lymphocytes and 2 per cent monocytes. The hematocrit was 31 per cent, the platelet count 61,000 per cu. mm. Examination of the bone marrow again showed only myeloid hyperplasia. The leukocyte alkaline phosphatase activity was normal. A skeletal muscle biopsy specimen showed mild interstitial infiltration with eosinophils, and a hepatic biopsy specimen was normal. The electrocardiogram showed normal sinus rhythm, frequent ventricular premature contractions, and QRS, T wave and S-T segment changes interpreted as indicating myocardial damage and ischemia (Fig. 2). Right heart catheterization disclosed the following pressures, in mm. Hg.: pulmonary trunk 25/10; right ventricle 25/0; right atrial a wave 15, v wave 15, mean 11; pulmonary artery wedge a wave 15, v wave 20, mean 14; and brachial artery, 135/80 (mean = 100). The arterial oxygen saturation was 91 per cent, and the resting cardiac output was 5.2 L. per minute, the cardiac index, 2.7 L. per minute per M^2. With exercise, the cardiac output rose to 7.0 L. per minute, and cardiac index to 3.7 L. per minute per M^2.

The patient remained in the hospital for the next four months, and despite intensive therapy remained in cardiac failure. Signs of digitalis toxicity developed even when small doses of the drug were administered. During this period the hemoglobin varied from 7.7 to 11.4 gm. per 100 ml., the white blood cell count from 7,400 to 35,000 per cu. mm., total eosinophil count from 5,000 to 15,000 per cu. mm., platelet count from 35,000 to 395,000 per cu. mm., reticulocyte count from 1.0 to 2.8 per cent, blood urea nitrogen from 9 to 21 mg. per 100 ml. and the uric acid from 9.0 to 12.1 mg. per 100 ml. Intermittent proteinuria and microscopic hematuria were found periodically, and a red blood cell cast was found in the urine sediment on one occasion. The patient was given Mapharsen® (total dose of 140 mg.) without noticeable benefit. He was discharged on February 20, 1958, and died suddenly on October 18, 1958, of severe congestive cardiac failure.

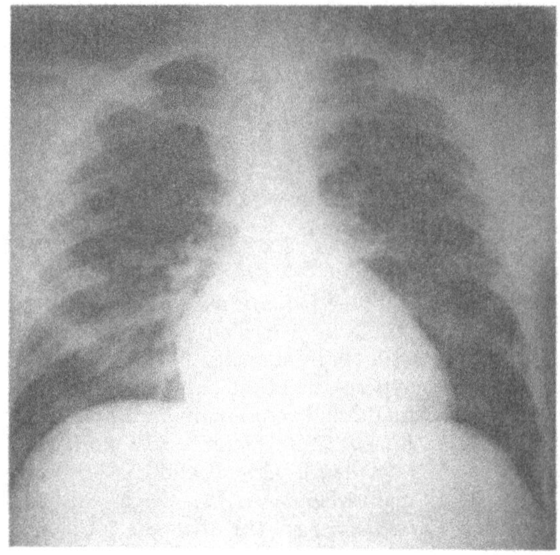

Fig. 1. Case 1. Chest roentgenogram showing generalized cardiomegaly.

An autopsy was performed at the local Air Force Hospital and subsequently fixed tissues, histologic sections and descriptions of the gross organs were submitted to the National Institutes of Health (A58-286). Necropsy disclosed edematous feet and ankles, serous pleural effusions (750 ml. each) and ascites (1,500 ml.).

The heart (Fig. 3 to 5) weighed 530 gm. Both ventricles were dilated and hypertrophied; the endocardium and subendocardium of the right ventricle was diffusely fibrotic, and that of the left ventricle was focally fibrotic. This thickened fibrous tissue was covered by recent and organizing thrombi. In addition, focal scars were present in the deeper portions of the walls of both ventricles and ventricular septum, and fibrin-platelet thrombi were present on the ventricular aspect of each of

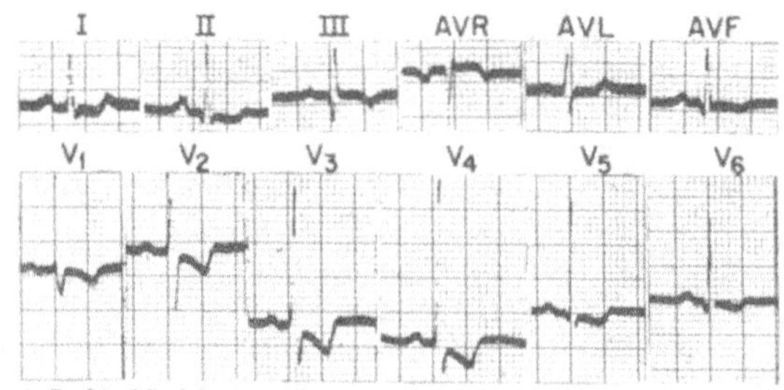

Fig. 2. Case 1. Electrocardiogram.

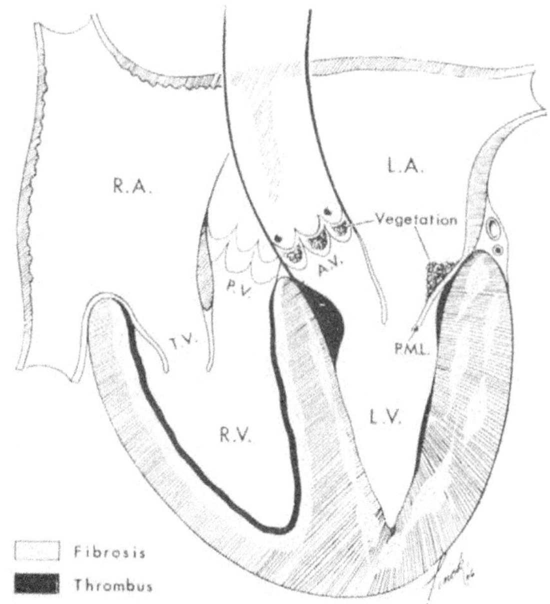

Fig. 3. Case 1. Diagrammatic representation of the cardiac lesions. All chambers are dilated and hypertrophied. The interior surface of the right ventricle is diffusely fibrotic, and the fibrous tissue is covered in most areas by fibrin-platelet thrombi. Focal mural thrombi also are present in the left ventricle. Areas of replacement fibrosis are present in the deeper portions of the ventricular walls, especially the left ventricle. Vegetative material is present on the atrial aspect of the posterior mitral leaflet and on the ventricular aspect of each of the three aortic valvular cusps, but no organisms were present.

the three aortic valvular cusps and on the atrial aspect of the anterior mitral leaflet. The valvular thrombi were devoid of bacteria (Brown and Brenn stain) and fungi (methenamine silver). The extramural coronary arteries had normal origins and courses and were free of luminal disease, but a few intramural coronary arteries showed evidence of recanalization (Fig. 6).

The liver (2,200 gm.) showed the typical changes of chronic cardiac failure, with sclerosis. The spleen (1,500 gm.) was the site of several small (<1 cm.) subcapsular infarcts, and its sinusoids contained many neutrophils, many of which were eosinophils. The bone marrow was hypercellular, the result of myeloid hyperplasia. Numerous mature eosinophils and some eosinophilic myelocytes and late promyelocytes were observed.

The left kidney weighed 160 gm., the right, 180 gm.; the surface of each was finely and uniformly pitted. The basement membranes of most glomeruli were thickened, the interstitial tissue contained an increased amount of fibrous tissue, infiltrated by inflammatory cells, mainly eosinophils. Some tubules were atrophied, and a rare arteriole and small muscular artery showed focal fibrinoid necrosis of its wall. An occasional tubule contained acute inflammatory cells. A few granulomatous lesions consisting of foreign-body type giant cells arranged circumferentially about radicular slit-like spaces were seen. No birefringent material was present.

Both left (775 gm.) and right (1,000 gm.) lungs were congested and edematous. Many alveoli were filled with erythrocytes, some with hemosiderin-laden macrophages, and some with necrotic material. A number of alveoli contained eosinophils. A rare small pulmonary artery showed evidence of recanalization (Fig. 6).

Case 2. A thirty-five year old engineer (W.D., 06-20-44) who died on November 19, 1965, had been well until December 1964 when he suffered from weakness and a recurring headache. Physical examination was unremarkable, but the peripheral white blood cell count was 14,000 per cu. mm., and the blood smear showed 70 per cent eosinophils. During the next several months he was anorectic and lost weight, periodically had fever (with tem-

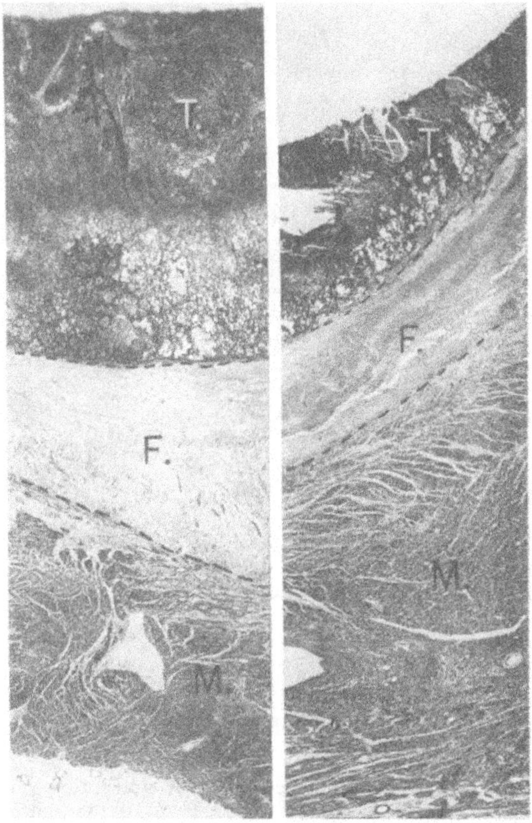

Fig. 4. Case 1. Photomicrographs of two sections extending through the entire right ventricular wall. The myocardium (M.) is covered by fibrous tissue (F.) which in turn is covered by fibrin-platelet thrombus (T.). Hematoxylin and eosin stain (left), phosphotungsten acid hematoxylin stain (right); original magnification, each × 10.

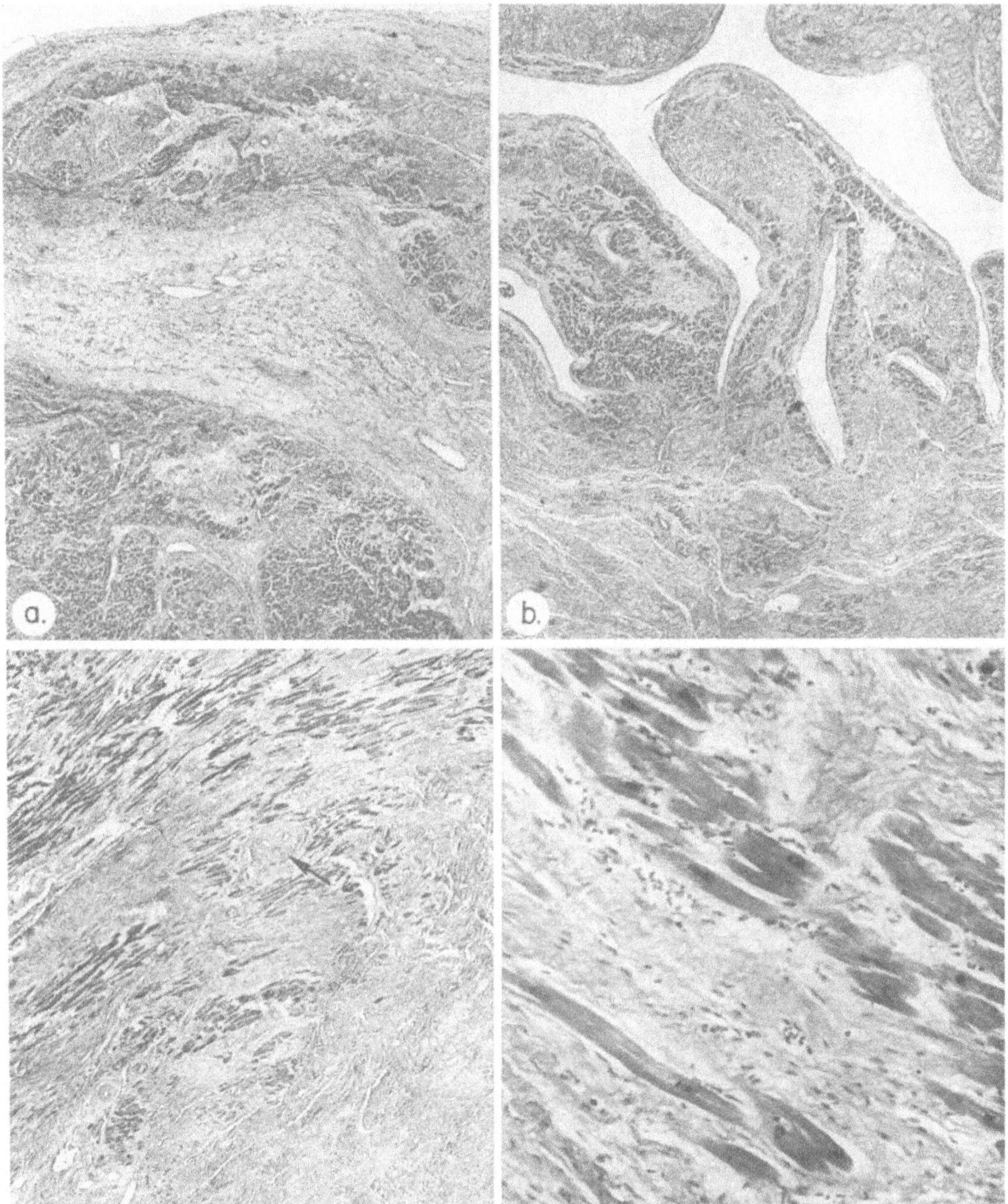

FIG. 5. Case 1. Histologic sections of myocardium and endocardium. *a*, right ventricle. Large amounts of fibrous tissue containing vascular channels covers the endocardium and large portions of myocardium are replaced by more dense fibrous tissue. Original magnification × 29. *b*, left ventricular trabecular carneae muscles. The endocardium is only mildly thickened, but much of the myocardium is replaced by fibrous tissue. Many of the myocardial fibers which remain are vacuolated. Original magnification × 29. *c*, extensive replacement fibrosis deep in the wall of the left ventricle. A small intramural coronary artery (arrow) contains four small channels, presumedly the result of recanalization of a thrombus. Original magnification × 29. *d*, close-up of left ventricular wall showing extensive fibrosis with hypertrophy of the remaining myocardial fibers. Original magnification × 170. Hematoxylin and eosin stains on each.

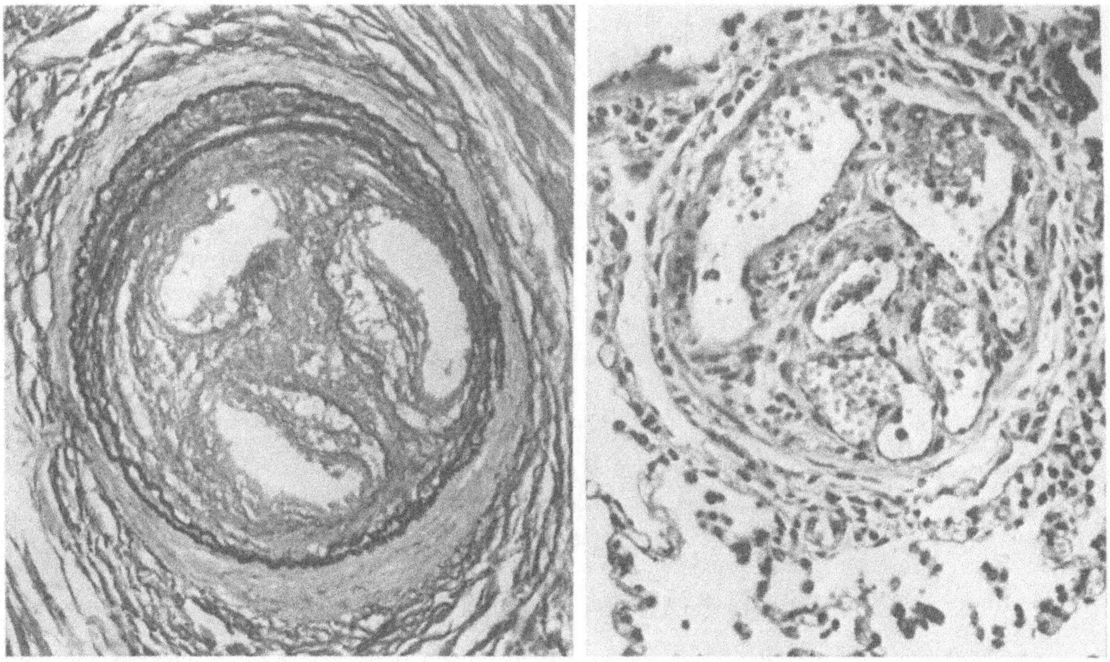

FIG. 6. Case 1. Recanalized left ventricular intramural coronary artery (left) and of a small pulmonary artery (right). Elastic van Gieson stain, original magnification × 170 (left); hematoxylin and eosin stain, original magnification × 250 (right).

peratures to 101°F.), a persistent headache, occasionally blurred vision, and in June 1965 was admitted to the National Institutes of Health. Examination disclosed an enlarged liver and spleen, dermal petechiae (chest), generalized muscle weakness, defective memory and poor interpretation of abstract concepts. The chest roentgenogram (Fig. 7) and electrocardiogram were normal. The hemoglobin was 9.1 gm. per 100 ml., white blood cell count 81,000 per cu. mm. with 80 per cent eosinophils, platelet count 158,000 per cu. mm., erythrocyte sedimentation rate 100 mm. in one hour, serum urea nitrogen 50 mg. per 100 ml. and urine sediment normal. The leukocyte alkaline phosphatase activity was 4 μM para-nitrophenol (PNP) per hour per 10^9 cells (normal 16 to 120). The intravenous pyelogram was normal. Skin, muscle and lymph node biopsy specimens revealed only infiltration with mature eosinophils. Examination of aspirated bone marrow showed eosinophilic hyperplasia without an increase in immature myeloid forms, but with hypersegmentation and cytoplasmic vacuolation of many eosinophils, and normal erythropoiesis and megakaryocytes. Drost chromosome studies of the marrow revealed a total of 36 analyzable metaphases. All had 46 chromosomes without the Philadelphia chromosome.

The patient was treated with prednisone (initially 60 mg. per day and later 40 mg. every other day), and the muscle strength, coordination and mentation improved. The urea nitrogen level dropped to normal, and the peripheral white blood cell count fell to a low of 10,000 per cu. mm. with 75 per cent eosinophils. The patient was discharged from the hospital on July 31, 1965. Two weeks later, however, headache, weakness, blurred vision and hepatosplenomegaly recurred, and the white blood cell count was 50,000 per cu. mm. with 70 per cent mature eosinophils. An electrocardiogram now showed frequent ventricular premature contractions. The dosage of prednisone was increased to 80 mg. per day but nevertheless the urea nitrogen level rose to 62 mg. per 100 ml. and "microscopic" hematuria appeared.

The symptoms persisted, the mental abnormalities reappeared and on October 18, 1965, the patient was rehospitalized. On examination the blood pressure was 136/70 mm. Hg. The face had a Cushingoid appearance, and a fine papulomacular rash was present over the trunk. The muscles in all extremities were weak, and the thenar and hypothenar musculature was atrophied. He demonstrated poor judgment, defective cognitive powers, ocular dysmetria, generalized hyperactive reflexes, including jawjerk and plantar extension on the left. The hemoglobin was 11.6 gm. per 100 ml., white blood cell count 43,000 per cu. mm. with 80 per cent eosinophils, platelet count 166,000 per

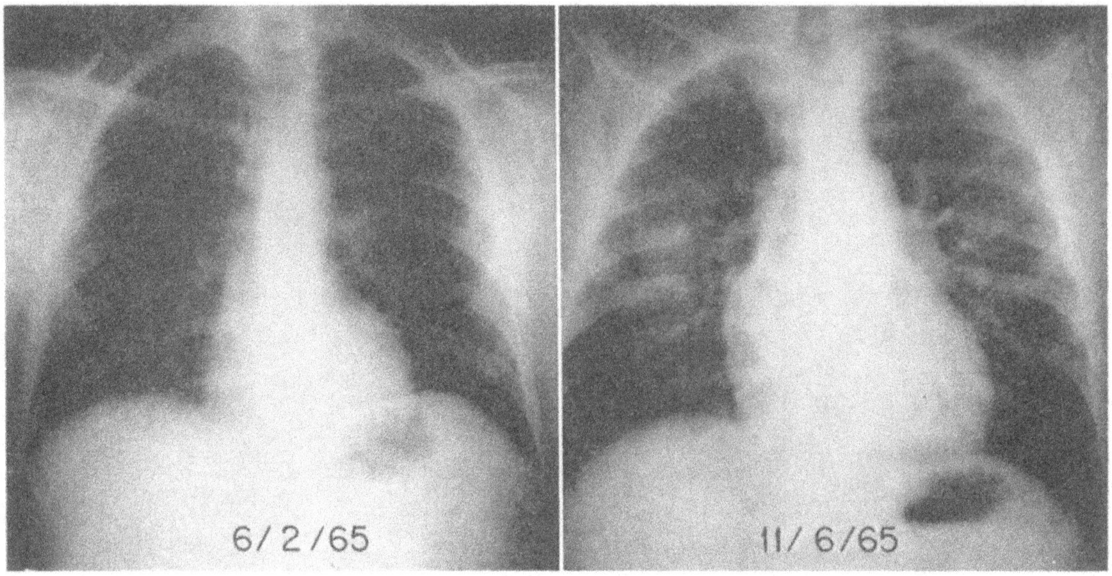

FIG. 7. Case 2. Chest roentgenograms showing progressive cardiomegaly.

cu. mm., erythrocyte sedimentation rate 80 mm. in one hour and reticulocyte count 2.3 per cent. An aspirate of the bone marrow again showed hyperplasia of the myeloid elements with an increased number of eosinophils. The urine contained 10 to 15 erythrocytes per high power field without casts. An electrocardiogram (Fig. 8) now showed left ventricular hypertrophy, and a chest roentgenogram revealed cardiomegaly. The cerebrospinal fluid was normal. The prednisone dosage was decreased and 6-mercaptopurine (200 mg. daily) was added. On November 1, 1965, overt cardiac failure developed, and the heart was larger on chest roentgenogram (Fig. 7). The heart failure was lessened by digitalis and diuresis therapy, but the patient became more confused and restless with myoclonic jerks, and finally comatose. The serum urea nitrogen level rose to 114 mg. per 100 ml., and the red blood cell and platelet counts fell. The white blood cell count dropped to 17,000 per cu. mm. 75 per cent mature eosinophils. During his last five days the patient received 2,000 mg. of prednisone. Two days before death, fever developed, Staphylococcus aureus was cultured from the blood, but despite methicillin and Keflin® therapy, the patient became hypotensive and died. At no time was precordial murmur audible, and numerous blood cultures taken before the last two days were negative.

At necropsy (A65-211) the heart (Fig. 9 to 12) weighed 430 gm. Mural thrombi were present in the apices of each ventricle and behind the posterior mitral leaflet adhering it to the markedly fibrotic endocardium covering the basilar portion of the left ventricular wall. Colonies of gram-positive cocci were present in the thrombotic material behind the posterior mitral leaflet, and culture of it and of the cardiac blood at necropsy yielded Staph. aureus. The atrial aspect of the posterior mitral leaflet was normal. Numerous abscesses, containing colonies of gram-positive cocci, were present in the myocardial walls of all four cardiac chambers. Similar abscesses, containing organisms, were found in the liver (1,800 gm.), spleen (480 gm.), kidneys (110 gm. each), brain, intestinal wall, pancreas, pituitary and adrenal glands, testes, skeletal muscle and lungs. The walls of occasional small arteries in these organs, including the heart, were infiltrated by polymorphonuclear cells and their lumens were plugged by necrotic debris, fibrin and

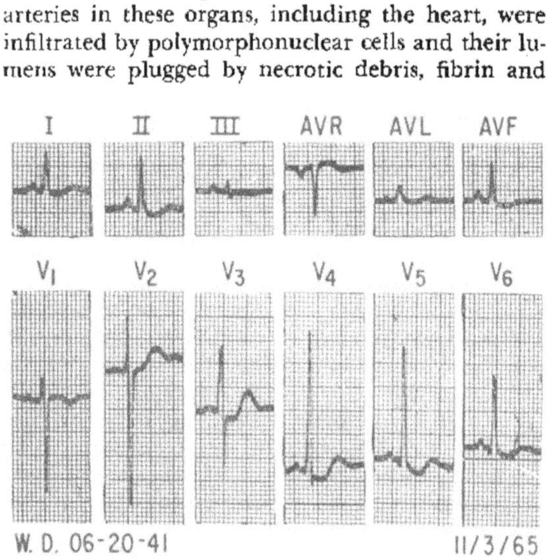

FIG. 8. Case 2. Electrocardiogram.

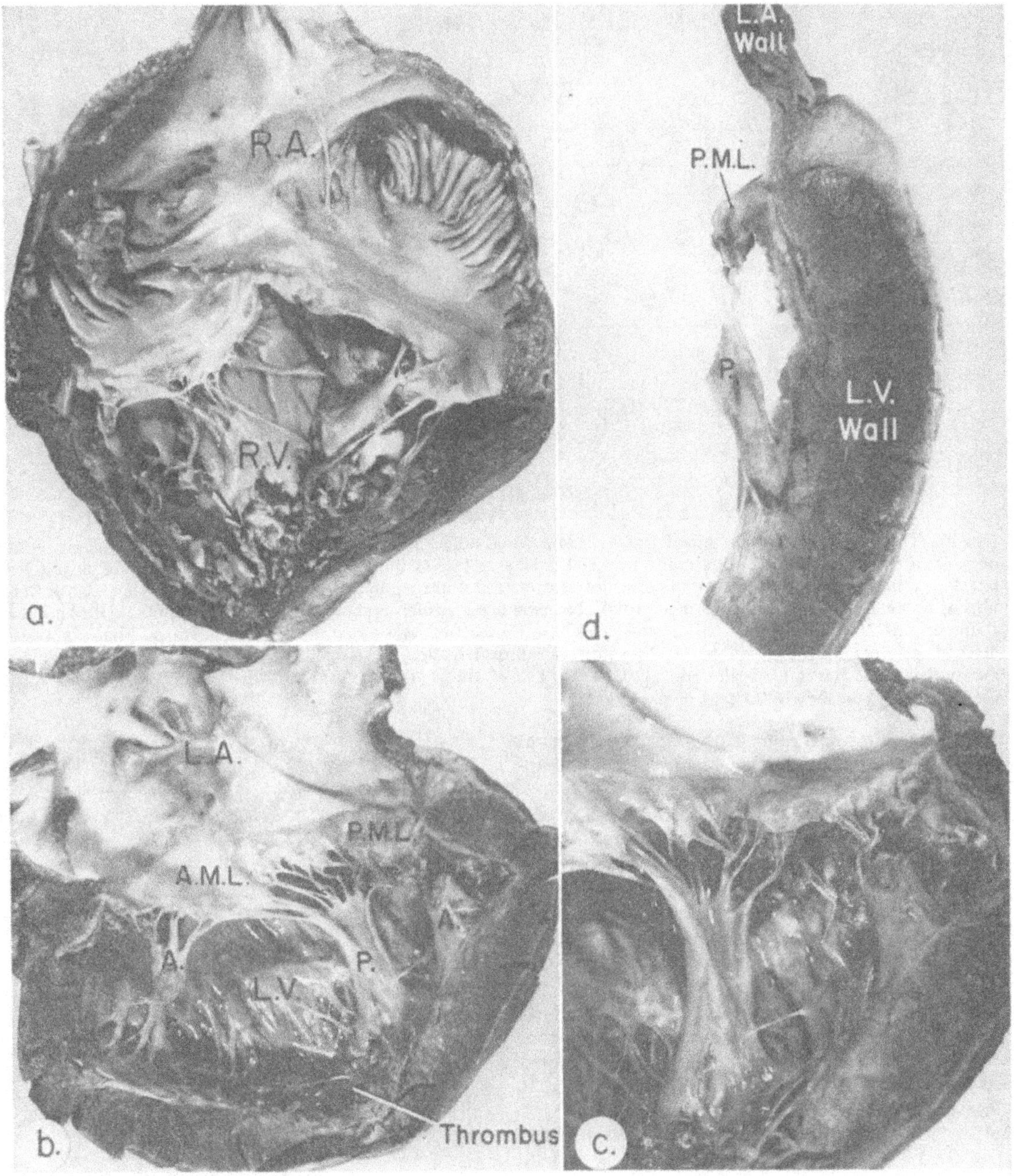

FIG. 9. Case 2. Interior of the heart. *a*, opened right atrium (R.A.), tricuspid valve and right ventricle (R.V.). Both chambers are dilated, and antemortum thrombus (arrow) is present in the apex of the ventricle. The endocardium of the right ventricle is more opaque than normal. *b*, opened left atrium (L.A.), mitral valve and left ventricle (L.V.). Both chambers are mildly dilated. The endocardium of the left ventricle is more opaque than usual, both the anterior (A.) and posterior (P.) papillary muscles, particularly the latter one, are severely scarred and atrophied, and thrombus is present at the apex and behind the posterior mitral leaflet (P.M.L.). A.M.L. = anterior mitral leaflet. A close-up view of the posterior mitral leaflet is shown in *c*. *d*, longitudinal section which includes the posterior mitral leaflet and the material behind it, left atrial (L.A.) wall, scarred posteromedial papillary muscle (P.) and left ventricular (L.V.) wall.

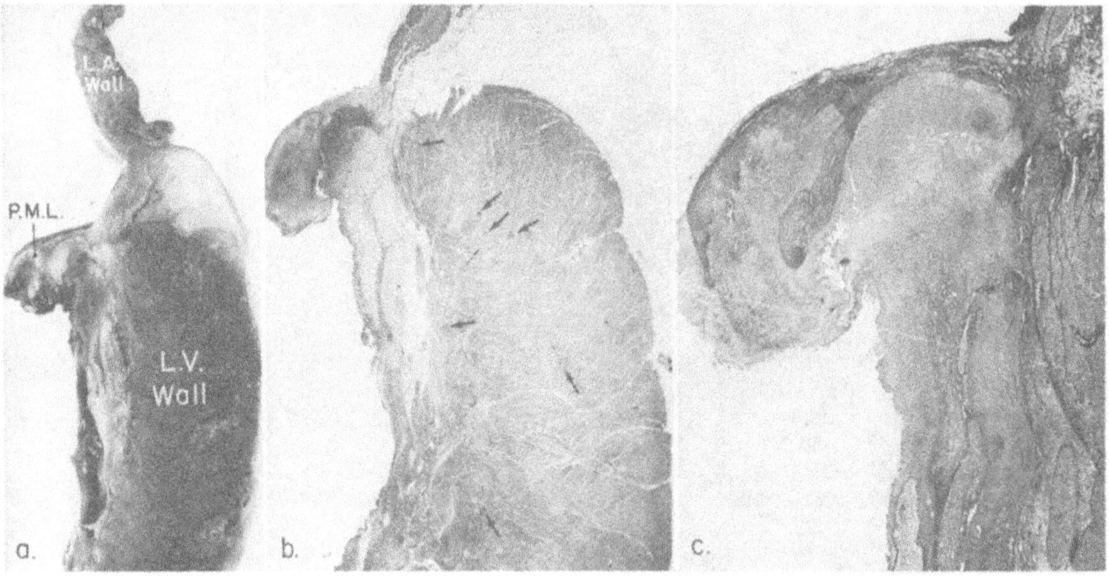

FIG. 10. Case 2. The posterior mitral leaflet (P.M.L.) and adjacent structures. *a*, gross section. *b*, histologic section of most of the area shown in *a*. Necrotic material (stains dark) lies immediately beneath the posterior mitral leaflet. The other excess tissue beneath this leaflet and on the mural endocardium of the left ventricle (L.V.) is dense fibrous tissue. The arrows point to myocardial abscesses, one of which is shown in Figure 11. Hematoxylin and eosin stain, original magnification × 4. *c*, same area but the section is stained for elastic fibers by the van Gieson method, original magnification × 11. The posterior mitral leaflet is well outlined. The fibrous tissue which is nearly devoid of elastic fibers lies entirely beneath, i.e., on the ventricular aspect, of the leaflet. Virtually no fibrous tissue is located on the atrial aspect of the leaflet.

platelets. Clumps of polymorphonuclear leukocytes also were present in the lumens of some renal tubules.

The bone marrow was hypercellular with a predominance of eosinophils. Sections of the abscesses in the various organs, with the exception of those in the kidneys, did not contain numerous eosinophils. Sections of the kidneys disclosed severe congestion, thickening of the basement membranes of many glomeruli, increased interstitial fibrous tissue, atrophy of some tubules and thickening of the walls, at times by fibrinoid change, of an occasional arteriole. The lumen of a rare renal arteriole contained fibrin material. Sections of lung disclosed several recanalized thrombi in the small muscular arteries.

CASE 3. A twenty-six year old man (F.M., 05-75-67) who died on April 6, 1965, had been well until February 1963 when he noted easy fatigability, myalgia and pain in the left upper abdominal quadrant. A blood smear at that time showed eosinophilia. In November 1963 exertional dyspnea and generalized weakness appeared, and he was hospitalized. Examination showed a grade 2/6 ejection-type systolic murmur over the precordium. Raynaud's phenomenon was demonstrated. The

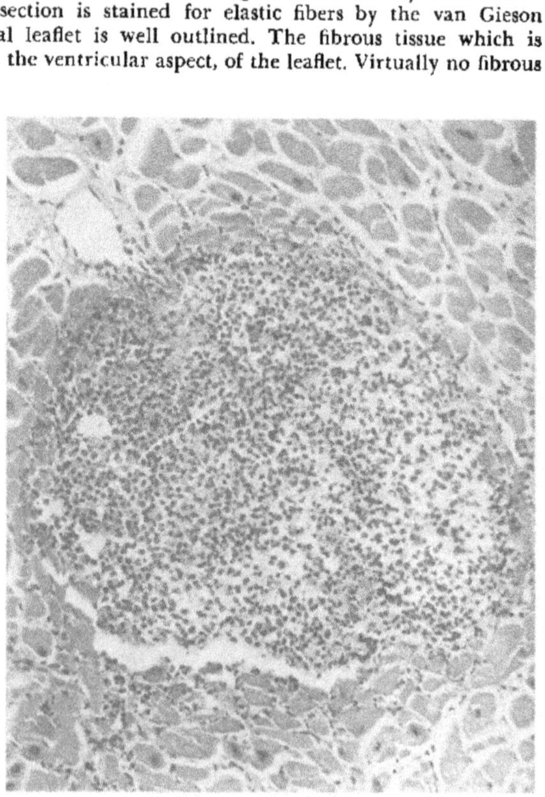

FIG. 11. Case 2. Myocardial abscess. Gram-positive organisms were present within it.

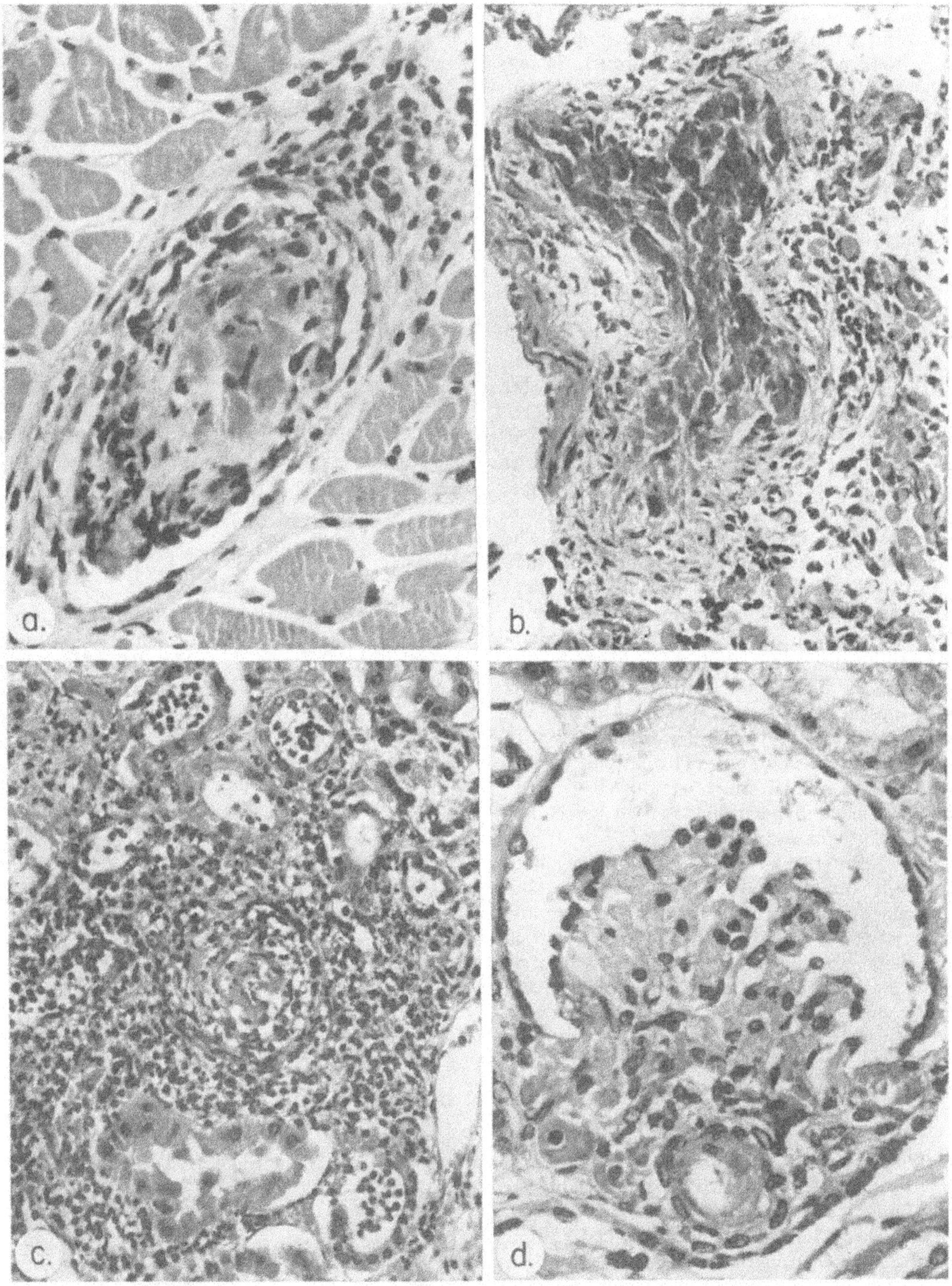

FIG. 12. Case 2. Small arterial disease. *a*, intramural coronary artery showing thrombotic material within the lumen and inflammatory cells in one portion of its wall. Original magnification × 400. *b*, pulmonary artery is occluded by thrombotic material. Original magnification × 251. *c*, small renal artery containing fibrin material in its lumen and its wall and adjacent structures are invaded by polymorphonuclear leukocytes. Original magnification × 251. *d*, renal glomerulus showing diffuse thickening of the capillary membranes and narrowing of the arteriole. Original magnification × 400. Hematoxylin and eosin stains on each.

white blood cell count was 27,000 per cu. mm. with 70 per cent mature eosinophils, hemoglobin 10.8 gm. per 100 ml. and serum urea nitrogen 24 mg. per 100 ml. The aspirated bone marrow was interpreted as showing myelocytic hyperplasia, with predominance of eosinophils. He received busulfan (12 mg. daily) from March 1964 through May 1964, and the white blood cell count dropped to 3,400 per cu. mm. with 30 per cent eosinophils. Hepatosplenomegaly, however, appeared, the dyspnea worsened and the heart enlarged.

On August 11, 1964, the patient was admitted to the Clinical Center. Since 1958 his fingers had intermittently become blue and ached when exposed to cold. The heart, liver and spleen were enlarged, a ventricular gallop was present, and the skin over the distal phalanges was blue, cold and taut.

The white blood cell count was 20,000 per cu. mm. with 80 per cent mature eosinophils, platelet count 20,000 per cu. mm. and hemoglobin 14.0 gm. per cent. The white blood cell alkaline phosphatase activity was 15 μM PNP per hour per 10^9 cells. The creatinine clearance (twenty-four hour urine sample) was 87 ml. per minute and the urine sediment was normal. The bone marrow showed eosinophilic hyperplasia with normal erythropoiesis and megakaryocytes. Chromosome studies on several occasions failed to disclose the Philadelphia chromosome. A muscle biopsy specimen was normal. Chest roentgenogram (Fig. 13) showed cardiomegaly with left ventricular prominence. The initial electrocardiogram was normal, but later showed evidence of left ventricular hypertrophy as well as changes in the S-T segment and T wave (Fig. 14).

Digitalis, diuretics and bed rest brought about considerable improvement in his symptoms, but the anemia worsened (to 8.0 gm. per 100 ml.) and the platelet count fell to 5,000 per cu. mm. so that almost daily platelet transfusions were required. The survival of infused Cr_{51}-labeled platelets was markedly shortened, and sequestration of radioactivity over the spleen was demonstrated as compared to ten normal volunteer subjects. Platelet isoantibodies could not be demonstrated. The patient was treated with prednisone (60 mg. daily for two weeks) with no perceptible change in red cell or platelet counts. Because of the persistence of thrombocytopenia and anemia despite prednisone therapy, splenectomy was performed (uneventfully) on November 24, 1964. The spleen weighed 235 gm. Histologic examination of the spleen showed numerous eosinophils and foci of fibrosis and necrosis, and biopsy specimens of the liver and abdominal lymph nodes revealed eosinophilic infiltration. The platelet count stabilized thereafter at about 70,000 per cu. mm.; the hemoglobin fluctuated between 10 and 14 gm. per 100 ml.

In December 1964 the patient became anorectic and jaundiced (serum total bilirubin 22.0 mg. per 100 ml.), and a diagnosis of serum hepatitis was made. In three weeks the jaundice and anorexia had nearly disappeared, and the patient went home. At the time of discharge the white blood cell count was 30,000 per cu. mm. with 70 per cent mature eosinophils, platelet count 64,000 per cu. mm. and hemoglobin 11.4 per 100 ml.

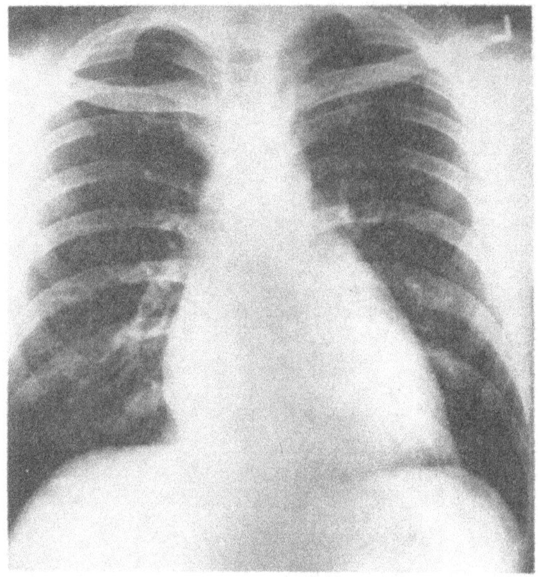

FIG. 13. Case 3. Chest roentgenogram taken five months before death.

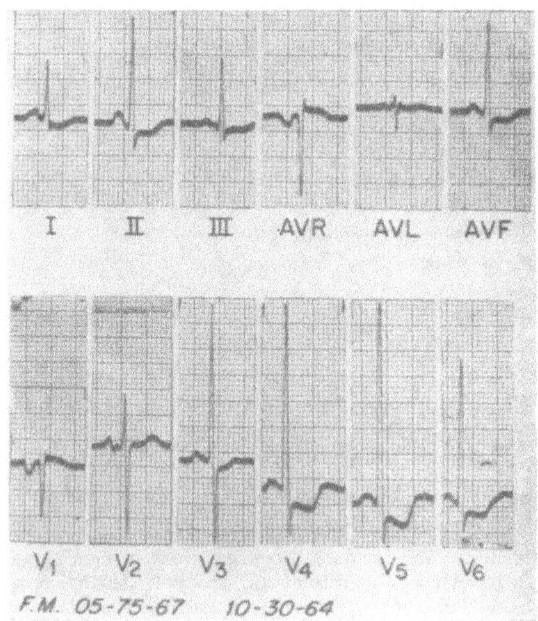

FIG. 14. Case 3. Electrocardiogram taken six months before death.

On February 11, 1965, the patient entered the Kansas City General Hospital and Medical Center in overt congestive cardiac failure. A grade 3/6 systolic murmur, loudest over the cardiac apex, and a ventricular gallop were described. He was jaundiced, the digits were cold and dusky, the legs edematous and the liver enlarged. The white blood cell count was 57,000 per cu. mm. with 77 per cent eosinophils, platelet count 19,000 per cu. mm. and hemoglobin 11.7 gm. per 100 ml. The serum total bilirubin was 6.0 mg. per 100 ml. with 3.1 mg. direct reacting. Bone marrow aspirate showed innumerable mature eosinophils. The test for cryoglobulin was positive. The electrocardiogram suggested left ventricular and left atrial enlargement and the QT interval was prolonged. The chest roentgenogram showed cardiomegaly, pulmonary congestion and a right pleural effusion. The signs and symptoms of cardiac failure gradually lessened following bed rest and diuretic therapy, but on April 6, 1965, the patient suddenly became unresponsive and died. The terminal event was believed to have been an intracerebral hemorrhage. One day earlier the hematocrit had been 35 per cent, white blood cell count 22,000 per cu. mm. with 38 per cent eosinophils and platelet count 57,000 per cu. mm. An autopsy was not performed.

COMMENTS

The three patients described had similar illnesses. Each was a young (aged twenty-five to thirty-five years) Caucasian man with leukocytosis (counts up to 81,000 per cu. mm), blood eosinophilia (up to 98 per cent), generalized cardiomegaly, intractable cardiac failure, renal dysfunction and a short illness (length of symptoms ranging from eleven to twenty-six months). Necropsy in two showed severe mural endocardial fibrosis with superimposed fibrin-platelet thrombi, myocardial scarring, vegetative valvular endocarditis, membranous glomerulopathy, eosinophilic hyperplasia of the bone marrow and spleen without abnormal or leukemic myeloblasts, and occasionally thrombosed small arteries in the heart, spleen, kidneys and lungs.

These features are similar to those in two patients described by Löffler in 1936 [*3*]. His patients, a forty-five year old woman and a thirty-seven year old man, died following illnesses of twelve and twenty-one months, respectively. Each of Löffler's patients had had evidence of severe right- and left-sided congestive cardiac failure, marked eosinophilia (up to 70 per cent), and mild leukocytosis. Necropsy in each showed the endocardium of both cardiac ventricles to be focally or diffusely thickened by fibrous tissue, which contained superimposed thrombi. The combination of the peculiar cardiac disease and eosinophilia was called by Löffler "fibroplastic parietal endocarditis with blood eosinophilia," and its etiology was unknown. Weiss-Carmine [*4*], from Löffler's department, summarized the findings in twenty-six necropsy patients with fibroplastic parietal endocarditis and eosinophila reported up to 1957, and Brink and Weber [*5*] five years later summarized the reported finding in eleven additional necropsy patients with this entity as well as in three patients studied by them. Several additional patients have been described subsequently [*6-10*]. Of the forty patients with Löffler's endocarditis described up to 1962, ten were women, thirty men; age range seven to sixty-five years, average thirty-four; with the exception of two patients, death occurred within two years following the onset of symptoms; nearly all had congestive cardiac failure, often with precordial murmurs suggesting mitral and/or tricuspid regurgitation; the white blood cell count was elevated (highest 165,000 per cu. mm.) at some time in all but four patients, two of whom had leukopenia; the heart weight was excessive in all but three patients; thirty-three of the forty subjects had thrombi superimposed on the thick fibrous endocardium of the right and/or left ventricle; thirty-two had fibrous scars in the myocardium in addition to the thickened endocardium; nearly all had eosinophils in some organs although sometimes the tissue eosinophilia was minimal; arterial lesions (fibrinoid necrosis, vasculitis, or intimal fibrous thickening) were seen in twenty-two of the forty subjects in the small vessels of one or more organs; and the liver and/or spleen was enlarged in about half of the patients. Of the forty patients, thirty were reported from Europe, seven from Africa and three from North America (U.S.A.). Each of the three patients described herein was a native of the United States.

The clinical and pathologic features listed are similar to those reported in patients with "eosinophilic leukemia." Bousser [*11*] summarized the clinical and pathologic findings in thirteen patients with "eosinophilic leukemia" reported between 1944 and 1956, and Odeberg [2] summarized the observations in twelve additional necropsy patients with "eosinophilic leukemia" reported between 1957 and 1963. These twenty-five patients ranged in age from seven to fifty-nine years (average thirty-two): eighteen were male and 7 female; all had blood eosinophilia (up to 98 per cent); only five patients survived longer than two years following the onset of symptoms, and death usually resulted from cardiac failure. At necropsy, over half of the subjects had extensive endomyocardial fibrosis with mural thrombosis, nearly all had infiltration by mature eosinophilis into one or more organs (usually spleen, liver, kidney, heart and/or lung), and occasional thrombi or other lesions in small arteries of one or more organs. Gruenwald and co-workers [12], however, described a patient who had blood eosinophilia, thrombophlebitis, splenomegaly and the Philadelphia (Ph 1) chromosome. This patient eventually had acute myeloblastic leukemia, which is usually associated with the terminal phases of chronic granulocytic leukemia, but at this stage the number of eosinophils in the peripheral blood was normal. Goh and co-workers [13] described two other patients with "eosinophilic leukemia" without the Ph 1 chromosome and one of them had increased numbers of blasts terminally. The heart in this latter patient was not mentioned in the autopsy description.

In none of the patients in the present report did increased numbers of abnormal or leukemic blasts develop during their illnesses. The fatal course in these three patients with "eosinophilic leukemia" cannot be disputed. Yet neoplastic proliferation of malignant eosinophils or myeloblastic precursors did not occur. We believe that the diagnosis of "eosinophilic leukemia" must be reserved for patients who eventually have abnormal myelopoiesis as well as eosinophilia with or without Ph 1 chromosome. Furthermore, the clinical and pathologic features of patients such as those described in the present report are indeed indistinguishable from those reported as having Löffler's endocarditis. Thus, it seems reasonable to conclude that they are indeed the same disease.

Patients described under a variety of other names have had clinical and pathologic features similar to those described in patients with Löffler's endocarditis and/or "eosinophilic leukemia." The disease described by Davies [14] in 1948 in West Africa and called "endocardial fibrosis" is characterized by marked thickening of the endocardium and scarring of the inner myocardium of the left and/or right ventricles, mainly the inflow portions. Clinically patients with this condition may show evidence of obstruction to filling of either or both ventricles; similar clinical features may occur in fibroplastic parietal endocarditis, as emphasized by Löffler [15]. Blood eosinophilia has only recently [16] been emphasized as a feature of endocardial fibrosis although in his initial report of thirty six patients Davies mentioned that "they sometimes show an eosinophilia for which none of the usual causes of eosinophilia account" [14]. Of forty necropsy patients with endocardial fibrosis studied by Ive and associates [16], seventeen (43 per cent) had eosinophilia (absolute count >1,000 per cu. mm. or differential count >20 per cent of the total white cell count). Davies speculated that the earliest lesion in endocardial fibrosis is infiltration of the myocardium by round cells and eosinophils leading to necrosis of the endocardium and subendocardial myocardium. Thrombi form over the necrotic areas. As the mural thrombi and necrotic cardiac tissue become organized the inflammatory cells disappear and finally only dense fibrous tissue remains. Gerbaux et al. [17] suggested in 1956 that endocardial fibrosis and Löffler's endocarditis were essentially the same disease. Gray [18] in 1951 described two white men in West Africa who had "endocardial fibrosis" and distinct blood eosinophilia (18 to 51 per cent). The cardiac lesions were similar to those of patients with Löffler's endocarditis or the endomyocardial fibrosis of Davies. Narrowing of small systemic arteries was observed in each of his patients, and was believed to be the result of emboli from the cardiac mural thrombi. McKusick and Cochran [19] in 1952 described severe endocardial thickening in a forty-seven year old white woman who had clinical features typical of constrictive pericarditis, but at thoracotomy the pericardium was normal. This patient had mild eosinophilia (7.5 per cent) and at necropsy endomyocardial thickening was observed in both ventricles. No tissue eosinophilia was found at autopsy, but the patient's clinical illness was relatively long (four years).

Actually, Löffler had appreciated the possible hemodynamic consequences of the ventricular endocardial thickening. In 1947 he wrote that the endocardial thickening "prevents normal diastolic relaxation of the ventricles" and the thrombotic masses decrease the capacity of the ventricles [*15*]. Thus, the clinical features may be the same as chronic constrictive pericarditis. It is "not the pericardium but the endocardium which prevents the normal diastolic relaxation of the ventricular myocardium" [*15*]. McNicol and associates [*20*] in 1953 described two white men, aged twenty-seven and thirty-four years, who had similar endomyocardial lesions, but there is no mention of examination of the peripheral blood for eosinophils. It is difficult to be certain whether the cardiac lesions in the South African patients described by Becker and colleagues [*21*] in 1953 with "cardiovascular collagenosis with parietal endocardial thrombosis" were similar to those in subjects with Löffler's endocarditis, since these investigators did not show gross photographs of the hearts, and the endocardium in some of their patients contained many elastic fibers. In twelve of their forty patients white blood cell counts were performed and leukocytosis was present at some time in at least nine of them. The number of patients who had blood smears for differential counts is not stated but at least two patients had eosinophilia; it was "marked" in one and "moderately elevated" in the other. The thirty-five year old white man described by Clark et al. [*22*] in 1956 had severe "endocardial fibrosis" and blood eosinophilia (56 per cent). This patient also underwent thoracotomy under the mistaken diagnosis of pericardial constriction, but the pericardium was normal. Cardiac catheterization in this patient had shown pressure tracings typical of those previously observed only in patients with constrictive pericarditis. At autopsy, this patient had severe endomyocardial fibrosis similar to that described in patients with Löffler's endocarditis or with the endomyocardial fibrosis of Davies.

It appears that some patients with endomyocardial fibrosis, of the type seen in Löffler's endocarditis or in Davies' endomyocardial fibrosis, may have eosinophilia and others may not. Löffler, in his initial report, emphasized that eosinophilia is inconstant and may disappear [*3*]. It is possible that the presence or absence of eosinophilia is dependent to some extent on the length of the illness. Patients with Löffler's endocarditis or eosinophilic leukemia usually die within two years from the onset of symptoms, whereas patients with endomyocardial fibrosis without eosinophilia may survive for longer periods.

The cause of the eosinophilia in patients with endomyocardial fibrosis is speculative. Löffler considered "the eosinophilia . . . to be the expression of an allergic reaction . . .," and a "phasic sign"—present only as long as the allergic condition is present [*15*]. Thus, when eosinophilia is present, a high degree of allergy is present in the body, and when eosinophilia is absent the allergic or anaphylactic stimulus has vanished. The healing of the eosinophilic inflammatory reaction in the meantime, however, has produced considerable scarring and when this occurs in the heart the damage is irreversible and fatal. In Löffler's endocarditis the allergic stimulus must be present for some time (months) in order to cause such extensive cardiac scarring. In transient eosinophilia, for example, the results of "tropical eosinophilia" or "Löffler's pneumonia," the stimulus to the production of eosinophilia is transient (days) or the amount of allergin is small. Consequently, permanent cardiac damage does not occur in either of these conditions, although transient electrocardiographic alterations are common [*23*]. Little anatomic information is available in patients with tropical eosinophilia or Löffler's pneumonia since these conditions are benign. One patient with Löffler's pneumonia died during an accident, and extensive eosinophilic infiltration of the ventricular endocardium was found [*24*].

The possibility that "Löffler's endocarditis," "eosinophilic leukemia" without abnormal myelopoiesis, "endomyocardial fibrosis" of Davies, "cardiovascular collagenosis with parietal endocardial thrombosis," "endocardial fibrosis" described by Gray, McKusick and Cochran, McNicol et al. and Clark et al. are the same disease seen simply at different stages of development is an attractive hypothesis. At one end of the spectrum may be patients with eosinophilia associated with a transient benign febrile illness such as tropical eosinophilia or Löffler's pneumonia. At the other end of the gamut may be patients with severe endomyocardial fibrosis with superimposed thrombi and no blood eosinophilia. Between these two extremes may be patients who still have eosinophilia but less extensive endomyocardial scarring and thrombi. The latter process is still active and thus eosinophilia is still present, but as the inflammatory process dies down cardiac scar tissue remains and eosinophilia disappears.

The occurrence of lesions in organs other than the heart has frequently been observed in patients reported to have Löffler's endocarditis and eosinophilic leukemia as well as in subjects reported to have other forms of endomyocardial disease [*2,4,21*]. The finding of "disseminated visceral lesions" in patients with Löffler's endocarditis and in two subjects studied by them prompted Engfeldt and Zelterstrom [*1*] to propose that Löffler's syndrome is related to periarteritis nodosa and should be considered a collagen disease. These investigators noted clinical and pathologic similarities between Löffler's endocarditis and eosinophilic leukemia and concluded that "it is highly doubtful whether real eosinophilic leukemia has ever been reported." Odeberg [*2*] and others [*25,26*] support this conclusion as well as the concept of "disseminated eosinophilic collagen disease." Small vascular lesions similar to those illustrated in the two necropsy patients described herein have been observed in a number of patients reported to have Löffler's endocarditis or eosinophilic leukemia [*1,2,4*]. Renal lesions have been observed in several patients [*3,27,28*]. Löffler in his first patient with fibroplastic parietal endocarditis found alterations in the kidney characteristic of Löhlein's nephritis [*3*]. Some of the small arterial occlusions observed in organs other than the heart in Löffler's endocarditis could, of course, represent emboli from the cardiac mural thrombi rather than manifestations of a systemic disease.

REFERENCES

1. Engfeldt, B. and Zetterström, R. Disseminated eosinophilic "collagen disease." *Acta med. scandinav.*, 153: 337, 1956.
2. Odeberg, B. Eosinophilic leukemia and disseminated eosinophilic collagen disease—a disease entity? *Acta med. scandinav.*, 177: 129, 1965.
3. Löffler, W. Endocarditis parietalis fibroplastica mit Bluteosinophilie. *Schweiz. med. Wchnschr.*, 66: 817, 1936.
4. Weiss-Carmine, S. Die endocarditis parietalis fibroplastica mit Bluteosinophilie (Löffler) und ihre Stellung im Rahmen der Parietalendokardfibrosen. *Schweiz. med. Wchnschr.*, 87: 890, 1957.
5. Brink, A. J. and Weber, H. W. Fibroplastic parietal endocarditis with eosinophilia. Löffler's endocarditis. *Am. J. Med.*, 34: 52, 1963.
6. André, R. and Duhamel, G. Sur un cas d'endocardite de Loeffler avec étude anatomique. *Bull. et mém. Soc. méd. hôp. Paris*, 115: 1215, 1964.
7. Waible, R. and Wichert, P. Endocarditis parietalis fibroplastica (Löffler). *Zentralbl. allg. Path.*, 108: 112, 1965.
8. Turiaf, J. Löeffler's fibroplastic parietal endocarditis with dominant extracardiai manifestations. *Poumon et Coeur*, 21: 819, 1965.
9. Löhr, K. and Jahnecke, J. Über einen Fall von Endocarditis parietalis fibroplastica mit Bluteosinophilie (Löffler) mit dem klinischen Bild einer "eosinophilen Leukämie." *Deutsches Arch. klin. Med.*, 210: 119, 1965.
10. Mautner, L. S. and Harris, F. Fibrosing endocarditis with eosinophilia: Loeffler's endocarditis parietalis fibroplastica. *Canad. M. A. J.*, 95: 1201, 1966.
11. Bousser, J. Eosinophilie et Leucémie. *Sang*, 28: 553, 1957.
12. Gruenwald, H., Kiossoglou, K. A., Mitus, W. J. and Dameshek, W. Philadelphia chromosome in eosinophilic leukemia. *Am. J. Med.*, 39: 1003, 1965.
13. Goh, K., Swisher, S. N. and Rosenberg, C. A. Cytogenetic studies in eosinophilic leukemia. The relationship of eosinophilic leukemia and chronic myelocytic leukemia. *Ann. Int. Med.*, 62: 80, 1965.
14. Davies, J. N. P. Endocardial fibrosis in Africans. *East African M. J.*, 25: 10, 1948.
15. Löffler, W. The pathogenetic significance of the so-called endocarditis parietalis fibroplastica. *Bull. schweiz. Akad. med. Wissensch.*, 2: 287, 1947.
16. Ive, F. A., Willis, A. J. P., Ikeme, A. C. and Brockington, I. F. Endomyocardial fibrosis and filariasis. *Quart. J. Med.*, 36 (n.s.): 495, 1967.
17. Gerbaux, A., de Brux, J., Bennaceur, M. and Lenègre, J. L'endocardite pariétale fibroplastique avec éosinophilie sanguine endocardite de Loeffler. *Bull. et mém. Soc méd. hôp. Paris*, 72: 456, 1956.
18. Gray, I. R. Endocardial fibrosis. *Brit. Heart J.*, 13: 387, 1951.
19. McKusick, V. A. and Cochran, T. H. Constrictive endocarditis. Report of a case. *Bull. Johns Hopkins Hosp.*, 90: 90, 1952.
20. McNicol, C., MacMahon, H. E., Benenson, A. S. and Winship, T. Recurrent parietal thromboendocarditis. *Circulation*, 7: 497, 1953.
21. Becker, B. J. P., Chatgidakis, C. B. and van Lingen, B. Cardiovascular collagenosis with parietal endocardial thrombosis. A clinicopathologic study of forty cases. *Circulation*, 7: 345, 1953.
22. Clark, G. M., Valentine, E. and Blount, S. G., Jr.

Endocardial fibrosis simulating constrictive pericarditis. Report of a case with determinations of pressure in the right side of the heart and eosinophilia. *New England J. Med.,* 254: 349, 1956.
23. VAKIL, R. J. Cardiovascular involvement in tropical eosinophilia. *Brit. Heart J.,* 23: 578, 1961.
24. BAYLEY, E. C., LINDBERG, D. O. N. and BAGGENSTOSS, A. H. Loeffler's syndrome: report of a case with pathologic examination of the lungs. *Arch. Path.,* 40: 376, 1945.
25. KARLE, H. and VIDEBAEK, A. Eosinophilic leukaemia or a collagen disease with eosinophilia. *Danish M. Bull.,* 13: 41, 1966.
26. PIERCE, L. E., HOSSEINIAN, A. H. and CONSTANTINE, A. B. Disseminated eosinophilic collagen disease. *Blood,* 29: 540, 1967.
27. ROULET, F. Beitrag zur Kenntnis der "Endocarditis parietalis fibroplastica mit Bluteosinophilie" (Löffler). *Schweiz. med. Wchnschr.,* 74: 427, 1944.
28. ZOLI, A. Parietal fibroplastic endocarditis with blood eosinophilia. *Cardiologia.,* 19: 139, 1951.

Papillary muscle fibrosis in primary myocardial disease

*Frank I. Marcus, M.D.**
*Lucia Gomez, M.D.***
*D. Luke Glancy, M.D.****
*Gordon A. Ewy, M.D.*****
*William C. Roberts, M.D.******
Washington, D. C., and Bethesda, Md.

Papillary muscle dysfunction due to coronary occlusive disease is now well recognized.[1-3] Other causes of dysfunction or fibrosis of the papillary muscles include origin of the left coronary artery from the pulmonary artery,[4] endocardial fibroelastosis,[5] and left ventricular hypertrophy of diverse etiology.[6,7] This report describes fibrosis of the posteromedial papillary muscle of the left ventricle of a 44-year-old Negro woman with primary myocardial disease.

Case report

S. A. was admitted to the Washington Hospital Center at the age of 39 because of an incomplete abortion. At that time she had no history, symptoms, or signs of heart disease. Her blood pressure was 120/80 mm. Hg, and the heart was of normal size on chest roentgenogram (Fig. 1, left). At the age of 41, she had the acute onset of pulmonary edema. Thereafter, she had repeated episodes of congestive heart failure, requiring many hospital admissions. At each hospital admission, the blood pressures were in the range of 120/90 to 130/100 mm. Hg. Invariably, atrial and ventricular diastolic gallops were heard. There was a Grade 3/6 or 4/6 pansystolic murmur heard best at the apex. On several occasions, during her last year of life, an additional pansystolic murmur could be identified. This murmur was heard maximally at the fourth left interspace and was considered to be a functional tricuspid murmur. Usually the intensity of the apical pansystolic murmur, interpreted as being due to mitral regurgitation, decreased with treatment to Grade 1/6 or 2/6. On several occasions, the apical systolic murmur was noted to end before the second sound closure. Electrocardiograms consistently showed sinus rhythm, left axis deviation, and an intraventricular conduction defect (Fig. 2). Despite salt restriction, diuretics, and digitalis, the heart remained large (Fig. 1, right).

Her last admission was at the District of Columbia General Hospital because of a generalized skin eruption and confusion. She was an alcoholic and had been admitted to another hospital 6 weeks before because of an epileptic seizure. Discharge medica-

From the Georgetown University Medical Division, District of Columbia General Hospital, the Washington Hospital Center, Washington, D. C.; and the Section of Pathology, Clinic of Surgery, National Heart Institute, National Institutes of Health, Bethesda, Md.

Received for publication March 18, 1968.

*Associate Professor of Medicine, Chief of Cardiology, Georgetown University Medical Division, District of Columbia General Hospital.
**Division of Cardiography, Georgetown University Hospital.
***Staff Associate, Section of Pathology, Clinic of Surgery, National Heart Institute, National Institutes of Health Bethesda, Md.
****Associate Cardiologist, Georgetown University Medical Division, District of Columbia General Hospital.
*****Chief, Section of Pathology, Clinic of Surgery, National Heart Institute, National Institutes of Health, Bethesda, Md.

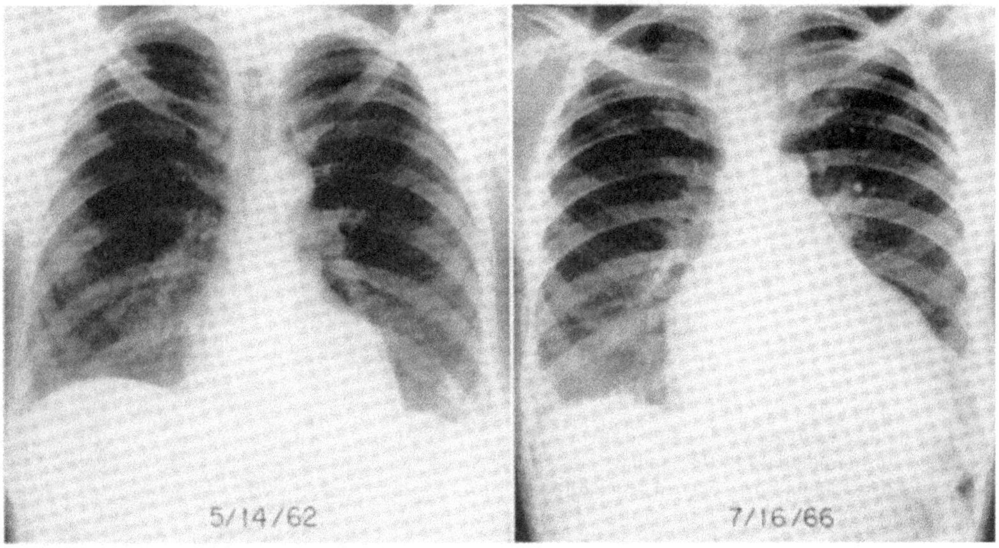

Fig. 1. Chest roentgenograms. *Left,* 5 years before death. There was no evidence of heart disease at that time. The cardiac size is normal. *Right,* 1 year before death. Marked cardiomegaly is present.

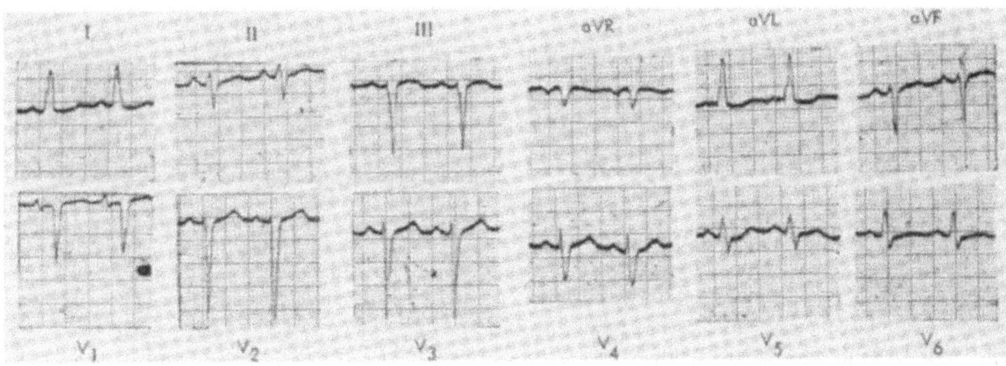

Fig. 2. Electrocardiogram recorded one year before death showing normal sinus rhythm, left axis deviation, and an intraventricular conduction defect.

tions had included diphenylhydantoin, phenobarbital, digitalis, and warfarin sodium. The skin eruption was believed to be secondary to one of these medications.

The blood pressure was 120/80 mm. Hg, pulse 120 per minute and regular, and temperature 103° F. The jugular venous pressure was normal. The left ventricular impulse was present at the fifth interspace in the anterior axillary line. The first and second heart sounds were single, and both atrial and ventricular gallops were heard. A Grade 2/6 systolic murmur was heard over the precordium. The white blood count was 11,200 per cubic millimeter, and the differential blood smear showed 40 per cent eosinophils. Cultures of sputum, blood, and urine were negative. Despite the withdrawal of all drugs, the fever and skin rash persisted and she died suddenly on the third hospital day.

Autopsy showed bronchopneumonia, pulmonary emboli to the small branches of the right lower lung, portal cirrhosis, and encephalomalacia of the right basal ganglia.

The heart weighed 350 grams. The pericardium, cardiac valves, and extramural coronary arteries were normal. The coronary arteries were entirely free of plaques. The right ventricular cavity was considerably dilated. The left ventricle was only mildly dilated. The atria were of normal size. The right ventricular wall measured up to 0.6 cm. and the left ventricular wall up to 0.9 cm. in thickness. The myocardium of the right ventricle was free of scars. The posteromedial papillary muscle of the left ventricle was atrophied and extensively scarred (Figs. 3, 4, and 5). The free wall of the left ventricle just beneath this papillary muscle was also focally fibrotic. In contrast, the anterolateral papillary mus-

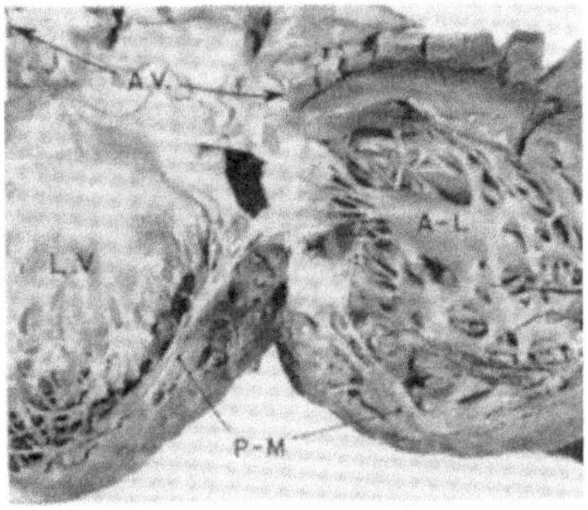

Fig. *3.* Opened left ventricle (*L.V.*) and aortic valve (*A.V.*). The posteromedial (*P-M*) papillary muscle is scarred and atrophied. In contrast, the anterolateral (*A-L*) papillary muscle is large and free of scars.

cle was large and free of scars (Figs. 3, 4, and 5). There was no evidence of fibrosis or mononuclear infiltrate in the remainder of the left ventricle.

Histologic examination of sections of heart disclosed large areas of interstitial and replacement fibrosis in the posteromedial papillary muscle and in the left ventricular free wall just beneath it. No inflammatory cells or Aschoff bodies were observed, and the intramural coronary arteries were normal.

Comments

This woman had myocardial disease of unknown origin (primary myocardial disease) for at least 3 years. The excessive intake of alcohol may have caused or contributed to the myocardial disease. The mild elevation of the diastolic blood pressure following the onset of cardiac symptoms appears to be of no etiologic significance. The blood eosinophilia, present terminally, is not believed to be related to the cardiac disease. Infiltrative myocardial diseases such as sarcoid, hemochromatosis, or amyloidosis were not found at autopsy, and both the extra- and intramural coronary arteries were entirely normal.

Pathological examination of the hearts of patients with primary myocardial disease usually show myocardial hypertrophy, varying degrees of interstitial myocardial fibrosis, and focal destruction of muscle fibers.[8-11] The fibrosis may produce intraventricular or bundle branch block.[8,9,11-17] The subject of this report had an intraventricular conduction defect. In addition, a large area of fibrosis involved the subendocardial portion of the left ventricle just beneath and including the posteromedial papillary muscle (Figs. 4 and 5). In contrast, the anterolateral muscle was large and free of scars (Figs. 4 and 5). Although papillary muscle fibrosis has been reported in Duchene's muscular dystrophy[17] and in sarcoid,[18] it has not previously been noted in idiopathic primary myocardial disease.

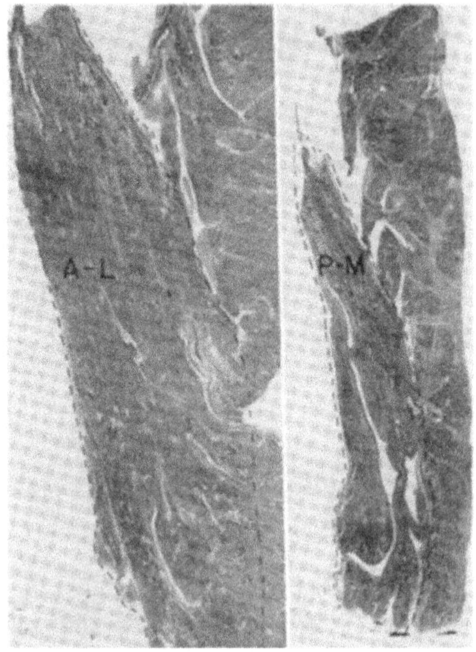

Fig. *4.* Photomicrographs, each taken at the same magnification (×3), of histologic sections through the thickest portions of the anterolateral (*A-L*) and posteromedial (*P-M*) papillary muscles (enclosed by dashed lines) of the left ventricle. The anterolateral muscle is twice as thick as that of the posteromedial. Only a portion of the free wall of the left ventricle beneath the anterolateral papillary muscle is included in the photomicrograph. In contrast, the entire free wall beneath the posteromedial papillary muscle is included in the photomicrograph. Hematoxylin and eosin sections on each.

In our patient, functional impairment of the posteromedial papillary muscle of the left ventricle appears to have been present and may have been responsible for the mitral regurgitation. Since mitral regurgitation is common in patients with primary myocardial disease in the absence of papillary muscle fibrosis,[8,9,11-13,15,16,19] the association between the pathological finding of papillary muscle fibrosis and clinical finding

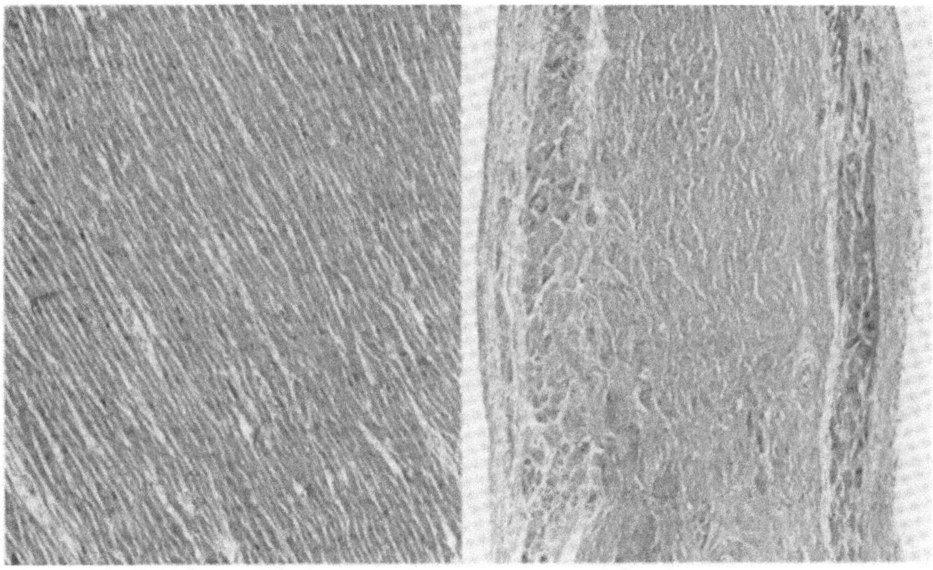

Fig. 5. Sections of portions of each of the papillary muscles. Each photomicrograph is taken at the same magnification (×65). *Left*, Portion of anterolateral papillary showing hypertrophy of the myocardial fibers but no scarring. *Right*, Portion of posteromedial papillary muscle showing extensive scarring. Most of the myocardial fibers which remain are located in the periphery of the papillary muscle. Hematoxylin and eosin stains on each.

of mitral regurgitation must remain speculative in our patient. Papillary muscle fibrosis nevertheless should be considered a possible cause of mitral regurgitation in patients with primary myocardial disease.

Summary

A 44-year-old woman with primary myocardial disease was found to have fibrosis of the posterior papillary muscle of the left ventricle. The fibrosis also involved the free wall of the left ventricle just beneath this papillary muscle. In patients with primary myocardial disease who have mitral insufficiency, papillary muscle fibrosis should be considered as a possible cause of this murmur.

We are indebted to Dr. James Bacos, Chief of Sub-Department of Cardiology, Washington Hospital Center, for permission to review the extensive hospital records of this patient. We wish to thank Mrs. Yvonne McIlwain for secretarial assistance and Mr. Bernard Salb of the Department of Medical Communications, Georgetown University Hospital.

REFERENCES

1. Heikkila, J.: Mitral incompetence complicating acute myocardial infarction, Brit. Heart J. **29**:162, 1967.
2. Bashour, F. A.: Mitral regurgitation following myocardial infarction: The syndrome of papillary mitral regurgitation, Dis. Chest. **48**:113, 1965.
3. Phillips, J. H., Burch, G. E., and DePasquale, N. P.: The syndrome of papillary muscle dysfunction, Ann. Int. Med. **59**:508, 1963.
4. Noren, G. R., Raghib, G., Moller, J. H., Amplatz, K., Adams, P., Jr., and Edwards, J. E.: Anomalous origin of the left coronary artery from the pulmonary trunk with special reference to the occurrence of mitral insufficiency, Circulation **30**:171, 1964.
5. Moller, J. H., Lucas, R. V., Jr., Adams, P., Jr., Anderson, R. C., Jorgens, J., and Edwards, J. E.: Endocardial fibroelastosis. A clinical and anatomic study of 47 patients with emphasis on its relationship to mitral insufficiency, Circulation **30**:759, 1964.
6. Arosemena, E., Moller, J. H., and Edwards, J. E.: Scarring of the papillary muscles in left ventricular hypertrophy, Am. Heart J. **74**:446, 1967.
7. Moller, J. H., Nakib, A., and Edwards, J. E.: Infarction of papillary muscles and mitral insufficiency associated with congenital aortic stenosis, Circulation **34**:87, 1966.
8. Massumi, R. A., Rios, J. G., Gooch, A. S., Nutter, D., DeVita, V. T., and Datlow, D. W.: Primary myocardial disease. Report of fifty cases and review of the subject, Circulation **31**:19, 1965.
9. Harvey, W. P., Segal, J. P., and Gurel, T.: The clinical spectrum of primary myocardial disease. Progr. Cardiovas. Dis. **7**:17, 1964.
10. Saphire, A.: Myocarditis. A general review, with

an analysis of two hundred and forty cases, Arch. Path. **32**:1000, 1941; **33**:88, 1942.

11. Fowler, N. O., Gueron, M., and Rowlands, D. J.: Primary myocardial disease, Circulation **23**:498, 1961.
12. Dye, C. L., Rosenbaum, D., Lowe, J. C., Behnke, R. H., and Genovese, P. D.: Primary myocardial disease. I—Clinical features, Ann. Int. Med. **58**:426, 1963.
13. Brigden, W.: Uncommon myocardial diseases. The non coronary cardiomyopathies, Lancet **2**:1179, 1243, 1957.
14. Marriott, H. J. L.: Electrocardiographic abnormalities, conductive disorders and arrhythmias in primary myocardial disease, Progr. Cardiovas. Dis. **7**:99, 1964.
15. Spodick, D. M., and Littman, D.: Idiopathic myocardial hypertrophy, Am. J. Cardiol. **1**:610, 1958.
16. Barritt, D. W., and Majeed, Al-Shammaá: Heart failure from unexplained cardiomyopathy, Brit. Heart J. **28**:674, 1966.
17. Perloff, J. K., Roberts, W. C., de Leon, A. C., and O'Doherty, D.: The distinctive electrocardiogram of Duchenne's progressive muscular dystrophy, Am. J. Med. **42**:179, 1967.
18. Scotti, T. M., and McKeown, C. E.: Sarcoidosis involving the heart, Arch. Path. **46**:289, 1948.
19. Wood, P.: Chronic constrictive pericarditis. Am. J. Cardiol. **7**:48, 1961.

Löffler's Fibroplastic Parietal Endocarditis, Eosinophilic Leukemia, and Davies' Endomyocardial Fibrosis: The Same Disease at Different Stages?

W. C. ROBERTS, L. M. BUJA, and V. J. FERRANS

Section of Pathology, National Heart and Lung Institute, National Institutes of Health, Bethesda, Md.

Between 1953 and 1969 three patients were referred to the Clinical Center of the National Institutes of Health because of 'eosinophilic leukemia'. Each was a young white man, each had large numbers of mature eosinophils in the blood, and each had severe, ultimately fatal, congestive cardiac failure. Necropsy in 2 of them disclosed extensive endomyocardial fibrosis with superimposed thrombi and small arterial and arteriolar lesions in several organs. A brief summary of the observations in these 3 patients and a discussion of their meaning are presented in the report which follows.

Patients Studied

Detailed descriptions of the 3 patients have been presented elsewhere [8]. Their ages were 25, 26 and 35 years. Length of symptoms varied from 12 to 26 months. Each had progressive cardiomegaly shown by chest roentgenogram. All were normotensive. Two had apical pansystolic blowing murmurs (grade 3/6 intensity) and ventricular gallops. Electrocardiograms showed sinus rhythm, premature ventricular contractions and non-specific ST-T wave changes in all 3 and evidence of left ventricular hypertrophy in 2. Each was anemic (hemoglobin 7.9–11.4 g/100 ml) and each had leukocytosis (14,000 to 108,000/cumm). Eosinophils varied from 30 to 80%. The highest blood urea nitrogen in the 3 patients was 21, 24 and 114 mg%. Two patients had 'microscopic' hematuria. Platelet counts in the 3 patients varied from 5,000 to 166,000/cumm. Each patient received prednisone without significant improvement.

Death in each resulted from progressive cardiac failure. Necropsy in 2 patients disclosed extensive endomyocardial fibrosis with superimposed thrombi in both ventricles (fig. 1 and 2), vegetative valvular endocarditis, membranous glomerulopathy, eosinophilic hyperplasia of the bone marrow and spleen without abnormal or leukemic myeloblasts, and occasionally thrombosed small arteries in the heart,

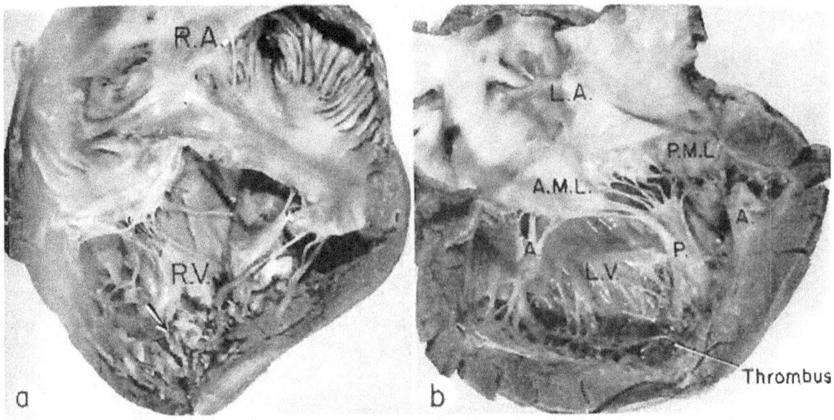

Fig. 1. Interior of the heart in 1 of the 3 patients. a, opened right atrium (RA), tricuspid valve and right ventricle (RV). b, opened left atrium (LA), mitral valve (AML = anterior mitral leaflet; PML = posterior mitral leaflet) and left ventricle (LV). The endocardium of both ventricles is extensively thickened and antemortum thrombus is present in both apices. Both left ventricular papillary muscles (A = anterolateral and P = posteromedial) are severely scarred and both extra- and intra-mural coronary arteries were normal. Both atria and ventricles are dilated.

spleen, kidneys, and lungs. The extra- and intra-mural coronary arteries in both patients were normal, but the left ventricular papillary muscles in each were severely scarred. The hearts weighed 530 and 430 g; the spleens, 1,500 and 480 g; and the livers, 2,200 and 1,800 g. Mature eosinophils were seen on histologic study in several organs of both patients.

Comments

The findings in the 3 patients presented are similar to those in patients with 'fibroplastic parietal endocarditis with blood eosinophilia', a condition originally described by LÖFFLER in 1936 [6]. Of 40 patients with Löffler's endocarditis described up to 1962 [2, 9], ten were women, 30 men; age range 7 to 65 years (average 34); with the exception of 2 patients, death occurred within 2 years after the onset of symptoms; nearly all had congestive cardiac failure, often with precordial murmurs suggesting mitral or tricuspid regurgitation or both; leukocyte counts were elevated (highest 165,000 per cu/mm) at some time in all but 4 patients; the heart weights were excessive in all but 3 patients; the endocardium of the right or left ventricle or both in all was thick and fibrous and 33 had super-

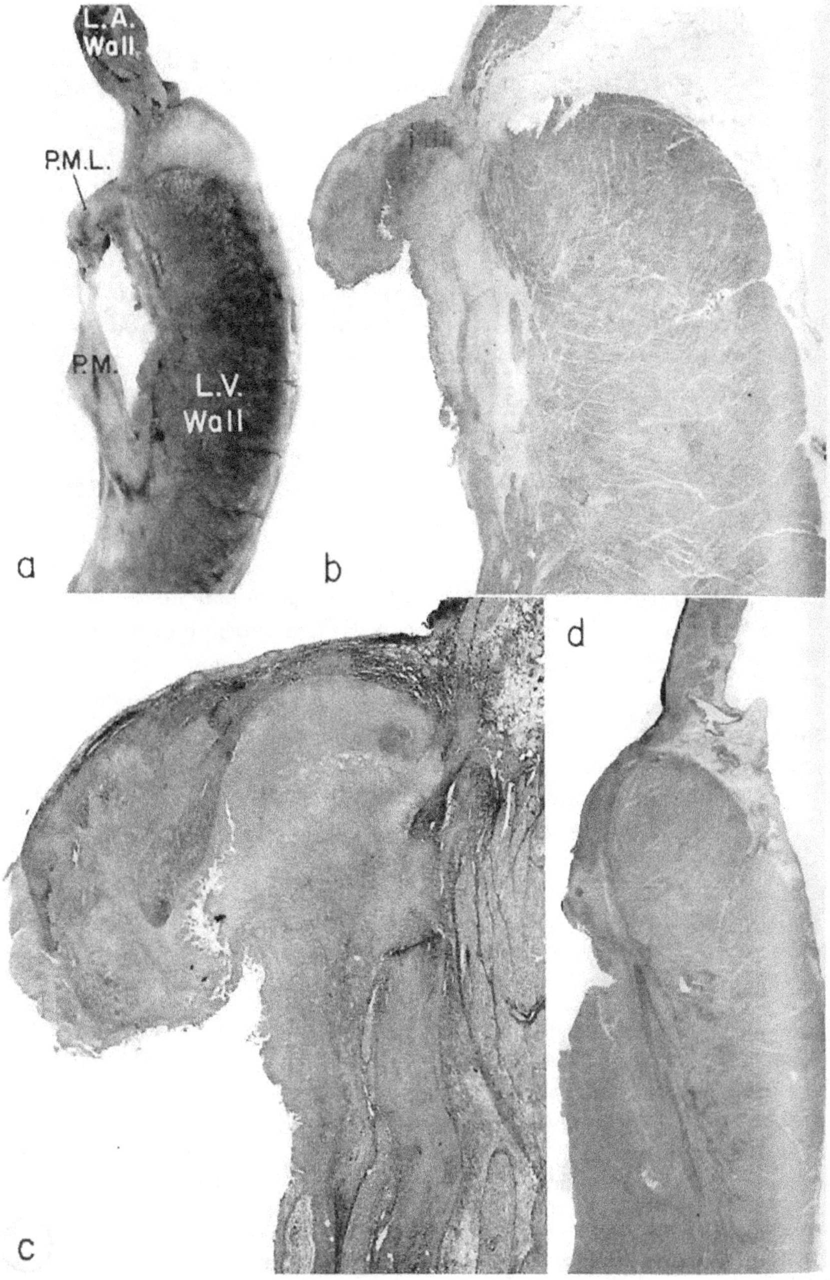
L.A.
Wall
P.M.L.
P.M.
L.V.
Wall
a
b
c
d

imposed thrombi; 32 had fibrous scars in the myocardium; nearly all had mature eosinophils in some organs although sometimes the tissue eosinophilia was minimal; fibrinoid necrosis, vasculitis, or intimal fibrous thickening occurred in small arteries of one or more organs in 22 patients; and the liver or spleen or both were enlarged in about half the patients. Of the 40 patients, 30 were reported from Europe, 7 from Africa, and 3 from North America (USA). Each of our 3 patients was a native of the United States.

The clinical and pathologic features listed above and in our 3 patients are similar to those reported in patients with 'eosinophilic leukemia'. The 23 autopsy patients reported with this condition up to 1963 [1, 7] ranged in age from 7 to 59 years (average 32); 18 were male, 7 female; all had blood eosinophilia (up to 98%); only 5 survived longer than 2 years after the onset of symptoms, and death usually resulted from cardiac failure; over half had extensive endomyocardial fibrosis with mural thrombosis; nearly all had infiltration by mature eosinophils into one or more organs and occasional thrombi or other lesions in small arteries of one or more organs. Thus, the clinical and pathologic findings in patients with 'eosinophilic leukemia' and Löffler's endocarditis are indistinguishable except for the extremely rare patient with malignant eosinophils or myeloblastic precursors with or without the Philadelphia chromosome. It seems reasonable to conclude that these 2 conditions are indeed the same disease.

Certain similarities also exist between endomyocardial fibrosis (EMF) [3, 4] of the African Negro and the condition described in our 3 white

---

Fig. 2. Posterior mitral leaflet (PML) and left atrial (LA) and left ventricular (LV) walls (a, b, c) in the patient whose heart is shown in figure 1, and a section of heart for comparison from a patient with Davies' endomyocardial fibrosis (EMF) (d). a, the endocardium of the mitral leaflet and the mural endocardium of the left ventricular free wall is very thick. The papillary muscle (PM) is severely scarred. b, section includes left atrial and left ventricular walls and posterior mitral leaflet. (Hematoxylin and eosin stain, × 4.) Compare this with section from similar area of heart in d, from a patient with EMF. The endocardium of each is severely thickened and there is superimposed thrombi in d. The posterior mitral leaflet is adherent to underlying fibrous tissue. (The section from the patient with EMF was given to me (W. C. R.) by Professor J. N. D. DAVIES and is from Mulago Hospital postmortum number 145/57, Kampala, Uganda.) c, close-up view of posterior mitral leaflet stained for elastic fibers, which are absent from the superimposed fibrous tissue. The posterior mitral leaflet and an attached chorda tendinea are clearly demarcated from the fibrous tissue. Elastic van Gieson stains; × 11 (b), × 2-½ (c).

men. In both conditions there is usually mural endocardial thickening of both ventricles. Blood eosinophilia has recently been emphasized as a feature of EMF although in his initial report of 36 patients DAVIES mentioned that 'they sometimes show an eosinophilia for which none of the usual causes of eosinophilia account' [3]. Of 40 patients with EMF studied by IVE and associates 17 or 43% had eosinophilia [5]. DAVIES speculated that the earliest lesion in EMF is infiltration of the myocardium by round cells and eosinophils leading to necrosis of the endocardium and subendocardial myocardium. Thrombi form over the necrotic areas. As the mural thrombi and necrotic cardiac tissue become organized the inflammatory cells disappear and finally only dense fibrous tissue remains.

It appears that some patients with endomyocardial fibrosis, of the type seen in Löffler's endocarditis or in Davies' EMF, may have eosinophilia and others may not. LÖFFLER, in his initial report, emphasized that eosinophilia is inconstant and may disappear. It is possible that the presence or absence of eosinophilia is dependent on the length of the illness.

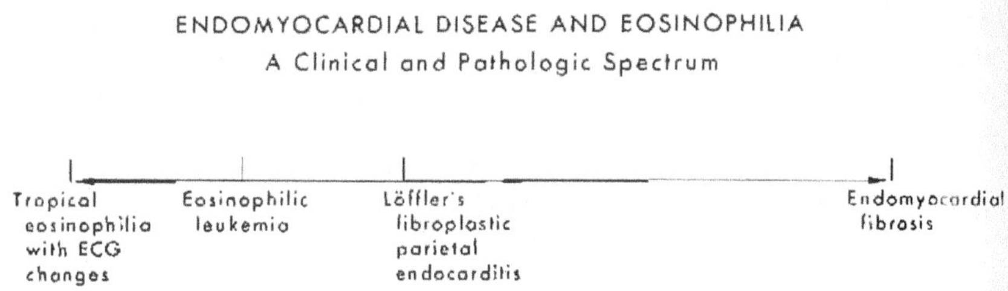

Fig. 3. See text.

The possibility that Löffler's fibroplastic parietal endocarditis, eosinophilic leukemia without abnormal myelopoiesis, and endomyocardial fibrosis of Davies are the same disease at different stages of development is an attractive hypothesis (fig. 3). Patients with eosinophilia associated with a transient benign febrile illness, such as tropical eosinophilia or Löffler's pneumonia, may represent one end of the spectrum. Patients with severe EMF and no blood eosinophilia may represent the other end. Between these 2 extremes there may be patients who still have eosinophilia but less extensive endocardial scarring. The latter process is still active and thus eosinophilia is still present, but as the inflammatory process dies down cardiac scar tissue remains and eosinophilia disappears.

Three patients with cardiomegaly, congestive cardiac failure and blood eosinophilia are described. Necropsy in 2 disclosed severe mural endocardial fibrosis with superimposed fibrin-platelet thrombi, myocardial scarring, eosinophilic hyperplasia of the bone marrow and spleen without abnormal or leukemic myeloblasts, and occasionally thrombosed small arteries in the heart, spleen, kidneys and lungs. These features are similar to those described in patients with Löffler's fibroplastic parietal endocarditis and in 'eosinophilic leukemia' without abnormal myelopoiesis. It is suggested that these two conditions are the same disease. It is also suggested that the predominantly African condition, endomyocardial fibrosis, may be a late or inactive stage of either Löffler's endocarditis or of 'eosinophilic leukemia' without abnormal myelopoiesis.

References

1. BOUSSER, J.: Eosinophilie et leucémie. Sang *28:* 553–580 (1957).
2. BRINK, A. J. and WEBER, H. W.: Fibroplastic parietal endocarditis with eosinophilia. Löffler's endocarditis. Amer. J. Med. *34:* 52–70 (1963).
3. DAVIES, J. N. P.: Endocardial fibrosis in Africans. East afr. med. J. *25:* 10–14 (1948).
4. DAVIES, J. N. P. and BALL, J. D.: The pathology of endomyocardial fibrosis in Uganda. Brit. Heart J. *17:* 337–359 (1955).
5. IVE, F. A.; WILLIS, A. J. P.; IKEME, A. C. and BROCKINGTON, I. F.: Endomyocardial fibrosis and filariasis. Quart. J. Med. *36* (n.s.): 495–516 (1967).
6. LÖFFLER, W.: Endocarditis parietalis fibroplastica mit Bluteosinophile. Schweiz. med. Wschr. *66:* 817–820 (1936).
7. ODEBERG, B.: Eosinophilic leukemia and disseminated eosinophilic collagen disease – a disease entity? Acta med. scand. *177:* 129–144 (1965).
8. ROBERTS, W. C.; LIEGLER, D. G. and CARBONE, P. P.: Endomyocardial disease and eosinophilia. A clinical and pathologic spectrum. Amer. J. Med. *46:* 28–42 (1969).
9. WEISS-CARMINE, S.: Die Endocarditis parietalis fibroplastica mit Bluteosinophilie (LÖFFLER) und ihre Stellung im Rahmen der Parietalendokardfibrosen. Schweiz. med. Wschr. *87:* 890–898 (1957).

Authors' address: Dr. WILLIAM C. ROBERTS; Dr. L. MAXIMILIAN BUJA; Dr. VICTOR J. FERRANS, Section of Pathology, National Heart and Lung Institute, National Institutes of Health, *Bethesda, Md.* (USA)

Iron in the Heart

Etiology and Clinical Significance

L. MAXIMILIAN BUJA, M.D.
WILLIAM C. ROBERTS, M.D.
Bethesda, Maryland

Nineteen of 135 patients (four with idiopathic hemochromatosis and 131 with chronic anemia) had cardiac iron deposits (CID). The ventricular CID were grossly visible in nine patients and microscopically visible only in ten patients. Atrial CID were extensive in six patients with extensive ventricular CID, but in the other thirteen patients atrial CID were minimal. Iron deposits in cardiac conduction tissue were minimal and always less than in working myocardium. Every patient who had iron in the myocardium also had iron in other organs and tissues. Nine patients had pigmentary cirrhosis which was associated with anemia and exogenously administered iron in six and unassociated with anemia in three (idiopathic hemochromatosis). Each of seven patients with extensive CID without other cardiac disease had clinical evidence of cardiac dysfunction, and five had chronic congestive cardiac failure. In contrast, cardiac failure, usually transient and mild, occurred in one of six patients with minimal CID and in eight of eighty-four patients without CID.

Of the nineteen patients with CID, three had idiopathic hemochromatosis; 16 had chronic anemia. Each anemic patient who received more than 100 units of blood had extensive CID unless chronic bleeding diatheses coexisted. Each anemic patient with extensive CID who received less than 100 units of blood had hepatic cirrhosis.

In conclusion (1) grossly visible CID are always associated with cardiac dysfunction and usually chronic cardiac failure; (2) CID, usually extensive, occur in patients with idiopathic hemochromatosis; (3) extensive CID occur in patients who receive more than 100 units of blood unless bleeding diatheses coexist; (4) patients with chronic anemia and hepatic cirrhosis who receive less than 100 units of blood also may have extensive CID; (5) CID initially occur in ventricular myocardium, and are usually more extensive in ventricular than in atrial myocardium; (6) CID are always more extensive in working than in conducting myocardium; (7) supraventricular arrhythmias correlate with the extent of CID in atrial myocardium. Thus, the iron heart is not a strong heart but a weak one.

From the Section of Pathology, National Heart and Lung Institute, Bethesda, Maryland 20014. Requests for reprints should be addressed to Dr. William C. Roberts, Section of Pathology, National Heart & Lung Institute, National Institutes of Health, Bethesda, Maryland 20014. Manuscript received August 7, 1970.

Iron deposits may occur in many tissues and organs in the body [1–3]. Deposits in some organs, such as liver, tend to produce reactive fibrosis and occasionally clinical features of hepatic dysfunction [4–7]. Iron deposits in other organs, such as kidney, although occasionally anatomically striking, do not cause dysfunction [8]. Controversy has existed concerning the functional significance of iron deposits in myocardium. Some studies [4,9,10] have indicated that cardiac iron deposits (CID) cause cardiac dysfunction, whereas others [2,3,11] have suggested that iron deposits in the heart are of no functional significance. This study was undertaken to reexamine the problem of whether or not cardiac iron deposits cause cardiac dysfunction. In addition, the etiologic factors related to myocardial iron deposition and the distribution of these deposits in the heart were determined.

PATIENTS STUDIED AND METHODS

The data in the 135 autopsy patients studied are summarized in Tables I through IV. Pigmentary cirrhosis in each of the four patients with idiopathic hemochromatosis was unrelated to anemia and was demonstrated before either blood transfusions or other iron therapy had been administered. Of the 131 patients with chronic anemia, 100 had chronic leukemia, one had acute leukemia, and thirty had chronic non-neoplastic anemia. Of the latter thirty patients, nineteen had aplastic anemia (with hypo- or hyperplastic bone marrow), six had myeloid metaplasia, two had hemolytic anemia, two had hemophilia and one had sickle cell anemia. The 135 patients included all patients with chronic leukemia, chronic non-neoplastic anemia and idiopathic hemochromatosis subjected to autopsy at the Clinical Center from 1953 through 1969 in whom pertinent anatomic and clinical data were available. In addition, one patient with acute leukemia and three patients (two with idiopathic hemochromatosis and one with sickle cell anemia) whose hearts and other tissues were submitted to the Section of Pathology, National Heart and Lung Institute, were included.

The clinical records and electrocardiograms of each patient were reviewed. The number of blood transfusions received by each patient was tabulated, and evidences of cardiac dysfunction were recorded. One histologic section of left ventricle and liver was stained for iron by the Perls' hydrochloric acid-potassium ferrocyanide method [12]. The iron deposits were identified by a positive Prussian blue reaction in histologic sections. The extent of iron deposition was graded as 3+ (massive), 2+ (extensive), 1+ (minimal) and 0. Selected sections of myocardium also were stained with the periodic acid-Schiff (PAS) method before and after digestion with diastase. The whole hearts and histologic sections of other organs of patients with stainable CID were reexamined. Quantitative analyses of the iron content of the left ventricle and liver of most patients with stainable CID were performed (Table II) by digesting aliquots of tissue, which included the full thickness of left ventricular wall of each heart, with a perchloric acid (20 ml/L) [13] and concentrated sulfuric acid (900 ml/L) mixture at 100°C and measuring the iron content of the supernate [14].

TABLE I Cardiac Iron Deposits (CID)

Clinical Diagnosis	Patients: No.	Patients: No. Without CID (%)	Patients: No. With CID (%)	Extent of CID: 1+	Extent of CID: 2+
Leukemia	101*	94 (93)	7 (7)†	6	1
Non-neoplastic anemia	30*	21 (70)	9 (30)‡	3	6
Idiopathic hemochromatosis	4	1 (25)	3 (75)§	1	2
Totals	135	116 (86)	19 (14)¶	10	9

* Four patients had cirrhosis at autopsy.

† Age range twenty to seventy-five years (average fifty years).

‡ Eight patients had aplastic anemia and one had sickle cell anemia; age range ten to sixty-two years (average thirty-five years).

§ Aged fifty-eight, sixty-nine and eighty-two years (average seventy years).

¶ Age range ten to eighty-two years (average forty-six years); eleven were women.

ANATOMIC FINDINGS

Nineteen of the 135 patients had CID (Tables I and II); certain findings in them are illustrated in Figures 1 to 7. Six patients had other associated cardiac diseases: coronary arterial luminal narrowing more than 75 per cent (two patients), cardiac infections (three patients) and valvular disease (one patient). The degree of iron deposition in the left and right ventricular myocardium was 1+ in ten patients and 2+ in nine patients. In patients with 2+ iron deposits, the myocardium grossly was rusty brown, whereas the iron deposits were visible only on microscopic examination in patients with 1+ iron deposits. In each patient the iron deposits were greatest in the epicardial third, intermediate in the subendocardial third and least in the middle third of the ventricular walls (Figure 2). In patients with 1+ CID, the deposits were located mostly in the perinuclear areas of the myocardial fibers and occupied small portions of myocardial fibers (Figure 1). In patients with 2+ CID, a greater number of myocardial fibers contained iron deposits, many iron deposits also were

TABLE II Clinical and Anatomic Findings in Nineteen Patients with Cardiac Iron Deposits

Case No.	Autopsy No.	Age (yr) and Sex	Diagnosis	Blood Transfused: No. Units	Blood Transfused: gm Iron*	Low Hemoglobin (gm %)	Abnormal Glucose Metabolism	CHF	Abnormal ECG	Other Heart Diseases	Liver Weight (gm)	mg Iron/gm Liver (Wet Weight)	Iron Content of Liver (gm)	Cirrhosis	Heart Weight (gm)	CID: LA	CID: RA	CID: SN	CID: AVB	mg Iron/gm LV: Wet Weight	mg Iron/gm LV: Dry Weight	Iron Content of Heart (gm)	Lesions: VW or VS	Lesions: PM
											Grossly Visible (2+) CID†													
1	A61-98	30,F	AA	247	62	5.5	+‡	C	+§	0	4,750	...	...	0	320	2+	2+	1+	...	0.60	3.5	0.19	0	0
2	A62-150	58,M	AA	197	49	7.9	+¶	C	+§	0	3,000	4.14	12.42	0	500	2+	2+	0	1+	0.67	...	0.34	+#	+**
3	A64-104	62,F	AA	92	23	7.0	+¶	T	+§	0	2,400	5.94	14.26	+	350	2+	2+	...	1+	0.91	...	0.32	0	+**
4	A65-95	21,M	AA	116	29	3.9	0	T	+	0	2,190	4.42	9.68	0	350	2+	2+	...	1+	0.70	...	0.25	0	+**
5	A66-3	19,F	AA	276	69	3.9	0	C	+§	0	2,470	3.87	9.56	0	400	2+	2+	1+	1+	1.02	6.9	0.41	+#	+**
6	A67-261	58,F	IH	0	0	11.0	0	C	+	0	1,700	...	...	+	380	1+	1+	...	...	...	...	...	+#	0
7	A68-327	42,F	SSA	359	90	5.0	+‡	C	+	0	...	...	...	+	420	2+	1+	...	1+	1.47	9.2	0.62	+#	+**
8	A57-16	69,M	IH††	36	8	4.8	+‡	C	+	+	1,800	2.35	4.23	+	370	2+	2+	...	1+	...	...	...	+‡‡	+‡‡
9	A59-45	75,F	CLL	52	13	2.8	+¶	C	+	+	1,450	...	...	+	340	1+	0	...	...	...	...	...	+‡‡	0
											Only Microscopically Visible (1+) CID§§													
10	A60-83	10,M	AA	92	23	6.6	+¶	0	0	0	850	0.23	0.20	0	200	0	0	...	...	...	...	...	0	0
11	A65-45	62,M	CLL	30	7.5	2.0	+¶	T	+	0	1,430	0.92	1.32	+	360	1+	0	...	...	0.24	...	0.09	0	+**
12	A66-164	21,F	AA	60	15	4.5	0	0	0	0	2,640	1.65	4.36	0	245	0	0	...	...	0.16	...	0.04	0	+**
13	A67-37	43,M	ALL	110	27.5	4.8	+¶	0	0	0	3,200	0.64	2.05	+	400	0	0	...	0	0.23	...	0.09	0	+**
14	A67-184	20,F	CML	82	20.5	3.1	+‡	0	0	0	1,900	2.48	4.71	0	200	1+	1+	...	...	0.32	...	0.06	0	0
15	A69-25	59,F	CML	38	9.5	6.7	0	0	0	0	2,700	1.17	3.16	0	340	0	0	...	...	...	...	...	0	+**
16	A65-194	42,M	CML	47	12	5.3	0	T	+	+	1,800	0.91	1.64	0	430	0	0	...	...	...	...	...	+‡‡	0
17	A68-275	47,F	CML	66	16.5	4.4	0	C	+	+	3,180	1.18	3.75	0	530	0	0	0	1+	...	...	...	+‡‡	0
18	A70-12	82,M	IH¶¶	65	16	4.8	0	C	+	+	1,956	0.67	1.31	+	500	1+	0	...	...	0.29	...	0.15	+‡‡	+‡‡
19	A70-96	59,F	AA	290	72.5	7.5	0	C	0	+	1,200	4.48##	5.38	+	310	1+	0	0	0	0.29	2.1	0.09	+‡‡	0

NOTE: AA = aplastic anemia; ALL = acute lymphocytic leukemia; AVB = atrioventricular bundle; C = chronic; CHF = congestive heart failure; CID = cardiac iron deposits; CLL = chronic lymphocytic leukemia; CML = chronic myelocytic leukemia; IH = idiopathic hemochromatosis; LA = left atrium; RA = right atrium; SN = sinus node; SSA = sickle cell anemia; T = transient; VW = ventricular walls; VS = ventricular septum; PM = papillary muscles.

* Each unit of blood (whole or packed erythrocytes) contained approximately 250 mg of iron.

† In Cases 1 through 7 cardiomegaly was evident on chest roentgenogram.

‡ Elevated fasting blood sugar only (two with 3+, one with 2+ and one with 1+ pancreatic iron deposits).

§ Supraventricular rhythm disturbance unassociated with other cardiac disease.

¶ Diabetes mellitus which required insulin or oral agents (1 with 3+ and 5 with 2+ pancreatic iron deposits); associated with corticosteroid therapy in 4 patients.

Focal interstitial fibrosis and/or dystrophic calcification, myocardial fibers.

** Focal replacement fibrosis or necrosis with or without apical calcific deposits.

†† Chronic leukemia and anemia subsequently developed.

‡‡ Extensive myocardial replacement fibrosis and/or necrosis.

§§ No patient had cardiomegaly on x-ray film.

¶¶ Hemolytic anemic (anti-e and anti-s antibodies) subsequently developed, and treated with transfusions and iron-depleting agents after IH was diagnosed.

30.5 mg/gm, dry weight.

TABLE III **Iron Deposits in Other Organs of Nineteen Patients with Cardiac Iron Deposits**

Organ	No. Patients (%)	Grade 1+	Grade 2+	Grade 3+
Liver	19 (100)*	0	9	10
Pancreas	19 (100)†	6	9	4
Spleen	14/14 (100)‡	7	5	2
Lymph nodes	19 (100)	9	5	5
Bone marrow	17/18 (94)§	14	3	0
Kidney	16 (84)	15	1	0
Adrenal cortex	15/18 (83)	12	3	0
Gastric mucosa	14/17 (82)	10	4	0
Thyroid	12/16 (75)	5	3	4
Ovary	5/7 (71)	4	1	0
Parathyroid	7/10 (70)	4	0	3
Salivary gland	2/3 (66)	2	0	0
Skeletal muscle	10/16 (62)	10	0	0
Pituitary gland	7/14 (50)	4	2	1
Breast	4/9 (44)	3	1	0

* Iron deposits were present in Kupffer and hepatic parenchymal cells and periportal connective tissue of each patient, and twelve also had iron deposits in epithelial cells of bile ducts.

† Iron deposits were present in the exocrine and islet cells of each patient. Mild, focal fibrosis was present in eight patients (two with 1+, four with 2+ and two with 3+ iron), including the three patients with hemochromatosis.

‡ Splenectomy performed in five patients.

§ Erythroid hypoplasia in fifteen patients, erythroid hyperplasia with abnormal erythropoiesis in two and bone marrow normal in one patient (idiopathic hemochromatosis).

located in the periphery of myocardial fibers, and the deposits occupied large portions of each myocardial fiber (Figure 1). In each of the nineteen patients iron deposits were present in both interstitial (connective tissue) cells of the myocardium and in myocardial fibers. The granular iron deposits in interstitial cells and myocardial fibers were periodic acid-Schiff–positive both before and after treatment of sections with diastase. Electron microscopic examination of myocardium in one patient showed that the CID consisted of granules which contained masses of electron-dense particles each of which measured approximately 60 Å in diameter, and that the deposits were located between myofibrils (Figure 6).

The extent of iron deposits in the ventricles was greater than that in the atria in thirteen of the nineteen patients, including the ten with 1+ CID, five of whom had no deposits in the atria, and three of nine with 2+ CID (Figure 3). In the other six patients with 2+ CID, the atria and ventricles both contained 2+ CID (Figure 3). The atrioventricular bundle of one patient (Case 5) was serially sectioned, and random sections of conduction tissue from nine other patients were examined. The conduction tissue contained 0 to 1+ CID in each patient (Figures 4 and 5). Epicardial nerves in two of nineteen patients contained iron deposits, but they were negligible.

In all nineteen patients with CID, iron deposits occurred in parenchymal cells of other organs (Table III) and in reticuloendothelial and connective tissue cells of many tissues. Iron deposits were present in the skin in the four patients with increased dermal pigmentation. Portal cirrhosis (severe scarring, loss of architecture and evidence of regeneration) occurred in nine of nineteen patients with CID, including three with idiopathic hemochromatosis (Figure 7). Mild to moderate periportal fibrosis without hepatic cirrhosis occurred in the other ten patients. Of the 116 patients without CID, ninety-three (79 per cent) had hepatic iron deposits (thirty-five, 1+; thirty-six, 2+; and twenty-two 3+), sixty-four had mild to moderate periportal fibrosis, and three additional patients had cirrhosis. Thus, twelve of the 135 patients had pigmentary cirrhosis. The etiology of the cirrhosis in the nine patients with CID is unclear: three patients, two of whom had idiopathic hemochromatosis, had historic or anatomic evidence, or both, of chronic alcoholism; one had serum hepatitis two years before death; no etiologic factors were identified in the other five patients. Two of the three patients with cirrhosis and no CID had common duct stones (one also had a history of chronic alcoholism), and one patient had idiopathic hemochromatosis.

TABLE IV **Relation of Cardiac Iron Deposits (CID) to Amount of Blood Transfused in 135 Patients**

Units of Blood	Patients: No. Patients	No. Without CID (%)	No. With CID (%)	Extent of CID 1+	Extent of CID 2+
0–25	71	70	1 (1.4)	0	1
26–50	35	31	4 (11)	3	1
51–75	14	10	4 (28)	3	1
76–100	5	2	3 (60)	2	1
101–200	5	2*	3 (60)	1*	2
201–300	3	0	3 (100)	1*	2
>300	2	1*	1 (50)	0	1
Totals	135	116	19 (14)	10	9

* Each had repeated massive bleeding episodes.

CLINICAL FINDINGS

These clinical findings are summarized in Table II. Each of the seven patients with 2+ CID and without other cardiac disease had clinical evidence of cardiac dysfunction which was unassociated with sepsis or pneumonia. Each of the five patients

Figure 1. *Longitudinal (**a** and **c**) and transverse (**b** and **d**) sections of myocardial fibers of left ventricle stained for iron. In **a** and **b** iron deposits are classified as 2+ and they occupy large portions of the hypertrophied myocardial fibers. When the iron deposits in individual myocardial fibers are this extensive they are present in nearly all fibers and therefore are grossly visible, imparting a rusty brown color. In **c** and **d** the iron deposits are limited to the central, perinuclear portions (arrows) of the myocardial fibers and are not visible grossly. Hence, they are classified in this study as 1+. Prussian blue stains, original magnification × 1,000.*

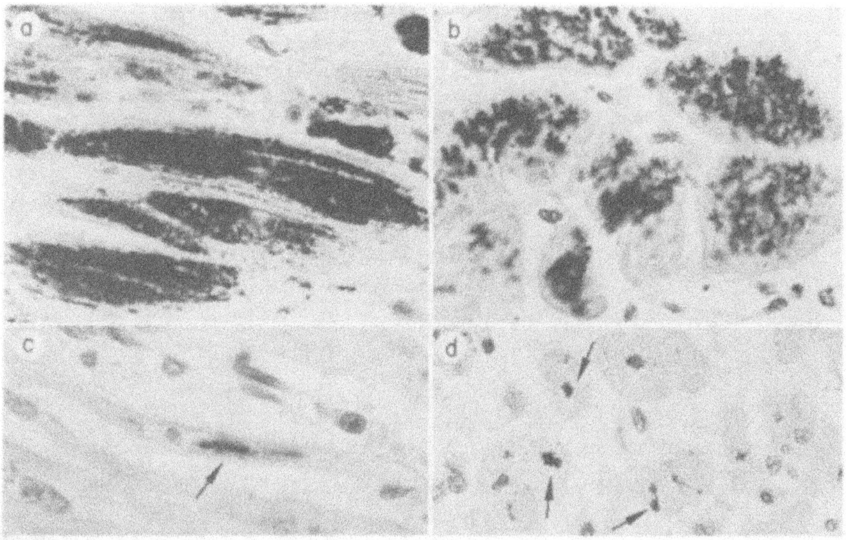

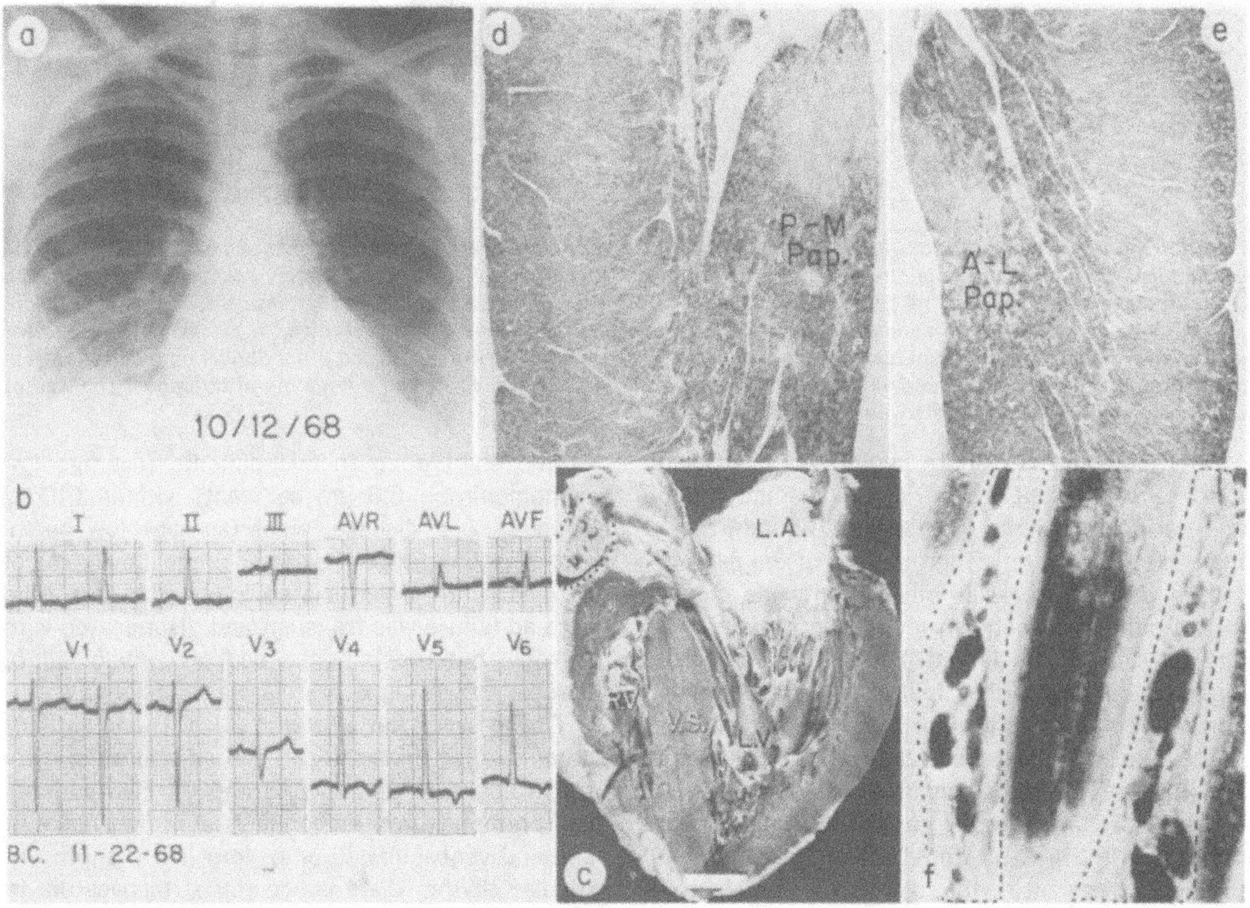

Figure 2. *Chest roentgenogram (**a**); electrocardiogram (**b**); opened heart (**c**); histologic sections of left ventricular wall with posteromedial (P-M) and anterolateral (A-L) papillary muscles (Pap.) (**d** and **e**); and close-up of subepicardial left ventricular myocardial fibers (**f**) of patient (Case 7) who died on November 23, 1968. The patient had sickle cell anemia and had received 260 units of blood when congestive cardiac failure developed six years before death. Chest roentgenograms showed cardiomegaly (**a**), and electrocardiograms, ischemic S-T segment and T wave changes. By the time of death she had received 359 units of blood (90 gm iron). At autopsy (A68-327), the walls of the right (R.V.) and left (L.V.) ventricles, left atrium (L.A.), and atrial and ventricular (V.S.) septums were rusty brown (**c**) due to extensive iron deposits. The right atrial wall (partially enclosed by dotted line), in contrast, was tan (**c**) and microscopically only minute particles of iron were present. Large areas of replacement fibrosis (pale areas) were present in both left ventricular papillary muscles (**d** and **e**). Severely degenerated myocardial fibers (enclosed by dotted lines) which also contained iron deposits were often found adjacent to viable myocardial fibers (**f**), Prussian blue stains, original magnification × 3 (**d**), × 2 (**e**), and × 628 (**f**).*

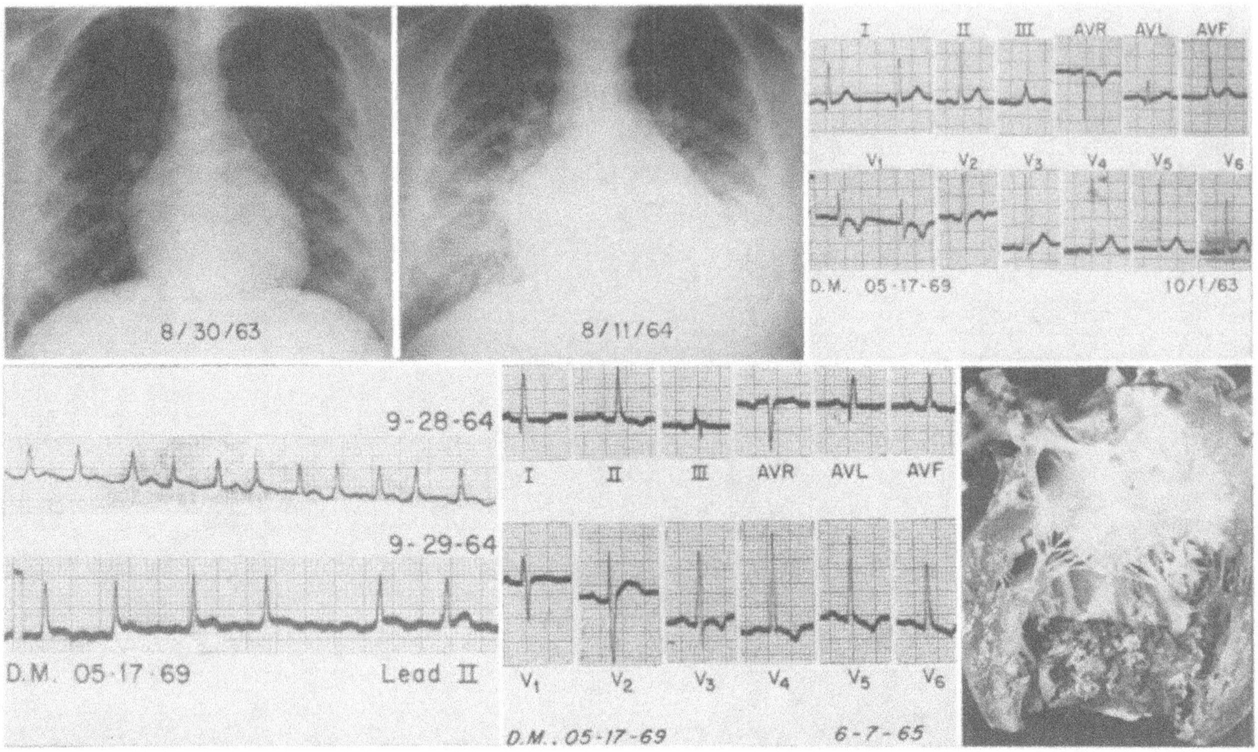

***Figure 3.** Chest roentgenograms (dates when taken are shown), electrocardiograms and opened heart of patient (Case 5) who died with aplastic anemia on January 5, 1966. Congestive cardiac failure with pulmonary edema and atrial fibrillation developed seventeen months before death. Shortly afterward, she had a cerebrovascular accident. The cardiac failure was partially alleviated by the administration of digitalis and bed rest, sinus rhythm returned, but ischemic S-T segment and T wave changes were present. One month before death cardiac failure worsened, and atrial fibrillation recurred. At autopsy (A66-3), the left atrium and ventricle were dilated; the left ventricle contained a large mural thrombus. The wall of each chamber contained extensive iron deposits.*

with chronic cardiac failure had severe exertional dyspnea, orthopnea, a ventricular diastolic gallop and peripheral edema (with serum albumin more than 3.0 gm/100 ml). The duration of the cardiac failure was two weeks in one patient, one month in two patients, seventeen months in one patient, and six years in one patient. Each patient received digitalis, but the cardiac failure in each was only partially or transiently alleviated. In one patient digitalis toxicity developed (atrial tachycardia with block). One patient had recurrent angina pectoris without coronary arterial narrowing. One of two patients with 2+ CID without chronic cardiac failure had a transient rhythm disturbance on electrocardiogram and transient acute pulmonary edema after transfusion which responded to digitalis. The seventh patient with 2+ CID had a transient ventricular diastolic gallop and transient ischemic T wave changes on electrocardiogram. Cardiac failure, as evidenced by a ventricular diastolic gallop, occurred in only one of six patients with 1+ CID unassociated with other heart disease. Of the eighty-four anemic patients (average low hemoglobin = 6.3 gm per cent) without CID or other cardiac disease, eight (average low hemoglobin = 6.0 gm per cent) had clinical evidence of cardiac failure unassociated with sepsis. In six the cardiac failure was transient and disappeared with therapy, but two patients died of cardiac failure associated with large pericardial effusions.

Of the seven patients with 2+ CID and without other cardiac disease each had an abnormal electrocardiogram (Figures 2, 3 and 4). Five patients had premature contractions (atrial in five, nodal in one and ventricular in one); four had a supraventricular rhythm disturbance (atrial tachycardia in two, atrial fibrillation in one, atrial flutter in one and sinus bradycardia with wandering atrial pacemaker in one); one had a P-R interval greater than 0.20 second transiently; and six had ischemic S-T segment and T wave changes. The only abnormality which occurred in the six patients with 1+ CID without other cardiac disease was premature atrial contractions in one patient. Thirty-five

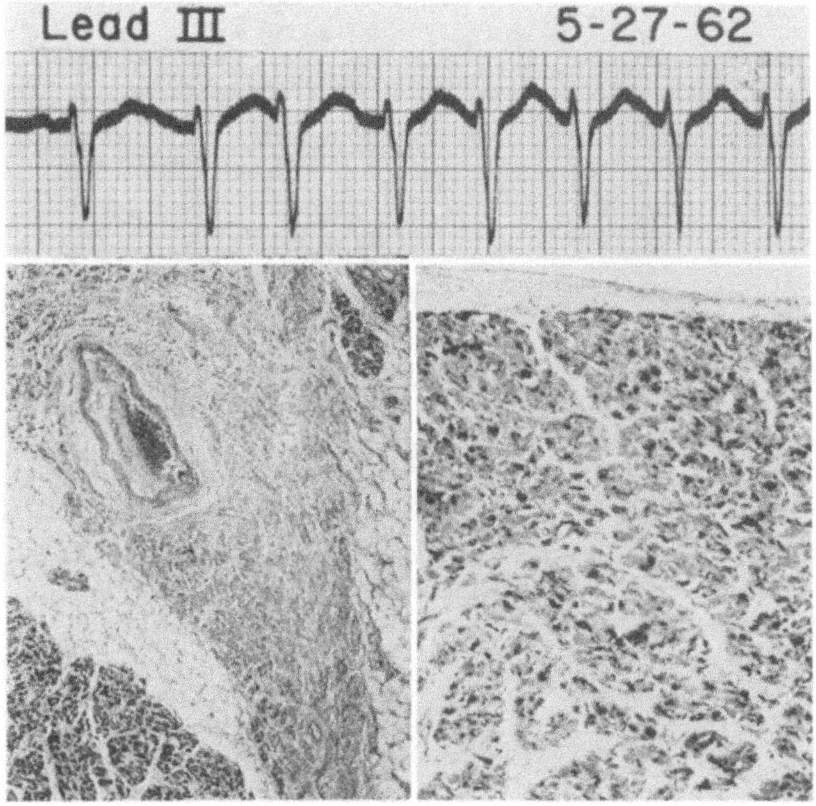

*Figure 4. Electrocardiogram, and histologic sections of sinus node (**lower left**) and right atrial wall (**lower right**) of patient (Case 2) who had aplastic anemia. The patient was hospitalized on May 26, 1962, because of syncope; electrocardiogram showed paroxysmal atrial tachycardia with normal atrioventricular conduction. He died on June 29, 1962, after a second syncopal episode. At autopsy (A62-150), the sinus node contained no iron deposits (**lower left**); the atrioventricular bundle, minimal deposits; but the working myocardial fibers of the atria (**lower right**) and ventricles contained extensive deposits. Prussian blue stains, original magnification × 46 (**lower left**) and × 133 (**lower right**).*

(57 per cent) of the sixty-one patients without CID or other cardiac disease had abnormal electrocardiograms, including low voltage (sum of QRS in leads I, II, III $\leq$ 1.5 mv) in thirteen, premature contractions in six, atrial tachycardia in two and S-T segment and T wave changes in fifteen (nonspecific in six, ischemic in seven and pericarditis-type in two).

Relationship of CID to Amount of Blood Transfused. These data are summarized in Table IV. In the patients with CID, the time interval between the transfusion of the first unit of blood and death varied from seven months to nineteen years, and was less than twelve months in only three patients (excluding the three with idiopathic hemochromatosis). Five of the nine patients with 2+ CID received more than 100 units of blood. The four patients with 2+ CID who received less than 100 units of blood had hepatic cirrhosis, including two with idiopathic hemochromatosis. Six (three with 1+ and three with 2+ CID) of the nineteen patients had taken iron preparations orally for brief periods of time. The three patients with cirrhosis and no CID received 0, 10 and 21 units, respectively.

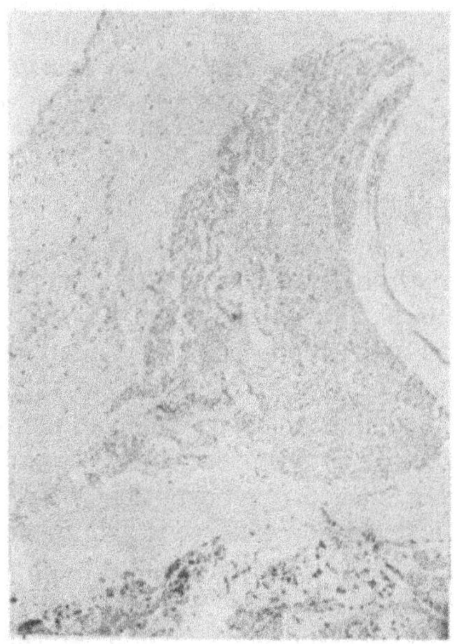

Figure 5. Histologic section of atrioventricular bundle of patient (Case 7, A68-327). The myocardial fibers of the bundle contain no iron deposits. Extensive iron deposits, however, are present in the working myocardial fibers below. Prussian blue stain, original magnification × 46.

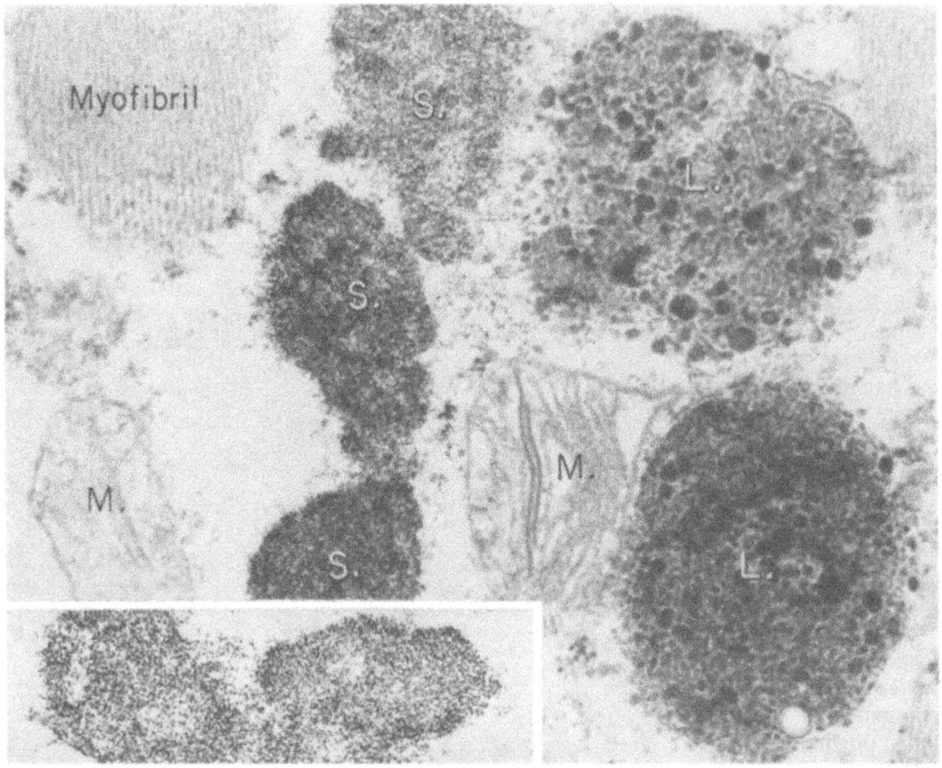

Figure 6. *Electron micrographs of portions of a left ventricular myocardial fiber of patient (Case 7, A68-327). Siderin (S.) and lipofuscin (L.) granules are present between the myofibrils. The siderin granules contain numerous iron particles, the electron-dense portions of which measure 60 Å in diameter (inset). The lipofuscin granules consist of masses of electron-dense material but contain no iron particles. M. = mitochondria. Formalin-fixed tissue, post-fixed in 3 per cent glutaraldehyde and 1 per cent osmium tetroxide (inset without osmium); embedded in Maraglas; counterstained with lead citrate and uranyl acetate (inset without counterstain); and examined in an RCA-3 electron microscope, original magnification × 46,865 and × 92,075 (inset).*

COMMENTS

Whenever iron deposits are present in myocardium, they are also always present in liver, spleen, pancreas and lymph nodes, and nearly always in bone marrow, stomach and various endocrine organs (Table III). Iron deposits limited to myocardial fibers have never been described to our knowledge. The occurrence of iron deposits in several body organs is commonly referred to as **iron storage disease** and its various causes are summarized in Table V [2–7, 15–20]. Any of the iron storage diseases may be associated with iron deposits in myocardium, but why some patients with heavy iron deposits in liver, spleen and bone marrow have iron deposits in the heart, and others with apparently similar quantities of iron in these other organs do not have iron in the myocardium is uncertain. We suspect (Table II) that the total body iron is greater in patients with CID than in those without CID but with iron deposits in many other organs. It is possible that iron is selectively deposited in liver and certain other organs, and that iron deposition in the heart does not occur until the other organs are saturated with iron. Cardiac muscle has a greater affinity for iron than does skeletal or smooth muscle (Table III).

Considerable controversy exists regarding the pathogenesis of iron deposition in any body organ. At least four factors appear important: cirrhosis, anemia, increased quantities of exogenous iron (oral and/or parenteral) and increased gastrointestinal absorption of normal dietary quantities of iron. Whether iron in the liver causes cirrhosis or whether hepatic iron is simply superimposed on an already cirrhotic liver still is debatable [2–7, 15,16]. Pigmentary cirrhosis (iron in the liver plus cirrhosis), which occurred in twelve of 135 patients studied by us, is of two types: (1) iron deposition in an otherwise normal liver which subsequently becomes cirrhotic, and (2) iron deposition in an already cirrhotic liver. Which of these types oc-

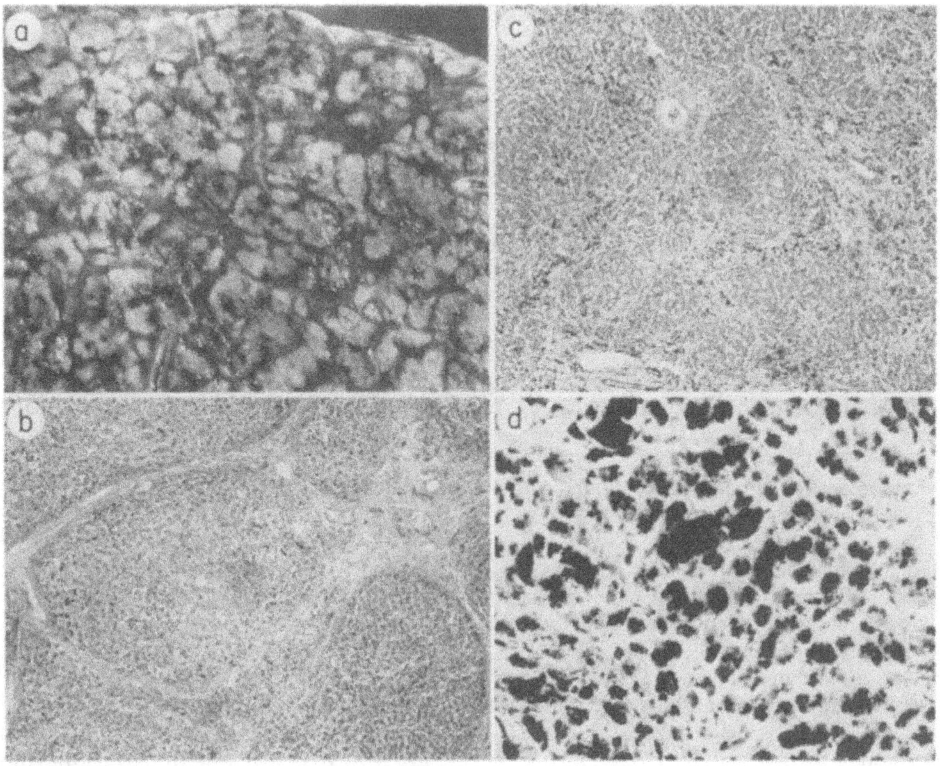

Figure 7. *Photograph of gross section (**a**) and photomicrographs of histologic sections (**b**, **c** and **d**) of liver from two patients with idiopathic hemochromatosis (**a**, Case 18, A70-12; **b**, Case 8, A57-16) and two patients with chronic anemia (**c**, Case 3, A64-104; **d**, Case 7, A68-327). Each patient had portal cirrhosis with extensive fibrosis, loss of normal hepatic architecture and nodular regeneration (**a**, **b** and **c**), and extensive iron deposits in hepatic parenchymal and Kupffer cells (**d**). Gross photograph, original magnification × 6 (**a**); hematoxylin and eosin stains, original magnification × 40 (**b** and **c**); Prussian blue stain, original magnification × 350 (**d**).*

curred in the twelve cirrhotic patients studied by us is uncertain. All but one of the 135 patients were anemic. Of the twelve patients with pigmentary cirrhosis, eight presented initially with anemia, but four had pigmentary cirrhosis before anemia developed (three patients), or without anemia (one patient). Whether the latter four patients had idiopathic hemochromatosis with a genetic defect in iron metabolism leading to increased gastrointestinal iron absorption [21–24] or whether increased iron deposition was superimposed on a preexisting cirrhosis is unknown [2,3,16]. Increased stores of iron have been demonstrated in many patients with alcoholic and other forms of cirrhosis, and in some the anatomic findings are identical with those in patients with idiopathic hemochromatosis [2,3,25–28]. In this study, patients with pigmentary cirrhosis unassociated with anemia were classified as having idiopathic hemochromatosis.

The role of anemia in iron storage disease also is controversial. In our anemic patients, the most important factor related to the deposition of iron in myocardium and other organs appeared to be the amount of exogenously administered iron in the form of blood transfusions. Iron storage disease in some previously described patients with anemia also can be explained by excess exogenous intake of iron, usually from blood transfusions [9,29–34]. Some of these patients, however, have been shown to have a significantly greater amount of stored iron than could be accounted for by the exogenously administered iron [1,5,9,35–39]. In addition, anemic patients with iron storage disease, including some with extensive CID, have been described who have received less than 25 units of blood [9]. Derangements of iron metabolism associated with anemia, therefore, may be as important in the development of excess iron storage as in the amount of exogenously administered iron [3,5–7,16,39].

Controversy has existed over the functional sig-

TABLE V Classification of Iron Storage Disease

A. **Hemochromatosis** (hepatic cirrhosis and increased iron deposits in many organs including liver and pancreas)
  I. Primary or idiopathic (genetic disorder causing increased gastrointestinal absorption of dietary iron; hepatic iron deposits produce cirrhosis unrelated to preexisting cirrhosis, anemia or increased exogenous iron)
  II. Secondary (increased iron deposits secondary to other diseases)
    (1) Preexisting cirrhosis (nutritional and other types)
    (2) Anemia (congenital or acquired defects of erythrocytes or erythrocyte production)
      (a) Factors associated with anemia (increased gastrointestinal absorption of dietary iron, decreased utilization of iron for erythropoiesis, hemolysis)
      (b) Excess exogenous intake of iron (blood transfusions or oral or parenteral iron therapy)
    (3) Excess oral iron
      (a) Hemochromatosis of the Bantu
      (b) Iatrogenic hemochromatosis

B. **Hemosiderosis** (increased iron deposits in many organs without cirrhosis)
  I. Malnutrition (folic acid deficiency, etc.)
  II. Anemia (with or without excess exogenous intake of iron)
  III. Excess oral iron

nificance of CID in patients with iron storage disease. Some workers have concluded that CID cause congestive cardiac failure. Finch and Finch [4] described eighty patients with idiopathic hemochromatosis and reviewed the findings in 1,018 other patients reported on up to 1954. Of the 1,098 patients with histologically-proved hemochromatosis, 31 per cent had fatal cardiac failure. The extent of CID or the presence of other cardiac disease in the 1,098 patients was not mentioned. Many individual patients with idiopathic hemochromatosis, extensive CID and congestive cardiac failure unassociated with other cardiac disease(s) have been described [22,40–51]. Engle and coworkers [9,10] studied forty-two patients with chronic anemia and clinical evidence of acquired iron storage disease: twenty-six had fatal congestive cardiac failure with cardiomegaly on chest roentgenogram and usually an abnormal electrocardiogram, and six other patients had cardiomegaly and an abnormal electrocardiogram without overt failure; each of fifteen patients subjected to autopsy had extensive, grossly visible CID, and quantitative studies performed on six hearts disclosed 0.9 to 3.1 mg of iron/gm of left ventricular myocardium (wet or dry weight not specified). Other patients with chronic anemia and acquired iron storage disease in whom cardiac failure developed associated with CID have been described [10,33–35]. None of the studies of iron storage disease associated with anemia, however, compared patients with CID with a control group of anemic patients without CID. In addition, indirect evidence of the adverse effects of CID has been provided by remission of cardiac failure and disappearance of electrocardiographic abnormalities following therapeutic procedures removing large quantities of systemic iron stores [15,22,52].

Some investigators have concluded that iron deposits in the heart do not cause cardiac failure. MacDonald and Mallory [2,3] studied 211 autopsy patients with iron storage disease, fifty-seven of whom they classified as having hemochromatosis (i.e., with cirrhosis), fifty with advanced hemosiderosis and 104 with simple (i.e., early) hemosiderosis. The incidence of CID in the three groups of patients was 100, 30 and 3 per cent, respectively, but the incidence of fatal cardiac failure in each group was approximately the same (18, 18 and 16 per cent). The authors concluded that CID were not clinically important since the presence of CID did not increase the incidence of cardiac failure. They did not separate, however, patients with and without other cardiac disease nor did they distinguish patients with minimal from those with extensive CID. Keschner [11] performed quantitative iron determinations on the hearts of eleven patients with hemochromatosis and reached the same conclusion as did MacDonald and Mallory. Of seven patients with extensive CID, only three had congestive cardiac failure and none had associated anatomic cardiac disease. The amount of CID in the patients with (3.54 to 5.50 mg/gm left ventricular myocardium, dry weight) and without (1.96 to 7.24 mg/gm left ventricular myocardium, dry weight) cardiac failure was similar.

The present study clearly shows that CID can cause congestive cardiac failure. All seven patients with grossly visible CID unassociated with other anatomic cardiac disease had clinical evidence of congestive cardiac failure, and none of the patients with only microscopically visible CID had cardiac dysfunction.

Electrocardiographic abnormalities occur frequently in patients with CID [4,9,10]. The most frequent abnormality previously reported was supraventricular arrhythmias, followed by disturbances of atrioventricular conduction and, much less frequently, ventricular arrhythmias. Supraventricular arrhythmias also were the most frequent rhythm or conduction disturbance observed in our patients with CID. None of our patients had a ventricular arrhythmia and only one had an abnormality of atrioventricular conduction (P-R interval more than 0.20 second).

Previous comparative electrocardiographic and pathologic studies of patients with CID have yielded contradictory results and have failed to correlate the presence or extent of iron deposits in the conduction system with the electrocardiographic abnormalities. James [53] found extensive iron deposits in the working myocardium and the atrioventricular node, but no deposits in the sinus node of five patients with CID. Schellhammer, Engle and Hagstrom [10] studied six patients with extensive iron deposits in the working myocardium. The sinus node contained light to moderate iron deposits in three and no deposits in three patients; the atrioventricular node and bundle, right and left bundle branches, and Purkinje fibers contained moderate to heavy iron deposits in five patients and light deposits in one patient; and the autonomic nerve fibers and ganglia showed negligible iron deposits in each patient. In neither study did the presence of a supraventricular arrhythmia (six of eleven patients) correlate with the extent of CID in the sinus node, nor did the presence of a disturbance of atrioventricular conduction (five of eleven patients) correlate with the extent of CID in the ventricular conduction tissue. Both previous studies, however, did not compare the extent of iron deposition in the atria and ventricles, nor did they attempt to correlate arrhythmias with the amount of atrial iron deposits. In our study, iron deposits in the conduction tissue were absent or minimal in the ten patients examined. The extent of atrial iron deposition, however, varied considerably in patients with extensive ventricular iron deposits. Four of five patients with extensive atrial iron deposits had supraventricular arrhythmias, whereas no patient with ventricular iron deposits and minimal (1+) atrial iron deposits had an arrhythmia.

Angina pectoris unrelated to coronary arteriosclerosis occurred in one of our patients and has been observed in patients with CID studied by others [48]. One patient with CID and features of constrictive cardiomyopathy or pericarditis has been described [54].

Cardiac hypertrophy and dilatation, degeneration of myocardial fibers and myocardial fibrosis also have been found in patients with CID [4,9,10, 33–35,40–55]. Chronic anemia may have contributed to these changes in some patients, but similar findings were observed in patients without anemia. In the present study lesions of the left ventricular papillary muscles occurred in patients both with grossly visible and only microscopically visible CID. Chronic anemia may well have played an important role in the development of lesions in the papillary muscles, which appear to be the last structure in the heart to be perfused with arterial blood. Degeneration, dystrophic calcification and loss of myocardial fibers and fibrosis in the free walls, however, most likely resulted primarily from the iron deposits because these lesions were observed only in hearts of patients with 2+ CID and they were located in areas of maximal iron deposition.

The distribution and nature of the iron deposits in the hearts of patients with CID has rarely been emphasized. We confirmed the observation of Cappell, Hutchinson and Jowett [1] that three zones of iron deposition occur in the myocardium and that the iron deposits are greatest in the subepicardial region, intermediate in the subendocardial region and papillary muscles, and least in the middle third of the ventricular myocardium. This pattern, however, was not apparent in atrial myocardium. Our data also indicate that iron is first deposited in ventricular rather than atrial myocardium and that atrial myocardium may contain small amounts of iron deposits when the ventricles contain large deposits. Iron deposition in our patients was always more extensive in working myocardium than in conducting myocardium. CID are localized mostly in siderin granules which contain numerous iron particles, the electron-dense portions of which average 60 Å in diameter, in an electronlucent, periodic acid-Schiff positive matrix [12,56–58]. Individual iron particles also may occur in sarcoplasm of myocardial fibers.

The pathogenesis of the anatomic and clinical cardiac abnormalities in patients with CID and iron storage disease is unclear. It has been suggested [59] that cardiac failure in these patients is secondary to multiple endocrine abnormalities. Although such abnormalities occur, a causal relationship with cardiac disease has not been proved [15,60]. Others have suggested that the rate of iron deposition in myocardium is of greater importance in the development of clinical cardiac disease than the amount of CID found at autopsy [49]. Our anatomic studies, however, indicate that cardiac dysfunction does depend upon the **quantity** of iron deposited in individual myocardial fibers and the **number** of fibers affected. Iron deposits are usually limited to the perinuclear areas of myocardial fibers and are present in relatively few fibers in patients with little or no evidence of cardiac dysfunction, whereas iron deposits occupy large areas of individual myocardial fibers and are present in many fibers of patients with significant cardiac dysfunction. Degeneration and loss of myocardial fibers with resultant fibrosis probably occurs when iron deposits replace many normal constituents of myocardial fibers and thereby prevent adequate cellular metabolism and function.

REFERENCES

1. Cappell DF, Hutchinson HE, Jowett M: Transfusional siderosis: the effects of excessive iron deposits in the tissues. J Path Bact 74: 245, 1957.
2. MacDonald RA, Mallory GK: Hemochromatosis and hemosiderosis; study of 211 autopsied cases. Arch Intern Med (Chicago) 105: 686, 1960.
3. MacDonald RA: Hemochromatosis and Hemosiderosis, Springfield, Ill, Charles C Thomas, 1964, pp 3, 94, 207.
4. Finch SC, Finch CA: Idiopathic hemochromatosis, an iron storage disease. Medicine (Balt) 34: 381, 1955.
5. Kent G, Popper H: Secondary hemochromatosis: its association with anemia. Arch Path (Chicago) 70: 623, 1960.
6. Kent G, Popper H: Liver biopsy in diagnosis of hemochromatosis. Amer J Med 44: 837, 1968.
7. Block M: Histopathologic studies in beta-thalassemia minor and intermedia. Ann New York Acad Sci 165: 126, 1969.
8. Roberts WC, Morrow AG: Renal hemosiderosis in patients with prosthetic aortic valves. Circulation 33: 390, 1966.
9. Engle MA, Erlandson M, Smith CH: Late cardiac complications of chronic, severe, refractory anemia with hemochromatosis. Circulation 30: 698, 1964.
10. Schellhammer PF, Engle MA, Hagstrom JW: Histochemical studies of the myocardium and conduction system in acquired iron-storage disease. Circulation 35: 631, 1967.
11. Keschner HW: The heart in hemochromatosis. Southern Med J 44: 927, 1951.
12. Lillie RD: Histopathologic Technic and Practical Histochemistry, 3rd ed, New York, McGraw-Hill, 1965, p 397.
13. Zak B, Willard HH, Myers GB, Boyle AJ: Chloric acid method for determination of protein-bound iodine. Anal Chem 24: 1345, 1952.
14. Giovanniello TJ, DiBenedetto G, Palmer DW, Peters T Jr: Fully automated method for the determination of serum iron and total iron-binding capacity, Technicon Symposia 1967, vol 1, White Plains, New York, Mediad Inc, 1968, p 185.
15. Charlton RW, Bothwell TH: Hemochromatosis: dietary and genetic aspects, Progress in Hematology, vol 5 (Brown EB, Moore CV, eds), New York, Grune & Straton, Inc, 1966, p 298.
16. MacDonald RA: Primary hemochromatosis: inherited or acquired? Progress in Hematology, vol 5 (Brown EB, Moore CV, eds), New York, Grune & Straton, Inc, 1966, p 324.
17. Lewis SM: Red-cell abnormalities and haemolysis in aplastic anaemia. Brit J Haemat 8: 322, 1962.
18. Case Records of Massachusetts General Hospital (Case 44131). New Eng J Med 258: 652, 1958.
19. Johnson BF: Hemochromatosis resulting from prolonged oral iron therapy. New Eng J Med 278: 1100, 1968.
20. Greenberg MS, Grace ND: Folic acid deficiency and iron overload. Arch Intern Med (Chicago) 125: 140, 1970.
21. Williams R, Scheuer PJ, Sherlock S: The inheritance of idiopathic hemochromatosis. Quart J Med 31: 249, 1962.
22. Perkins KW, McInnes IWS, Blackburn CRB, Beal RW: Idiopathic hemochromatosis in children. Report of a family. Amer J Med 39: 118, 1965.
23. Balcerzak SP, Westerman MP, Lee RE, Doyle AP: Idiopathic hemochromatosis. Amer J Med 40: 857, 1966.
24. Sinniah R: Environmental and genetic factors in idiopathic hemochromatosis. Arch Intern Med (Chicago) 124: 455, 1969.
25. Butt EM, Nusbaum RE, Gilmour TC, DiDio SL: Trace metal patterns in disease states. III. Hepatic and pancreatic cirrhosis in alcoholic patients, with and without storage of iron. Amer J Clin Path 42: 437, 1964.
26. Zimmerman HJ, Chomet B, Kulesh MH, McWhorter CA: Hepatic hemosiderin deposits. Incidence in 558 biopsies from patients with and without intrinsic hepatic disease. Arch Intern Med (Chicago) 107: 494, 1961.
27. Williams R, Williams HS, Scheuer PJ, Pitcher CS, Loiseau E, Sherlock S: Iron absorption and siderosis in chronic liver disease. Quart J Med 36: 151, 1967.
28. Pascal RR, Einspruch BC: Hemochromatosis secondary to liver disease and iron ingestion. New York J Med 63: 2825, 1963.
29. Norris RP, McEwen FJ: Exogenous hemochromatosis following multiple blood transfusions. JAMA 143: 740, 1950.
30. Aufderheide AC, Horns HL, Goldish RJ: Secondary hemochromatosis. I. Transfusion (exogenous) hemochromatosis. Blood 8: 824, 1953.
31. Wallerstein RO, Robbins SL: Hemochromatosis after prolonged oral iron therapy in a patient with chronic hemolytic anemia. Amer J Med 14: 256, 1953.
32. Pletcher WD, Brody GL, Meyers MC: Hemochromatosis following prolonged iron therapy in patient with hereditary nonspherocytic hemolytic anemia. Amer J Med Sci 246: 27, 1963.
33. Frumin AM, Waldman S, Morris P: Exogenous hemochromatosis in Mediterranean anemia. Pediatrics 9: 290, 1952.
34. Howell J, Wyatt JP: Development of pigmentary cirrhosis in Cooley's anemia. Arch Path (Chicago) 55: 423, 1953.
35. Goldish RJ, Aufderheide AC: Secondary hemochromatosis. II. Report of a case not attributable to blood transfusions. Blood 8: 837, 1953.
36. Zeltmacher K, Bevans M: Aplastic anemia and its association with hemochromatosis. Arch Intern Med (Chicago) 75: 395, 1945.
37. Schwartz SO, Blumenthal SA: Exogenous hemo-

chromatosis resulting from blood transfusions. Blood 3: 617, 1948.

38. Muirhead EE, Crass G, Jones F, Hill JM: Iron overload (hemosiderosis) aggravated by blood transfusions. Arch Intern Med (Chicago) 83: 477, 1949.
39. Butt EM, Nusbaum RE, Gilmour TC, DiDio SL: Trace metal patterns in disease states. I. Hemochromatosis and refractory anemia. Amer J Clin Path 26: 225, 1956.
40. Althausen TL, Kerr WJ: Hemochromatosis. II. A report of three cases with endocrine disturbances and notes on a previously reported case. Discussion of etiology. Endocrinology 17: 621, 1933.
41. Murray Lyon RM: Haemochromatosis: A report on three cases. Brit Med J 1: 1297, 1936.
42. Blumer G, Nesbit RR: Case of hemochromatosis with degeneration of the heart muscle and death from congestive heart failure. New Eng J Med 218: 295, 1938.
43. Bloom N: Hemochromatosis—a study of three cases. Virginia Med Monthly 66: 79, 1939.
44. Petit DW: Hemochromatosis with complete heart block, with discussion of cardiac complications. Amer Heart J 29: 253, 1945.
45. Tucker HStG Jr, Moss LF, Williams JP: Hemochromatosis with death from heart failure. Amer Heart J 35: 993, 1948.
46. Horns HL: Hemochromatosis. Cardiac failure associated with extensive hemosiderosis of the myocardium. Amer J Med 6: 272, 1949.
47. Griffin WR, Nelson HG, Seal JR: Hemochromatosis with auricular fibrillation: a case report. Amer Heart J 39: 904, 1950.
48. Swan WGA, Dewar HA: The heart in haemochromatosis. Brit Heart J 14: 117, 1952.
49. Bothwell TH, van Lingen B, Alper T, du Preez ML: Cardiac complications of hemochromatosis. Report of a case including radioiron studies and a note on etiology. Amer Heart J 43: 333, 1952.
50. Levin EB, Golum A: The heart in hemochromatosis. Amer Heart J 45: 277, 1953.
51. Lewis HP: Cardiac involvement in hemochromatosis. Amer J Med Sci 227: 544, 1954.
52. McAllen PM, Coghill NF, Lubran M: The treatment of haemochromatosis, with particular reference to the removal of iron from the body by repeated venesection. Quart J Med 26: 251, 1957.
53. James TN: Pathology of the cardiac conduction system in hemochromatosis. New Eng J Med 271: 92, 1964.
54. Wasserman AJ, Richardson DW, Baird CL, Wyso EM: Cardiac hemochromatosis simulating constrictive pericarditis. Amer J Med 32: 316, 1962.
55. Kleckner MS Jr, Baggenstoss AH, Weir JF: Hemochromatosis and transfusional hemosiderosis: a clinical and pathologic study. Amer J Med 16: 382, 1954.
56. Richter GW: A study of hemosiderosis with the aid of electron microscopy. With observations on the relationship between hemosiderin and ferritin. J Exp Med 106: 203, 1957.
57. Richter GW, Bessis MC: Commentary on hemosiderin. Blood 25: 370, 1965.
58. Linder E: Der elektronenimkroskopische Nachweis von Schwermetallen. Acta Histochem (Jena) suppl 3, p 98, 1963.
59. Gennes deL, Delarue J, DeVericourt R: Le syndrome endocrino-hepato-cardiaque. Presse Med 1: 377, 1936.
60. Bannerman RM, Keusch G, Kreimer-Birnbaum M, Vance VK, Vaughan S: Thalassemia intermedia with iron overload, cardiac failure, diabetes mellitus, hypopituitarism and porphyrinuria. Amer J Med 42: 476, 1967.

PATHOLOGIC ANATOMY OF THE CARDIOMYOPATHIES

Idiopathic Dilated and Hypertrophic Types, Infiltrative Types, and Endomyocardial Disease with and without Eosinophilia

*William C. Roberts, M.D.,**
and Victor J. Ferrans, Ph.D., M.D.†

Abstract

This presentation summarizes necropsy observations in patients with three types of cardiomyopathy: idiopathic, infiltrative, and endomyocardial disease. The idiopathic variety is subdivided into two types depending on the size of the ventricular cavity. In the dilated ventricular type the left ventricular wall is frequently less than 1.5 cm. thick, intracardiac thrombi are common, the atrioventricular valve rings usually are mildly dilated, and focal myocardial and endocardial scars are common. In the nondilated type (hypertrophic cardiomyopathy), the ventricular septum is usually thicker than the left ventricular free wall, which also is thick (> 1.5 cm.). When the septum is similar in thickness to the left ventricular free wall (symmetric), left ventricular outflow obstruction does not occur. When the septum is thicker than the left ventricular free wall (asymmetric), left or right ventricular outflow obstruction may or may not be present. The orientation of myocardial fibers one to another in the ventricular septum in the nondilated (hypertrophic) type is abnormal, whereas it is normal in the dilated ventricular type. Intracardiac thrombi are rare and atrioventricular valve rings are never dilated in the nondilated type of idiopathic cardiomegaly.

The infiltrative types of cardiomyopathies include iron, calcium, lipids, mucopolysaccharides, granulomas, amyloid, and neoplasms. The first four usually are located within myocardial cells and the latter three, between myocardial cells. It is probable that all these myocardial infiltrates are capable of producing cardiac dysfunction, primarily on a restrictive basis.

Endomyocardial disease may or may not be associated with eosinophilia. When the latter occurs, the eosinophils are structurally normal. Death is related to congestive cardiac failure. This category in actuality also is idiopathic.

---

*Clinical Professor of Pathology and Medicine (Cardiology), Georgetown University, Washington, D.C. Chief, Section of Pathology, National Heart and Lung Institute, National Institutes of Health, Bethesda, Maryland.

†Senior Investigator, Section of Pathology, National Heart and Lung Institute, National Institutes of Health, Bethesda, Maryland.

TABLE 1. Hypertrophic Cardiomyopathy: Clinical and Necropsy Observations in 40 Patients

Groups	No. pts.	FH of HD	Ages (yr.) Range (avg.)	Sex F	Sex M	Systemic hyper-tension[a]	LV-SA PSG (mm. Hg) (rest)	LV-SA PSG (mm. Hg) (provo-cation)	Heart weight (gm.) Range (avg.)	VS > LVFW[h]	"Small" or normal sized RV and LV cavities	Endo. plaque LVO	Thick mitral valve	LVFW behind PML normal thick-ness	Di-lated left atrium	Normal aortic valve	No. pts. with CA >50% narrowed
I. With sub-aortic stenosis	20	6	18–70 (43)	12	8	7	8–170 (85)	56–140[b] (100)	390–1250 (654)	17	20	19	19	0	20	18	7[c]
II. Without subaortic stenosis	13	9[d]	9–55 (28)	6[e]	7	1	0	0–150[f]	350–1020 (683)[g]	10	13	6	6	11	13	13	0
III. No catheteri-zation	7	0	49–78 (67)	5	2	5	-	-	430–710 (518)	6	7	4	4	0	7	7	0
TOTALS	40	15	9–78 (42)	23	17	13	0–170	0–150	350–1250 (634)[g]	33[h]	40	29	29	11	40	38	7[c]

[a]Systemic blood pressure by cuff > 140 systolic or > 90 mm. Hg diastolic or both.
[b]The PSG increased in each of the 11 patients provoked (by isoprotorenol or Valsalva maneuver).
[c]Transmural left ventricular fibrosis in only one patient.
[d]No information available in two patients.
[e]Two patients were asymptomatic. One died suddenly; the second committed suicide.
[f]Of 10 patients provoked, PSG remained zero in four and increased to 10–150 mm. Hg in seven. In only one of the latter was the PSG with provocation > 32 mm. Hg.
[g]Heart weights of four children are excluded. The hearts of the 22 women averaged 551 gm.; those of the 14 men, 759 gm.
[h]Defined as thickest portion of ventricular septum > thickest portion of left ventricular free wall.
Abbreviations: CA = coronary artery; Endo = endocardial; FH = family history; HD = heart disease; LV = left ventricle; LVFW = left ventricular free wall; LV = left ventricular outflow tract; PML = posterior mitral leaflet; PSG = peak systolic gradient; SA = systemic artery; VS = ventricular septum; RV = right ventricle.

Although much has been written about the various cardiomyopathies, surprisingly few reports have focused on the pathologic anatomy of these conditions. This communication focuses on the structural alterations in the heart in the dilated and nondilated (hypertrophic) types of idiopathic cardiomyopathy, in the infiltrative types of cardiomyopathy, and in endomyocardial disease with and without eosinophilia (Table 1). The secondary cardiomyopathies, those associated with known conditions (collagen diseases, endocrine disorders, generalized infections, metabolic and neurologic disorders, physical forces, drugs, and metals), are not included. Concrete data from patients studied at necropsy by the authors are presented in addition to information derived from reports of others.

IDIOPATHIC CARDIOMYOPATHY

Dilated Ventricular Type (Congestive Type, Primary Myocardial Disease)

We have studied at necropsy 64 patients with idiopathic cardiomegaly of the dilated type (Figs. 1 to 11). In each, the ventricles were dilated, the coronary arteries were free of significant luminal narrow-

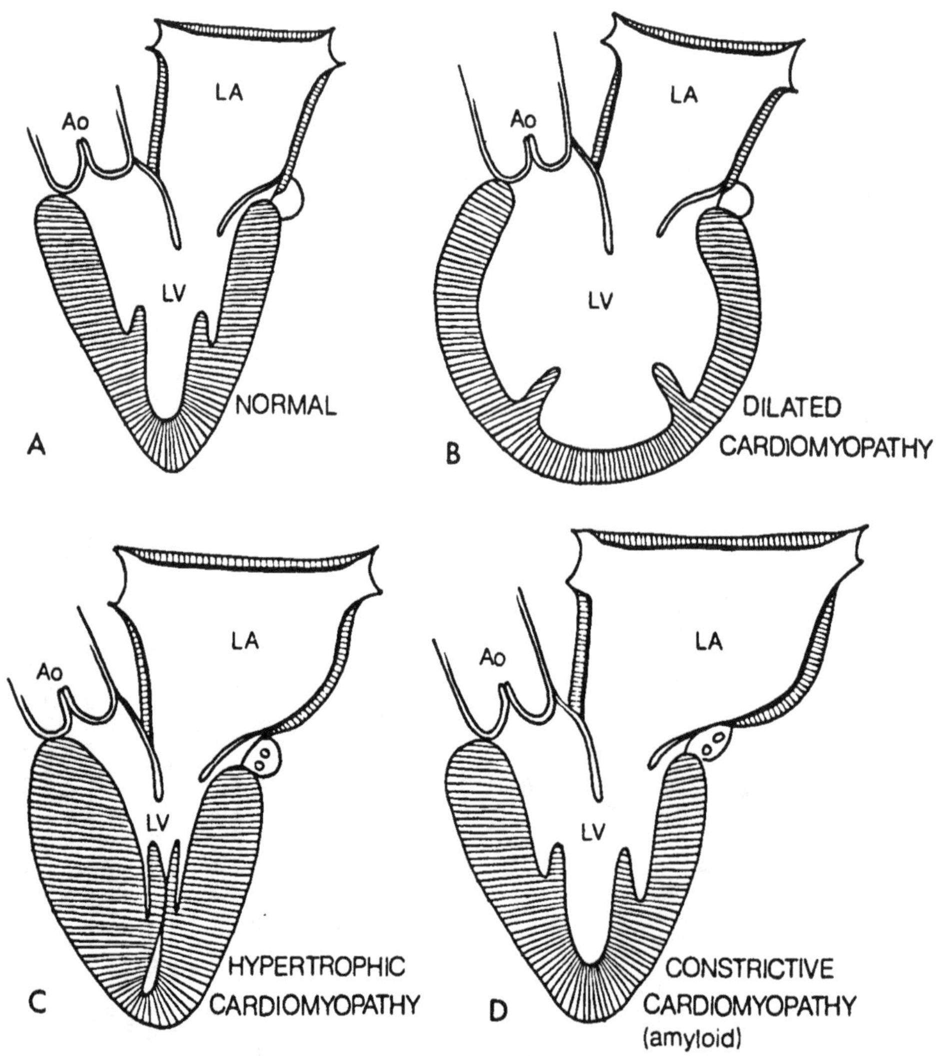

Figure 1. Diagram illustrating the various types of cardiomyopathies, compared to the normal, discussed herein. In the hypertrophic type of cardiomyopathy the left ventricular cavity is small, and in the constrictive variety, as illustrated by amyloidosis, the left ventricular cavity is of normal size. In the dilated type the largest circumference of the left ventricle is not at its base but midway between the apex and base.

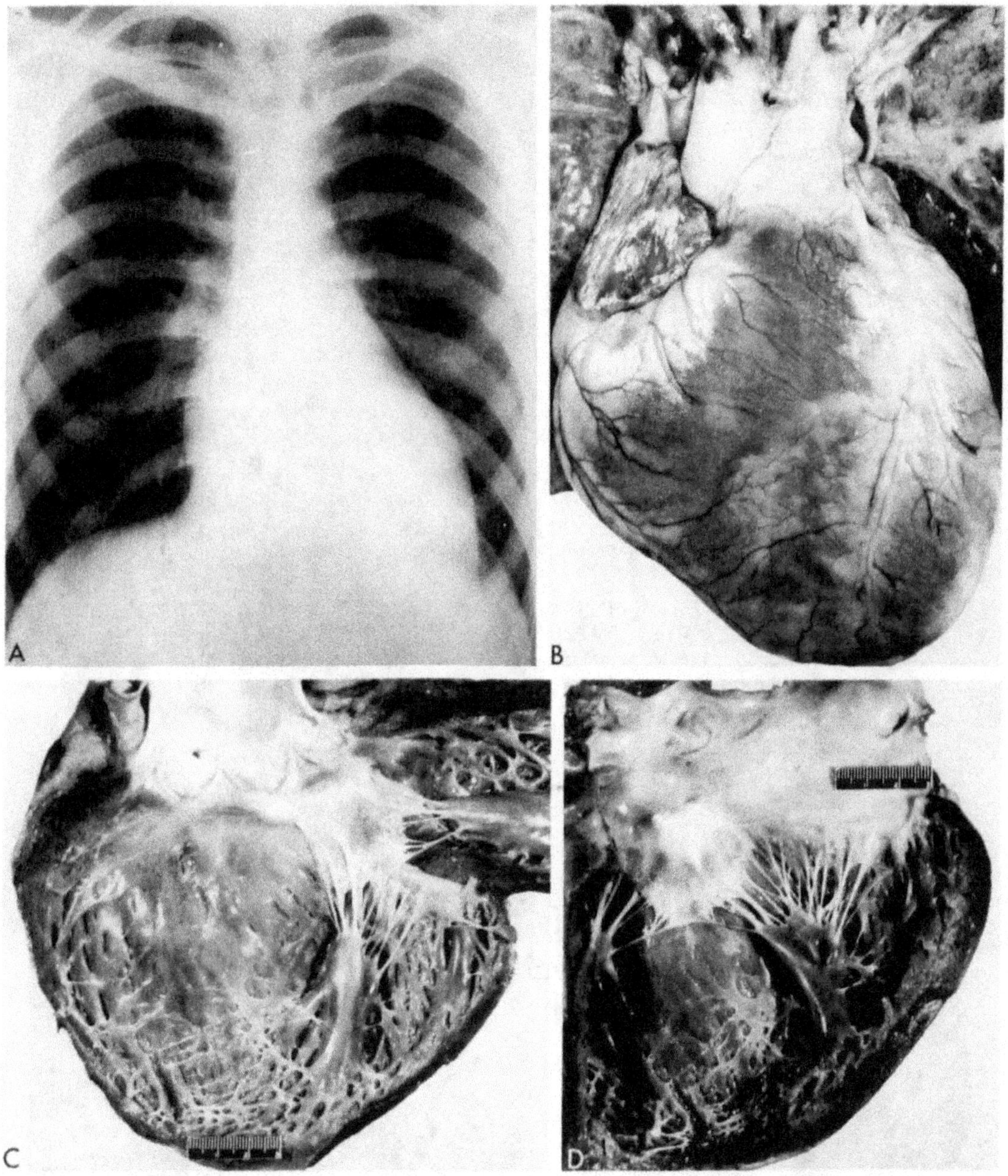

Figure 2. Idiopathic dilated cardiomegaly in a 22 year old white man (A61–56) who had been well until age 17 (five years before death), when the onset of a pleuritic type of pain was followed by congestive cardiac failure. The electrocardiogram showed nonspecific T wave changes. After a four month hospitalization, he was entirely well until two months before death when an upper respiratory infection resulted in overt congestive heart failure. Thereafter the heart failure progressively worsened and the heart enlarged. A grade 2/6 apical systolic murmur appeared. At necropsy the heart weighed 570 gm. and*both ventricles were very dilated. The valves and coronary arteries were normal. Histologic sections of left ventricular wall showed only mild interstitial fibrosis. *A*, Chest roentgenogram during last week of life. *B*, Anterior aspect of heart. The pericardial sac contained 50 ml. of serous fluid. *C*, Opened left ventricle, aortic valve, and aorta. Small focal endocardial thickenings are present. *D*, Opened left atrium, mitral valve, and left ventricle. The mitral anulus is not dilated.

ing, the valves were normal except for occasional focal thickening of the atrioventricular valve leaflets, and there was not significant or prolonged systemic hypertension. The ages of the 64 patients ranged from 13 to 96 years (average, 46): the 43 males averaged 44 years and the 21 females, 49 years. Forty patients were black.

Twenty-three of the 64 patients were known to be chronic alcoholics. Twelve patients (seven women) had had documented systemic hypertension at some time (systolic pressure > 140 mm. Hg or diastolic pressure > 90 mm. Hg, or both). In most the blood pressure elevation was associated with congestive cardiac failure, but in at least one patient hypertension, which had been present for many years, disappeared when congestive failure appeared. In five patients other family members also had a cardiomyopathy: in two of the five the cardiomyopathy in other family members

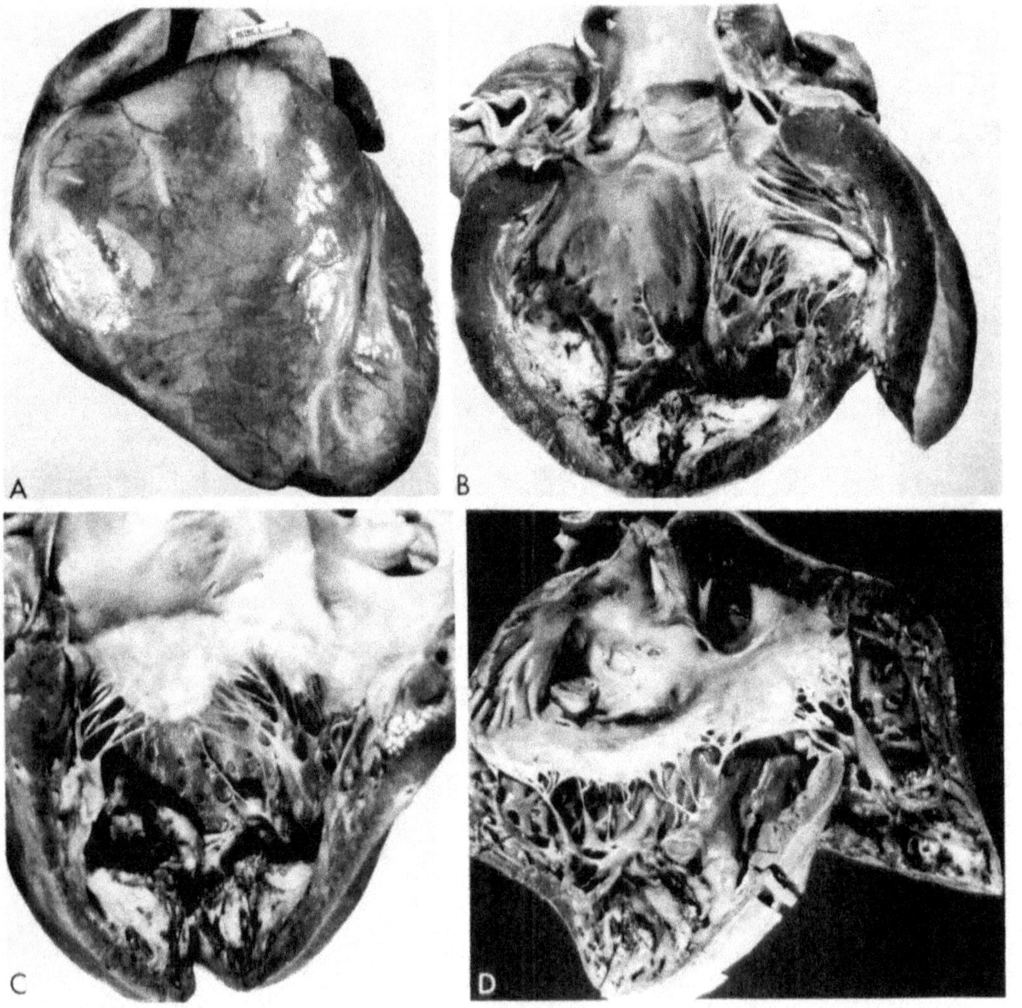

Figure 3. Idiopathic dilated cardiomegaly in a 36 year old black man (A69-199), a chronic alcoholic who had been well until two years before death, when evidence of congestive cardiac failure appeared. The latter gradually worsened and various arrhythmias also appeared. Finally pulmonary infiltrates, proved to be secondary to pulmonary emboli, precipitated death. By radiography the heart was markedly enlarged. An electrocardiogram showed low voltage, Q and T wave changes suggesting old infarction, and an intraventricular conduction defect. He never had chest pain, hypertension, or a precordial murmur. At necropsy the heart with the intracardiac thrombi weighed 750 gm. "Milk spots" were present over the anterior surface of the right ventricle and at the left ventricular apex *(A)*. Thrombi were present in the apex of both ventricles *(B, C, D)* and in the right atrial appendage *(D)*. Histologically, large foci of replacement and interstitial fibrosis were seen in the left ventricular wall. Both left ventricular papillary muscles were atrophied and severely scarred. *A*, Heart as viewed anteriorly. This is better seen in Figure 4. The notch present at the junction of the left ventricular apices was considered at one time to be diagnostic of the African condition, endomyocardial fibrosis, but this is not the case as shown by this patient. *B*, Opened left ventricle, aortic valve, and aorta showing the large apical thrombus. *C*, Opened left atrium, mitral valve, and left ventricle. The mitral anulus is not dilated. *D*, Open right atrium, tricuspid valve, and right ventricle showing a thrombus at the apex of the ventricle.

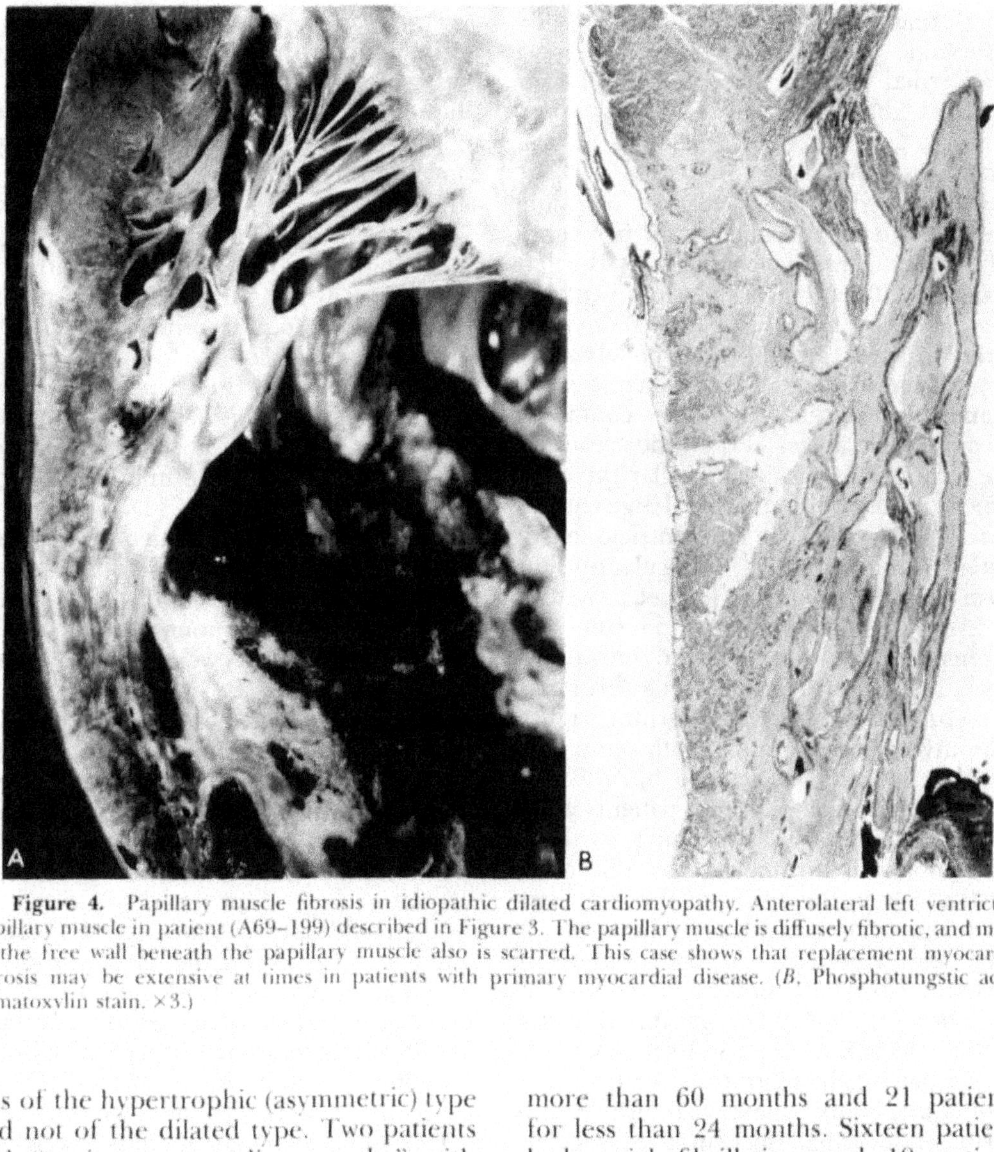

Figure 4. Papillary muscle fibrosis in idiopathic dilated cardiomyopathy. Anterolateral left ventricular papillary muscle in patient (A69–199) described in Figure 3. The papillary muscle is diffusely fibrotic, and much of the free wall beneath the papillary muscle also is scarred. This case shows that replacement myocardial fibrosis may be extensive at times in patients with primary myocardial disease. (*B*, Phosphotungstic acid-hematoxylin stain, ×3.)

was of the hypertrophic (asymmetric) type and not of the dilated type. Two patients had "peripartum cardiomyopathy" with the onset of congestive cardiac failure one and three months, respectively, after delivery. Eight patients had diabetes mellitus (adult onset type). Eleven patients had episodic chest pains, four of whom clinically were believed to have had acute myocardial infarcts in the past. At necropsy six of the 11 had left ventricular scars, but each was small. One patient, a 30 year old man, died suddenly and unexpectedly without previous symptomatic evidence of cardiac dysfunction. His heart weighed 780 gm. and was known to have been enlarged for 16 years. All remaining 63 patients had evidence of cardiac dysfunction (congestive cardiac failure) ranging from one to 240 months (average, 47); 12 patients had had evidence of congestive cardiac failure for more than 60 months and 21 patients, for less than 24 months. Sixteen patients had atrial fibrillation and 19 patients had complete bundle branch block (left in 13, right in two, and indeterminate in four). Death in most patients was the result of progressive congestive cardiac failure, but at least 15 patients died suddenly without apparent worsening of the congestive cardiac failure.

At necropsy the hearts ranged in weight from 350 to 860 gm. (average, 597): the hearts of the 21 females ranged from 350 to 860 gm. (average, 576) and those of the 43 males from 400 to 830 gm. (average, 610). All four cardiac chambers were dilated in all 64 patients. In some patients the left ventricular walls were more than 1.5 cm. thick, and in others the walls were of normal thickness. The greater the dilatation of the left ventricle, the less the likelihood that the walls were thickened. By histiologic examination, however, most myocardial cells in the walls of all four cardiac chambers appeared hypertrophied; a few fibers in the walls of all four chambers appeared atrophied.

Intracardiac fibrin-platelet thrombi were found in 36 patients (56 per cent). The most common location was the left ventricle (30 patients). The right ventricle contained thrombi in 16 patients, the right atrial appendage in 14, and the left atrial appendage in eight. In 22 patients more than one cardiac chamber contained thrombi. The apices of the ventricles were the locations of most ventricular thrombi, which usually were multiple. Huge thrombi were present in the left ventricle in two patients, and in one left ventricular outflow obstruction (24 mm. Hg peak systolic pressure gradient) appeared to result from extension of the thrombus into the outflow tract. In only one patient was a thrombus present in the body of an atrium (right). The myoendocardium beneath some ventricular thrombi was scarred but this was not always the case. In 12 patients focal endocardial fibrous thickening, without superimposed thrombus, was observed, particularly in the apices of the ventricles or in the atrial appendages. These lesions may have resulted from organization of thrombi. If these lesions are interpreted as evidence of "healed" or organized endocardial thrombi, then 48 (75 per cent) of the 64 patients had intracardiac thrombi at some time. Many patients had diffuse, uniform, endocardial thickening of the left ventricle, usually of a minimal degree, and occasionally also of the right ventricle.

Foci of intramural fibrosis were observed grossly in the left ventricular walls in 23 patients. The scarring was most frequent in one or both left ventricular papillary muscles and, next, in the subendocardial portions of the free wall. In seven patients the scarring was transmural. By histologic examination, however, foci of fibrosis, mainly interstitial (intermyocardial and perivascular) rather then replacement, were observed in the walls of all four cardiac chambers of virtually every heart. Foci of myocardial necrosis and inflammatory cell infiltrates were absent in the cardiac walls of all 64 patients. In most patients the extramural coronary arteries grossly were free of atherosclerotic plaques or other lesions. In the patients in whom some atherosclerotic plaques were observed, the lumens in none were narrowed more than 50 per cent. No significant abnormality of intramural coronary arteries was observed by histologic examination in any patient.

Except for focal fibrous thickening of one or more leaflets of the tricuspid or mitral valves or both, the valves were normal. The minimal focal scarring was of no functional significance. In most patients the circumferences of the tricuspid and mitral valve anuli were mildly dilated. The tricuspid anuli ranged from 10.5 to 16.5 cm. (average, 13.0) and the mitral anuli from 9.0 to 12.5 cm. (average, 11). Normally the tricuspid anulus in adults averages 11.0 cm. (range, 8.5 to 13.5) and the mitral anulus, 9.0 cm. (range, 7.0 to 10.5). The circumferences of the pulmonary trunk and ascending aorta usually were normal (< 8 cm.). The circumference of the base of the left ventricle (this excludes the distance of the basal attachment of the anterior mitral leaflet) and the longitudinal distances between the bases of the aortic valve (or the base of the posterior mitral leaflet) and the left ventricular apex were increased in all patients.

In addition to studying 64 necropsy patients with idiopathic cardiomegaly of the dilated type, we examined by electron microscopy biopsy specimens of ventricular myocardium (obtained either with a Konno catheter or with a Menghini needle[1]) from 31 living patients with the same condition.[2] Three main findings were observed (Figs. 8 to 11):

1. Interstitial fibrosis, i.e., increased numbers of mature and developing collagen fibrils in interstitial spaces.

2. Cellular hypertrophy, consisting of increased transverse diameters of the muscle cells; increased size of nuclei and Golgi complexes; and increased numbers of mitochondria, myofibrils, glycogen granules, and free and membrane bound ribosomes.

3. Changes considered as probably degenerative, such as cellular edema; increased numbers of lipid droplets, lysosomes, and lipofuscin granules; dilatation of tubules of the sarcoplasmic reticulum and the T system; myofibrillar damage; and various mitochondrial alterations, in-

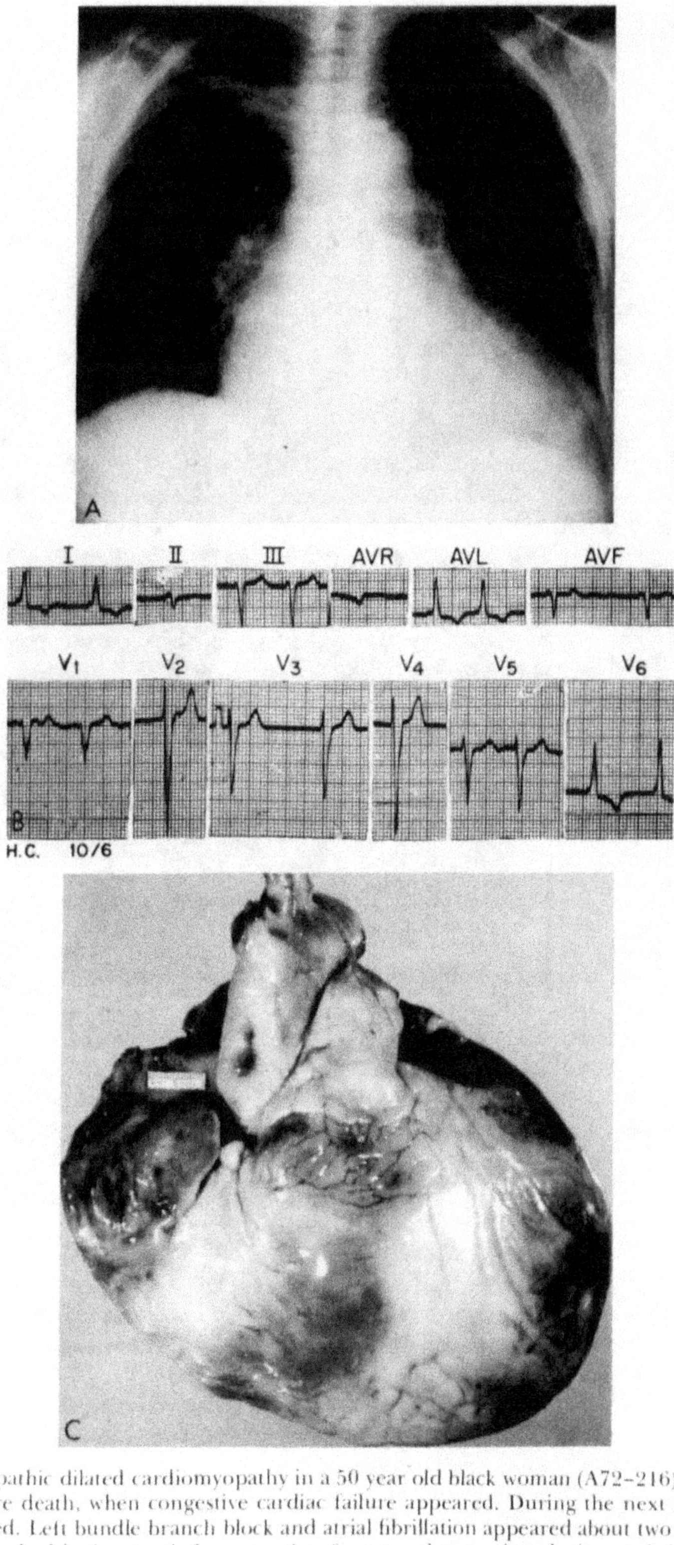

Figure 5. Idiopathic dilated cardiomyopathy in a 50 year old black woman (A72–216) who had been well until five years before death, when congestive cardiac failure appeared. During the next five years the heart progressively enlarged. Left bundle branch block and atrial fibrillation appeared about two years before death. It was stated that she had had systemic hypertension for several years, but during each hospitalization most blood pressure recordings were normal. On admission to the National Heart and Lung Institute she was in severe congestive cardiac failure (functionally class IV [New York Heart Association]). Grade 3/6 pansystolic blowing murmurs were present: one over the apex and another along the lower left sternal border. The latter murmur increased with inspiration. At catheterization the pressures in mm. Hg were: pulmonary artery 70/40, right ventricle 70/24, right atrium m26 v30, left ventricle 100/30, and brachial artery 110/75. Left ventricular cineangiogram showed a severely dilated, poorly contracting ventricle, 3^+ to 4^+ mitral regurgitation, and a large

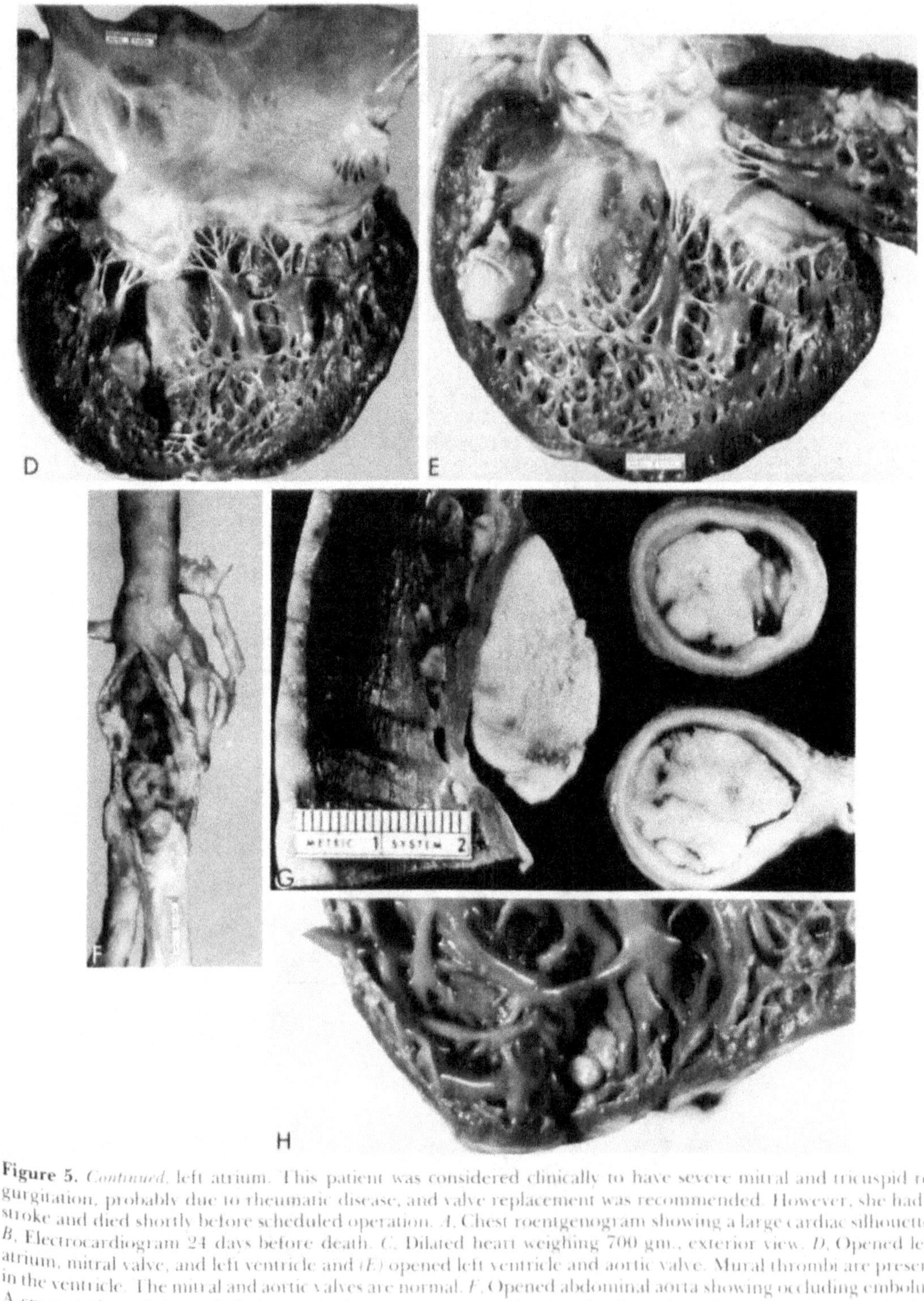

Figure 5. *Continued,* left atrium. This patient was considered clinically to have severe mitral and tricuspid regurgitation, probably due to rheumatic disease, and valve replacement was recommended. However, she had a stroke and died shortly before scheduled operation. *A*, Chest roentgenogram showing a large cardiac silhouette. *B*, Electrocardiogram 24 days before death. *C*, Dilated heart weighing 700 gm., exterior view. *D*, Opened left atrium, mitral valve, and left ventricle and *(E)* opened left ventricle and aortic valve. Mural thrombi are present in the ventricle. The mitral and aortic valves are normal. *F*, Opened abdominal aorta showing occluding embolus. A cross section of the occluded aorta is shown in *G* along with a longitudinal view of the thrombus attached to the wall of the left ventricle. The material in the aorta is identical to that in the left ventricle. A small mural thrombus also is present in the apex of the right ventricle *(H)*.

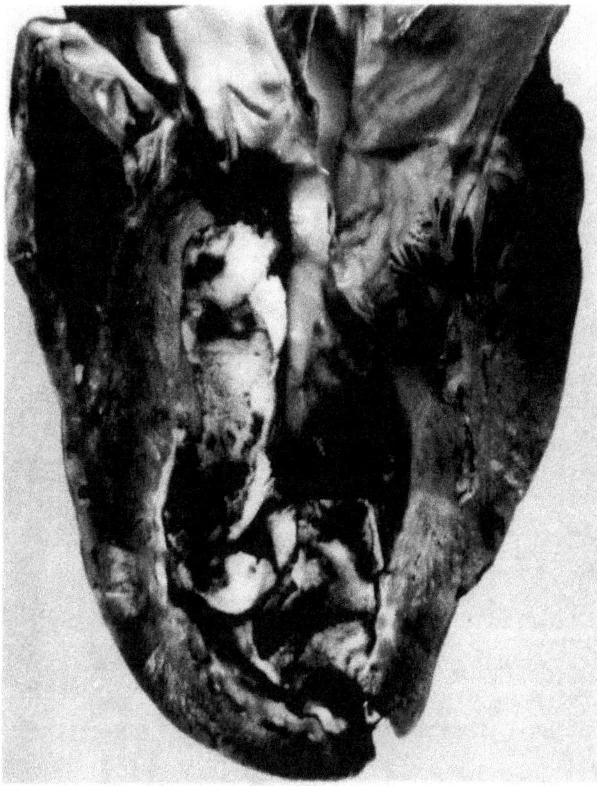

Figure 6. Idiopathic dilated cardiomyopathy. Posterior half of both ventricles exposed to show a huge left ventricular thrombus extending from the apex to just below the aortic valve in a 31 year old black man (DCGH 71A-273) who had had evidence of congestive cardiac failure with cardiomegaly for eight years. A grade 2/6 pansystolic apical murmur was present. Electrocardiogram disclosed left ventricular hypertrophy with ischemia. At catheterization, pullback pressures from the left ventricle to the ascending aorta were 126/26 and 102/67 mm. Hg, respectively. The 24 mm. Hg peak systolic pressure gradient probably resulted from the large thrombus that extended into the left ventricular outflow tract. Pulsus alternans was noted in the left ventricular and aortic pressure tracings. The patient died of pulmonary infarction from emboli. At necropsy the heart weighed 550 gm. and the left ventricular thrombus weighed 50 gm. The coronary arteries and valves were normal.

cluding mitochondrial swelling, intramitochondrial concentric lamellae, and loss of mitochondria cristae.

In addition, the mitochondria in most patients showed wide ranges in size, frequently with a predominance of mitochondria that were smaller than normal. No viral particles were observed. Abnormalities of myofibrillar orientation were observed in biopsy specimens from three of the 31 patients and were minimal. Edematous and damaged myocardial capillaries were observed in nine patients. Morphologic findings in patients with histories of chronic alcoholism were indistinguishable from those in patients without chronic alcoholism. The degree to which degenerative changes occurred in individual biopsy specimens generally correlated with the duration and severity of symptoms of cardiac dysfunction.

Comments on Idiopathic Cardiomegaly of the Dilated Type. By definition, the cause of the dilated type of cardiomyopathy is uncertain. If a viral etiology or other etiology is established as the cause, the cardiomyopathy is no longer "idiopathic" and with time it is hoped that the number of cases in the idiopathic category will decrease. This diagnosis is made by exclusion both clinically and at necropsy. Although valvular regurgitation (tricuspid or mitral or both) may occur, the valvular leaflets and chordae are normal except for occasional minimal focal thickening. Furthermore, although chest pain and electrocardiographic changes consistent with healed myocardial infarction may occur in this cardiomyopathy, the extramural coronary arteries are free of "significant" luminal narrowing. But how much coronary arterial luminal narrowing is permissible before a diagnosis of idiopathic cardiomegaly is permitted? We have chosen 50 per cent luminal narrowing as the upper limit. The presence of chronic pulmonary parenchymal disease, other than pulmonary infarction from emboli or of congenital cardiac malformations, even one such as atresia of the ostium of the coronary sinus,[3] also disallows a diagnosis of primary myocardial disease.

The level of the systemic blood pressure obviously is an essential piece of in-

(Text continued on page 302.)

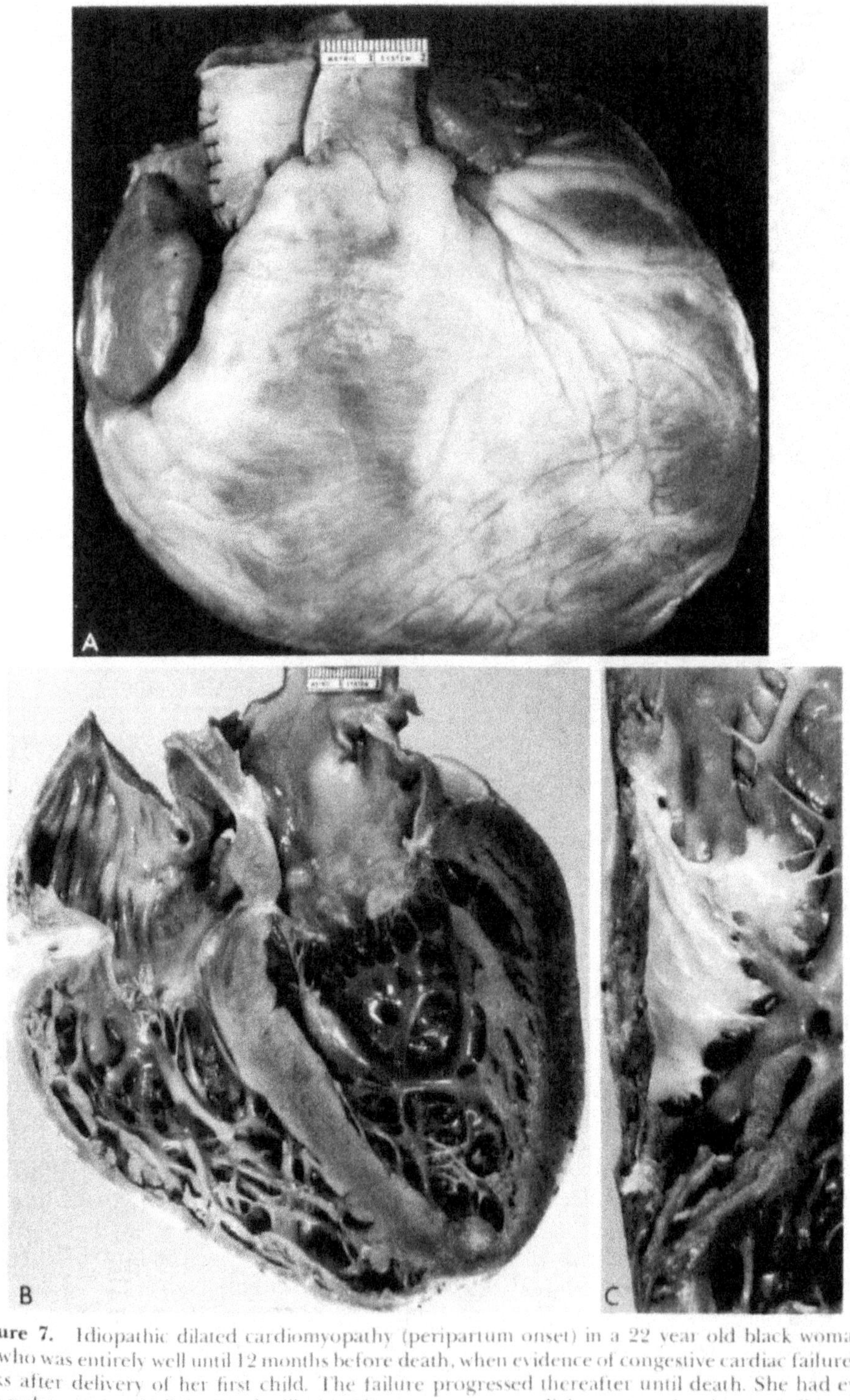

Figure 7. Idiopathic dilated cardiomyopathy (peripartum onset) in a 22 year old black woman (DCGH 73A–2) who was entirely well until 12 months before death, when evidence of congestive cardiac failure appeared six weeks after delivery of her first child. The failure progressed thereafter until death. She had evidence of multiple pulmonary emboli during the illness. There was no precordial murmur. An electrocardiogram showed ST-T wave changes and right atrial abnormality. *A*. The heart weighed 440 gm. All four chambers are dilated. The mitral anular circumference is considerably less than the circumference of the midportion of the left ventricle (*B*). The mural endocardium in the right ventricle is focally thickened (*C*). This lesion probably results from the organization of thrombus.

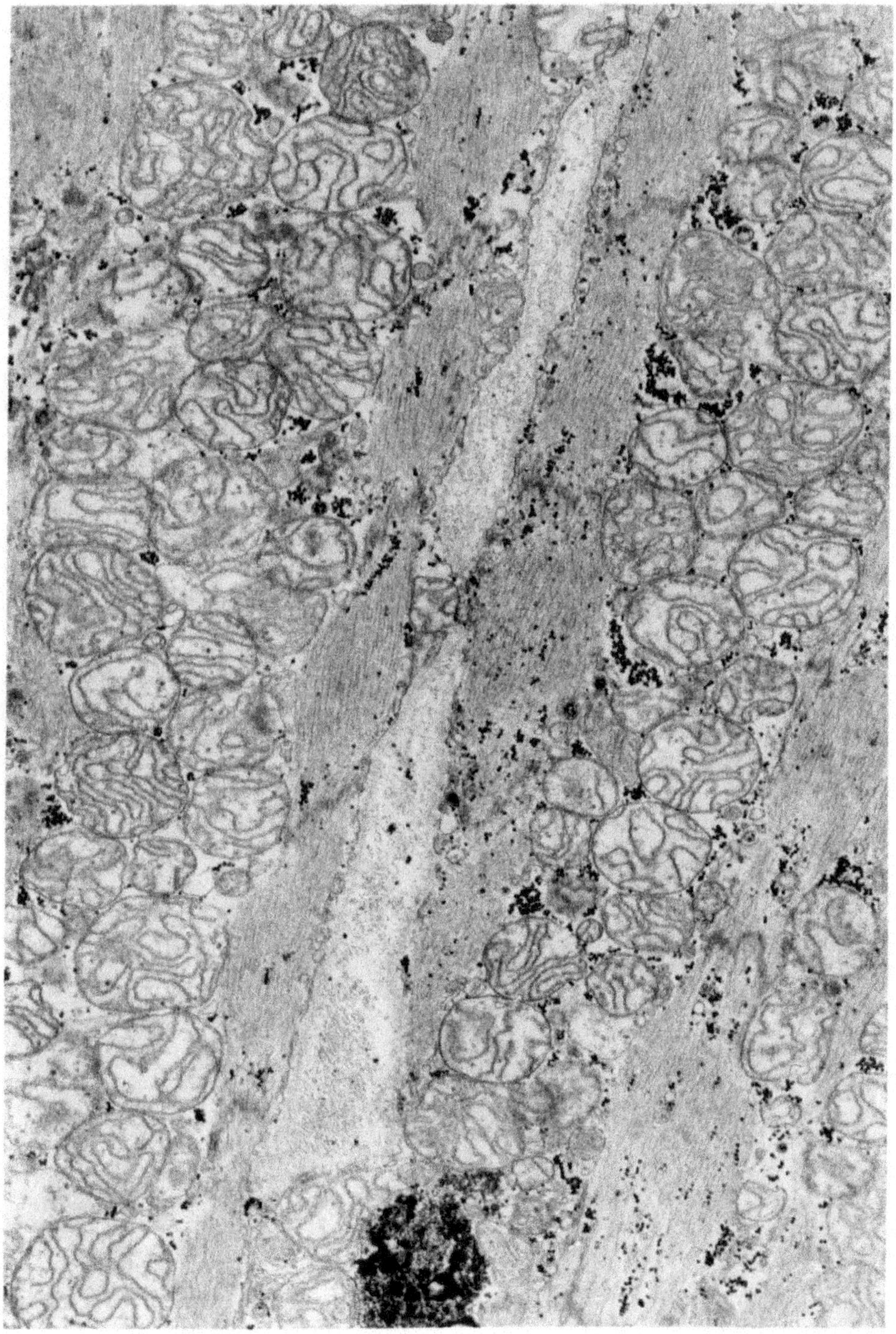

Figure 8. Dilated cardiomyopathy in a 25 year old man. Mitochondria in two adjacent cardiac muscle cells show swelling, clearing of matrix, and reduction in the numbers of cristae. (× 20,000.)

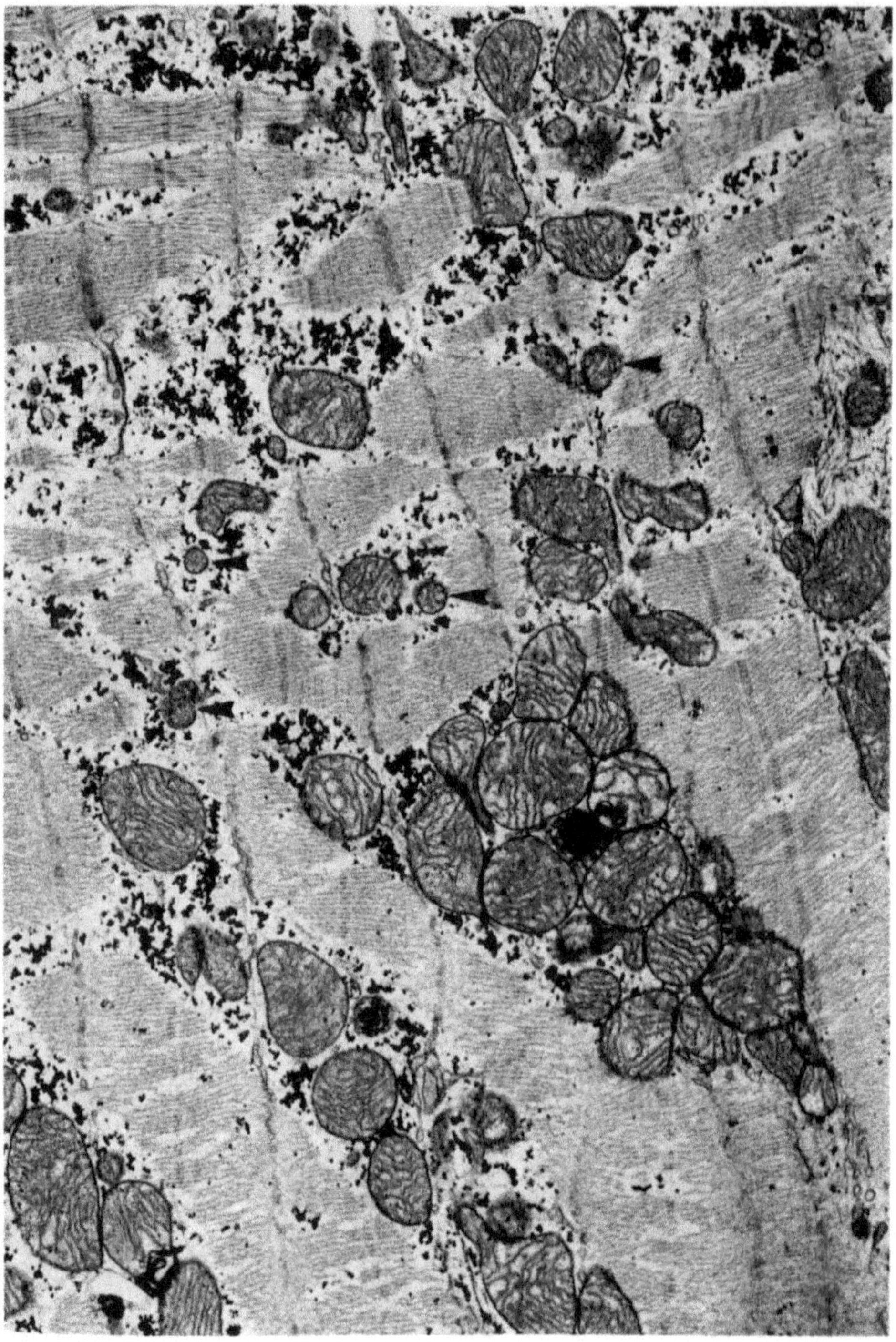

Figure 9. Dilated cardiomyopathy in a 28 year old man. The mitochondria in this cardiac muscle cell vary in size from very small (arrowheads) to normal. (× 17,000.)

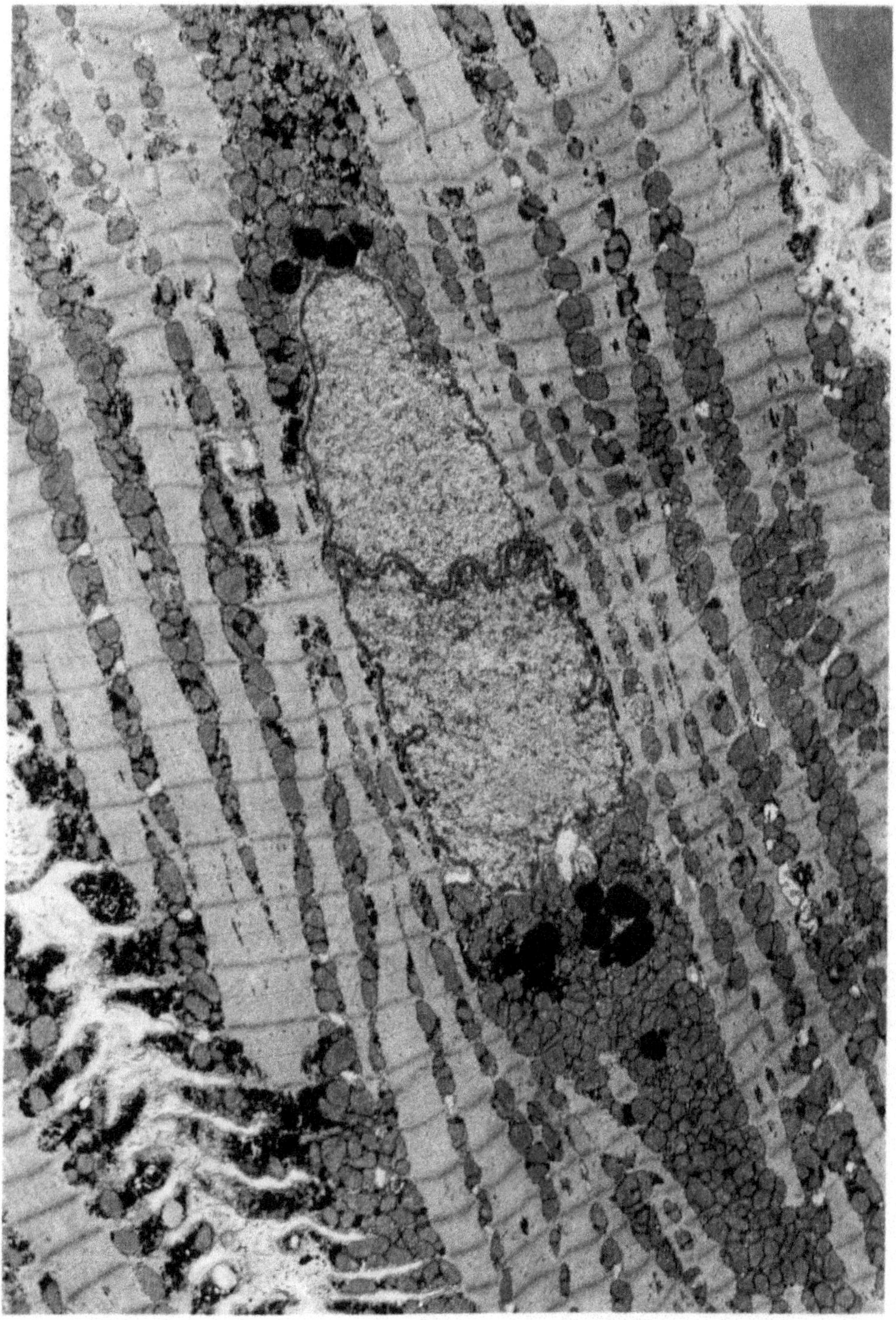

Figure 10. Dilated cardiomyopathy in a 43 year old man. The hypertrophied cardiac muscle cell has two nuclei, large perinuclear zones filled with mitochondria and a few lipofuscin granules, and normally arranged myofibrils. (× 6200.)

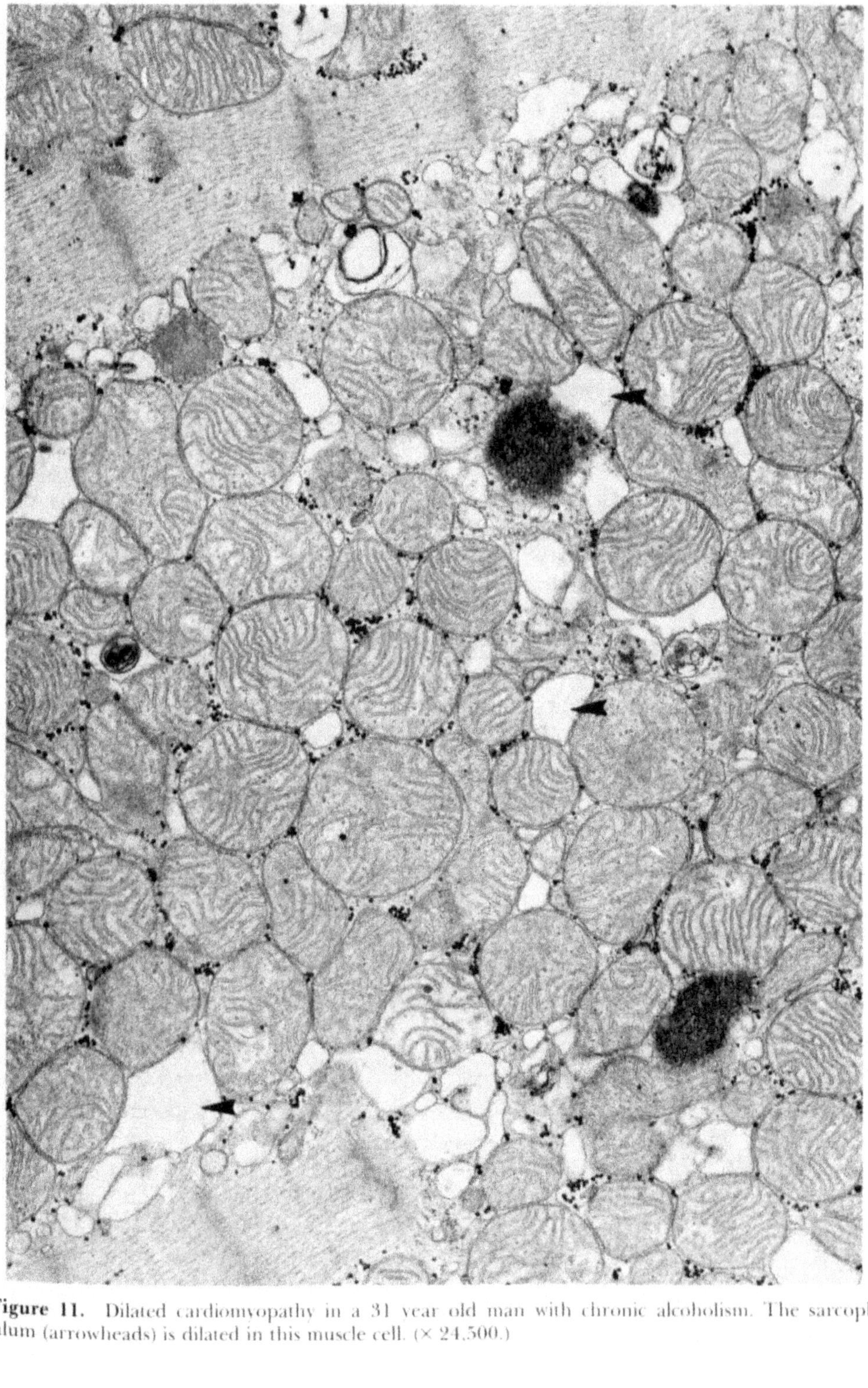

Figure 11. Dilated cardiomyopathy in a 31 year old man with chronic alcoholism. The sarcoplasmic reticulum (arrowheads) is dilated in this muscle cell. (× 24,500.)

formation. At necropsy, the heart of a hypertensive patient with fatal chronic congestive cardiac failure may simulate the heart of a patient with idiopathic cardiomegaly of the dilated type. It is probable that a number of patients considered to have idiopathic cardiomegaly, particularly those in older age groups may have had normal blood pressures during their symptomatic illness but elevated pressures years earlier. Eight of our 64 patients were known to have had systemic hypertension several years before presenting with normal blood pressure and severe congestive cardiac failure; four others had mild systolic systemic hypertension during their terminal illnesses. Although elevations of blood pressure may occur in idiopathic cardiomegaly, and may be of importance in its pathogenesis, it is unlikely that hypertension plays a major role in causing fatal congestive cardiac failure in primary myocardial disease, and consequently these 12 patients were included in our study. None had morphologic evidence of chronic hypertension in the kidney or spleen.

The inclusion in this study of a 96 year old patient might raise questions as to proper diagnosis. This patient had had evidence of congestive cardiac failure for about six months without chest pain or previously known systemic hypertension. Although the clinical diagnosis was coronary heart disease, at necropsy the coronary arteries were wide open, actually dilated; the four valves were normal, the myocardial walls were free of fibrosis or necrosis except for scarring of the papillary muscles, and the heart weighed 630 gm. Thus, by exclusion, this patient is included. Of the 64 patients, only three were more than 65 years of age and two were less than 21 years of age.

Study of the myocardium in these

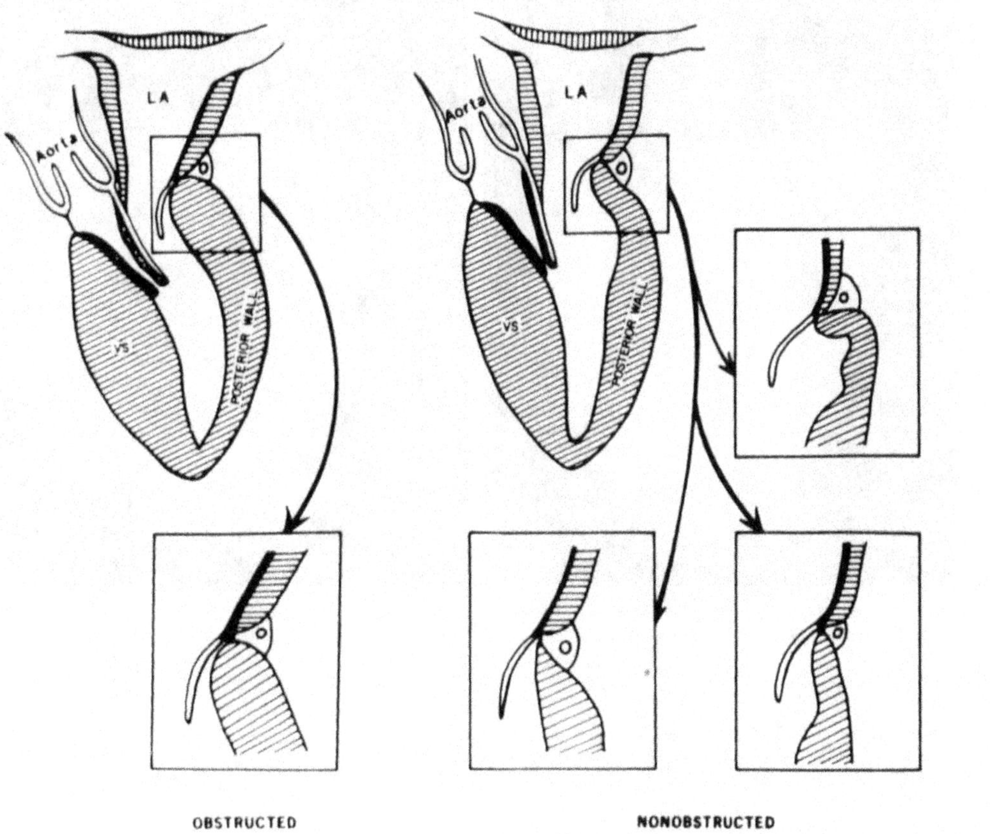

Figure 12. Diagram depicting the configuration and thickness of the left ventricular free wall behind the posterior mitral leaflet in obstructive and nonobstructive types of hypertrophic cardiomyopathy. In the obstructive form the most basal portion of the free wall is rounded and thick. In the nonobstructive form the most basal portion of the left ventricular free wall is pointed, or thin, or arched. In each type the ventricular septum is much thicker than the left ventricular free wall; the mural endocardium in the left ventricular outflow tract and the anterior mitral leaflet in apposition to it are thickened.

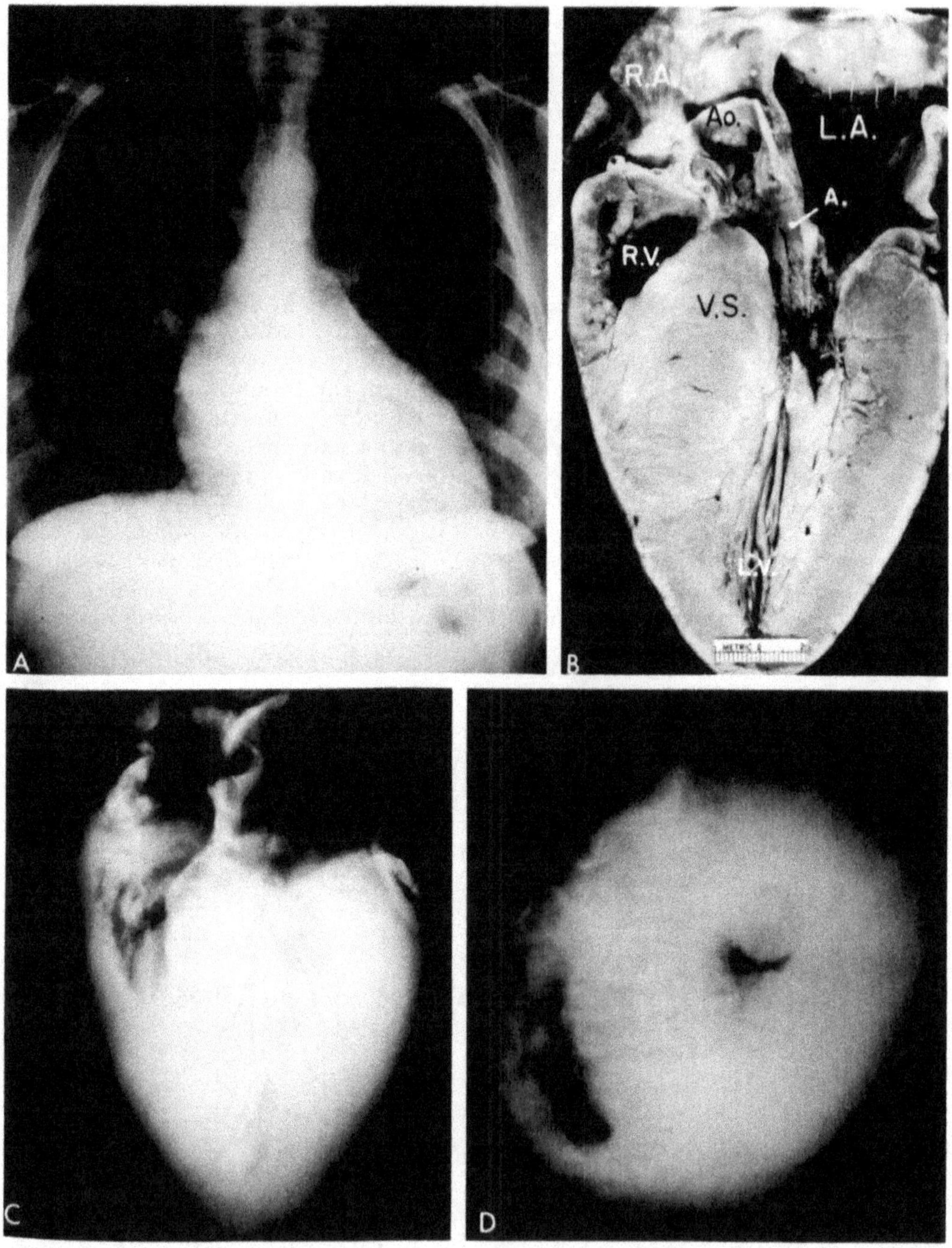

Figure 13. Hypertrophic asymmetric obstructive cardiomyopathy. This 36 year old woman (A67-121) developed congestive cardiac failure during her second pregnancy at age 32. When studied at age 34, she had a grade 3/6 precordial systolic murmur, loudest over the apex, and audible third and fourth heart sounds. An electrocardiogram showed bilateral bundle branch block with left axis deviation and prolongation (0.23 sec.) of the P-R interval. Catheterization disclosed a 75 mm. Hg peak systolic pressure gradient at rest between the left ventricle (160/18) and femoral artery (85/50) and a 125 mm. Hg gradient with provocation (Valsalva). The premature ventricular response was positive for idiopathic hypertrophic subaortic stenosis. She died during an episode of rapid heart action. She was known to have had multiple premature ventricular contractions on occasion. At necropsy the heart was enlarged *(A)*, weighing 450 gm., the left ventricular cavity was small *(B, C, D)*, and the ventricular septum was much thicker than the left ventricular free wall. There was little room in the left ventricular cavity for the mitral leaflets, and contact lesions (fibromas) were present on the ventricular aspect of the anterior mitral leaflet and on the adjacent left ventricular mural endocardium *(B)*. This is the typical "muscle bound" heart in which the ventricular cavities are minute in comparison to the mass of ventricular muscle. Both atria are dilated.

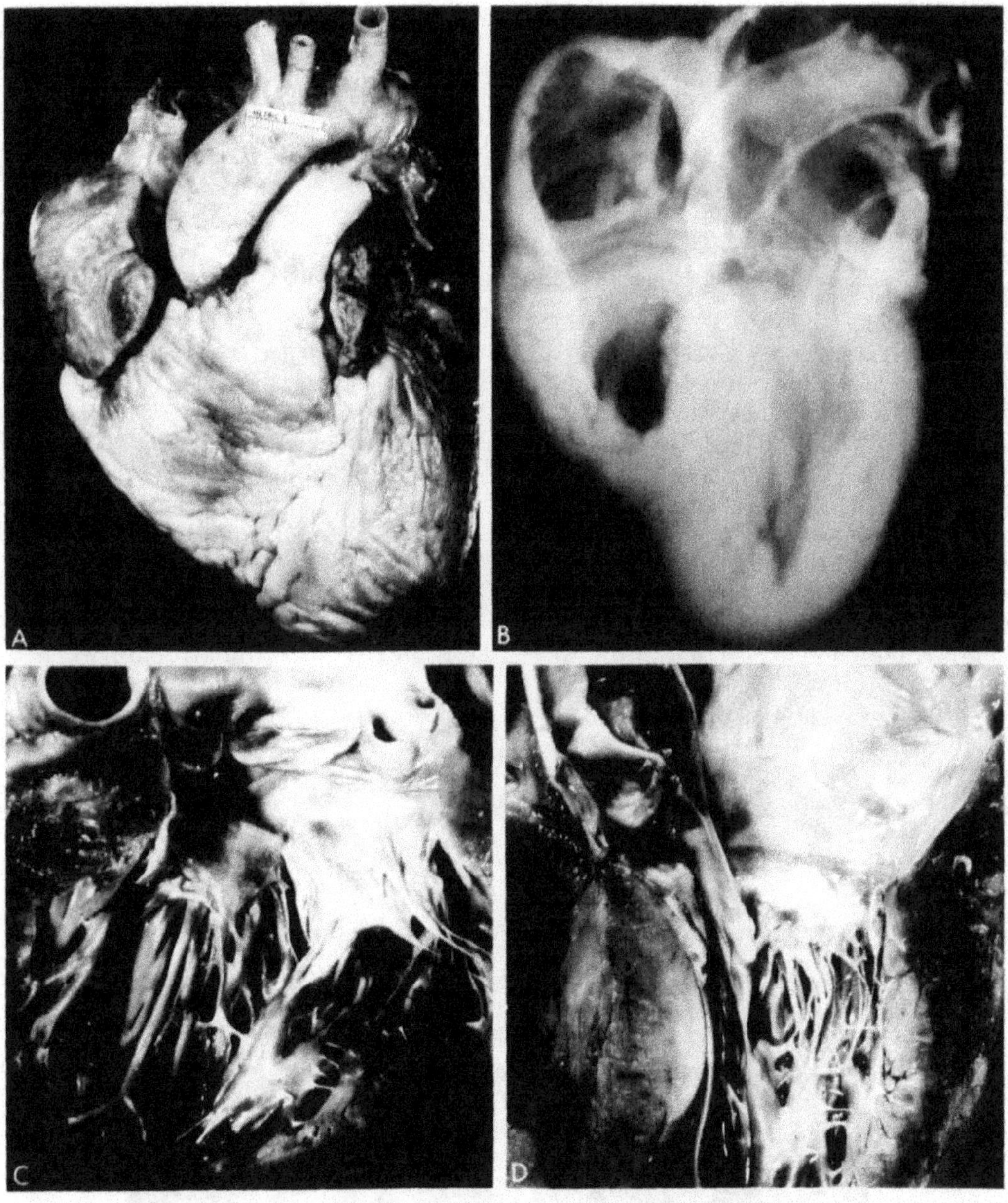

Figure 14. Hypertrophic asymmetric nonobstructive cardiomyopathy. This 33 year old man (A68–185) had no systolic pressure gradient at rest between the left ventricle and brachial artery, but a 33 mm. Hg gradient was provoked by isoproterenol. He died of sudden unilateral hemiparesis, which appeared six days after the catheterization. He had been asymptomatic when examined at age 26, when a grade 2 to 3/6 precordial systolic murmur, loudest at the apex, was heard. Catheterization at that time showed a 30 mm. Hg peak systolic gradient at rest between the left ventricle and brachial artery, and it rose to 85 mm. Hg with ouabain provocation. He became symptomatic (exertional and nocturnal dyspnea) six months before death, when atrial fibrillation appeared. The precordial murmur then was only intermittently audible. At necropsy the heart weighed 450 gm.; both atria were dilated but neither ventricle was dilated *(A)*. The ventricular septum was thicker than the left ventricular free wall *(B)*. A mural endocardial plaque was present in the left ventricular outflow tract, and the corresponding anterior mitral leaflet was thickened (*C*, *D*). The longitudinal cut of the heart in *D* clearly shows that the ventricular septum is thicker than the left ventricular free wall.

patients either by light or by electron microscope discloses only nonspecific findings. It is disappointing that the electron microscope has not been more useful from a diagnostic standpoint in this condition. Electron microscopic observations in the dilated type of idiopathic cardiomegaly, however, have been limited, and therefore it is possible that more specific findings will be appreciated with further study. Our knowledge of myocardial changes in the early stages of primary myocardial disease is limited. It is apparent, however, that once myocardial degeneration occurs, it can lead to a vicious cycle of further cardiac failure and further degeneration. Progression of degenerative changes in cardiac muscles may be responsible for the clinical deterioration and therapeutic unresponsiveness of patients with advanced stages of idiopathic cardiomegaly of the dilated type. There is not enough scarring in the walls of these hearts to account for the poor cardiac function.

Intracardiac mural thrombi in the idiopathic dilated type of cardiomyopathy probably represent anatomic manifestations of relative stasis of blood within the heart as a result of an extremely depressed cardiac output. The areas of greatest stasis appear to be the apices of the ventricles and the atrial appendages. On rare occasion left ventricular thrombi may be large enough to obstruct the blood flow within this chamber.

Although the typical heart in idiopathic cardiomyopathy of the dilated type has greatly dilated ventricles and ventricular walls of normal thickness, some patients with this condition have relatively thick ventricular walls and only mildly dilated cavities. The size of the left ventricular cavity appears to be roughly proportional to the severity and duration of symptomatic congestive heart failure; the larger the cavity, the longer the duration of symptoms and vice versa.

The myocardium in patients with the dilated type of cardiomyopathy occurring in the puerperium appears to be similar to that in patients with idiopathic dilated cardiomyopathies occurring in nonpuerperal states.[4,5] Fatty change in cardiac muscle cells, however, a common finding in pa-

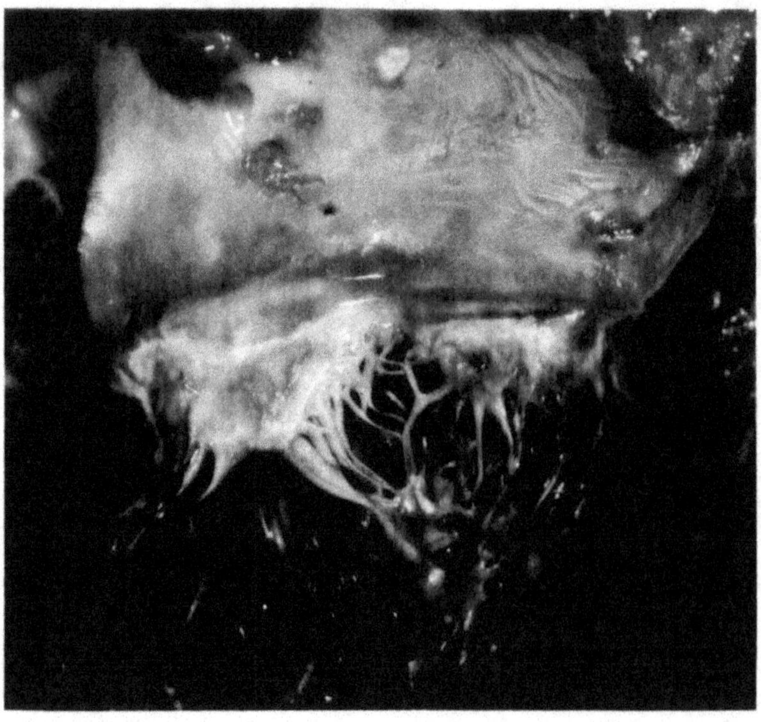

Figure 15. Hypertrophic asymmetric obstructive cardiomyopathy. Opened mitral valve showing that both posterior and anterior leaflets are thickened in the patient described in Figure 14 (A68–185). This type of leaflet thickening is typical of hypertrophic cardiomyopathy.

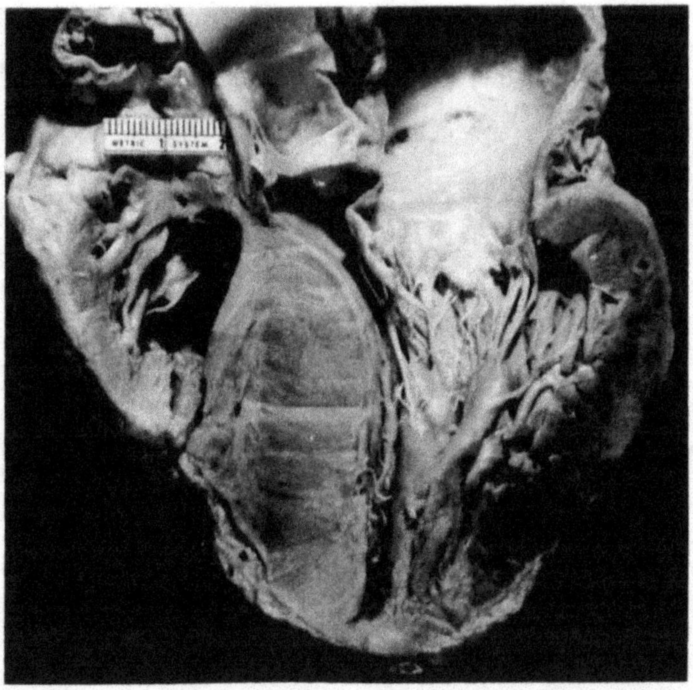

Figure 16. Hypertrophic asymmetric nonobstructive cardiomyopathy. This 33 year old woman (A67–70) became mildly symptomatic when she was 15 years of age. She had three pregnancies without difficulty, but during the fourth she had overt congestive cardiac failure. When admitted to the National Heart and Lung Institute at age 28, she had exertional dyspnea, chest pain, and occasional episodes of dizziness. Several other family members had idiopathic hypertrophic subaortic stenosis. A grade 2/6 precordial systolic murmur, loudest at the apex, and a fourth heart sound were audible. An electrocardiogram showed left bundle branch block and premature ventricular contractions. The cardiac silhouette was enlarged by radiography. No systolic gradient was present between the left ventricle (108/34 mm. Hg) and the brachial artery (114/64 mm. Hg) at rest. By age 30, the angina, dyspnea, and dizziness were more frequent and worse; the syncope had occurred once. On repeat catheterization there was still no systolic gradient present between the left ventricle (97/30 mm. Hg) and the femoral artery (102/58) at rest, but a 9 mm. Hg gradient was provoked by isoproterenol. The premature ventricular contraction response was normal. Repeat catheterization two years later yielded virtually identical findings. The left ventricular angiocardiogram was interpreted as showing "cavity obliteration." She was found dead in bed at home four months later. At necropsy the heart weighed 430 gm. The ventricular septum was much thicker than the left ventricular free wall, which was of normal thickness. The mitral leaflets were only slightly thickened and no endocardial mural plaque was present in the left ventricular outflow tract. Both atria were dilated. This case is typical of the nonobstructive variety of hypertrophic asymmetric cardiomyopathy and is characterized by normal thickness of at least the basal portion of the left ventricular free wall.

tients with nonpuerperal dilated cardiomyopathy and chronic alcoholism,[6,7] may be less frequent in puerperal cardiomyopathy.

Nondilated (Hypertrophic) Cardiomyopathy

This section summarizes observations in 40 patients with hypertrophic cardiomyopathy studied at necropsy by the authors (Figs. 12 to 28). The findings in some of these patients have been described previously.[8–11] The 40 patients ranged in age from nine to 78 years (average, 42): 23 were women and 17 were males. Other family members of 15 patients had similar cardiac conditions. Thirteen patients had systemic hypertension; five, anemia (blood hematocrit < 35 per cent); nine, atrial fibrillation; nine, bundle branch block (left in three, indeterminate in five, and bilateral in one); and one, complete heart block (the latter was preceded by left bundle branch block). Eighteen patients died naturally of the cardiac condition (13 suddenly, five in progressive congestive cardiac failure), nine after cardiac operations, three of complications of cardiac catheterization, one of acute myocardial infarction, and nine of noncardiac causes.

The 40 patients were divided into three groups on the basis of documentation by cardiac catheterization of the presence or absence of peak systolic pressure gradients

Figure 17. Hypertrophic asymmetric obstructive cardiomyopathy in a 20 year old woman (A72–197). A precordial murmur had been heard at age 11, and symptoms (exertional dyspnea and palpitations) appeared at age 12 years. Catheterization at age 14 disclosed a 50 mm. Hg peak systolic pressure gradient between the left ventricle (158/10) and the brachial artery (108/57) and an abnormal premature ventricular response. A left ventricular cineangiocardiogram was consistent with idiopathic hypertrophic subaortic stenosis and showed considerable mitral regurgitation. The left ventricular cavity was small. From age 14 to 20 she had no overt congestive cardiac failure, but there were episodic palpitations and rarely chest pain relieved by rest. During this time she was functionally class II (New York Heart Association). Three months before death she had clinical, electrocardiographic, and enzymatic changes typical of acute transmural (anterolateral wall) myocardial infarction. During the period of infarction there was evidence of congestive cardiac failure. After discharge she continued to have mild dyspnea and episodic chest pain. She died shortly after the sudden appearance of features of acute pulmonary edema. The radiographs shown here were taken four years before death (age 16 years). The cardiac silhouette is massively enlarged. At necropsy the heart weighed 1250 gm. and she weighed only 47 kg. This may be one of the largest hearts ever recorded in a woman.

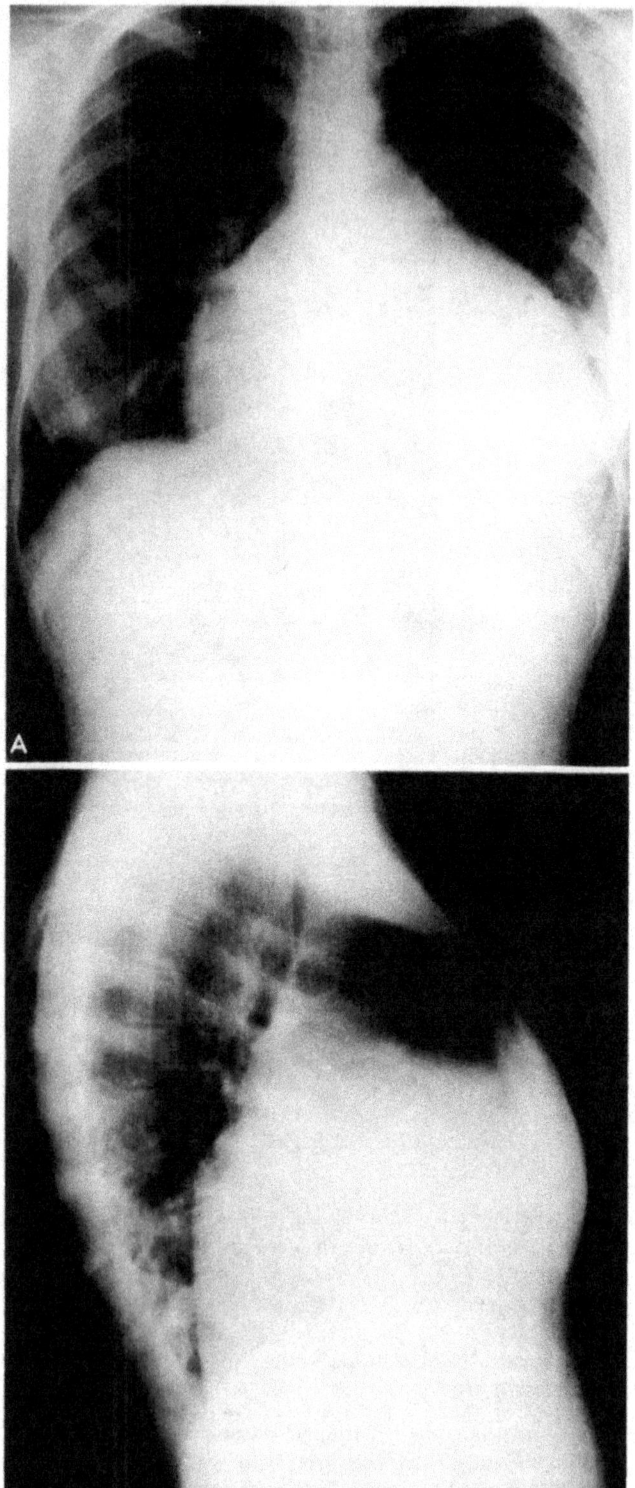

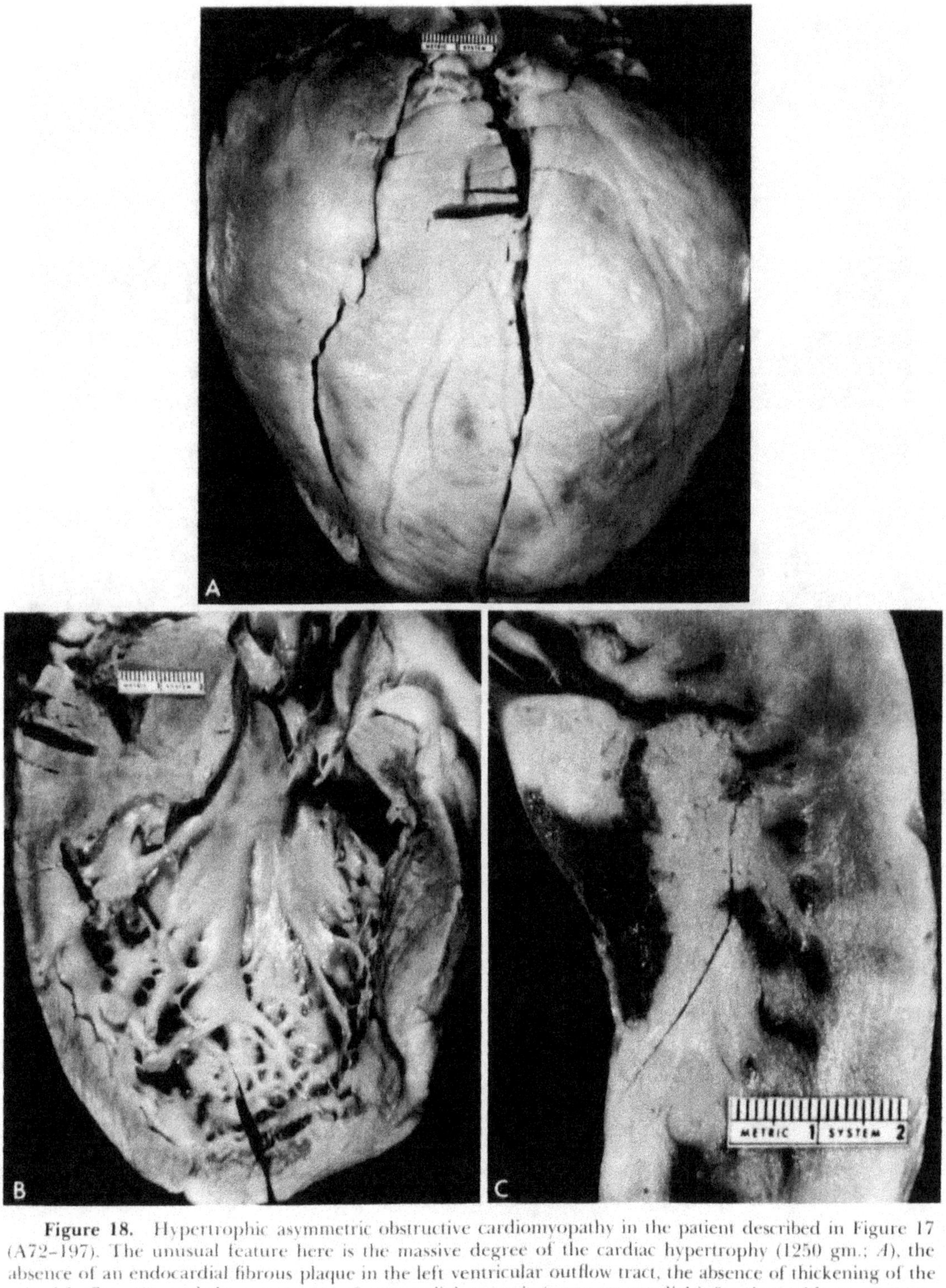

Figure 18. Hypertrophic asymmetric obstructive cardiomyopathy in the patient described in Figure 17 (A72-197). The unusual feature here is the massive degree of the cardiac hypertrophy (1250 gm.; *A*), the absence of an endocardial fibrous plaque in the left ventricular outflow tract, the absence of thickening of the mitral leaflets *(B)*, and the occurrence of myocardial necrosis (acute myocardial infarction) without coronary arterial luminal narrowing. The ventricular septum is enormously thickened. Both the anterior and the posterior left ventricular free walls are thinned, presumably a result of the acute myocardial infarction three months before death. A longitudinal section showing necrosis in one left ventricular papillary muscle is shown in *C*. The left ventricular cavity in this patient is dilated *(B)*, but the dilatation is probably the result of the myocardial infarction rather than idiopathic hypertrophic subaortic stenosis, because a left ventricular angiogram several years before the infarction had shown a "small" left ventricular cavity.

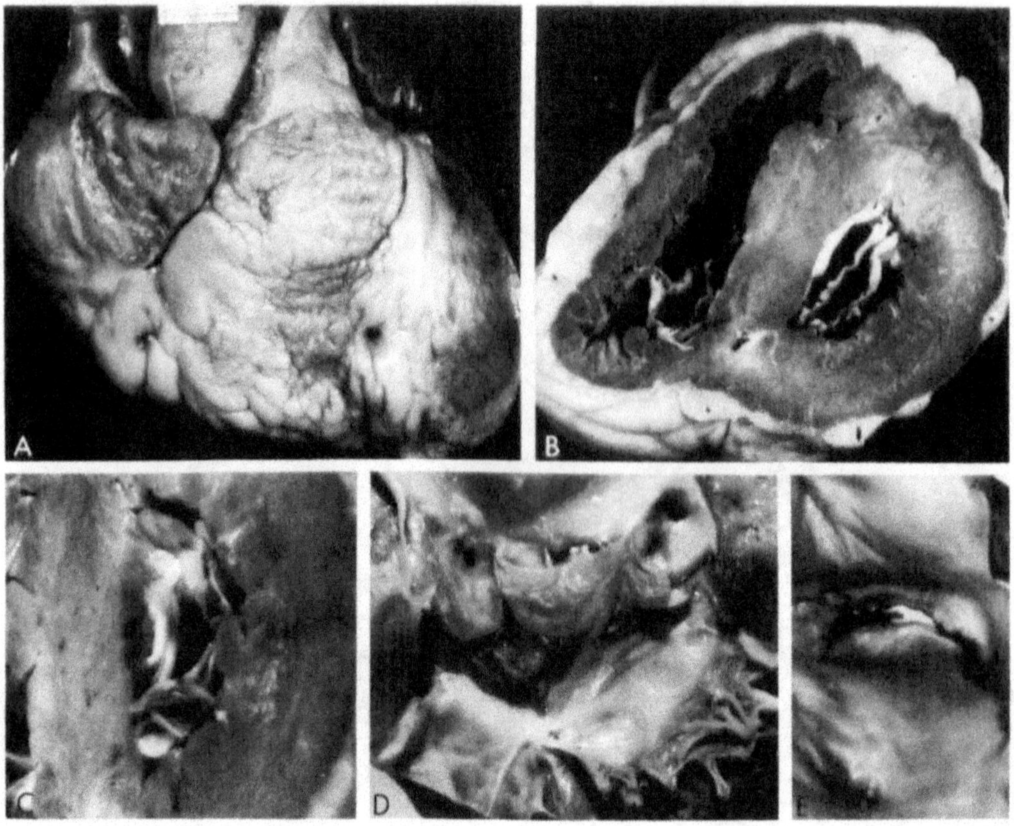

Figure 19. Hypertrophic symmetric (nonobstructive) cardiomyopathy. This 46 year old woman (A72–15), who was noted to have a precordial murmur at age 16, was asymptomatic until age 29, when features of congestive cardiac failure appeared. At age 36 she was studied at the National Heart and Lung Institute. Her father had died of heart disease at age 42, and two siblings in their 30's had had heart disease of an unknown type. A grade 4/6 precordial systolic murmur, loudest at the apex, and a fourth heart sound were audible. An electrocardiogram showed left axis deviation, atrial abnormality, and left ventricular hypertrophy. At catheterization the pressures (in mm. Hg) were: pulmonary artery 36/16; right ventricle 42/4; left atrium m14, a24, v15, and simultaneous left ventricle and brachial artery 162/16 and 96/60, respectively, giving a 66 mm. Hg peak systolic gradient. This gradient increased with isoproterenol infusion. The typical premature ventricular beat response of idiopathic hypertrophic subaortic stenosis was present. A left ventricular cineangiocardiogram was diagnostic of idiopathic hypertrophic subaortic stenosis. From age 36 to 44 she did well and at age 43 could swim, hike two miles, and climb one flight of stairs with difficulty. At age 44 exertional dyspnea became bothersome again, and intermittent claudication of the right leg appeared. At age 45 episodic tachycardia and angina pectoris appeared, and six months before death she had two episodes of syncope, one followed by transient hemiplegia. She was readmitted to the National Heart and Lung Institute one month before death and was functionally class III (New York Heart Association). Examination showed that now no precordial murmur was present, but loud third and fourth heart sounds were audible. The liver was enlarged and all pulses in both legs were absent. Electrocardiogram showed sinus rhythm, a prolonged P-R interval (>0.20 sec.), left axis deviation, low voltage, and Q waves in II, III, and AVF. Radiography showed enlargement of both the left atrium and the left ventricle. The serum cholesterol and triglyceride levels were normal. During the first several days in the hospital she lost 5 kg. and felt better. Shortly thereafter, however, she became febrile and had a grand mal seizure. Her course thereafter was progressively downhill, characterized by complete heart block, atrial fibrillation, low urine output, and hypotension. It is likely that no outflow gradient was present during her last year of life because during this period no precordial murmur was heard. At necropsy the atria were dilated, the ventricular cavities were not dilated, and the ventricular septum was identical in thickness to the left ventricular free wall (*A*, *B*). An endocardial mural plaque was present in the left ventricular outflow tract (*C*, *D*) and the ventricular aspect of the anterior mitral leaflet was thickened. *A*, View of heart from anterior aspect. The atria are prominent. *B*, Transverse section of ventricles. The mural endocardial plaque in the left ventricular outflow tract is apparent. *C*, Close-up view of endocardial plaque. *D*, Opened left ventricular outflow tract. *E*, Mitral orifice viewed from left atrium. This orifice is always "small" in hypertrophic cardiomyopathy because the left ventricular cavity is not dilated.

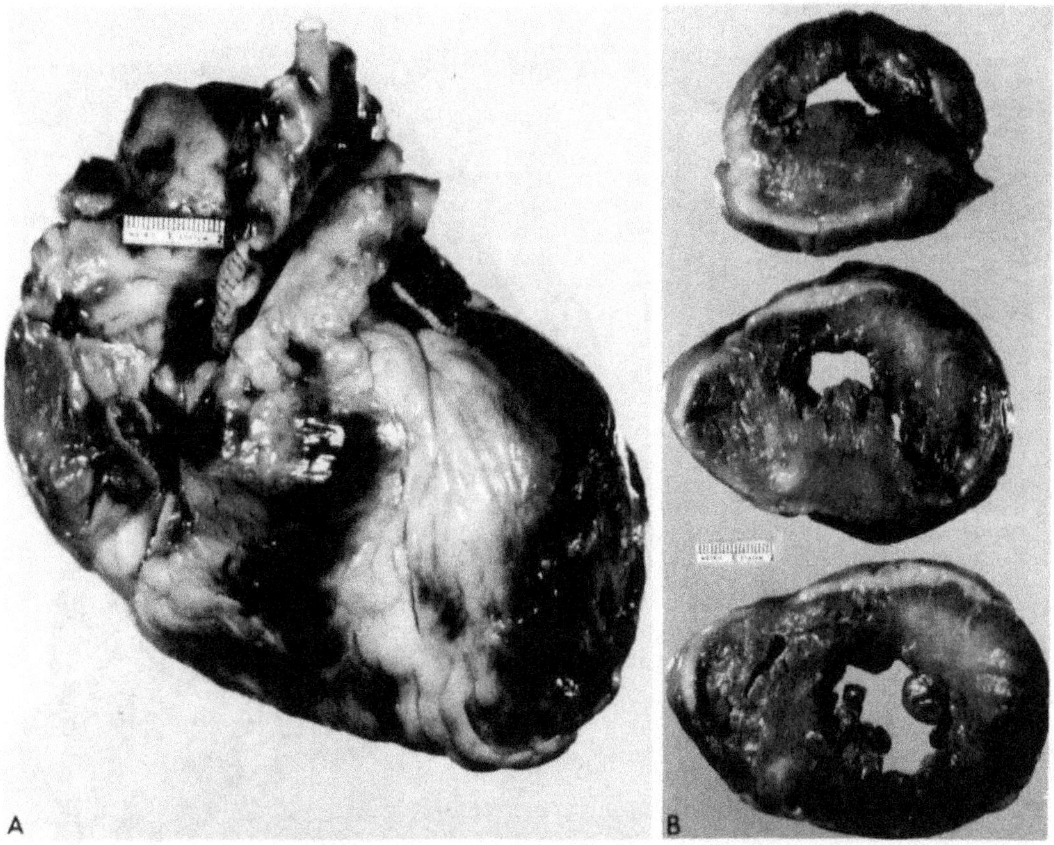

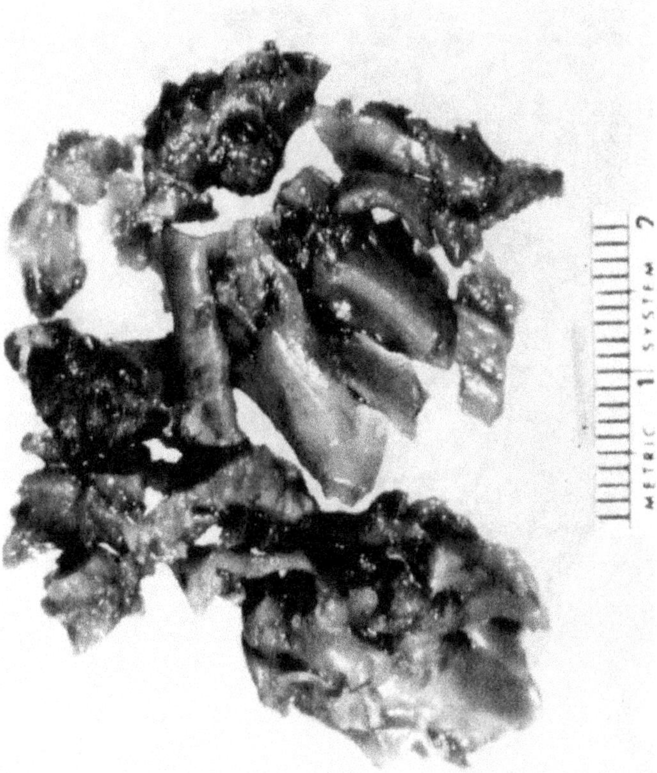

Figure 20. Hypertrophic symmetric (nonobstructive) cardiomyopathy. This 25 year old woman (A72–200) developed exertional dyspnea at age 21. During the next four years congestive heart failure progressed and angina pectoris appeared. She had a grade 2 to 3/6 precordial systolic murmur, loudest at the apex, and the murmur was increased in intensity by the Valsalva maneuver. Catheterization at age 23 disclosed no systolic pressure gradient between the left ventricle (124/25 mm. Hg) and the femoral artery (125/83). A repeat study at age 25 (10 months before death) was similar: left ventricle 130/38 and femoral artery 130/80 mm. Hg. On cineangiocardiography the left ventricular cavity was minute and there was mild mitral regurgitation. Because of a lack of improvement with propanolol therapy, a left ventricular myotomy and myectomy was performed. Because the aorta was so small, the resection had to be carried out via a left ventriculotomy incision. Approximately 8 gm. of myocardium was excised (*C*). *A*, Anterior view of heart. *B*, Transverse sections of ventricles. The top one is near the apex and the bottom one near the base. The anterior free wall near the apex and the posterior free wall near the base are of normal thickness.

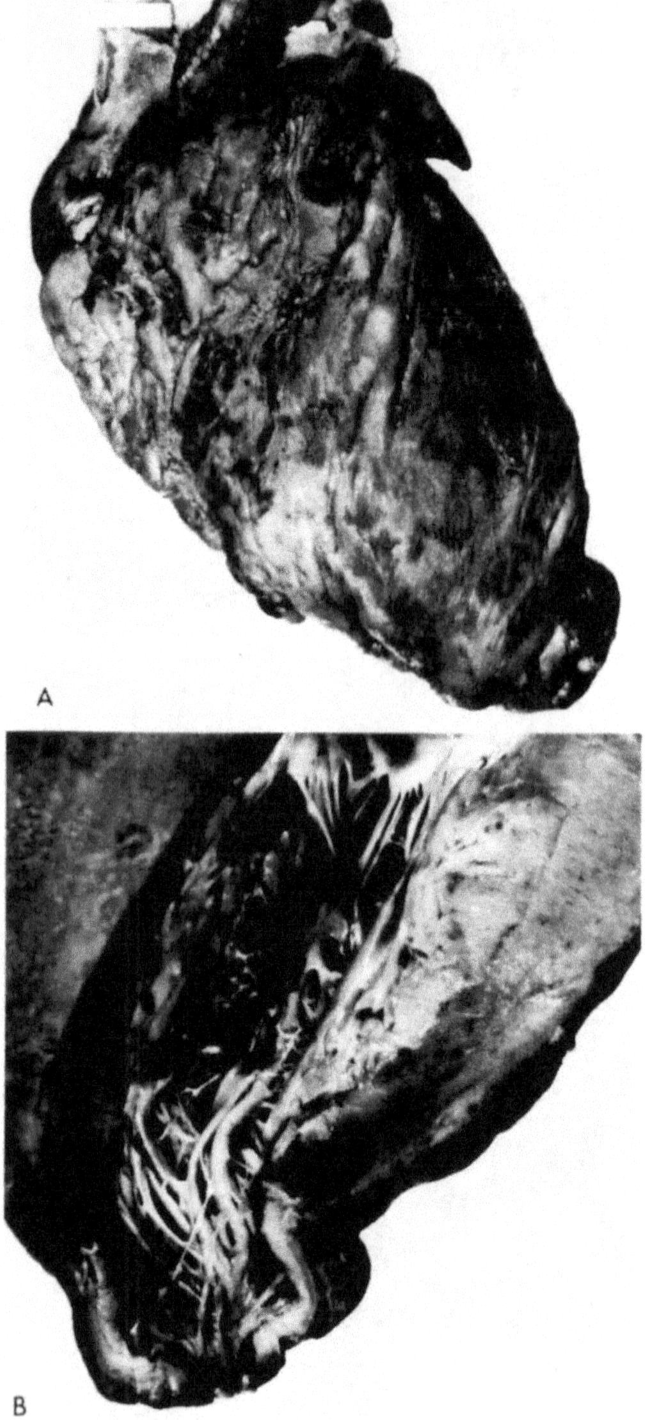

A

B

Figure 21. Hypertrophic asymmetric obstructive cardiomyopathy. This 19 year old girl (A70–278), who was found to have a precordial murmur at age six, was asymptomatic until age 19 (22 months before death), when she developed fever, supraventricular arrhythmias, and alpha streptococcal septicemia two months after some dental work. Because of a marked deterioration in effort tolerance, cardiac catheterization was performed (16 months before death). A peak systolic pressure gradient of 162 mm. Hg was recorded between the left ventricle (260/20) and the ascending aorta (98/75), and a 38 mm. Hg gradient between the right ventricle (62/12) and the pulmonary trunk (28/20). A left ventricular cineangiocardiogram was typical of idiopathic hypertrophic subaortic stenosis. Mitral regurgitation was trivial. The apical portion of the left ventricle was not visualized on angiography. The coronary arteries appeared normal following aortic root injection. An electrocardiogram showed biventricular hypertrophy. At an operation (left ventricular outflow myotomy and myectomy) performed nine days before death a left ventricular apical aneurysm, noted here, was observed. A left ventricular aneurysm is indeed rare in idiopathic hypertrophic subaortic stenosis except after left ventricular incision during operative therapy. This aneurysm is unique in that its wall consists of myocardium similar to that in other portions of the left ventricular free wall. (Most aneurysms at this site obviously consist entirely of fibrous tissue, the result of healing of an acute myocardial infarction, and myocardial fibers are infrequently observed in the aneurysmal wall.) The mechanism of formation of this "myocardial aneurysm" is uncertain. It might be reasoned that the extremely high left ventricular systolic pressure (260 mm. Hg) simply caused bulging of the thinnest portion of the left ventricular free wall, i.e., the apex. Because left ventricular outflow was obstructed, this high pressure was exerted onto the apex with resulting aneurysmal formation. This high a systolic left ventricular pressure in idiopathic hypertrophic subaortic stenosis is unusual at any age but particularly so in childhood, and the latter in some way also may have been a factor. At autopsy the heart weighed 730 gm. and the ventricular septum was disproportionally hypertrophied. The left ventricular cavity was minute. The apical aneurysm was free of thrombus; its wall consisted of myocardial fibers, many of which had been made necrotic by the ligature that had been placed about the base of the aneurysm at operation nine days earlier.

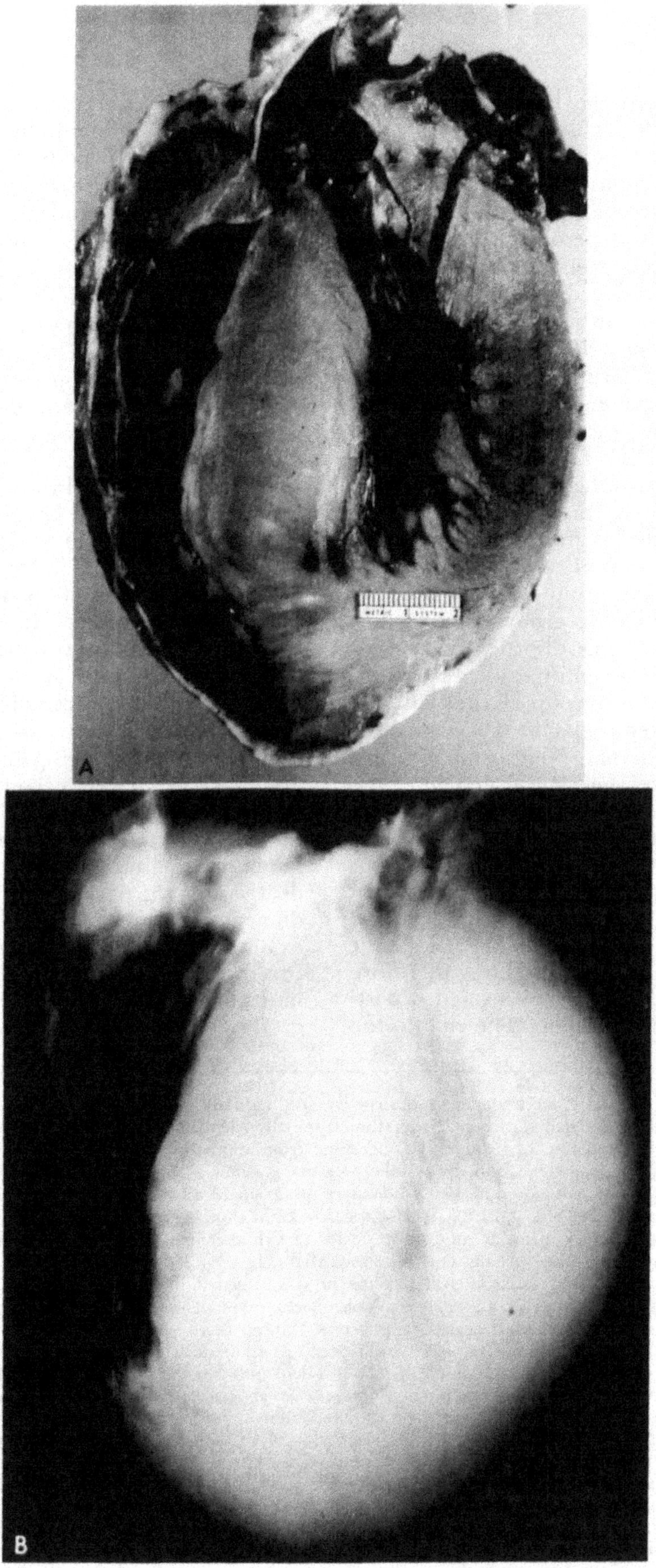

Figure 22.

at rest between the left ventricle and a systemic artery (Table 1). Twenty patients had subaortic stenosis with a peak systolic pressure gradient at rest of 20 to 170 mm. Hg (average, 93; group I). Thirteen patients with zero pressure gradients at rest comprise group II; provocation in 11 patients produced gradients (range, 10 to 150 mm. Hg) in seven. In only one patient was the provoked peak systolic pressure gradient greater than 32 mm. Hg. The seven patients in whom cardiac catheterization was not performed comprise group III. The diagnosis of idiopathic hypertrophic subaortic stenosis was established preoperatively in 19 of 20 patients in group I, in 11 of 13 patients in group II, and in only two of seven patients in group III. The only undiagnosed patient in group I was studied in 1956 before this disorder was recognized as a distinct entity. The two undiagnosed patients in group II clinically had pure mitral regurgitation, believed to be on a rheumatic basis, but again each was studied before the clinical and hemodynamic features of idiopathic hypertrophic subaortic stenosis were well recognized; one died in 1961 and the second in 1963.

At planned mitral valve replacement in one, the left ventricular wall was found to be thick and the cavity, small; idiopathic hypertrophic subaortic stenosis therefore was suspected and later confirmed at postoperative catheterization. The clue to the proper diagnosis in each of the two patients in group II was the rapidly rising systemic arterial pulses. An additional clue in one patient was the increased intensity of the precordial systolic murmur during beats following premature ventricular contractions.[9] The diagnosis of idiopathic hypertrophic subaortic stenosis in each of the eight patients in whom this diagnosis was not established clinically was made at necropsy by observing anatomic cardiac findings identical to those in patients in whom the diagnosis was established by clinical means.

The 20 patients in group I averaged 43 years of age; the 13 in group II, 28 years; and the seven in group III, 67 years. All patients in group I had symptoms of cardiac dysfunction; two patients in group II and four in group III were asymptomatic. Whereas only six patients in group I had histories of similar heart disease in other family members, nine patients in group II had positive histories. Precordial systolic murmurs ranging in intensity from grades 3/6 to 5/6 were present at some time in all 20 patients in group I. In one patient, however, a grade 3/6 systolic precordial murmur was audible eight years before death when the peak systolic pressure gradient was 70 mm. Hg, but when she was examined during the last year of life, no precordial murmur was audible. Similar murmurs occurred in 11 of 13 patients in group II, but the intensity was less (grade

Figure 22. Hypertrophic asymmetric obstructive (right sided) cardiomyopathy. This 18 year old boy (A72-78), described in detail elsewhere,[12] was studied initially when he was asymptomatic at age eight years because his brother had just died suddenly at age nine from idiopathic hypertrophic subaortic stenosis (left sided obstruction). At catheterization, no systolic pressure gradient was observed between the left ventricle and the systemic artery, but a 35 mm. Hg systolic pressure gradient was recorded between the right ventricle (56/5) and the pulmonary artery (21/9). An electrocardiogram showed right axis deviation, right ventricular hypertrophy, and a right ventricular conduction delay. The child remained asymptomatic until age 12, when he developed chest pain while playing football. Precordial pain recurred frequently thereafter and was precipitated by exertion of decreasing intensity so that he was forced to limit his activities to a sedentary level. When he was restudied at age 13, a grade 4/6 systolic ejection type of precordial murmur was heard, loudest along the left sternal border. Electrocardiography now showed more severe right ventricular hypertrophy. Catheterization showed a 118 mm. Hg peak systolic pressure gradient between the right ventricle (135/7) and pulmonary artery (17/7) and there was no systolic gradient between the left ventricle (108/4) and the brachial artery (108/63 mm. Hg). Resection of the right ventricular outflow myocardium with insertion of a patch at the right ventriculotomy was performed, and catheterization seven months postoperatively showed virtually no systolic pressure gradient between the right ventricle (30/4 mm. Hg) and the pulmonary artery (28/12). He was asymptomatic. Electrocardiography now showed a right bundle branch block. This boy apparently remained asymptomatic until the day of death, when he felt faint while driving a car. He pulled over to the side of the road and collapsed. No anatomic explanation for death was provided by necropsy. His heart weighed 660 gm. The right ventricular outflow tract was wide open. The ventricular septum was much thicker than the left ventricular free wall (4.0 compared to 1.9 cm.), and the right ventricular wall was of normal thickness. The endocardium of the left ventricular outflow tract was not thickened and the mitral valve was normal. Mild interstitial fibrosis involved the ventricular septum. *A*, A longitudinal section of the ventricles shows the disproportional ventricular septal hypertrophy. The right ventricular cavity is larger than the left. *B*, The radiograph of the heart was taken before it was opened.

3/6 in three patients, grade 2/6 in five, grade 1/6 in three). Systolic murmurs were audible in six (grade 4/6 in one, grade 3/6 in four) of seven patients in group III. Four of 20 patients in group I, two of 12 in group II, and one of seven in group III had atrial fibrillation. Of 15 patients in group I in whom left ventricular angiographic studies were performed, seven had mitral regurgitation; of nine patients in

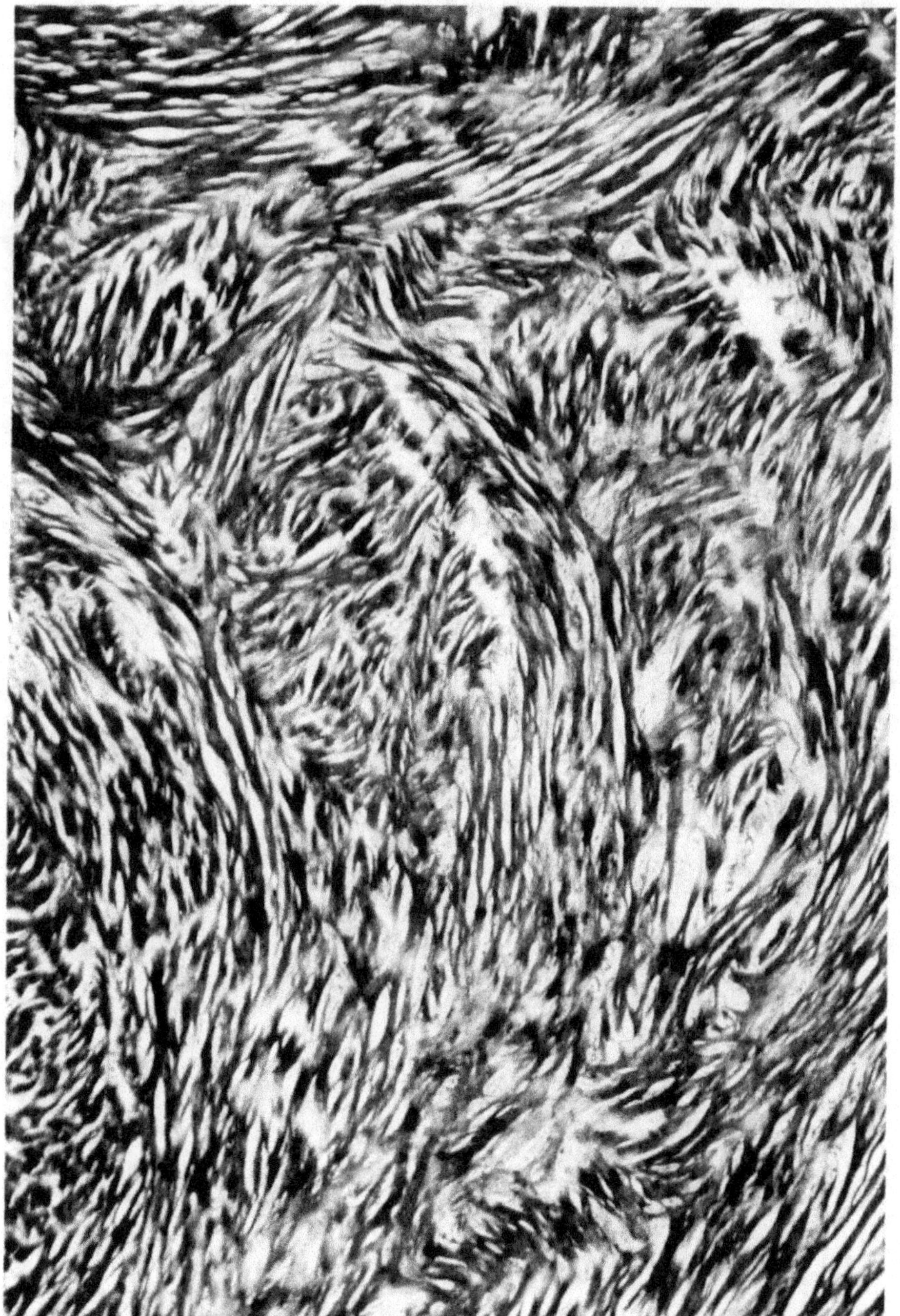

Figure 23. Histologic section of ventricular septal myocardium from 19 year old man with hypertrophic obstructive cardiomyopathy. The bundles of muscle cells are irregularly arranged and course in various directions. (Masson stain. × 60.)

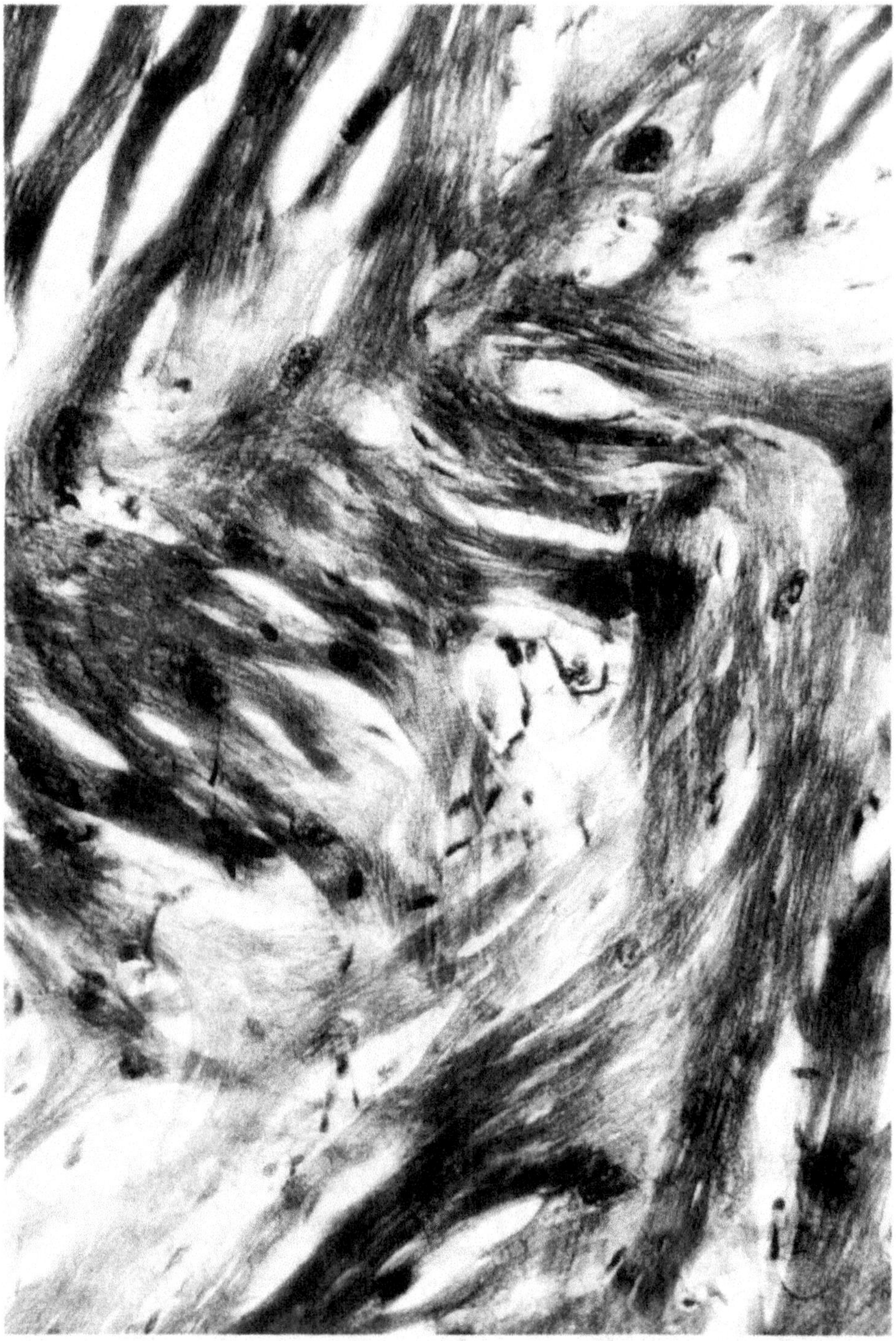

Figure 24. High power view of same tissue as in Figure 23, showing marked divergence in the orientation of adjacent muscle cells. (Masson stain. × 300.)

group II with left ventricular angiograms, five had mitral regurgitation. Seven patients in group I and four in group II had systolic pressure gradients between the right ventricle and pulmonary trunk. One of the latter patients had a 128 mm. Hg peak systolic pressure gradient between the right ventricular body and pulmonary trunk and none between the left ventricle and systemic artery.[12] His brother, how-

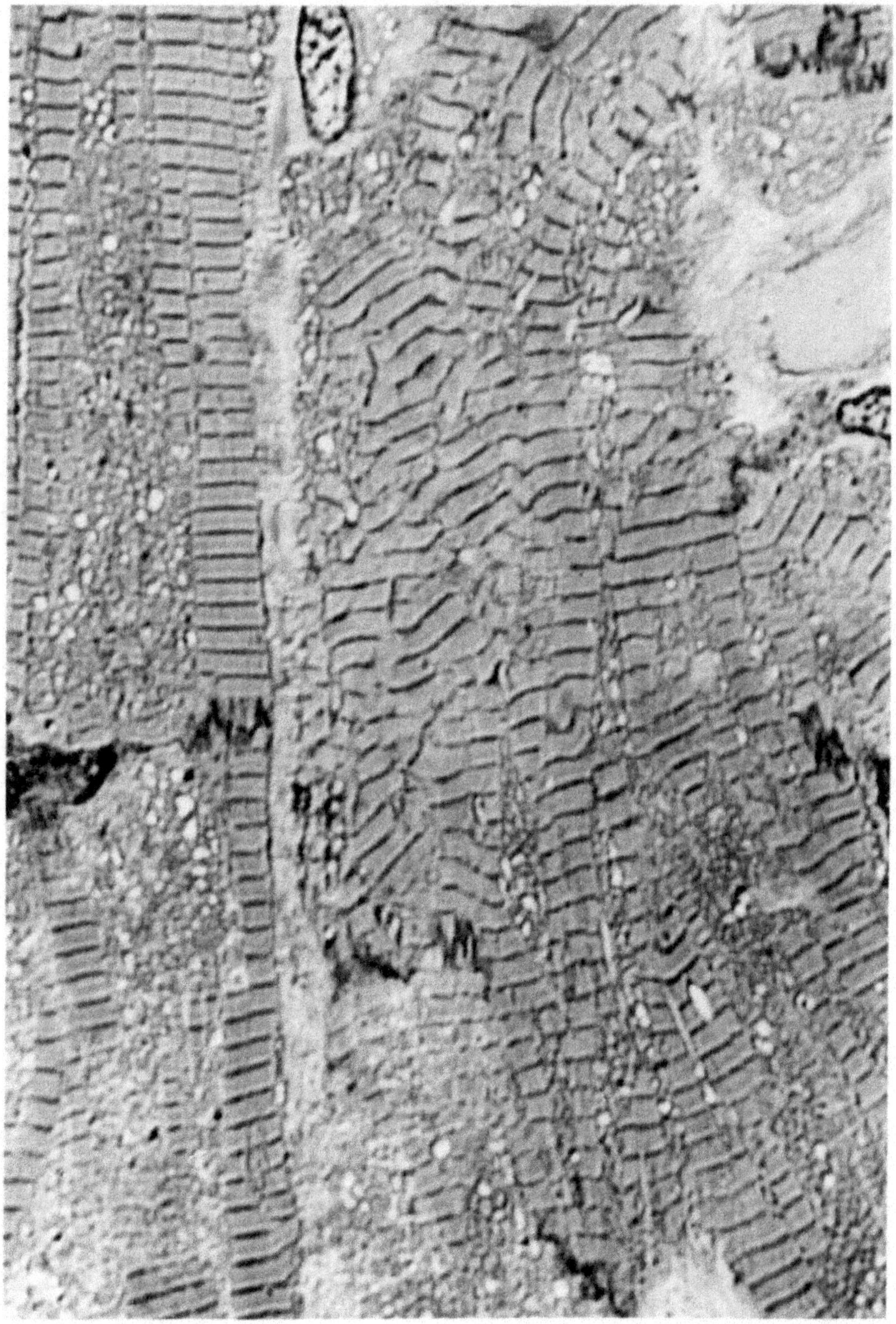

Figure 25. Some muscle cells in the ventricular septum of a patient with hypertrophic obstructive cardiomyopathy show pronounced irregularity in alignment and orientation of myofibrils; two other cells have normally aligned myofibrils. One micron thick section of plastic-embedded tissue. (Nomarski interference contrast optics. × 2000.)

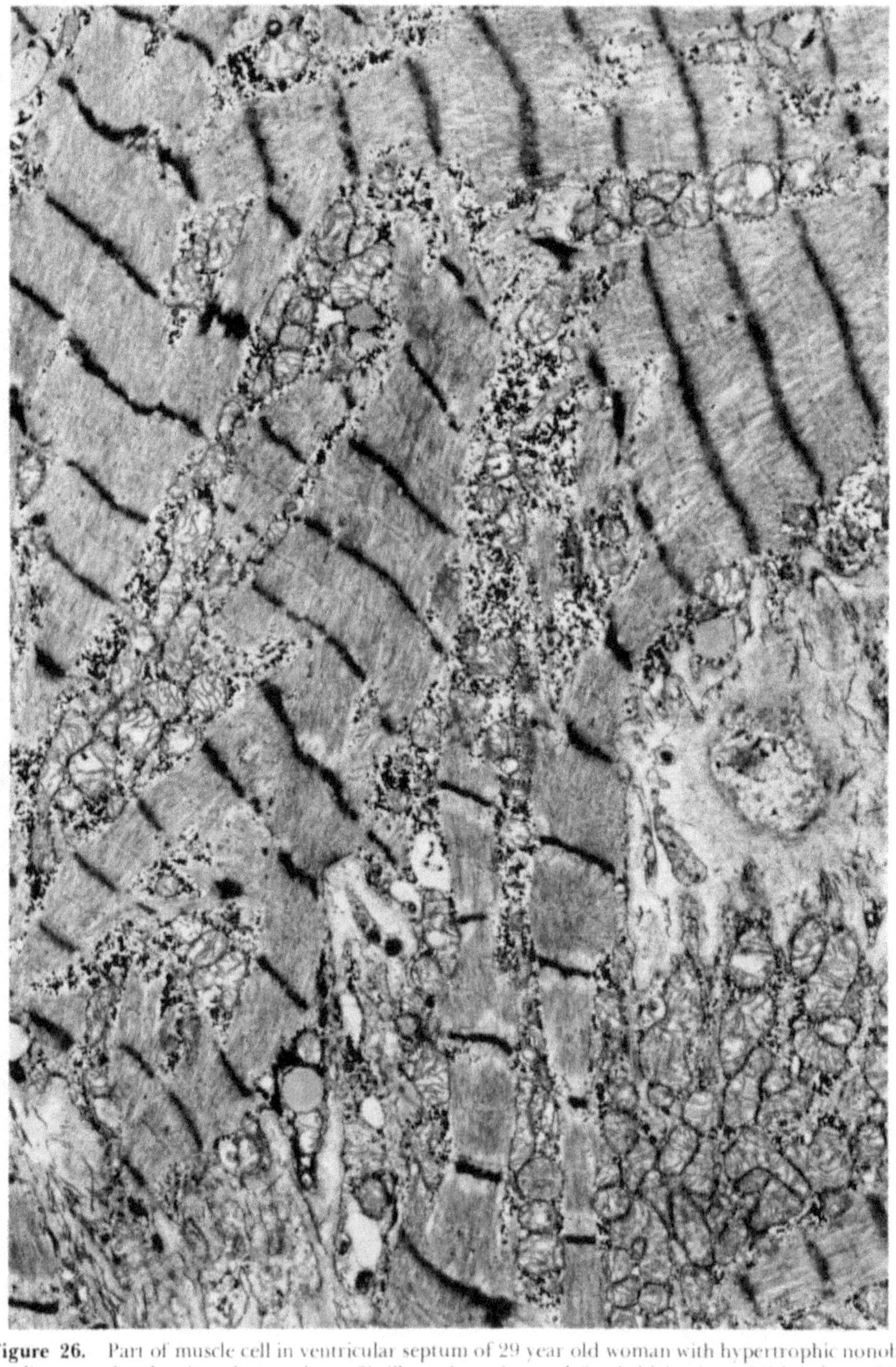

Figure 26. Part of muscle cell in ventricular septum of 29 year old woman with hypertrophic nonobstructive cardiomyopathy showing abnormal myofibrillar orientation and focal thickening of Z bands. (× 8000.)

ever, had typical left sided idiopathic hypertrophic subaortic stenosis. Four patients in group I and five in group II had pulmonary hypertension; in two patients the pulmonary systolic pressure was greater than 50 mm. Hg. Six of 11 patients in group I and seven of nine patients in group II had elevated left atrial pressures; all 12 patients with elevated left atrial pressures had either mitral regurgitation or elevated left ventricular end diastolic pressures. Twelve patients in group I and nine in group II had elevated (≥ 12 mm. Hg) left ventricular end diastolic pressures.

The necropsy cardiac observations in 40 patients are summarized in Table 1. The hearts of the 40 patients ranged from 350 to 1250 gm. (average, 634). In 33 patients the ventricular septa were unequivocally thicker than the thickest portion of left ventricular free wall. In all 20 patients with documented left ventricular outflow obstruction at rest, the left ventricular free walls (anterior, lateral, and posterior) were hypertrophied and to similar degrees at all corresponding levels (Fig. 15). In contrast, the left ventricular free walls behind the posterior mitral leaflets were not thickened in 11 of 13 patients without obstruction at rest, and in two of them the entire free wall was of normal thickness. In 40 patients both ventricular cavities appeared smaller than normal or normal in size. The mural endocardium of the left ventricular outflow tract in apposition to the anterior mitral leaflet was thickened in 29 patients. The mitral valve leaflets, particularly the anterior ones, were thickened by fibrous tissue in 29 patients. Both left and right atria were dilated in 40 patients. Except for fibromas in two patients, the aortic valve cusps were normal. Foci of fibrosis were observed grossly in the left ventricular papillary muscles in 38 patients, and these structures appeared smaller than normal in all of them. Other subendocardial scars were present grossly in most patients. Only one had a transmural scar and it was small. Excluding the nine patients who died during or soon after cardiac operations, foci of myocardial necrosis were present in only one patient. She was a 21 year old woman who had an acute myocardial infarct beginning three months before death. The coronary arteries were normal, but her heart weighed 1250 gm. (body weight, 47 kg.). Histologic examination of sections of the left ventricular free wall and of the ventricular septum disclosed interstitial fibrosis of varying degrees in all patients and, usually, small foci of replacement fibrosis as well. Varying degrees of disorientation of myocardial fibers were observed in histologic sections of ventricular septa in all 40 patients. The intramural coronary arteries in the ventricular septae appeared increased in number and their walls were thick in one patient.

The myocardium in the left ventricular outflow tract of patients with idiopathic hypertrophic subaortic stenosis is distinctive by light and electron microscopy. Ferrans et al.[13] studied by electron microscope the operatively excised left ventricular outflow tract muscle in 14 patients with this disorder. Distinctive abnormalities were found in each patient. Bundles of muscle cells were severely disorganized with cells running in different directions instead of in parallel. Muscle cells were wider and shorter than in hypertrophy due to other causes and showed increased cellular branching, extensive side-to-side intercellular junctions, widened Z bands, and evidence of formation of new sarcomeres. Some myofibrils were oriented obliquely or perpendicular to the longitudinal axes of the cells, and some myofilaments that originated from a single Z band inserted into the Z bands of other myofibrils. Examination of the left ventricular apical myocardium in two of the 14 patients disclosed hypertrophied but normally arranged muscle cells. The abnormal architecture of the muscle cells appears to be a unique feature of hypertrophic cardiomyopathy.

Comments on Idiopathic Cardiomyopathy of the Hypertrophic Type. Study of our patients with hypertrophic cardiomyopathy disclosed several characteristic anatomic features of this entity: disproportional hypertrophy of the ventricular septum, small or normal sized left and right ventricular cavities, endocardial mural plaque of the left ventricular outflow tract, thickened mitral valve, dilated atria, hypertrophied (focal or diffuse) free walls of all four cardiac chambers, normal or nearly normal aortic valve cusps, normal sized ascending aorta, and severe abnormalities involving the organization of mus-

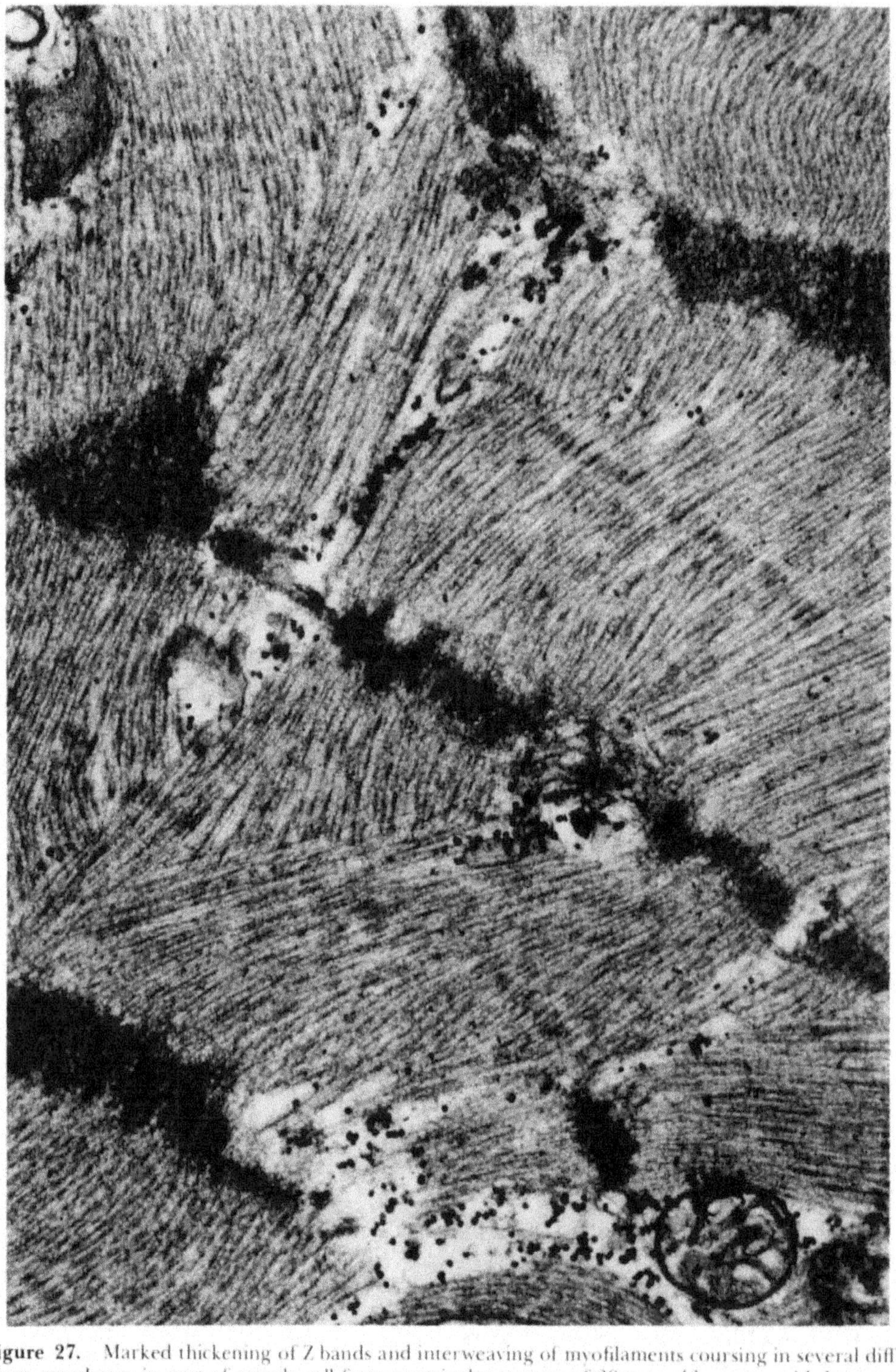

Figure 27. Marked thickening of Z bands and interweaving of myofilaments coursing in several different directions are shown in part of muscle cell from ventricular septum of 39 year old woman with hypertrophic obstructive cardiomyopathy. (×47,000.)

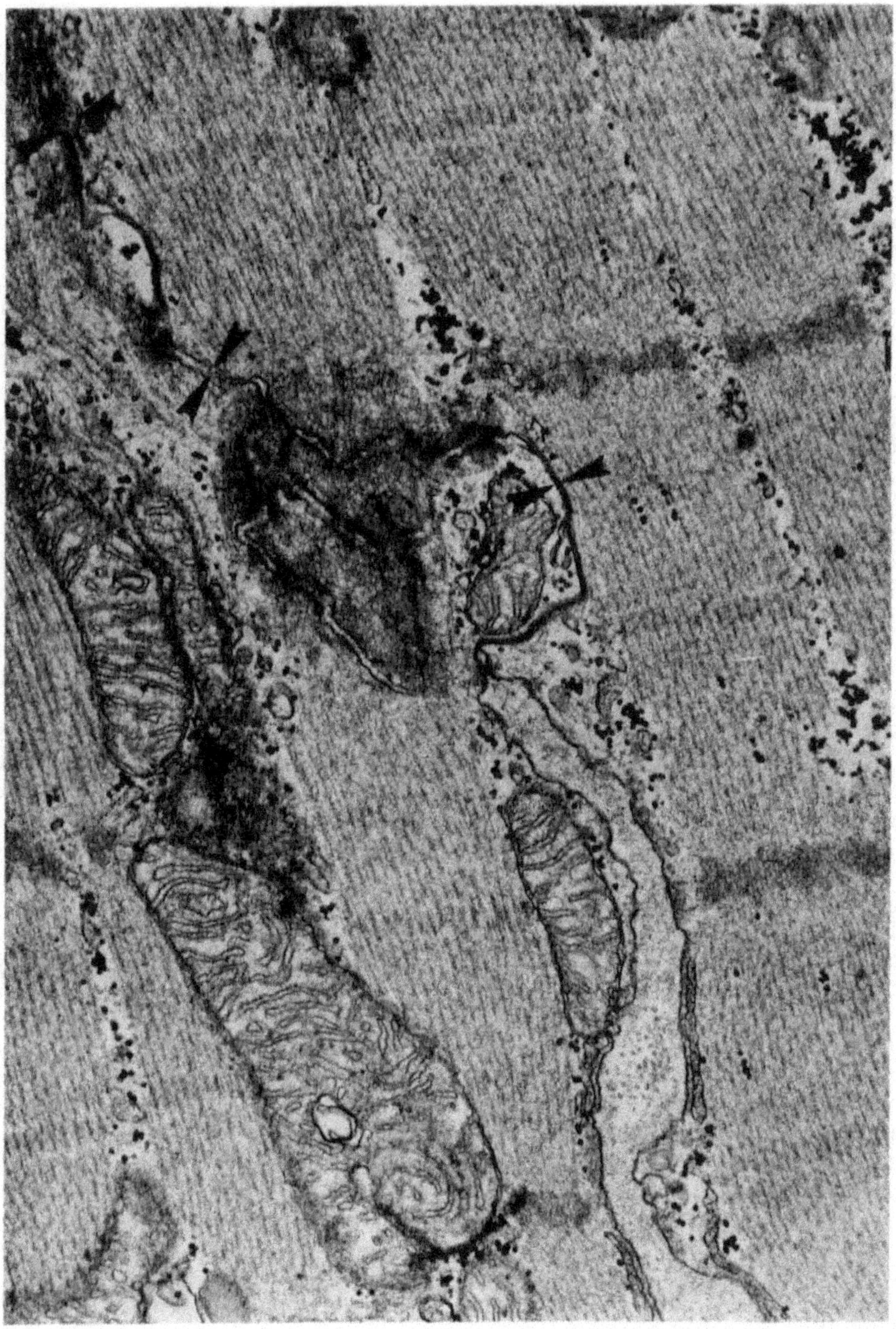

Figure 28. Area of side-to-side junction (arrowheads) between two adjacent muscle cells in ventricular septum of 30 year old man with hypertrophic obstructive cardiomyopathy. (× 40,000.)

cle cell bundles and the arrangement and orientation of myofibrils and myofilaments of individual muscle cells in the ventricular septum.

The major gross anatomic feature of hypertrophic cardiomyopathy is disproportional hypertrophy of the ventricular septum; i.e., the ventricular septum is thicker than the left ventricular free wall. Normally, at all ages, the ventricular septum and left ventricular free wall are equal in thickness. Disproportional or asymmetric septal hypertrophy is the characteristic anatomic feature of hypertrophic cardiomyopathy. Disproportional septal hypertrophy and disorganization of the septal muscle fibers are probably the only anatomic features of hypertrophic cardiomyopathy present from birth. The other features appear to be secondary to these basic defects and are acquired later. Originally it was believed that the thickest portion of the ventricular septum in this condition was that portion just below the aortic valve. Study of our 40 necropsy patients, however, clearly demonstrates that the thickest portion of the septum is about midway between the base of the aortic valve cusps and the apex of the left ventricle. The thickest portion of the septum also is usually just opposite the apex of the right ventricle. Thus, an adequate myotomy or myectomy in idiopathic hypertrophic subaortic stenosis must include interruption or excision of the myocardium located in the middle third of the septum and not just that portion close to the aortic valve.

Six of the 40 patients had symmetric rather than asymmetric hypertrophic cardiomyopathy. By definition, the thickest portion of the ventricular septum was equal in thickness to the thickest portion of the left ventricular free wall. In all six patients, however, that free wall immediately behind the posterior mitral leaflet was thinner than the thickest portion of the ventricular septum. It is probable that typical asymmetric septal hypertrophy had been present at one time in four of them, because each had mural endocardial fibrous plaques in the left ventricular outflow tract and correspondingly thickened anterior mitral leaflets. One (a 46 year old woman) of these three had had a 70 mm. Hg peak systolic pressure gradient between the left ventricle and a systemic artery and a loud systolic murmur eight years before death, but no murmur was audible during her last several months of life. It is possible that the ventricular septum thinned and outflow obstruction (and the murmur) disappeared as a consequence.

Another (a 62 year old woman) of these three patients had systemic hypertension, and a huge (170 mm. Hg) peak systolic pressure gradient was measured shortly before operation. Also preoperatively, an echocardiogram showed no disproportional septal hypertrophy. At operation disproportional septal hypertrophy was not observed, and pressure recordings in the operating room showed no systolic gradient between the left ventricle and the systemic artery. The third patient (a 53 year old man) had had systemic hypertension for years, and at catheterization at age 46 the peak systolic pressure gradient between the left ventricle and the systemic artery at rest was 8 mm. Hg and with provocation, 56 mm. Hg. The last of these four patients (a 65 year old woman) also had systemic hypertension but never underwent catheterization. The fifth patient (a 25 year old woman) with symmetric hypertrophy had no mural or valvular endocardial thickening and no peak systolic pressure gradient between the left ventricle and the systemic artery at rest or after provocation. The sixth patient (a nine year old boy) had massive cardiomegaly (670 gm. heart) and he weighed less than 50 kg. Injection of contrast material into the right and left ventricles at the same time showed that the ventricular septum was not disproportionally hypertrophied. This child died suddenly.

In addition to the six patients with symmetric hypertrophic cardiomyopathy already discussed, three others at necropsy also had ventricular septa identical in thickness to the left ventricular free walls. Each of them, however, had undergone left ventricular myotomy and myectomy (septectomy) for idiopathic hypertrophic subaortic stenosis 31 to 57 months earlier. One of them died of suicide, another of acute myocardial infection from severe coronary disease, and the third of progressive congestive cardiac failure. With the exception of the latter patient, not only had the ventricular septa returned to normal thickness but the ventricular cavities had dilated to normal dimensions. The heart of the patient dying of congestive failure looked like the heart in the dilated type of cardiomyopathy—the ventricular cavities were quite dilated and the ventricular septum was of the same thickness as the left ventricular free wall.

The presence or absence of hypertrophy of the left ventricular free wall is helpful in separating patients with the obstructive type from those with the nonobstructive type of hypertrophic cardiomyopathy.[14, 15] The left ventricular free wall was uniformly hypertrophied in all 20 patients with hypertrophic cardiomyopathy and subaortic stenosis at rest (true idiopathic hypertrophic subaortic stenosis). In contrast, the most basal portion of the left ventricular free wall (i.e., that portion immediately behind the posterior mitral leaflet) was of normal thickness in 11 of the 13 patients with hypertrophic cardiomyopathy and no subaortic stenosis. In two of the latter patients the entire left ventricular free wall was of normal thickness. The absence of hypertrophy in the left ventricular free wall behind the posterior mitral leaflet is detectable by echocardiogram, and thus has made possible the clinical separation of nonobstructive from obstructive patients with hypertrophic cardiomyopathy by this noninvasive technique.[14, 15]

The small systolic pressure gradients between the right ventricular body and the pulmonary trunk in some patients with hypertrophic cardiomyopathy almost certainly result from severe hypertrophy of the ventricular septum, because these gradients often disappear after left ventricular myotomy with or without myectomy. The cause of the hypertrophy of the right ventricular free wall in patients with idiopathic hypertrophic subaortic stenosis without right ventricular systolic hypertension or outflow obstruction is uncertain.

Both ventricular cavities in hypertrophic cardiomyopathy are smaller than normal or are normal in size. Most commonly the left ventricular cavity is slitlike with an S-shaped configuration. The papillary muscles probably contact one another during ventricular systole as do the anterior mitral leaflet and the mural endocardium in the outflow tract. Fibromas, which appear to result from abnormal contact of surfaces during ventricular contraction, were present in two of our patients. A saccular aneurysm was present at the apex of the left ventricle in one patient, a 19 year old girl with a 162 mm. Hg outflow tract gradient (Fig. 21). It consisted entirely of myocardium, but its thickness was considerably less than that of the wall in other areas.

The small left ventricular cavity appears to be responsible for the thickening of the mural endocardium in the left ventricular outflow tract and also for the fibrous thickening of the mitral leaflets. It is important to recall that the mitral valve resides in the left ventricle, which being relatively small in hypertrophic cardiomyopathy, causes abnormal contact of the mitral leaflets with each other and causes the anterior leaflet to contact the mural endocardium in the left ventricular outflow tract. The caudal margin of the mural endocardial plaque corresponds precisely to the distal margin of the anterior mitral leaflet. The focal fibrous thickening of the posterior leaflet probably results from contact of the mitral leaflets during ventricular systole, because there is not enough room in the left ventricular cavity to accommodate the leaflets and chordae easily. The ventricle and mitral leaflets in this respect may be regarded as being similar to an accordion. The mitral leaflet thickening in hypertrophic cardiomyopathy is somewhat analogous to that which occurs normally as a consequence of aging. With aging the left ventricular cavity becomes smaller, presumably in response to the lowered cardiac output; the mitral leaflets, thicker; and the left ventricular muscle, less compliant. The left atrium dilates in response to the increased work required to fill the small left ventricle. Similar mechanisms appear to be accelerated in idiopathic hypertrophic subaortic stenosis.

Most patients with hypertrophic cardiomyopathy have some degree of mitral regurgitation. It is not related to anular dilatation because the mitral anulus in this condition is not dilated. Furthermore, the leaflet thickening is not extensive enough to cause valvular regurgitation. The most likely explanation appears to be abnormal bending of the papillary muscles, particularly the anterolateral one.[16, 17] These structures may be bent abnormally by the bulging ventricular septum with resulting excessive tension on the chordae tendineae, preventing closure of the mitral orifice. Although usually present in hypertrophic cardiomyopathy, focal papillary muscle scarring cannot account for the regurgitation. Mitral regurgitation, usually mild, may be the predominant clinical feature of this condition. Mitral valve replacement in idiopathic hypertrophic subaortic stenosis, despite contrary views,[18] is hazardous because the small left ventricular cavity is rarely capable of freely accommodating a prosthesis.[19]

The aortic valve cusps are usually normal in patients with hypertrophic cardiomyopathy. By contrast, in discrete subaortic stenosis they are the sites of jet lesions produced by blood being ejected under high force and velocity through the area of narrowing, which is only about 1 cm. below the base of the aortic cusps. In hypertrophic obstructive cardiomyopathy (idiopathic hypertrophic subaortic stenosis) the area of obstruction is farther down in the left ventricular cavity, almost certainly at the caudal margin of the left ventricular outflow endocardial plaque, which corresponds to the distal margin of the anterior mitral leaflet. This site is considerably below the aortic valve cusps, so that if a jet is produced it is diffused before reaching the valve cusps.

The recent electron microscope studies of Ferrans et al.[13] clearly demonstrate distinctive morphologic abnormalities in hypertrophic cardiomyopathy. They consist of severe disorganization of the bundles of muscle cells and of the architecture of individual muscle cells in the ventricular septum. Similar findings are rare in the left ventricular free wall in patients with idiopathic hypertrophic subaortic stenosis or in the crista supraventricularis muscle of patients with the tetralogy of Fallot. Abnormalities of the organization of muscle bundles and muscle cells were observed in only 10 per cent of the patients with idiopathic cardiomegaly of the dilated type and were minimal in degree and uncommon.[2] The biopsy specimens in the latter patients, however, were from the caudal portion of the right ventricle or from the left or right ventricular free walls, and not from the cephalad portion of the ventricular septum as in the patients with idiopathic hypertrophic subaortic stenosis. The disorganization of the muscle fibers in the latter disorder also can be appreciated by light microscopic examination, by which method disorganization is infrequent in subjects with idiopathic cardiomegaly of the dilated type and is virtually always present in patients with idiopathic hypertrophic subaortic stenosis.

INFILTRATIVE CARDIOMYOPATHIES

The infiltrative cardiomyopathies include various infiltrates into the walls of the cardiac chambers. The infiltrates may be localized to the myocardial interstitium (amyloid, granulomas, neoplasms, acid mucopolysaccharides), or they may be within myocardial cells (calcium, iron, glycogen, and lipids). Some infiltrates, such as calcium, may involve both interstitium and myocardial fibers.

Amyloid

We have studied at necropsy 18 patients with cardiac amyloidosis extensive enough to cause cardiac dysfunction during life (Fig. 29). Fifteen were described elsewhere.[20] The 18 patients ranged in age from 21 to 89 years (average, 59): 12 were men and six were women. Fifteen patients had congestive cardiac failure; in none was the failure lessened by the administration of digitalis. Conduction disturbances or arrhythmias developed in 11 patients—in 10 of them while they were receiving digitalis. All three patients without congestive cardiac failure had gastrointestinal disturbances and peripheral neuropathy. Congestive cardiac failure was the cause of death in 15 of the 18 patients. Although three had had a history of elevated blood pressure in the past, no patient had systemic hypertension during the last three months of life. Electrocardiograms disclosed low voltage (sum of the total R and S wave voltage in leads I, II, and III $\leq$ 1.5 millivolts) in 15 patients and patterns simulating old anterior (poor R wave progression in leads V_1-V_3) or posterior (Q wave in leads II, III, and aVF) myocardial infarction in 12 patients. Chest roentgenograms showed cardiomegaly in 15 patients. None, how-

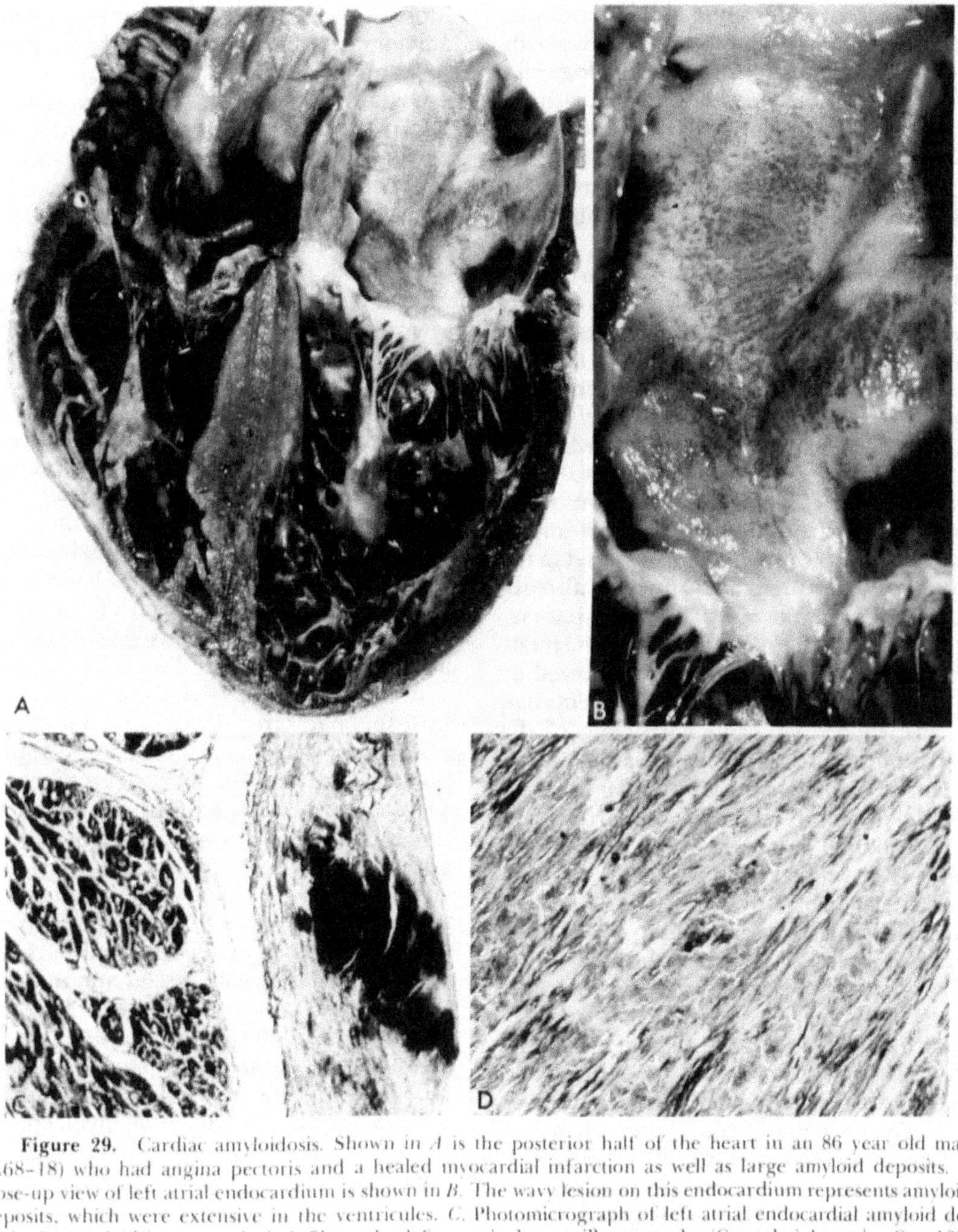

Figure 29. Cardiac amyloidosis. Shown in *A* is the posterior half of the heart in an 86 year old man (A68–18) who had angina pectoris and a healed myocardial infarction as well as large amyloid deposits. A close-up view of left atrial endocardium is shown in *B*. The wavy lesion on this endocardium represents amyloid deposits, which were extensive in the ventricules. *C*, Photomicrograph of left atrial endocardial amyloid deposit. *D*, Amyloid has extensively infiltrated a left ventricular papillary muscle. (Crystal violet stain. *C*, × 107. *D*, × 32.)

ever, had massive enlargement. Two patients had clinical and hemodynamic findings suggesting constrictive pericarditis and one underwent thoracotomy for planned pericardiectomy.

In 14 patients amyloidosis was not associated with another systemic disease (primary amyloidosis), and in four patients another systemic disease (multiple myeloma) was present (secondary amyloidosis). In 16 patients amyloid was present in many body orgăns (systemic amyloidosis) and in two patients amyloid was present only in the heart (isolated amyloidosis). In four patients more than one family member had amyloidosis (familial amyloidosis); each had peripheral neuropathy and three had vitreous opacities. The diagnosis of amyloidosis was established during life by biopsy in 13 of the 16 patients with systemic amyloidosis.

At necropsy the hearts weighed 370 to

700 gm. (average, 498). The ventricular myocardium in each patient was firm, rubbery, and noncompliant. Histologically, amyloid was present between many myocardial cells in each heart. Focal small deposits of amyloid, replacing areas of myocardium, also were found in most hearts. Both left ventricular papillary muscles in all 18 patients contained amyloid. The sinus node or atrioventricular bundle or both showed amyloid in five of eight patients in whom these tissues were examined. Tan, waxy appearing, focal deposits of amyloid were visible grossly in the endocardium of both the right and left atria of every patient and also in the ventricular endocardium in 12 patients. One or more cardiac valves in each patient contained amyloid, but in no patient did the deposits appear to impair valvular function. Amyloid occurred in the adventitia and media of intramural coronary arteries and veins in every patient, and in half of them the lumens of the intramural coronary vessels were narrowed by intimal amyloid deposits. Four patients had severe (> 75 per cent) narrowing of the extramural coronary arteries by old atherosclerotic plaques, but in none were intimal amyloid deposits found in these arteries. In two patients, however, small amyloid deposits were observed in the media of extramural coronary arteries. In Congo red preparations the amyloid deposits stained orange and showed green birefringence. The deposits were metachromatic when stained by crystal violet. By electron microscopy (one patient) the cardiac amyloid deposits consisted of nonbranching fibrils 80 to 130Å in diameter (average, 100).

The foregoing data and those of others indicate that amyloid in the heart must be extensive in order to produce cardiac dysfunction. The hearts that function improperly because of amyloid infiltration have firm, rubbery, noncompliant ventricular walls. Although the ventricular walls are firm, the ventricular cavities are usually not dilated.* The atria, however, usually are dilated, and the enlargement of the cardiac silhouette in this condition may well be related to the atrial dilatation rather than to the ventricular wall thickening. Most patients with symptomatic cardiac amyloidosis have congestive cardiac failure unresponsive to digitalis therapy, electrocardiographic low voltage, and conduction or rhythm disturbances. The latter are particularly common after digitalis administration, which may be contraindicated in this condition. A diagnosis of clinically significant cardiac amyloidosis should be questioned in the absence of congestive cardiac failure and electrocardiographic low voltage.

*Cardiac amyloidosis thus joins hypertrophic cardiomyopathy and constrictive pericarditis as a cause of congestive cardiac failure not associated with ventricular dilatation.

Granuloma (Giant Cell Myocarditis)

Granulomas with giant cells have been observed in the myocardium in a number of conditions (Table 2). We found giant cells in the myocardium at necropsy in 16 patients, excluding those with acute rheumatic fever (Table 3; Figs. 30 to 32). Four patients had sarcoidosis. Each of them had granulomas in other body organs as well as in the myocardium. Two other patients with numerous myocardial granulomas also probably had sarcoidosis, but other organs and tissues were not available for examination. In each of these six patients the granulomatous inflammation in the myocardium was widespread, always involving the entire thickness of the right and left ventricular walls at some sites (transmural; Figs. 30, 31). In one of the six patients the granulomas completely replaced both left ventricular papillary muscles and much of the free wall beneath them (Fig. 30). This patient presented shortly before death with mitral regurgitation from papillary muscle dysfunction.[16] Each of these six patients died as a result of myocardial involvement:

TABLE 2. Conditions Associated with Giant Cells in Myocardium

1. Infection
    A. Tuberculosis
    B. Parasites
    C. Fungi
    D. Spirochetes (syphilis)
2. Systemic noninfectious diseases
    A. Sarcoidosis
    B. Wegener's granulomatosis
    C. Panarteritis (pulseless disease)
3. Rheumatic heart disease or acute rheumatic fever
4. Rheumatoid arthritis
5. Coronary heart disease
6. Hypertensive heart disease
7. Thymoma or myasthenia gravis or myositis
8. Idiopathic

TABLE 3. Giant Cell Myocarditis: Data in 16 Necropsy Patients

Patient	Age (years)	Race	Sex	Associated disease	CHF	ECG	Mode of death	Myocardial giant cells (1+–4+)	Extracardiac giant cells
1	48	W	F	–	+	–	CHF Arrhythmia	++++	–
2				–	+	CHB	CHF	+++	–
3	40	W	F	Sarcoid	+	LVH	RF CHF	+++	+ (liver)
4	26	B	F	Sarcoid	+	CHB	Arrhythmia CHF	++++	+ (liver, L, LN)
5	44		F	Sarcoid	+	SB ↑ G-T	Arrhythmia****	++++	+ (liver, L, LN, spleen)
6	30	B	M	Sarcoid	0	RBBB	Arrhythmia****	+++	+ (liver, L, LN)
7	26	B	M	IE (active)	+	AMI	AMI 2° embolus	+***	0
8	17	W	F	IE (active)	+	RVH, RAD	CHF	+	0
9	42	W	M	IE (healed)	+	AF, LVH	CHF	+	0
10	10	W	F	IE (healed)*	+	–	CHF	++	+ (L)
11	65	W	F	RA	+	LBBB ↑ P-R	CHF	++	+ (L, SC)
12	73	B	M	RA	+	LAD	Sudden	++	+ (SC)
13	15	B	M	Panarteritis	0	PVC	Operation	+**	+ (arteries)
14	38	B	M	CAD	+	IVCD	CHF	+	+ (liver, L)
15	50	W	M	CAD	+	OMI	Operation	+	0
16	61	W	F	HCVD Cancer, uterus	0	LVH	Shock	+	0

Abbreviations:
+ = positive; 0 = negative; – = information not available; ↑ = increased; AF = atrial fibrillation; AMI = acute myocardial infarction; CAD = coronary heart disease; CHB = complete heart block; CHF = congestive heart failure; ECG = electrocardiogram; HCVD = hypertensive cardiovascular disease; IE = infective endocarditis; IVCD = intraventricular conduction defect; LAD = left axis deviation; LBBB = left bundle branch block; L = lung; LN = lymph nodes; OMI = old myocardial infarction; P-R = P-R interval; PVC = premature ventricular contractions; RA = rheumatoid arthritis; RAD = right axis deviation; RBBB = right bundle branch block; RF = renal failure; RVH = right ventricular hypertrophy; SB = sinus bradycardia; SC = subcutaneous tissue.

* = complex congenital malformation of heart and great vessels also.
** = giant cell arteritis also involved the coronary arteries but produced no significant obstruction.
*** = septic coronary embolus occluding left anterior descending artery.
**** = paroxysmal ventricular tachycardia several times in past.

all had either episodic arrhythmias, usually ventricular in origin, or severe congestive cardiac failure or both.

The numbers of multinucleated and mononucleated inflammatory cells in the myocardium in the other 10 patients was minimal compared to that observed in the six with definite or probable sardoidosis (Table 3). Four had infective endocarditis.[21–23] In these patients the granulomas may represent organization of septic coronary emboli. Two patients had rheumatoid arthritis with rheumatoid nodules (which contain giant cells) in the myocardium and endocardium.[24, 25] Another had giant cell arteritis of the aorta and its major branches, leading to absent pulses (pulseless disease).[26] Foci of granulomatous inflammation containing giant cells were present in the left ventricular wall. Their etiology is uncertain, but presumably the aortitis and the myocarditis have the same cause. The origin of the myocardial giant cells in the two patients with fatal coronary atherosclerosis and in the one patient with fatal hypertension also is uncertain. The giant cells in these three patients were located in areas of myocardial fibrosis.

It is evident from this and other reports that there are many causes of giant cell formation in the myocardium. Idiopathic giant cell myocarditis affects all ages without predilection for sex or race. Congestive cardiac failure, arrhythmias, and sudden death are common, and often the conducting as well as the working myocardium is extensively damaged. At the other end of the spectrum are patients who die from other conditions and at necropsy are found to have giant cells in the myocardium. The number of myocardial giant cells in the latter group of patients is usually small and of no functional significance. Patients with giant cells in the myocardium often also have giant cells in other organs or tissues.

It is difficult to distinguish idiopathic giant cell myocarditis with extracardiac involvement from sarcoidosis involving the heart and other organs. Although it rarely causes death, cardiac involvement occurs in about 20 per cent of the patients with sarcoidosis.[27] The noncaseating granulomas are usually located in the ventricular septa and free walls and occasionally in the pericardium. The myocardial granulomas may progress to fibrous scar formation without residual granulomatous inflammation, as in two other patients studied by us (Fig. 32). Degeneration of myocardial cells may occur also.[28] Arrhythmias, conduction disturbances, and sudden death occur. Probably some patients previously reported as having idiopathic giant cell myocarditis actually had sarcoidosis.

Giant cell myocarditis has a varied etiology and probably represents an unusual reaction of the myocardium to antigens or stimuli of varying types. Clinically the diagnosis of giant cell myocarditis cannot be established without myocardial biopsy and a negative biopsy report does not rule out this entity.

Neoplasm

Neoplastic disease of the heart has received through publications (many of which

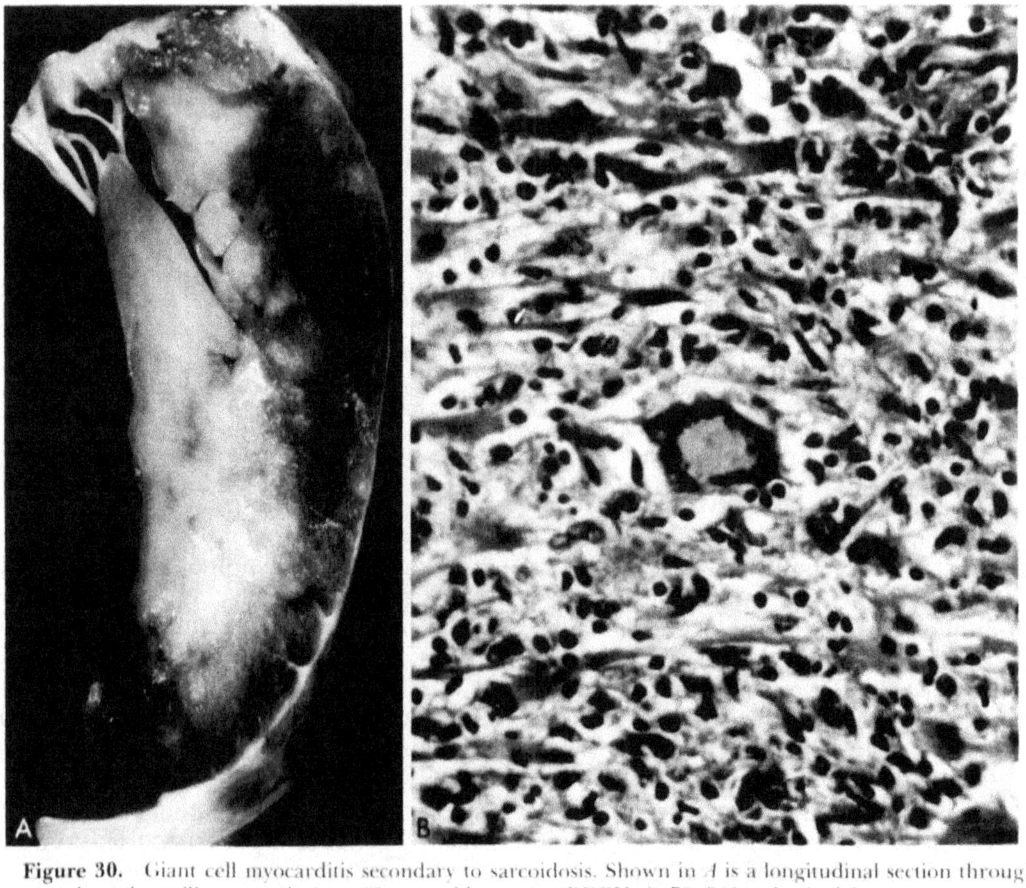

Figure 30. Giant cell myocarditis secondary to sarcoidosis. Shown in *A* is a longitudinal section through an anterolateral papillary muscle in a 26 year old woman (PGGH A–70–541) who had been asymptomatic until 10 days before death, when dyspnea appeared. The dyspnea rapidly worsened, and when hospitalized on the day of death she was in acute pulmonary edema. The blood pressure was 80/70 mm. Hg, the heart rate 160 beats per minute; a grade 3-4/6 pansystolic blowing murmur radiated to the axilla. Chest roentgenography showed congested lungs, cardiomegaly, and prominent hilar adenopathy. An electrocardiogram showed nonspecific ST-T wave changes and atrial hypertrophy. She developed complete heart block and died shortly thereafter. At necropsy large firm white deposits were present in the walls of all four cardiac chambers and completely replaced both left ventricular papillary muscles (*A*). On histologic section the firm white areas represented hard granulomas typical of sarcoidosis (*B*). Similar hard granulomas were present in lymph nodes, liver, spleen, and lung. Stains for acid-fast organisms; other bacteria, and fungi were negative. (*B*, Hematoxylin and eosin stain. × 400.)

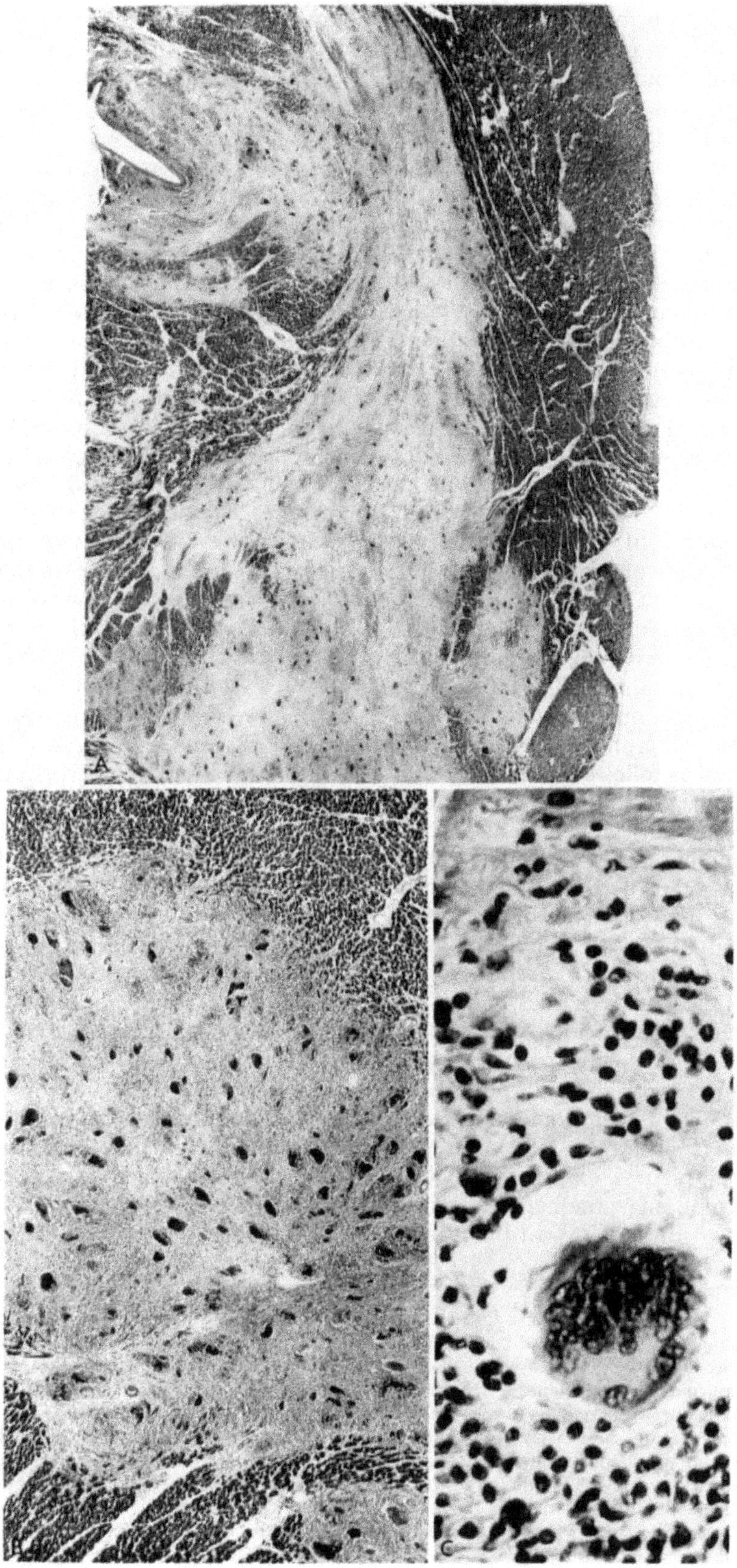

Figure 31.

are case reports) far more attention than it deserves. Most tumors in the heart represent metastases from primaries elsewhere, the most common being the lung and breast. The majority of secondary tumors invade only the epicardium (tumors limited to parietal pericardium should not be considered as involving the heart) and relatively few of them penetrate into the myocardium. Secondary tumors, which initially attach to the endocardium and then invade the myocardium, are far less frequent, although this pathway is the usual one for tumors originating in the kidney or adrenal gland. Primary tumors of the heart more often originate from the endocardium, the most frequent one being myxoma, which is benign. Primary malignant tumors of the heart are rare indeed and usually are sarcomas (Fig. 33).

One of us (WCR) has examined at necropsy the hearts of 686 patients who died of acute leukemia (420 patients),[29] or lymphoma (196 patients),[30] or malignant melanoma (70 patients).[31] Several observations that resulted from these studies may be summarized as follows. Although metastases to the heart in these three malignant disorders were relatively frequent (64 per cent in melanoma; 37 per cent in acute leukemia; 24 per cent in lymphoma), symptoms of cardiac dysfunction were infrequent. Indeed, in the case of leukemia and lymphoma, the frequency of dyspnea, chest pain, effusions into body cavities, precordial murmurs, ventricular gallops, edema, and electrocardiographic disturbances was similar in patients with and in those without cardiac leukemia or lymphoma, and these clinical findings most often were the result of mediastinal, pleural, or pulmonary leukemia or lymphoma, anemia, hypoalbuminemia, or an underlying cardiac condition. Electrocardiograms were abnormal in 61 per cent of 33 patients with cardiac lymphoma and in 62 per cent of 104 patients with lymphoma but without tumor nodules in the heart.

Controls of this type for patients with secondary cardiac neoplasms were not found in previous reports of cardiac metastases. Signs or symptoms of cardiac dysfunction could be attributed to lymphomatous involvement of the heart in only five of the 48 patients with cardiac lymphoma and in less than 20 of the 156 patients with cardiac leukemia cell infiltrates. Most patients with cardiac symptoms had extensive neoplastic involvement with hemorrhage in the pericardium or huge tumor deposits within a chamber or a cardiac wall. Most often, however, even huge tumor nodules in a cardiac chamber or wall were clinically silent. It is possible, however, that cardiac symptoms were masked or overshadowed by clinical manifestations of tumor deposits in other body organs or tissues.

The foregoing three reports are discussed because they were the first to our knowledge in which necropsy data were obtained by re-examination of the hearts, both grossly and histologically, by only one or two observers, rather than by accepting the information listed in the autopsy protocols. Moreover, the clinical data were obtained in patients with the same neoplasm but no cardiac metastases as well as in patients with cardiac metastases. These studies also demonstrated that many previously proposed criteria for clinically determining the presence of cardiac metastases were unreliable. In a patient with a malignant neoplasm and without previous cardiac disease, the following clinical findings strongly suggest the presence of cardiac metastases: acute pericarditis, cardiac tampon-

Figure 31. Giant cell myocarditis, idiopathic type, in a 49 year old obese Indian woman who had been well until two months before death, when syncope appeared. When she was hospitalized, an electrocardiogram disclosed complete heart block with a ventricular rate of 32 beats per minute. The blood pressure was 140/70 mm. Hg. No murmurs were audible. A chest radiograph showed moderate cardiomegaly. One month after the episode of syncope, acute pneumonia developed, followed shortly by evidence of congestive cardiac failure. Three days before death, substernal chest pain occurred and the electrocardiogram then showed changes consistent with acute myocardial infarction. Congestive heart failure persisted. Cardiac arrest followed a seizure. At necropsy the heart weighed 430 gm. Large white firm infiltrates were present in the cephalad portion of the muscular ventricular septum and in the anterolateral papillary muscle of the left ventricle. Histologic examination of the infiltrates disclosed them to be composed of fibrous tissue containing numerous giant cells and some mononuclear cells (*A* to *C*). Special strains for acid fast organisms, other bacteria, and fungi were negative. The heart was the only organ containing granulomas. *A*, Full thickness of ventricular septum showing the extensiveness of the infiltrates. *B* and *C*, Progressive higher power photomicrographs of the giant cell infiltrates. Some of the giant cells contained over 50 nuclei. (Hematoxylin and eosin stain. *A*, × 11. *B*, × 35. *C*, × 85.)

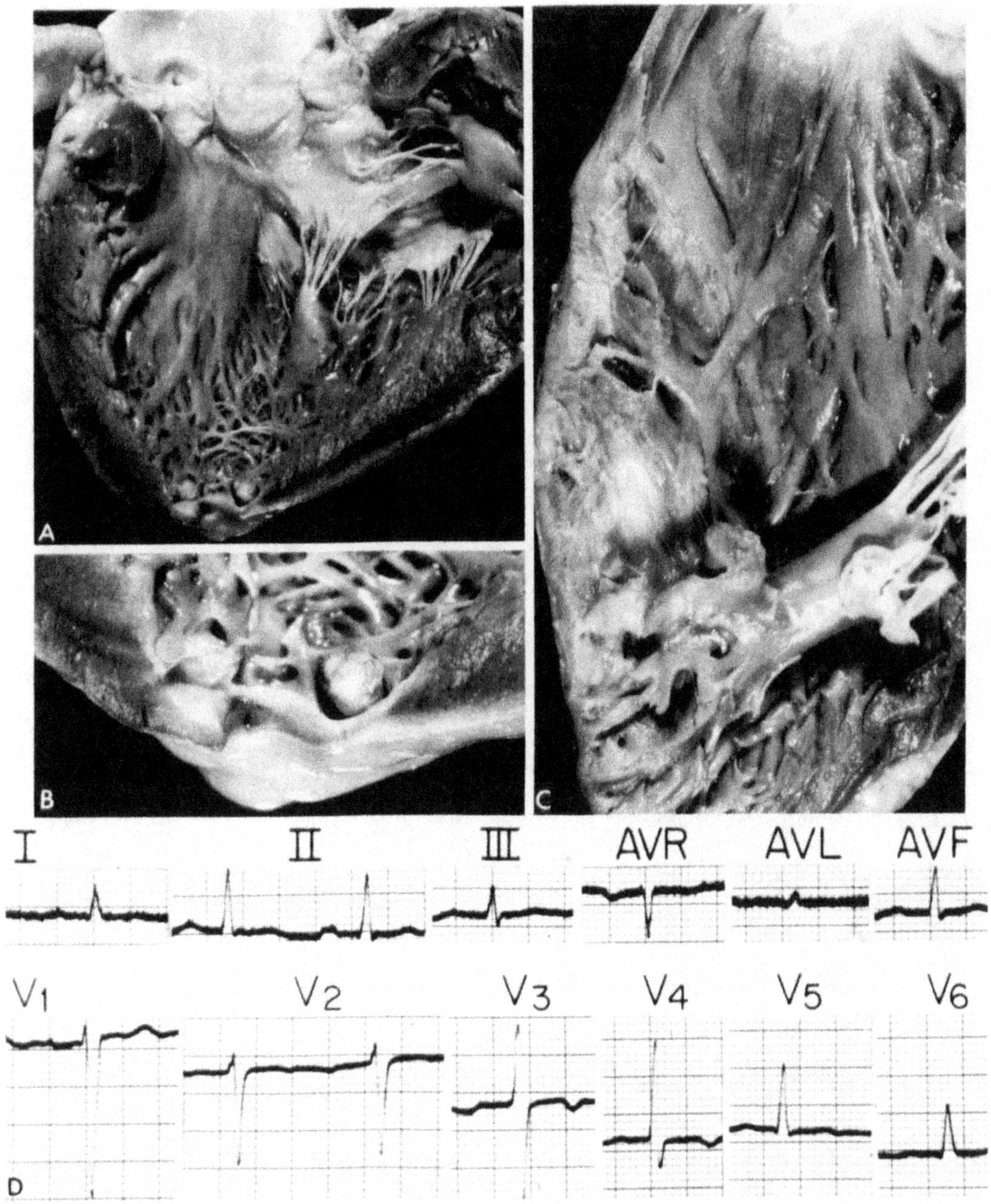

Figure 32. Sarcoid heart disease. This 34 year old man (A68–10) noted a swelling in his neck at age 29. Biopsy of the excised lump at age 30 disclosed that it consisted of lymph nodes infiltrated by hard granulomas. A diagnosis of sarcoidosis therefore was made. The liver was normal on biopsy at age 31. Chest radiography showed prominent bilateral hilar adenopathy, and prednisone therapy (10 to 20 mg. daily) was begun and continued thereafter until death. Five months later cryptococcal meningitis developed, but it was cured by amphoterin therapy. One year before death he developed marked hypercalcemia. About one month before death he developed a high degree of atrioventricular block, which at times progressed to complete heart block. He died of complications of peptic ulcer perforation. At necropsy the heart weighed 320 gm. Both ventricular cavities were mildly dilated. Mural thrombi were present at the apices of both ventricles. The apical left ventricular wall beneath the thrombi was fibrotic, a small area of scarring was present in the basal anterior left ventricular wall, and the anterior right ventricular wall was focally scarred. Histologic study of the scarred areas disclosed some mononuclear cells but no giant cells. The area of the atrioventricular node and bundle was serially sectioned: considerable scarring with some mononuclear cells was present in the conduction tissue, but the node and bundle and proximal bundle branches were not interrupted at any point. Although no granulomas were observed in this patient's heart, it is nevertheless highly likely that the myocardial scars were the result of "healed" sarcoid granulomas. The myocardial scarring, for example, was similar to that observed in the lymph nodes, and the coronary arteries were normal. The healing appears to have been the result of steroid therapy given for three years. *A*, Opened left ventricle. At the apex is a thrombus, better seen in *B*. The myocardium beneath the thrombus is scarred. *C*, Right ventricular wall showing severe focal scarring. The electrocardiogram was recorded three days before death.

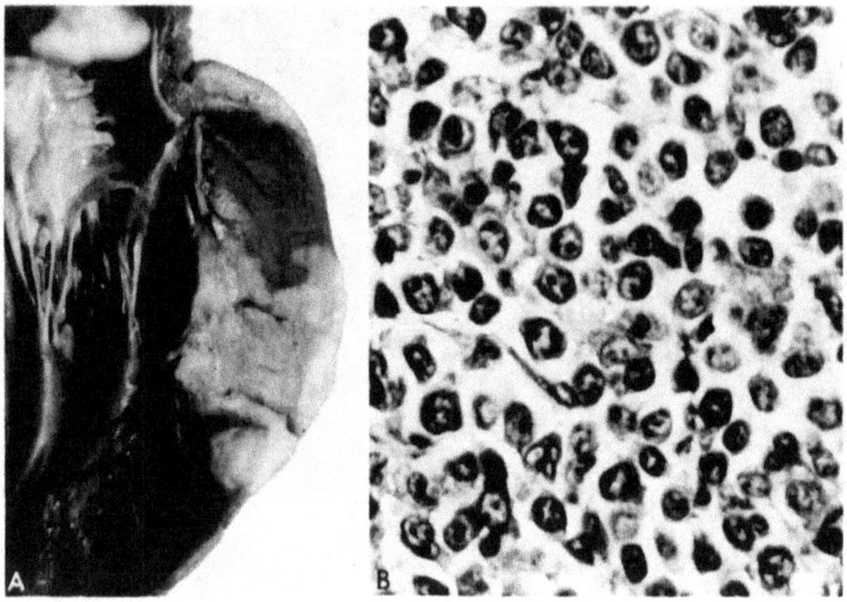

Figure 33. Secondary tumor (undifferentiated lymphoma) to heart in a 59 year old woman (A63–119) who had extensive deposits of tumor in the right atrium, left ventricle, and pericardium but no signs or symptoms of cardiac dysfunction. Tumor was present at necropsy in 16 organs and tissues. *A*, Longitudinal section of portions of left ventricular wall showing a through-and-through tumor deposit. *B*, Photomicrograph of an area of tumor nodule. (Hematoxylin and eosin stain, × 628.)

ade or constriction, rapid increase in the size of the cardiac silhouette by roentgenogram, onset of ectopic tachycardia, development of second or third degree atrioventricular block, and onset of unequivocal cardiac failure. Cytologic examination of the pericardial fluid and angiography obviously increase the ability to diagnose cardiac metastases.

Calcium

Calcium is most commonly observed in the heart in the coronary arteries, mitral anulus, aortic and scarred mitral valve cusps, large myocardial scars, and pericardium. In these circumstances the calcific deposits are extracellular. This discussion, however, concerns calcific deposits within individual myocardial fibers, also a frequent occurrence. Focal calcific deposits in myocardial cells are frequently observed in patients dying after periods of prolonged shock or in renal failure.[32] We have observed this lesion most frequently in patients dying soon after cardiac operations (Fig. 34).[33] Its cause is uncertain, although severe hypoxia is the most likely explanation and the lesion may be produced experimentally by this means.[34] High serum levels of calcium also may be a factor. The fibers infiltrated by calcium are always necrotic. Probably normal myocardial cells will not calcify. Thus, so-called metastatic calcification of the heart does not occur. Deposition of calcium salts into individual myocardial cells represents dystrophic calcification. When the lesions are extensive, it is probable that cardiac dysfunction may result. We have observed the heart of a patient who died with severe uremia in whom nearly every myocardial fiber was calcified. The myocardium felt like shark's skin. We also have observed huge deposits of calcium throughout the left ventricular wall in a 19 year old man from Uganda; the cause was unknown. Massive myocardial calcification has been reported by others.[35]

Iron

It is now clear that extensive iron deposits in myocardial cells cause cardiac dysfunction (Fig. 35). Buja and Roberts[36] studied 19 patients with cardiac iron deposits: the ventricular iron deposits were visible grossly in nine patients and by light

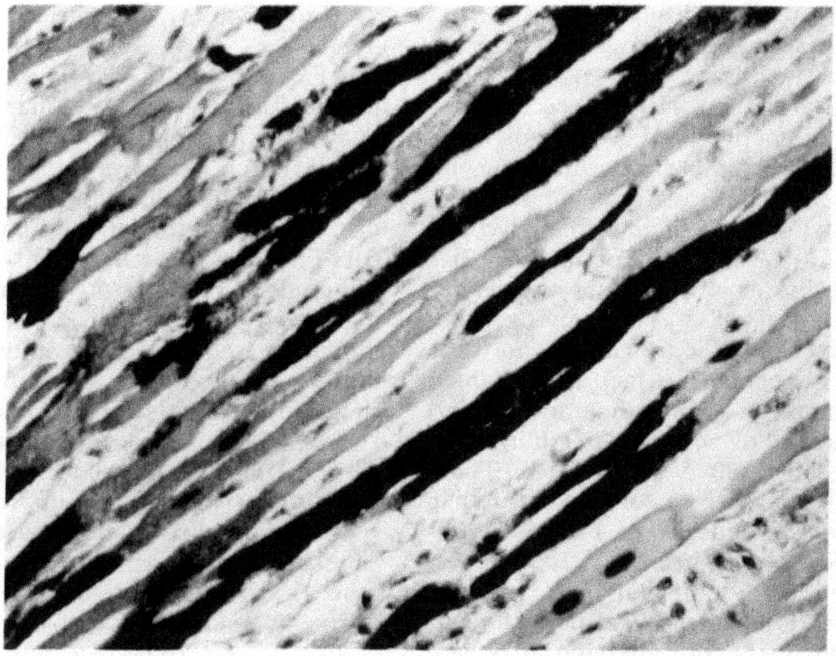

Figure 34. Myocardial fiber calcification in a 46 year old woman (A66–146) who died 20 days after replacement of stenotic mitral and incompetent tricuspid valves with prostheses. Postoperatively she had evidence of severely low cardiac output. Calcification of individual myocardial fibers was widespread at necropsy. The cause of this lesion is uncertain, but hypoxia probably plays a role in its formation. (Hematoxylin and eosin stain. ×200.)

microscopy only in the other 10. Each of the nine patients with grossly visible iron had clinical evidence of cardiac dysfunction (congestive cardiac failure in seven), whereas none of the 10 with only microscopically visible iron had cardiac dysfunction. All nine patients with grossly visible iron had abnormal electrocardiograms, mainly arrhythmias and conduction disturbances. Cardiac iron deposits were not distributed uniformly. The deposits were always most extensive in ventricular myocardium, less in atrial myocardium, the least in conducting as contrasted to working myocardium. The patients with supraventricular arrhythmias, however, had the largest atrial deposits of iron. Extensive cardiac iron deposits occurred not only in patients with idiopathic hemochromatosis but also in patients who received more than 100 units of whole blood (500 ml. per unit), unless bleeding diatheses coexisted, and in patients with chronic anemia and hepatic cirrhosis receiving less than 100 units of blood. The iron heart is not a strong heart but a weak one.

Glycogen

A deficiency of one or more of the enzymes involved in the biosynthesis and degradation of glycogen produces glycogen storage disease, of which at least eight types have been described.[37] Cardiac involvement occurs in types II, III, and IV. Most cases of glycogen storage disease causing cardiomegally belong to type II (Pompe's disease), caused by a deficiency of α-1,4-glucosidase, a lysosomal enzyme that hydrolyzes glycogen to glucose. The glycogen within the cardiac muscle cells is biochemically and morphologically normal (β particles, 250 to 400 Å in diameter), but is present in excessive amounts both within lysosomes and free in the cytoplasm.[38,39] As a result the heart enlarges, sometimes to a marked degree, and congestive cardiac failure supervenes. Survival rarely extends beyond infancy or early childhood.

Microscopically the muscle cells show a characteristic lacework pattern, with large clear central spaces (which represent the sites of glycogen deposition) and a peripheral rim of compressed cytoplasm. Endocardial fibroelastosis of at least the left ventricle usually is present also.[40] Although the deposits of glycogen usually involve all myocardial cells relatively uniformly, on occasion the fibers in the ventricular septum may contain disproportionately excessive quantities of glycogen and lead to subaortic stenosis.[41]

Myocardial involvement occurs to a variable extent in type II glycogenosis (glycogen debranching enzyme deficiency).[37] In type IV glycogenosis (branching enzyme deficiency) deposits of abnormal glycogen are found free in the cytoplasm of cardiac muscle cells, hepatocytes, and a variety of other types of cells.[42] These glycogen deposits are basophilic (in contrast to those in other glycogenoses, which are unstained in hematoxylin-eosin preparations) and are composed of nonbranching fibrils that measure 40 to 80 Å in diameter. These fibrils resemble those of the basophilic carbohydrate deposits in basophilic degeneration of the heart.[43,44] It has been suggested that congenital rhabdomyoma of the heart, in which the tumor cells contain large amounts of glycogen, may be a localized form of glycogen storage disease.[45] Small foci of basophilic degeneration of the heart are common findings at necropsy, particularly in the older age group. Extensive basophilic degeneration is found frequently in myxedema and occasionally in congestive and hypertrophic cardiomyopathy. Its functional significance is unknown.

In addition to the observations mentioned, glycogen deposits have been reported in cardiac muscle cells in idiopathic cardiomyopathy in infants[46] and in adults with beer drinker's cardiomyopathy[47] or in familial cardiomyopathy.[48] Except in the latter patients, the glycogen deposits were localized within myocardial cell mitochondria. Recently Buja et al.[49] showed that intramitochondrial glycogen deposits develop in canine myocardium as a delayed response to prolonged periods (30 to 45 minutes) of anoxic cardiac arrest. Furthermore, we have observed intramitochondrial glycogen in the myocardium of patients with Fallot's tetralogy. It would appear, therefore, that such deposits in cardiac muscle cells represent a type of response to injury rather than a specific type of cardiomyopathy.

Lipids and Mucopolysaccharides

Infiltration of the cytoplasm of cardiac muscle cells by lipid droplets (fatty degeneration) occurs as a nonspecific finding in a great variety of disorders, including hypoxia.

Fabry's disease (angiokeratoma corporis diffusum universale) may be singled out among the lipid storage diseases as the one in which extensive and clinically significant (cardiomegaly and congestive cardiac failure) accumulation of glycolipid occurs in cardiac muscle cells.[50] In this condition glycolipid deposits also are present in the endothelium and vascular smooth muscle as well as in most other tissues of the body. The disease results from a deficiency of ceramide trihexosidase, an enzyme that hydrolyzes ceramide trihexoside. This glycolipid accumulates in the form of birefringent granules composed of concentric or parallel lamellae spaced 40 to 65 Å apart. In ordinary histologic preparations the deposits are dissolved and the cardiac muscle cells resemble those in type II glycogenosis. In cardiac muscle cells of a patient with Hurler's disease we also observed small lipid deposits composed of parallel or concentric lamellae. The deposits, the composition of which is unknown, were extensive in the smooth muscle cells of coronary arteries also.

ENDOMYOCARDIAL DISEASE

A cardiomyopathy of unknown etiology characterized by severe focal endocardial fibrosis of one or both ventricles, with underlying subendocardial fibrosis and with or without associated eosinophilia is discussed under this heading. We have studied at necropsy eight patients with extensive ventricular endomyocardial fibrosis associated with severe blood eosinophilia (Figs. 36 to 39). Two of the eight patients were described earlier.[51,52] Five patients were diagnosed as having eosinophilic leukemia. One patient had a positive Philadelphia chromosome. We prefer to call this condition endomyocardial disease with eosinophilia. All eight patients were males, aged 13 to 52 years. Each had symptoms for 11 to 44 months (average, 29). The highest leukocyte counts ranged from 79,000 to 150,000 per cu. mm. and the highest percentage of eosinophils on differential smears of the peripheral blood ranged from 19 to 90 per cent. Although greatly increased in number, the eosinophils appeared structurally normal in each patient. Each patient had overt right and left sided congestive cardiac failure, which was the dominant clinical feature and usually the cause of death.

At necropsy the hearts weighed 420 to 530 gm. (average, 472). All four cardiac chambers were mildly dilated and the walls of all four chambers were mildly thickened. The endocardium in the left ventricular inflow tract and apex was markedly thickened by dense fibrous tissue in each patient, and this fibrosis, devoid of elastic fibrils, was overlain by fibrin-platelet-leukocyte-erythrocyte thrombi in all but one pa-

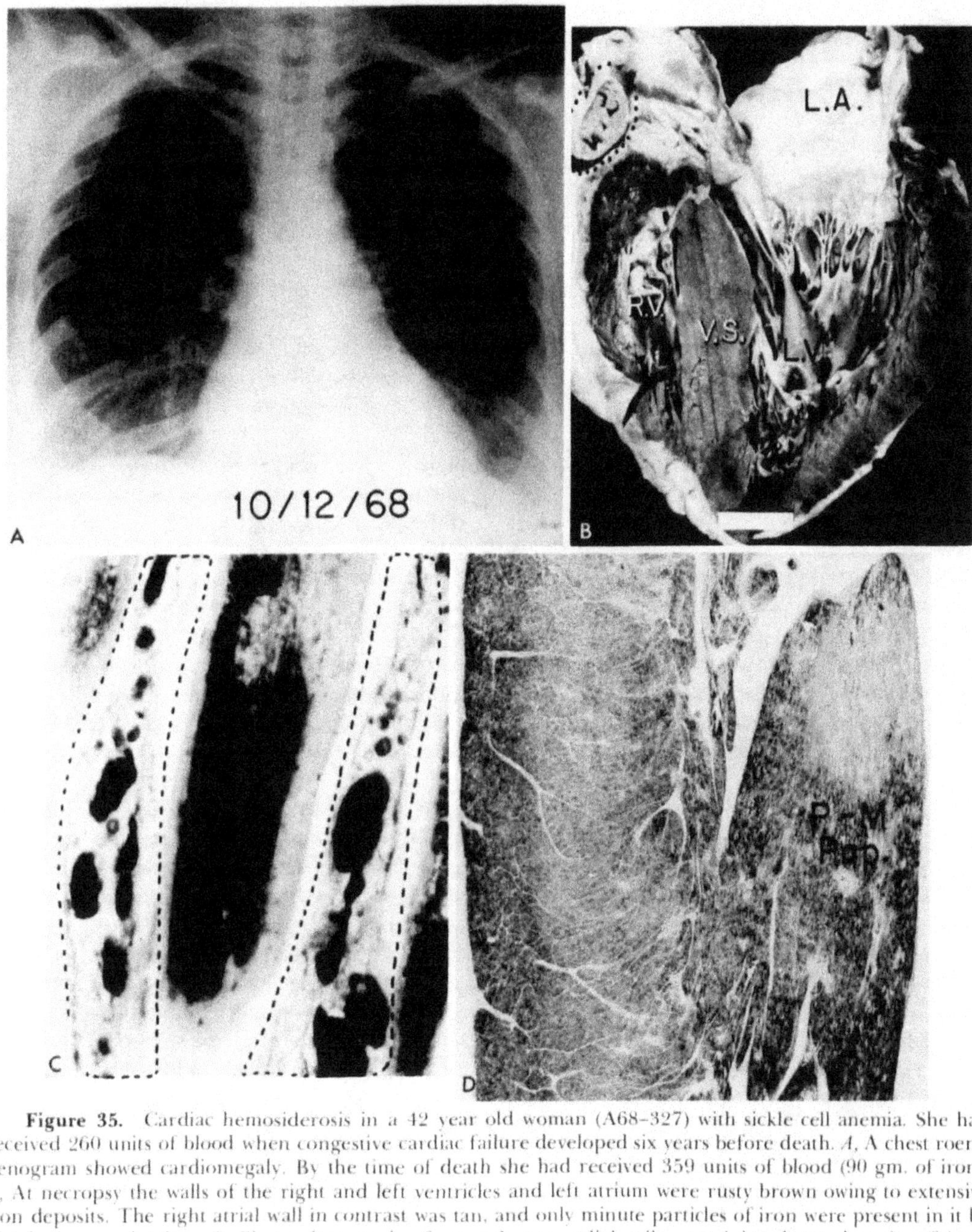

Figure 35. Cardiac hemosiderosis in a 42 year old woman (A68–327) with sickle cell anemia. She had received 260 units of blood when congestive cardiac failure developed six years before death. *A*, A chest roentgenogram showed cardiomegaly. By the time of death she had received 359 units of blood (90 gm. of iron). *B*, At necropsy the walls of the right and left ventricles and left atrium were rusty brown owing to extensive iron deposits. The right atrial wall in contrast was tan, and only minute particles of iron were present in it by histologic examination. *C*, Photomicrograph of several myocardial cells containing huge deposits of iron. Despite large deposits of iron in the working myocardium, no iron deposits were observed in the conducting myocardium. Longitudinal sections of left ventricular walls, including posteromedial (P-M) and anterolateral (A-L) papillary muscles, are shown in *D* and *E*, respectively. Foci of necrosis and fibrosis are present in each papillary muscle. These necrotic and fibrotic areas probably are anatomic indicators of chronic myocardial hypoxia, a result of the chronic anemia. (Prussian blue iron stains. *C*, × 628. *D*, × 3. *E*, × 2.)

tient. Right ventricular apical endocardial scars were present in all but one patient, and in two they extended cephalad toward the tricuspid valve in the inflow portion of this chamber. Mural thrombi overlay these right ventricular fibrous plaques in two patients. The left ventricular myocardium immediately beneath the fibrous plaques showed some degree of replacement and interstitial fibrosis in each patient, but in all the myocardial scarring was limited to the inner half of the wall (subendocardium). No right ventricular myocardial scarring was observed. Eosinophilic leukocytes, usually few in number, were found in sections of heart. In two patients several intramural coronary arteries were plugged by fibrin-platelet thrombi with resulting foci

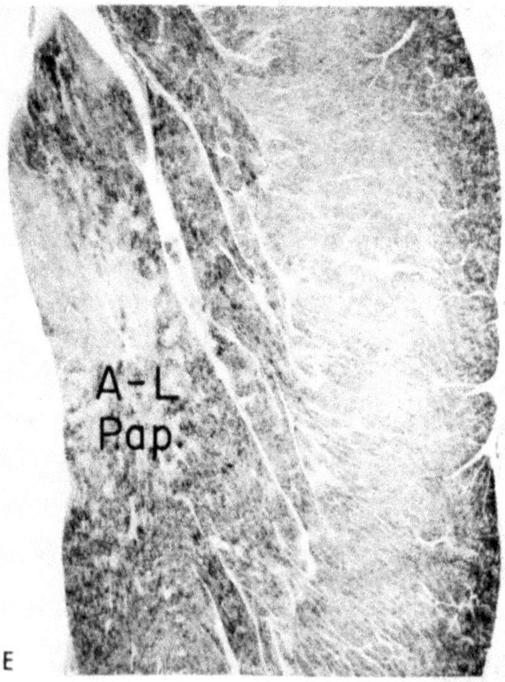

E

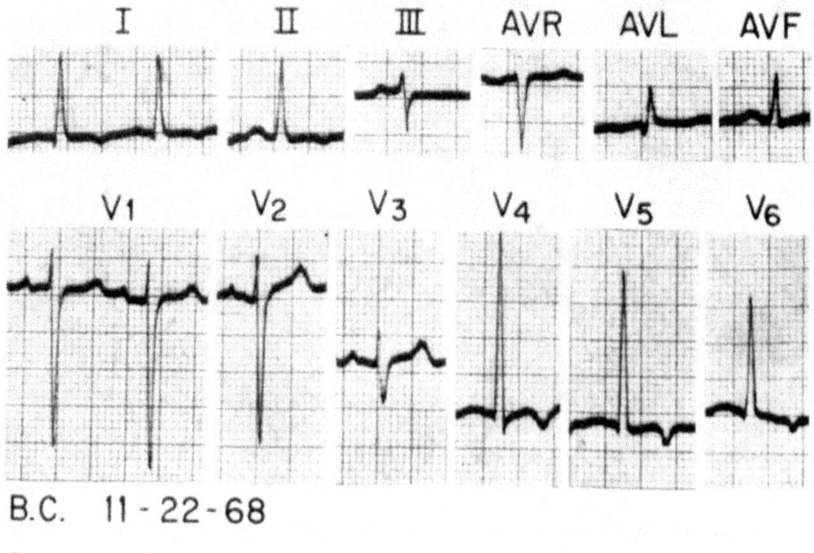

F

Figure 35. *Continued.*

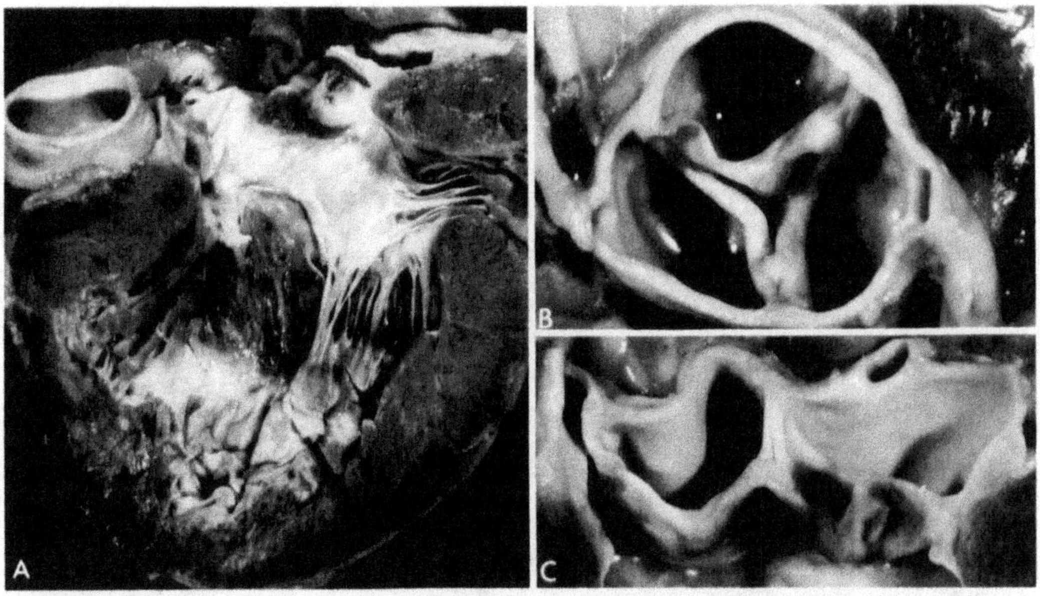

Figure 36. Endomyocardial disease and eosinophilia. Opened left ventricle in a 46 year old man (A71-250) who died after a complicated illness of 42 months. He had progressive congestive cardiac failure, leukocytosis (96,000 white blood cells per cu. mm.) with 90 per cent eosinophils on peripheral blood smear. He also had murmurs typical of aortic stenosis and regurgitation. At necropsy the heart weighed 520 gm., and large endocardial plaques were present in the apex of left ventricle (*A*) and small ones in apex of right ventricle. No intracardiac thrombi were present. *B*, Aortic valve from above, showing thickened cusps and fusion of two of the three commissures. *C*, Opened aortic valve showing fibrin material at the site of the fused commissure. The cause of the aortic valve disease is uncertain, but presumably it was caused by the same process affecting the mural endocardium in the apex of the left ventricle.

of myocardial necrosis. Except for one patient with extensive coronary arterial atherosclerosis, the extramural coronary vessels were normal. No patient had had clinical evidence of acute myocardial infarction, but one patient had had systemic hypertension at one time. The liver (1800 to 2800 gm. [average, 2200]) was enlarged in all eight patients but the lymph nodes were not prominent. Splenic weights, available in three patients (splenectomies elsewhere in two), were 480, 560, and 1500 gm. The weights were definitely larger than those in patients with idiopathic cardiomegaly of either the dilated or hypertrophic type. Several body organs, including lung, contained emboli with infarcts.

In addition to the eight American patients with endomyocardial disease and eosinophilia just described, one of us (WCR) has examined* the hearts of 24 patients who died in Kampala, Uganda, with endomyocardial fibrosis without significant eosinophilia. To our knowledge, none had peripheral blood eosinophilia (> 15 per cent). Their ages (known in 17 of the 24) ranged from three to 50 years (average, 27); three patients were over age 40 and six, under age 21 years. Of 16 patients in whom the sex was known, 11 were males and five were females. The duration of symptoms of cardiac dysfunction (known in 16 patients) ranged from two weeks to 24 months (average, seven months).

At necropsy the hearts were usually only mildly increased in weight, ranging from 370 to 500 gm. Endocardial plaquing (fibrous tissue devoid of elastic fibers) was present in the left ventricle in all 24 patients: in 14 it was severe, in five moderate, and in five minimal. Right ventricular endocardial plaquing was present in 18 and absent in six patients: in nine it was severe, in two moderate, and in seven minimal. Thus, endocardial fibrosis involved both ventricles in 18 (75 per cent) of the 24 patients. The endocardial fibrosis was located almost exclusively in the inflow tracts of the ventricles, and when the plaquing was severe it extended from the ventricular apices to beneath the posterior mitral or

*Through the courtesy of Doctors J. N. P. Davies and Monica Bishop at Albany, New York. Professor Davies, whose name should be attached to this entity,[53] brought these specimens to Albany when he moved there from Kampala, Uganda.

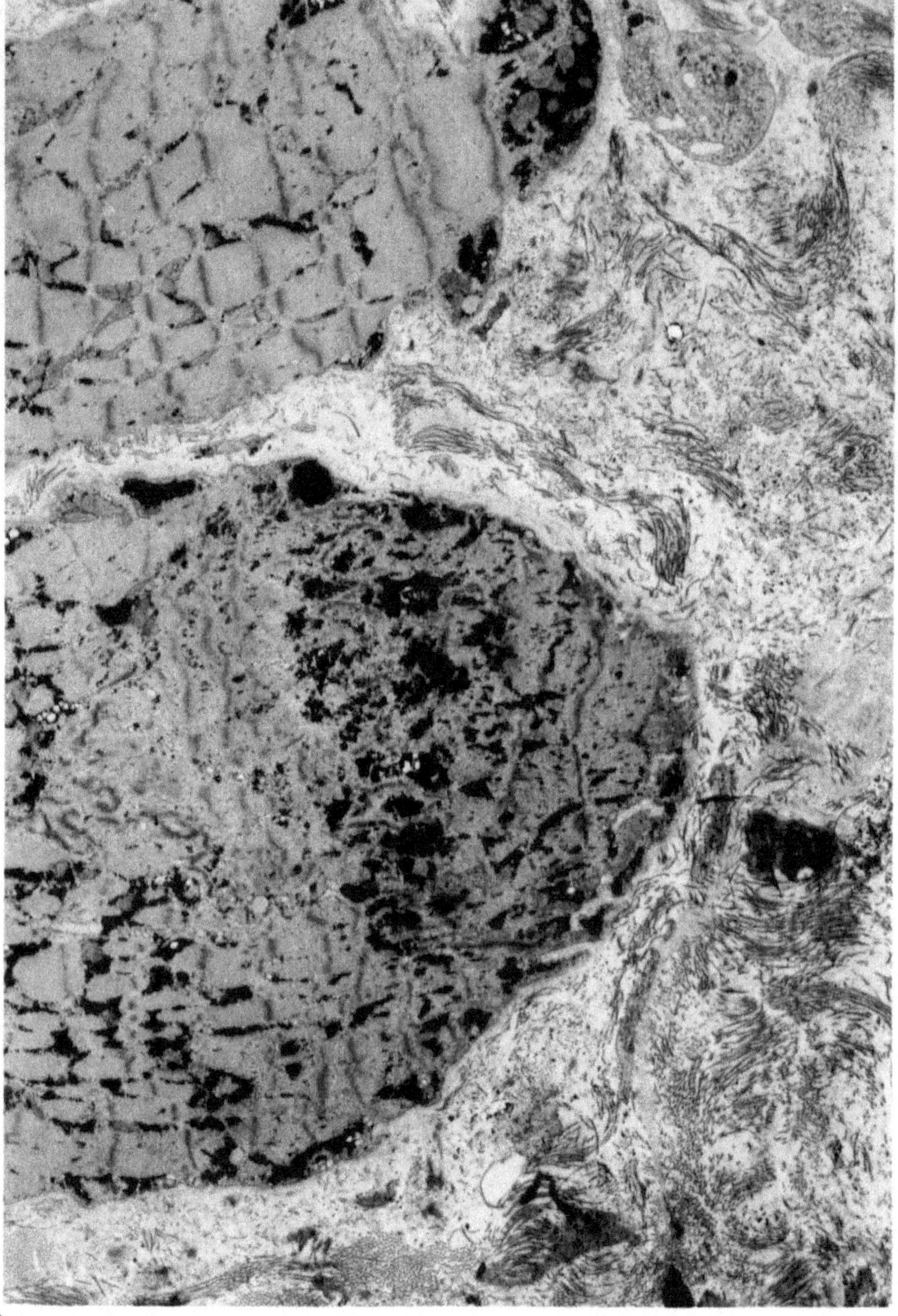

Figure 37. Muscle cells are surrounded by dense collagenous bundles in the right ventricular subendocardium of a man with eosinophilia and endomyocardial fibrosis. (× 5000.)

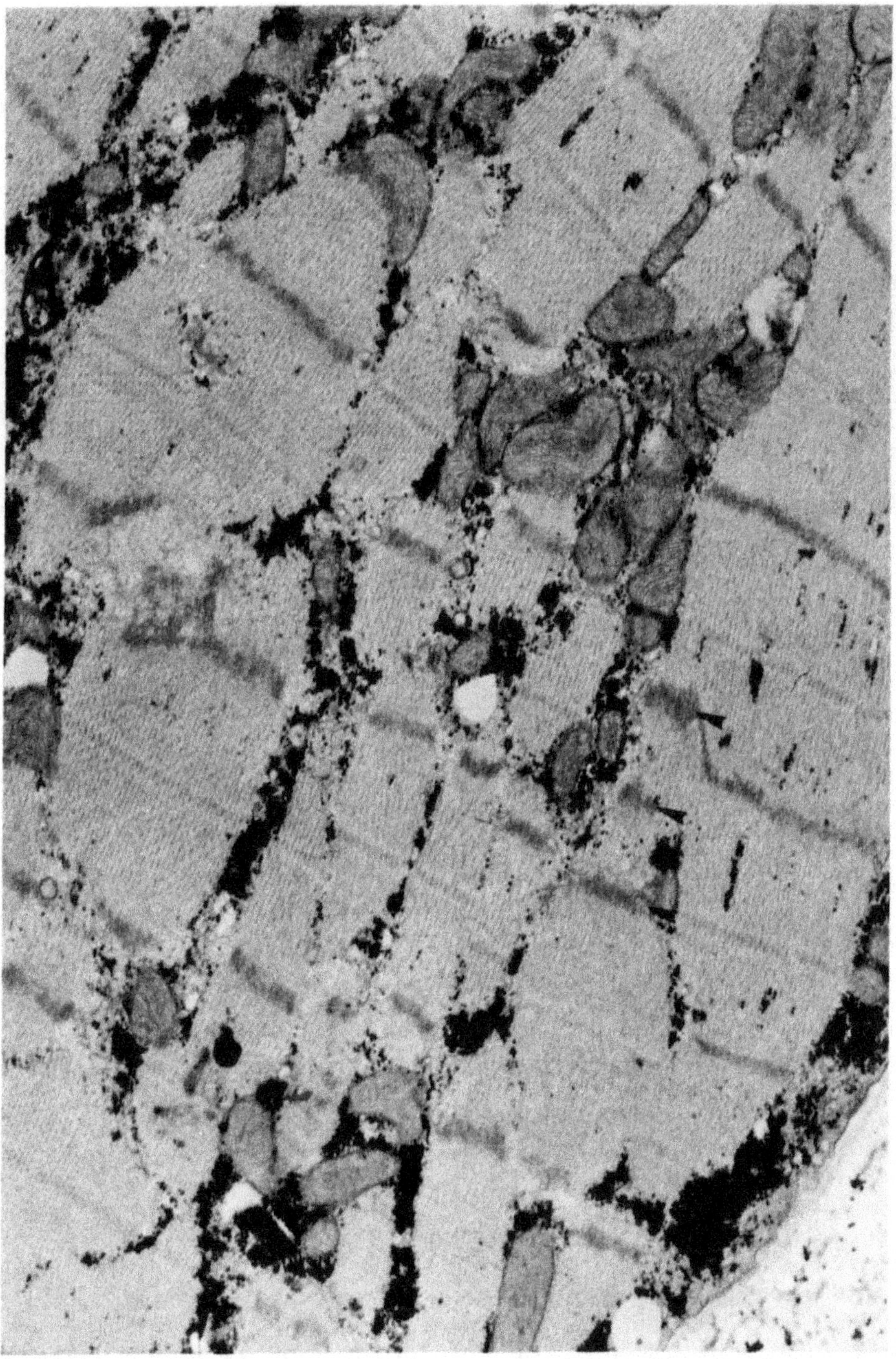

Figure 38. Myofibrils in cardiac muscle cell in a man with eosinophilia and endomyocardial fibrosis, showing loss of registration and focal widening of Z bands. Small sarcomeres (arrowheads) are considered to be in process of formation. (× 21,000.)

posterior and septal tricuspid valve leaflets. When the endocardial scars were mild, they were usually limited to the ventricular apices. The configuration of the heart (i.e., the size of the various cardiac chambers and of the pulmonary trunk) depended primarily on which ventricle contained the largest deposits of endocardial scar tissue or superimposed thrombi. When the amount of endocardial plaquing was severe in the left ventricle and absent, mild, or moderate in the right ventricle, the heart

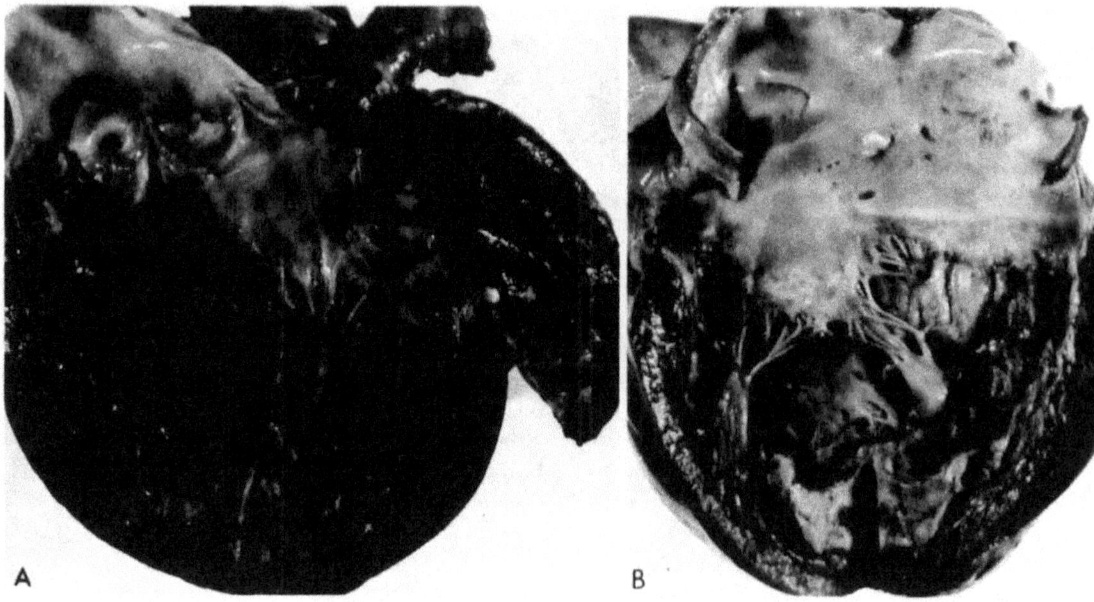

Figure 39. Davies' endomyocardial fibrosis in a Uganda native. *A*, Opened left ventricle, aortic valve, and aorta. *B*, Opened left atrium, mitral valve, and left ventricle. A large thrombus is present over the left ventricular apex, and the posterior mitral leaflet is adherent to the underlying mural endocardium. The process involves the endocardium of the entire inflow portion of the left ventricle. The presence of the large thrombus and the absence of dense endocardial fibrous tissue probably indicate that the process in this patient was of relatively recent onset. (The photographs were given to WCR by Dr. Gregory T. O'Connor, who spent two years in Kampala, Uganda.)

usually had the appearance of a mitral stenotic heart; i.e., the left atrium, pulmonary trunk, right ventricle and right atrium were dilated and the left ventricular cavity was small, being constricted by the extensive endocardial scarring. The left ventricle in this situation appears to be noncompliant and acts to some extent as an impediment to flow. The mitral lesion in this circumstance, however, is not stenotic unless another disease (e.g., rheumatic) coexists, but the mitral orifice in endomyocardial fibrosis is frequently made incompetent by the mural endocardial fibrosis, which adheres to the undersurface of the posterior mitral leaflet, causing the latter to be immobile. When the right ventricular endocardial scarring is more severe than that in the left ventricle, the right ventricle acts as an impediment to flow. The right atrium dilates, at times even to giant proportions as it did in one of the 24 patients; the right ventricle is usually constricted, and the left atrium and left ventricle remain more or less normal in size. This type of heart may be viewed as the tricuspid incompetent one. When the amount of endocardial plaquing is similar in both ventricles, each atrium becomes quite dilated and the ventricular cavities usually remain small or at least not dilated.

Although it is usually confined to the inflow tract, the ventricular endocardial plaquing in endomyocardial fibrosis on rare occasion may extend into the left ventricular outflow tract as it did in one of the 24 patients, and it also may be present in the atria. Also in one of the 24 patients both atria contained large endocardial plaques. Infective endocarditis appears to be a frequent complication in endomyocardial fibrosis. Three of the 24 patients had superimposed bacterial endocarditis of the mitral valve causing rupture of several chordae tendineae in each patient.

Comments on Endomyocardial Fibrosis with and without Eosinophilia. Löffler[54] in 1936 described two patients with "fibroplastic parietal endocarditis with blood eosinophilia." During his lifetime Löffler saw two patients with this condition, which bears his name. From 1936 to 1957, 24 other patients with this condition were reported,[51] and in the same year Bousser[55] summarized the clinical and pathologic findings in 13 patients with "eosinophilic leukemia" reported between 1944 and

1956. Since then many other patients with Löffler's "fibroplastic parietal endocarditis with blood eosinophilia" and "eosinophilic leukemia" have been described.[56] Each of these conditions is characterized by endocardial fibrosis of one or both ventricles and severe blood eosinophilia. Death is usually the result of congestive cardiac failure. From examination of previous reports and of our eight necropsy cases, it appears that the clinical and pathologic findings in patients with eosinophilic leukemia and Löffler's endocarditis are similar and that these two conditions are indeed the same disease. Whether this entity deserves to be called leukemia remains unclear. One of our eight patients had the Philadelphia (Ph 1) chromosome, a finding believed to be diagnostic of chronic granulocytic leukemia. Although greatly increased in number, the eosinophils in all eight patients appeared normal morphologically, an observation quite at variance with the usual concept of leukemia. The enlargement of the liver and spleen in these cases, however, is out of proportion to that found in most patients with congestive cardiac failure and tends to support the concept that this entity is in the leukemic category.

Certain similarities also exist between endomyocardial fibrosis of the African variety and endomyocardial fibrosis with eosinophilia, described by others as Löffler's endocarditis or eosinophilic leukemia. The mural endocardial thickening in the ventricles is seen in both conditions. Blood eosinophilia recently has been emphasized as a feature of endomyocardial fibrosis. Davies[57] in his initial report of 36 patients mentioned that "they sometimes show an eosinophilia for which none of the causes of eosinophilia account." Of 40 necropsy patients with endomyocardial fibrosis studied by Ive and associates,[58] 17 (43 per cent) had eosinophilia (absolute count > 1000 per cu. mm. or a differential count > 20 per cent of the total leukocyte count). Davies speculated that the earliest lesion in endomyocardial fibrosis is infiltration of the myocardium by round cells and eosinophils leading to necrosis of the endocardium and subendocardial myocardium. Thrombi form over the necrotic areas. As the mural thrombi and necrotic cardiac tissue become organized, the inflammatory cells disappear and only dense fibrous tissue remains.

In a recent study by Conner et al.[53] of the hearts of 16 patients dead from endomyocardial fibrosis, excessive amounts of acid mucopolysaccharide were found in the endocardium and inner myocardium, and these authors suggested that this was "a fundamental and possibly unique change" in endomyocardial fibrosis. These authors did not mention eosinophilic cell infiltration in endomyocardial fibrosis, but indeed these cells may be absent or rare in cases of Löffler's endocarditis or eosinophilic leukemia.[51, 52, 54]

It appears that some patients with endomyocardial fibrosis may have eosinophilia and that others may not. Löffler, in his initial report, emphasized that eosinophilia is inconstant and may disappear. It is possible that the presence or absence of eosinophilia is dependent on the length of the illness.

The possibility that Löffler's fibroplastic parietal endocarditis, eosinophilic leukemia (without abnormal myelopoiesis), and endomyocardial fibrosis of Davies are the same disease at different states of development is an attractive hypothesis. Patients with eosinophilia associated with a transient benign febrile illness, such as tropical eosinophilia or Löffler's pneumonia, may represent one end of the spectrum. Patients with severe endomyocardial fibrosis and no blood eosinophilia may represent the other end. Between these two extremes there may be patients who still have eosinophilia but less extensive endocardial scarring. The latter process is still active and thus eosinophilia is still present, but as the inflammatory process dies down, cardiac scar tissue remains and eosinophilia disappears.

REFERENCES

1. Ali, N., Ferrans, V. J., Roberts, W. C., and Massumi, R. A.: Clinical evaluation of transvenous catheter technique for endomyocardial biopsy. Chest, *63*:399–402, 1973.
2. Ferrans, V. J., Massumi, R. A., Shugoll, G. I., Ali, N., and Roberts, W. C.: Ultrastructural studies of myocardial biopsies in 45 patients with obstructive or congestive cardiomyopathy. *In* Bajusz, E., et al. (Editors): Recent Advances in Studies on Cardiac Structure and Metabolism: Cardiomyopathies. Baltimore, University Park Press, 1973, Vol. 2, pp. 231–272.
3. Falcone, M. E., and Roberts, W. C.: Atresia of the right atrium ostium of the coronary sinus unas-

sociated with persistence of the left superior vena cava: a clinicopathologic study of four adult patients. Am. Heart J., *83*:604–611, 1972.
4. Walsh, J. J., Burch, G. E., Black, W. C., Ferrans, V. J., and Hibbs, R. G.: Idiopathic myocardiopathy of the puerperium (post-partal heart disease). Circulation, *32*:19–31, 1965.
5. Demakis, J. G., and Rahimtoola, S. H.: Peripartum cardiomyopathy. Circulation, *44*:964–968, 1971.
6. Hibbs, R. G., Ferrans, V. J., Black, W. C., Weilbaecher, D. G., Walsh, J. J., and Burch, G. E.: Alcoholic cardiomyopathy: an electron microscopic study. Am. Heart J., *69*:766–779, 1965.
7. Bulloch, R. T., Pearce, M. B., Murphy, M. L., Jenkins, B. J., and Davis, J. L.: Myocardial lesions in idiopathic and alcoholic cardiomyopathy. Study by ventricular septal biopsy. Am. J. Cardiol., *29*:15–25, 1972.
8. Morrow, A. G., Roberts, W. C., Ross, J., Jr., Fisher, R. D., Behrendt, D. M., Mason, D. T., and Braunwald, E.: Obstruction to left ventricular outflow. Current concepts of management and operative treatment. Ann. Intern. Med., *69*:1255–1286, 1968.
9. Ewy, G. A., Marcus, F. I., Bohajalian, O., Burke, H. L., and Roberts, W. C.: Muscular subaortic stenosis. Clinical and pathologic observations in an elderly patient. Am. J. Cardiol., *22*:126–132, 1968.
10. Roberts, W. C.: Valvular, subvalvular, and supravalvular aortic stenosis: morphologic features. Cardiovas. Clin., *4*:98–126, 1973.
11. Roberts, W. C., Dangel, J. C., and Bulkley, B. H.: Nonrheumatic valvular cardiac disease: a clinicopathologic survey of 26 different conditions causing valvular dysfunction. Cardiovas. Clin., *5*:333–446, 1973.
12. Morrow, A. G., Fisher, R. D., and Fogarty, T. J.: Isolated hypertrophic obstruction to right ventricular outflow. Clinical, hemodynamic, and angiographic findings before and after operative treatment. Am. Heart J., 77:814–817, 1969.
13. Ferrans, V. J., Morrow, A. G., and Roberts, W. C.: Myocardial ultrastructure in idiopathic hypertrophic subaortic stenosis. A study of operatively excised left ventricular outflow tract muscle in 14 patients. Circulation, *45*:769–792, 1972.
14. Abbasi, A. S., MacAlpin, R. N., Eber, L. M., and Pearce, M. L.: Echocardiographic diagnosis of idiopathic hypertrophic cardiomyopathy without outflow obstruction. Circulation, *46*:897–904, 1972.
15. Henry, W. L., Clark, C. E., and Epstein, S. E.: Asymmetric septal hypertrophy. Echocardiographic identification of the pathognomonic anatomic abnormality of IHSS. Circulation, *47*:225–233, 1973.
16. Roberts, W. C., and Cohen, L. S.: Left ventricular papillary muscles. Description of the normal and a survey of conditions causing them to be abnormal. Circulation, *46*:138–154, 1972.
17. Perloff, J. K., and Roberts, W. C.: The mitral apparatus. Functional anatomy of mitral regurgitation. Circulation, *46*:227–239, 1972.
18. Cooley, D. A., Leachman, R. D., and Wukasch, D. C.: Diffuse muscular subaortic stenosis: surgical treatment. Am. J. Cardiol., *31*:1–6, 1973.
19. Roberts, W. C.: Operative treatment of hypertrophic obstructive cardiomyopathy. The case against mitral valve replacement. Am. J. Cardiol., *32*:377–381, 1973.
20. Buja, L. M., Khoi, N. B., and Roberts, W. C.: Clinically significant cardiac amyloidosis. Clinicopathologic findings in 15 patients. Am. J. Cardiol., *26*:394–405, 1970.
21. Buchbinder, N. A., and Roberts, W. C.: Active infective endocarditis confined to mural endocardium. A study of necropsy patients. Arch. Path., *93*:435–440, 1972.
22. Roberts, W. C., and Buchbinder, N. A.: Right-sided valvular infective endocarditis. A clinicopathologic study of twelve necropsy patients. Am. J. Med., *53*:7–19, 1972.
23. Buchbinder, N. A., and Roberts, W. C.: Left-sided valvular active infective endocarditis. A study of forty-five necropsy patients. Am. J. Med., *53*:20–35, 1972.
24. Carpenter, D. F., Golden, A., and Roberts, W. C.: Quadrivalvular rheumatoid heart disease associated with left bundle branch block. Am. J. Med., *43*:922–929, 1967.
25. Roberts, W. C., Kehoe, J. A., Carpenter, D. F., and Golden, A.: Cardiac valvular lesions in rheumatoid arthritis. Arch. Intern. Med., *122*:141–146, 1968.
26. Roberts, W. C., and Eibin, E. A.: Idiopathic panaortitis, supra-aortic arteritis, granulomatous myocarditis and pericarditis. A cause of pulseless disease and possibly left ventricular aneurysm in the African. Am. J. Med., *41*:453–461, 1966.
27. Ghosh, P., Fleming, H. A., Gresham, G. A., and Stovin, P. G. I.: Myocardial sarcoidosis. Brit. Heart J., *34*:769–773, 1972.
28. Ferrans, V. J., Hibbs, R. G., Black, W. C., Walsh, J. J., and Burch, G. E.: Myocardial degeneration in cardiac sarcoidosis: histochemical and electron microscopic studies. Am. Heart J., *69*:159–172, 1965.
29. Roberts, W. C., Bodey, G. P., and Wertlake, P. T.: The heart in acute leukemia. A study of 420 autopsy cases. Am. J. Cardiol., *21*:388–412, 1968.
30. Roberts, W. C., Glancy, D. L., and Devita, V. T., Jr.: Heart in malignant lymphoma (Hodgkin's disease, lymphosarcoma, reticulum cell sarcoma and mycosis fungoides). A study of 196 autopsy cases. Am. J. Cardiol., *22*:85–107, 1968.
31. Glancy, D. L., and Roberts, W. C.: The heart in malignant melanoma. A study of 70 autopsy cases. Am. J. Cardiol., *21*:555–571, 1968.
32. Terman, D. S., Alfrey, A. C., Hammond, W. S., Donndelinger, T., Ogden, D. A., and Holmes, J. H.: Cardiac calcification in uremia. A clinical, biochemical and pathologic study. Am. J. Med., *50*:744–755, 1971.
33. Roberts, W. C., and Morrow, A. G.: Causes of early postoperative death following cardiac valve replacement. Clinico-pathologic correlations in 64 patients studied at necropsy. J. Thorac. Cardiovasc. Surg., *54*:422–437, 1967.
34. Buja, L. M., Levitsky, S., Ferrans, V. J., Souther,

S. G., Roberts, W. C., and Morrow, A. G.: Acute and chronic effects of normothermic anoxia on canine hearts. Light and electron microscopic evaluation. Suppl. to Circulation *43* & *44*:I-44-I-50, 1971.

35. Testelli, M. R., and Pilz, C. G.: Massive calcification of the myocardium. A report of two cases, one associated with nephrocalcinosis. Am. J. Cardiol., *14*:407–414, 1964.
36. Buja, L. M., and Roberts, W. C.: Iron in the heart. Etiology and clinical significance. Am. J. Med., *51*:209–221, 1971,
37. Howell, R. R.: The glycogen storage diseases. *In* Stanbury, J. B., Wyngaarden, J. B., and Fredrickson, D. S. (Editors): The Metabolic Basis of Inherited Disease. Ed. 3. New York, McGraw-Hill Book Company, 1972, pp. 149–173.
38. Garancis, J. C.: Type II glycogenosis. Biochemical and electron microscopic study. Am. J. Med., *44*:289–300, 1968.
39. Bordiuk, J. M., Legato, M. J., Lovelace, R. E., and Blumenthal, S.: Pompe's disease. Electronmyographic, electron microscopic, and cardiovascular aspects. Arch. Neurol., *23*:113–119, 1970.
40. Ruttenbert, H. D., Steidl, R. M., Carey, L. S., and Edwards, J. E.: Glycogen-storage disease of the heart. Hemodynamic and angiocardiographic features in 2 cases. Am. Heart J., *67*:469–480, 1964.
41. Ehlers, K. H., Hagstron, J. W. C., Lukas, D. S., Redo, S. F., and Engle, M. A.: Glycogen-storage disease of the myocardium with obstruction to left ventricular outflow. Circulation, *25*:96–109, 1962.
42. Reed, G. B., Dixon, J. F. T., Neustein, H. B., Donnell, G. N., and Landing, B. H.: Type IV glycogenosis. Patient with absence of a branching enzyme α-1, 4-glucan; α-1, 4-glucan 6-glycosyl transferase. Lab. Invest., *19*:546–557, 1968.
43. Rosai, J., and Lascano, E. F.: Basophilic (mucoid) degeneration of myocardium. A disorder of glycogen metabolism. Am. J. Path., *61*:99–116, 1970.
44. Kosek, J. C., and Angell, W.: Fine structure of basophilic myocardial degeneration (BMD). Arch. Path., *89*:491–499, 1970.
45. Hudson, R. E. B.: Cardiovascular Pathology. Baltimore, The Williams & Wilkins Co., 1965, pp. 1581–1586.
46. Auger, C., and Chenard, J.: Quebec beer-drinkers' cardiomyopathy; ultrastructural changes in one case. Can. Med. Assoc. J., *97*:916–921, 1967.
47. Alexander, C. S.: Cobalt-beer cardiomyopathy. A clinical and pathologic study of twenty-eight cases. Am. J. Med., *53*:395–417, 1972.
48. Battersby, E. J., and Glenner, G. G.: Familial cardiomyopathy. Am. J. Med., *30*:382–391, 1961.
49. Buja, L. M., Ferrans, V. J., and Levitsky, S.: Occurrence of intramitochondrial glycogen in canine myocardium after prolonged anoxic cardiac arrest. J. Molec. Cell. Cardiol., *4*:237–254, 1972.
50. Ferrans, V. J., Hibbs, R. G., and Burda, C. D.: A histochemical and electron microscopic study of the heart in Fabry's disease. Am. J. Cardiol., *24*:95–110, 1969.
51. Roberts, W. C., Liegler, D. G., and Carbone, P. P.: Endomyocardial disease and eosinophilia. A clinical and pathologic spectrum. Am. J. Med., *46*:28–42, 1969.
52. Roberts, W. C., Buja, L. M., and Ferrans, V. J.: Löffler's fibroplastic parietal endocarditis, eosinophilic leukemia, and Davies' endomyocardial fibrosis: the same disease at different stages? Path. Microbiol., *35*:90–95, 1970.
53. Conner, D. H., Somers, K., Hutt, M. S. R., Manion, W. C., and D'Arbela, P. G.: Endomyocardial fibrosis in Uganda (Davies' disease). An epidemiologic, clinical, and pathologic study. Am. Heart J., *74*:687–709, 1967; *75*:107–124, 1968.
54. Löffler, W.: Endocarditis parietalis fibroplastica . mit Bluteosinophile. Schweiz. Med. Wschr., *66*: 817–820, 1936.
55. Bousser, J.: Eosinophilie et leucémie. Sang, *28*: 553–580, 1957.
56. Odeberg, B.: Eosinophilic leukemia and disseminated eosinophilic collagen disease—a disease entity. Acta Med. Scand., *177*:129–144, 1965.
57. Davies, J. N. P.: Endocardial fibrosis in Africans. East Afr. Med. J., *25*:10–14, 1948.
58. Ive, F. A., Willis, A. J. P., Ikeme, A. C., and Brockington, I. F.: Endomyocardial fibrosis and filariasis. Quart. J. Med., *36*:495–516, 1967.

Section of Pathology
National Heart and Lung Institute
Building 10A, Room 3E-30
National Institutes of Health
Bethesda, Maryland 20014 (Dr. Roberts)

Massive myocardial hemosiderosis: A structure-function conference at the National Heart and Lung Institute

Ernest N. Arnett, M.D.
Arthur W. Nienhuis, M.D.
Walter L. Henry, M.D.
Victor J. Ferrans, M.D., Ph.D.
David R. Redwood, M.D.
William C. Roberts, M.D.
Bethesda, Md.

Dr. William C. Roberts: In this conference a patient with massive myocardial iron deposition will be described and discussed. Dr. Arnett will present the patient's story.

Dr. Ernest N. Arnett: This 23-year-old black man was found to have *Blackfan-Diamond anemia* at 2 weeks of age, and he was tranfusion-dependent thereafter. At *age 10 years,* he received his first course of chelation therapy. At *age 12,* hypocalcemia was noted for the first time, and a diagnosis of *hypoparathyroidism* was made. At *age 15,* he received chelation therapy for 8 months with removal of approximately 8 Gm. of iron. By age 21, he was requiring 5 units (250 ml.) of packed erythrocytes every 3 weeks. Splenectomy during that year reduced the transfusion requirement to 2 units every 3 weeks.

At *age 22 years,* he was first admitted to NIH for chelation therapy. He had mild exertional dyspnea and easy fatigability when his blood hematocrit was in the low 20 per cent range. He had no orthopnea, nocturnal dyspnea, edema, or palpitations, and had never received digitalis or diuretics. It was estimated that he had received 500 units of packed erythrocyte transfusions, equivalent to 125 Gm. of iron, during his lifetime. The blood pressure was 90/60 mm. Hg. His neck was short. Both eyelids drooped. The cardiac apical impulse was normally located. The cardiac sounds were normal, and no precordial murmur was heard. The liver was firm. There was scant axillary and pubic hair and no subcutaneous edema. The hematocrit was 22 per cent, hemoglobin 7.7 Gm. per 100 ml., white blood cell count 10,800 per cubic millimeter with normal differential, reticulocyte count 0, serum iron 188 μg per 100 ml., and total iron-binding capacity 200 μg per 100 ml. (94 per cent saturation). The electrocardiogram (ECG) (Fig. 1) showed sinus rhythm, prolonged P-R interval, increased QRS voltage, and ST-T abnormalities. Chest roentgenograms (Fig. 2) disclosed a globular-shaped heart, prominent pulmonary vasculature, and diffuse reticulonodular pulmonary infiltrates. He remained in hospital for 5 months, during which time he received many transfusions and chelation therapy. Desferal (kindly supplied by Dr. John Zacchio of Ciba-Geigy Co.) was administered as part of a metabolic balance study.

Three weeks after discharge he noted mild exertional dyspnea and re-examination disclosed a Grade 3/6 systolic ejection-type mumur at the lower left sternal border, and pedal edema. An S_3 was now audible. The hematocrit was 19 per cent and with three transfusions rose to 29 per cent.

Following an episode of loss of consciousness at home, he was readmitted to NIH a month later. The hematocrit then was 17 per cent and an ECG showed multifocal premature ventricular beats, prolonged P-R interval, and nonspecific ST-T wave changes. The premature beats appeared to decrease after three transfusions. While sitting,

From the Section of Pathology, Molecular Hematology and Cardiology Branches, National Heart & Lung Institute, National Institutes of Health, Bethesda, Md. 20014.

Received for publication April 8, 1975.

Reprint requests: William C. Roberts, Bldg. 10A, Rm. 3E30, NIH, Bethesda, Md. 20014.

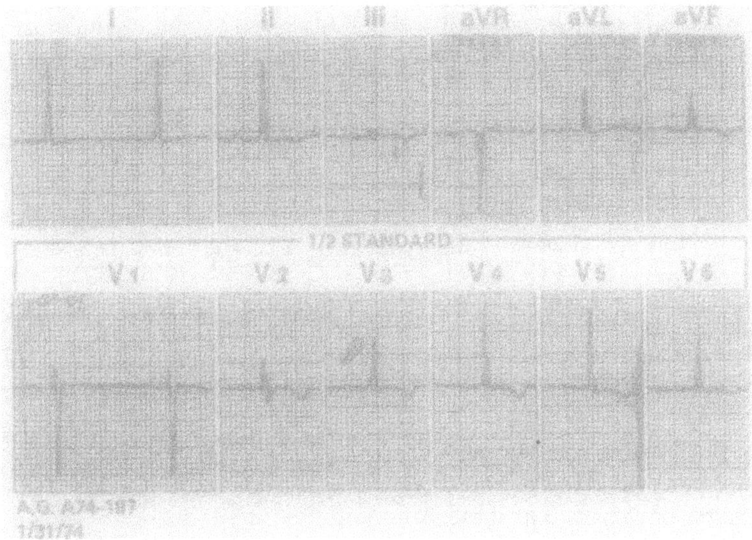

Fig. 1. ECG 7 months before death and before the onset of symptoms of cardiac dysfunction. It shows prolonged P-R interval and diffuse ST-T abnormalities.

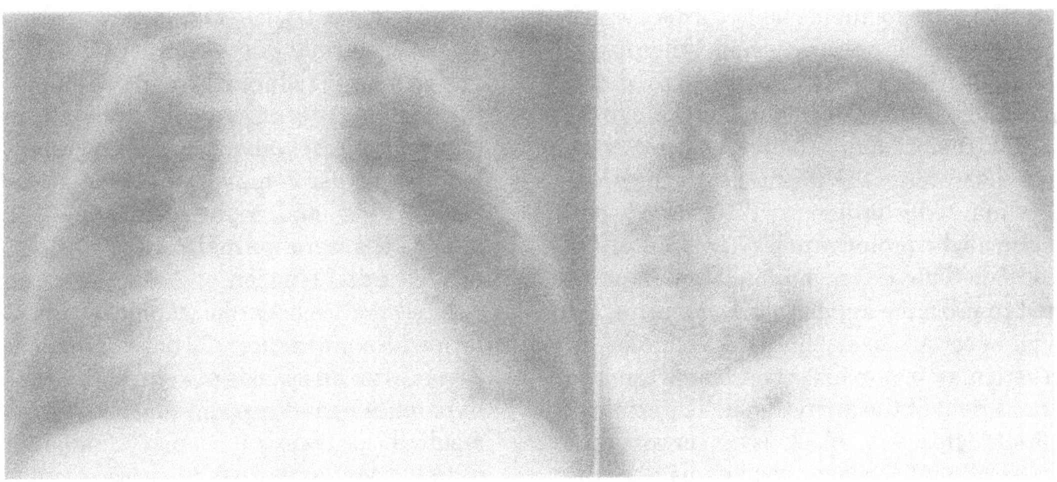

Fig. 2. Posteroanterior (left) and lateral (right) chest roentgenograms 7 months before death and before the onset of symptoms of cardiac dysfunction.

he had a grand mal seizure preceded by dizziness and palpitations. This episode was believed to be caused by ventricular tachycardia. Upon awakening, the blood pressure was 95/60 mm. Hg, an S_3 was audible, and the murmur was unchanged. The hematocrit was 29 per cent. The ECG was unchanged. He was monitored by telemetry, and given quinidine gluconate. Nausea and vomiting on the fourth hospital day prompted discontinuation of quinidine. Premature supraventricular beats with aberrancy, premature ventricular beats, and recurrent runs of ventricular tachycardia continued. On day 7, a sustained run of ventricular tachycardia (Fig. 3) led to hypotension and another grand mal seizure. He was treated with assisted ventilation and closed-chest cardiac massage, and sinus rhythm returned. From day 7 to day 26 he had frequent multifocal premature ventricular beats, daily episodes of ventricular tachycardia, and increasing subcutaneous edema. On day 26, a sustained run of ventricular tachycardia required electroversion. Chest radiograph revealed increasing congestion. During the remainder of his life the arrhythmias persisted. Serum potassium was frequently elevated, and on day 41 he became comatose, presumably because of severe hypoglycemia (30 mg. per 100 ml.). On day 47, ventricular fibrilla-

Table I. Echocardiographic observations

Time before death	7 months	23 days	4 days
LV transverse dimension (diastole)	50	62	63
LV transverse dimension (systole)	34	52	58
Septum	14	14	12
LV posterior wall	14	14	12
LV mass	368	516	430
Ejection fraction	69	41	22
Left atrium	31	46	41
Aortic root	23	23	22
Heart rate	74	86	88
Mitral diastolic closing rate	90	135	124
Pericardial effusion	None	None	Present

tion occurred, and resuscitation was successful. The hematocrit was 33 per cent. He died on day 61 because of recurrence of ventricular fibrillation.

DR. ROBERTS: Dr. Redwood could you discuss the His bundle electrogram?

DR. DAVID R. REDWOOD: On day 57, because of persistent runs of ectopic tachycardia which proved refractory to antiarrhythmic therapy, a His bundle electrogram was recorded to determine the origin of the ectopic beats. As can be seen in Fig. 4, the normally conducted beats show prolonged (300 msec.) PR interval; the A-H interval is markedly prolonged (210 msec.), and there is also slight prolongation (70 msec.) of the H-V interval. The latter prolongation can be attributed to procaine amide therapy. During the short burst of ectopic beats, no His spike preceded each ventricular complex, thus confirming a ventricular origin of the arrhythmia. The etiology of the first-degree A-V block is uncertain, but may have resulted from structural damage to the A-V node by iron deposits. It is unlikely that it can be attributed entirely to the pharmacologic effects of digoxin (0.125 mg. daily) or of procaine amide (2,000 mg. daily). The repeated runs of ventricular tachycardia are entirely consistent with myocardial damage from iron deposition.

DR. ROBERTS: This patient had three echocardiograms during his last 7 months of life. Dr. Henry, could you summarize your echocardiographic observations?

DR. WALTER L. HENRY: The first echocardiographic study was performed 7 months before death when the patient clinically had no symptoms of cardiac dysfunction except for exertional

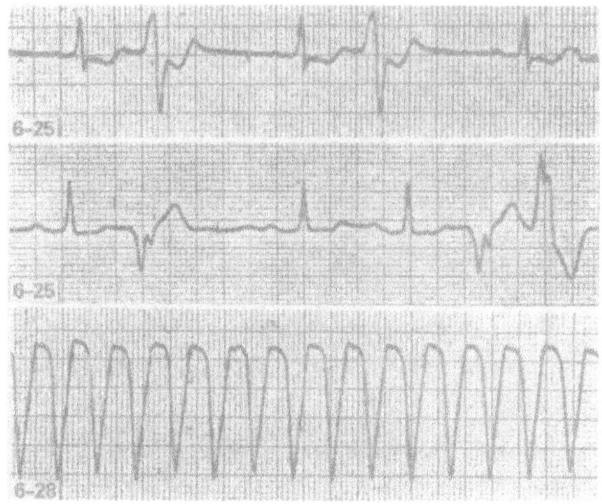

Fig. 3. ECG "rhythm strips" 2 months before death showing premature supraventricular beats with aberrancy, multifocal premature ventricular beats, and ventricular tachycardia.

dyspnea and easy fatigability when his hematocrit was below 25 per cent. This initial study demonstrated a nondilated concentrically thickened left ventricle (Fig. 5). Systolic function appeared normal (ejection fraction = 69 per cent) but a mildly reduced rate (90 mm. per second [normal = 110]) of early diastolic closure of the anterior mitral valve leaflet suggested reduced left ventricular compliance (Table I). Left atrial, aortic root, and right ventricular transverse dimensions were normal. There was no evidence of pericardial effusion.

A second echocardiographic study was performed 6 months later (23 days before death), and 2 days after an episode of ventricular tachycardia, hypotension, and a grand mal seizure, which had resulted in transient coma. Compared to the initial study, a marked decrease in ejection fraction (69 to 41 per cent) and increase in diastolic left ventricular transverse dimension and left atrial transverse dimension (31 to 46 mm.), had occurred (Fig. 5).

The final echocardiographic study was performed 4 days before death. The major change from previous studies was a further reduction in ejection fraction and perhaps a decrease in septal and posterior wall thicknesses.

The echocardiographic assessment of cardiac structure and function obtained in this patient are of particular interest in that they document the striking cardiac changes that may occur in some patients during the end stage of a chronic

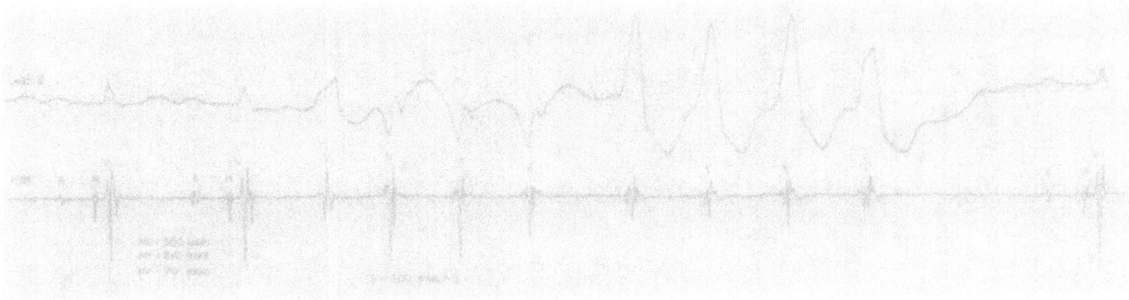

Fig. 4. Recording of His bundle bipolar electrogram (HBE) and standard ECG, Lead II. The normally conducted beats show prolonged AH and HV times. The ectopic beats show ventricular complexes that are not preceded by His bundle spikes, thus demonstrating their ventricular origin.

myocardial disease. In this patient, the initial echocardiographic assessment of cardiac structure revealed a nondilated, concentrically thickened left ventricle. Systolic function appeared to be reasonably well preserved; left ventricular compliance appeared mildly reduced. At this time (i.e., 7 months before death), the echocardiographic measurements were similar to those obtained from patients with infiltrative cardiomyopathies due to a variety of systemic diseases.

Six months later, however, a marked reduction in systolic function and marked left ventricular dilatation had occurred. Whether such striking changes preceded the patient's cardiac arrhythmias and hypotension or were at least in part due to these episodes cannot be determined. What is important, however, is that the final echocardiographic assessment and necropsy examination were consistent in that they both revealed a grossly dilated left ventricle whose walls were not particularly thickened. Thus, if the necropsy examination and the final echocardiographic study were the only information available, one would likely conclude that iron overload due to chronic transfusion therapy primarily produced a decrease in systolic function and marked ventricular dilatation, changes similar to those seen in patients with idiopathic cardiomyopathy of the ventricular dilated type ("congestive cardiomyopathy"). The echocardiographic studies from asymptomatic and minimally symptomatic patients with infiltrative cardiomyopathies as well as the initial echocardiographic study in the present patient, however, indicate that systolic dysfunction usually occurs only in the end stage of the disease process and that the initial changes that can be detected echocardiographically are a concentric increase in left ventricular mass without systolic dysfunction.

Dr. Roberts: This patient was studied by Dr. Nienhuis and his colleagues. Dr. Nienhuis, could you discuss the Blackfan-Diamond anemia, the possible effect on the heart of 23 years of severe anemia, and your hopes with chelation therapy as far as cardiac iron is concerned?

Dr. Arthur W. Nienhuis: Blackfan-Diamond syndrome, or *constitutional hypoplastic anemia,* is a congenital disorder characterized by the complete absence of red cell precursor in the bone marrow and of reticulocytes in the peripheral blood. In five reported families two siblings were affected, suggesting a hereditary basis with inheritance possibly as an autosomal recessive.[1] Onset may be shortly after birth, as in this patient, or may be delayed for several months. Partial or complete remission has occurred in response to corticosteroid therapy, although only if treatment is instituted shortly after the onset of the disease.[2,3] Androgen has been tried with little success in an attempt to stimulate the bone marrow. In contrast to erythroid hypoplasia in adults, there is no apparent association of Blackfan-Diamond syndrome with thymoma, nor have inhibitors to erythroid growth been found in the plasma. Thus, constitutional hypoplastic anemia appears to be a primary disorder of erythroid tissue rendering the patient dependent on blood transfusions to sustain life.

Cardiac disease in this patient reflects the combined effects of chronic anemia and progressive iron deposition in the myocardium. An important pathogenic role for the iron is suggested by the fact that most patients with severe—but non-transfusion-dependent—anemia do not develop symptoms of cardiac dysfunction. Recently, desferrioxamine has been shown to retard hepatic iron deposition and prevent fibrosis in patients with thalassemia major, indicating

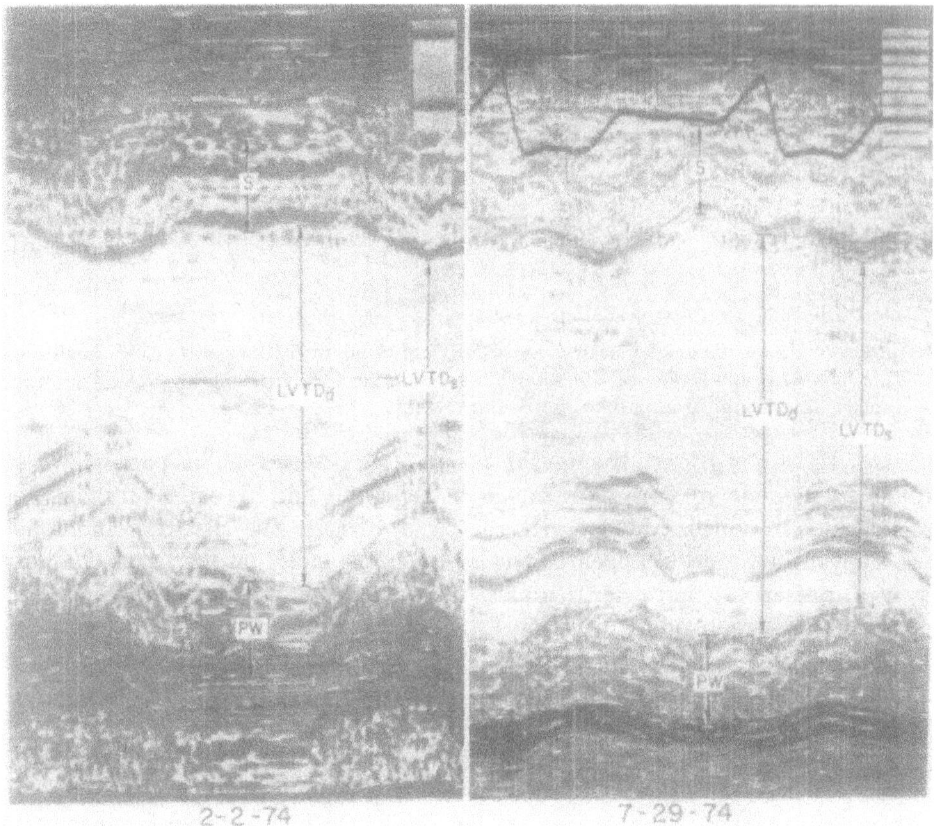

Fig. 5. Echocardiographic records obtained 7 months before death (left) when the patient was asymptomatic and again 1 month before death (right) after an episode of ventricular tachycardia and hypotension. The wall thicknesses that are labeled were confirmed in the damped portions of the echocardiographic tracings that are not shown in this figure. The 1 cm. calibration markers are shown in the upper right corner of each panel. (Note: the record in the right panel of this figure was obtained with an ultrasound instrument containing circuits especially designed to highlight the epicardial-lung interface). S = thickness of ventricular septum; PW = thickness of left ventricular posterior wall; $LVTD_s$ = internal dimension of left ventricular cavity at end-systole.

that chelation therapy may be useful in preventing tissue damage from iron in patients requiring transfusions.[4] Whether myocardial iron deposition also can be prevented remains to be determined. Daily administration of Desferal to this patient resulted in excretion of 35 to 45 mg. of iron per day. This amounts to 1.0 to 1.3 Gm. per month, exceeding that given by transfusions during the period of treatment. Nonetheless, serious cardiac disease was not prevented, indicating that irreversible myocardial iron accumulation already had occurred.

Dr. Roberts: Dr. Arnett could you summarize your finding at necropsy in this patient?

Dr. Arnett: At necropsy, serous effusions were present in the pericardial (230), pleural (right = 800 ml.; left = 50 ml.), and peritoneal cavities (1,200 ml.). Iron deposits were present, usually in huge amounts, in virtually every body organ (Table II). The liver was cirrhotic, portal type. The thyroid gland, pancreas, testes, and parathyroid glands were considerably scarred in addition to containing heavy iron deposits.

The heart weighed 320 grams, and all four chambers were dilated (Fig. 6). Neither ventricular wall was thickened (right 0.4 and left 1.4 cm.). The myocardium, except that of the right atrium, was rusty brown (Fig. 6). There were no gross myocardial scars. The only sites of myocardial necrosis, and these were only foci of myocytolysis, were the left ventricular papillary muscles (Fig. 7). The four cardiac valves were normal. The left ventricular endocardium was mildly thickened. Except for focal iron deposits in the internal elastic membrane, the extramural coronary arteries were normal.

Histologic sections of ventricular and left atrial myocardium revealed heavy iron deposits in

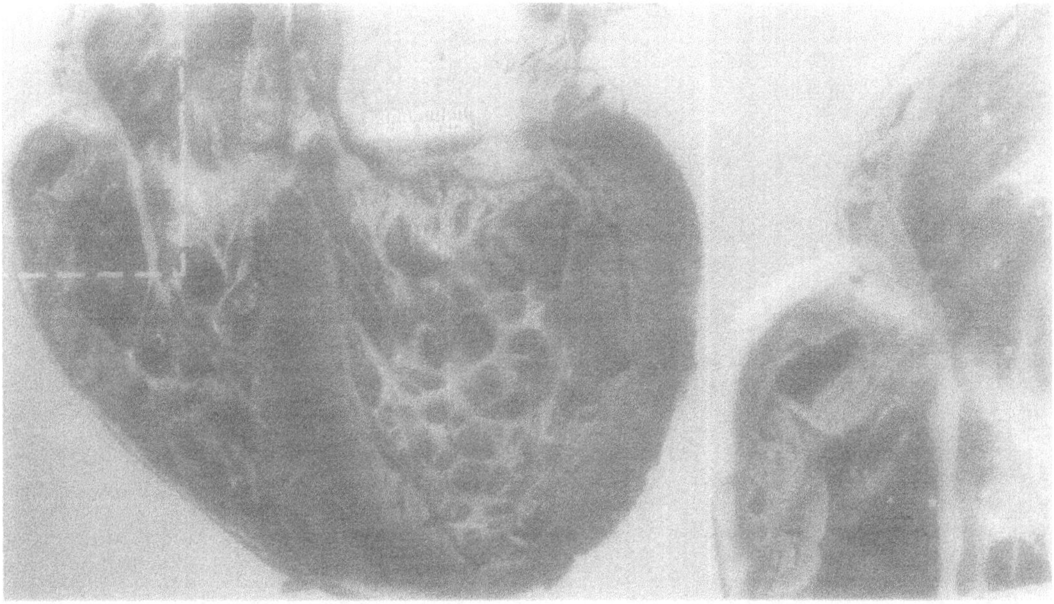

Fig. 6. Interior of the heart. Left: Longitudinal section showing relative sizes of the chambers and their walls. The myocardium of the ventricles, left atrium, and atrial septum is dark brown, whereas that of the right atrium is much lighter, indicating far fewer iron deposits. Right: A close-up of the junction of right atrium with right ventricle to demonstrate the light color of the atrial wall in comparison to the ventricular wall.

Table II. Presence and amount of iron in various body organs or tissues

Organ	*0-4+*
Myocardium	++++
Liver (1,220 Gm.)	++++
Pancreas	++++
Spleen (730 Gm.)	++++
Lymph node	++++
Pituitary gland	++++
Thyroid gland (10 Gm.)	++++
Parathyroid gland	++++
Adrenal gland	++++
Testis	++++
Prostate gland	++++
Stomach	++++
Kidney	++
Lung	++
Skeletal muscle	+
Esophagus	0
Small intestine	0
Large intestine	0
Central nervous system	0

virtually every working myocardial cell (Fig. 8). Iron deposits were greatest in the epicardial third and papillary muscles, intermediate in the endocardial third, and least in the middle third of the left ventricular wall. Focal myocytolysis was extensive in the papillary muscles; these collections of myocardial cells consisted only of nuclei,

Table III. Myocardial iron content

	μg/Gm.
Right atrium	119
Right ventricle	1,891
Left atrium	254
Left ventricle (LV)	2,362
Endocardial ½ of LV	1,409
Epicardial ½ of LV	3,498
Ventricular septum	2,192

sarcolemmal sheaths, and intracellular iron; the myofibrils and other organelles had vanished (Figs. 9 and 10). In preserved myocardial cells, iron deposits were heaviest around the nucleus, but filled a large part of many cells (Fig. 10). Sections of right atrial myocardium revealed only scattered, small, iron deposits (Fig. 11). Serial sections of A-V node, A-V bundle, and the proximal right and left bundle branches revealed only small, focal, iron deposits in the conducting cells (Fig. 12) as contrasted to the heavy deposits in the contracting myocardial cells. Iron, primarily in alveolar spaces, accounted for the reticulonodular pattern of the lung by chest roentgenogram (Fig. 13).

Iron content of myocardium from the walls of all four chambers was determined by atomic absorption spectrophotometry. This analysis

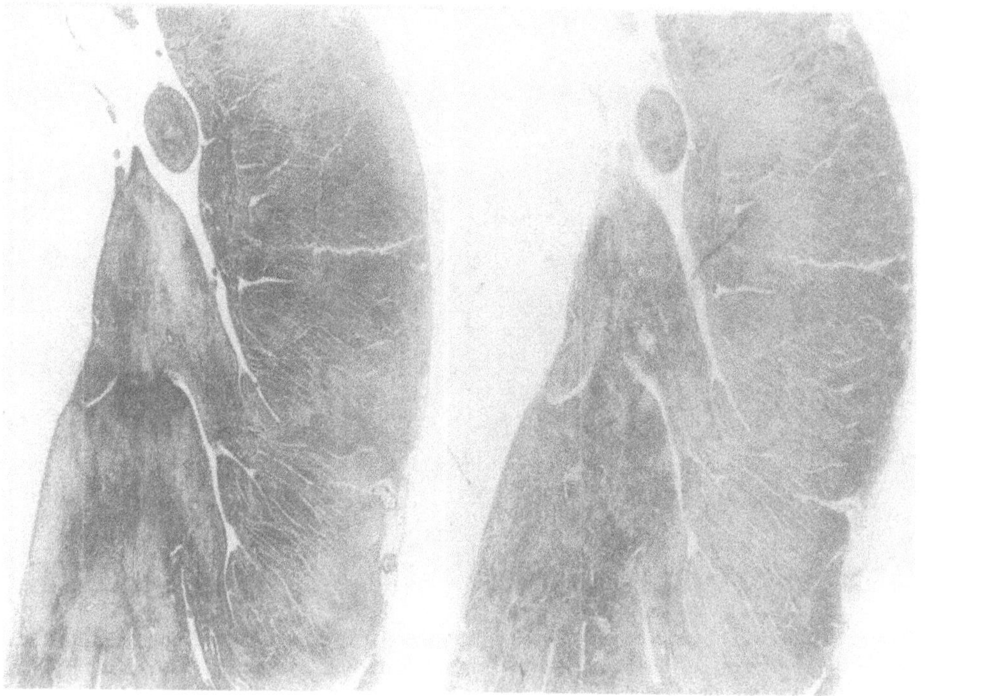

Fig. 7. Histologic sections of left ventricular wall and papillary muscle. Left: Hematoxylin and eosin stain showing extensive areas (pale) of myocytolysis in papillary muscle. Right: Iron stain showing the heavy deposition of iron in the papillary muscle and the epicardial third of free wall.

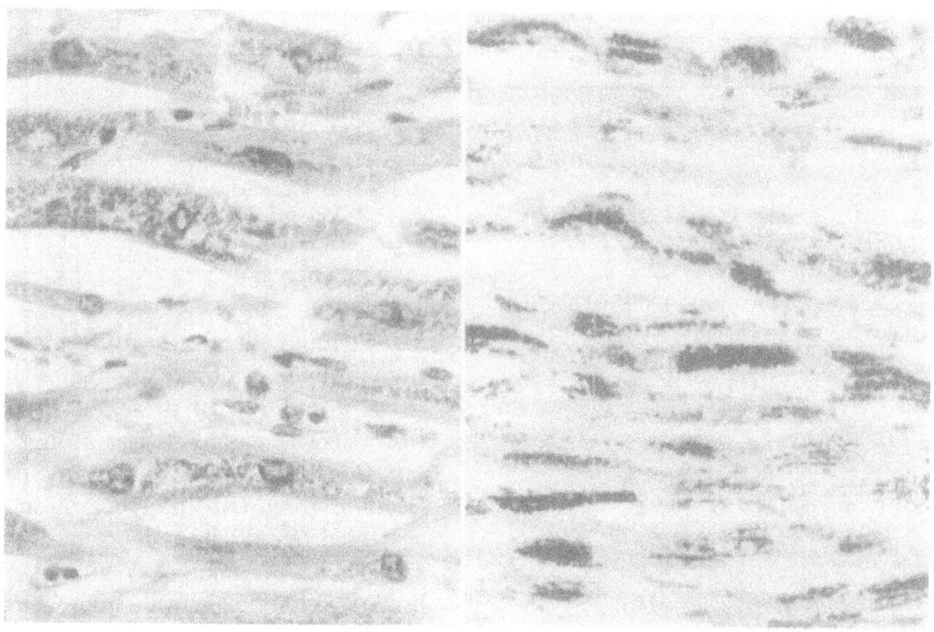

Fig. 8. Histologic sections of left ventricular myocardium showing extensive iron depositions. Left: Hematoxylin and eosin stains. Right: Iron stain. (Each ×560.)

again disclosed that the deposition of iron was least in the right atrial myocardium, and that within the left ventricular wall iron was more heavily deposited in the epicardial half than in the endocardial half (Table III).

DR. ROBERTS: Electron microscopic examination of myocardial cells was performed by Dr. Ferrans, who will summarize his observations.

DR. VICTOR J. FERRANS: The left ventricular myocardial cells examined ultrastructurally con-

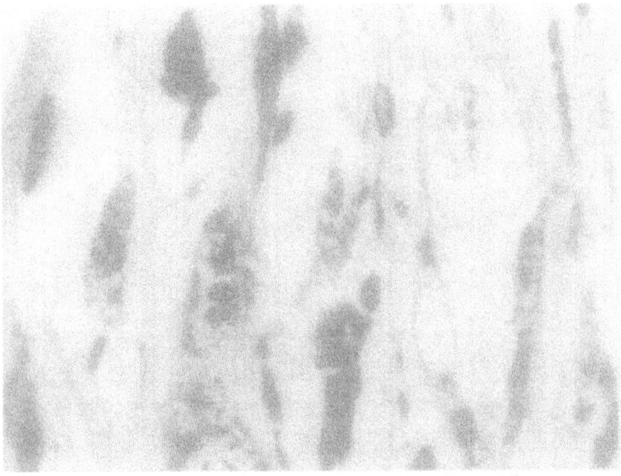

Fig. 9. Histologic section of left ventricular papillary muscle showing degenerated myocardial cells, consisting only of sarcolemmal sheaths, nuclei, and heavy iron deposits. (Hematoxylin and eosin stain; ×880.)

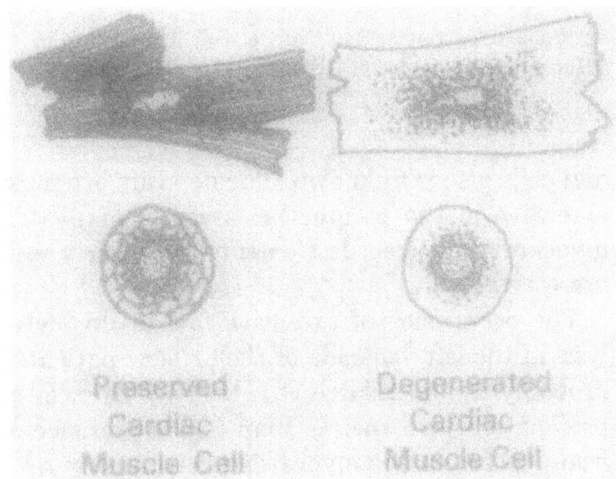

Fig. 10. Diagram showing both preserved and degenerated cardiac muscle cell containing iron deposits. Relatively few severely degenerated muscle cells were observed in comparison to the preserved cells. The amount of iron deposition in each appeared to be similar, suggesting that another factor, possibly anemia, was responsible for the disappearance of the myocardial fibers and filaments in the degenerated cell rather than the iron deposition.

tained large numbers of aggregates of iron particles, decreased numbers of mitochondria and myofibrils, and scattered concentric lamellae, presumed to be derived from products of mitochondrial breakdown (Fig. 14).

Dr. Roberts: Until recent years there was considerable debate whether or not infiltration of iron into myocardial cells could cause them to function abnormally. It is now clear beyond any reasonable doubt that myocardial hemosiderosis can cause myocardial dysfunction.[5] Whether or not dysfunction results is dependent on the

Fig. 11. Histologic sections of atrial walls. Left: Right atrium containing few iron deposits. Right: Left atrium containing heavy iron deposits. (Each ×54.)

Fig. 12. The conducting tissue (as shown on right) contained much less iron than the working myocardium (as shown on the left). The conducting tissue shown here is a portion of the His bundle. (Hematoxylin and eosin stain; ×140.)

amount of iron entering the myocardial cells: huge amounts, as occurred in the patient described herein, may produce congestive cardiac failure and arrythmias; small amounts of myocardial iron cause no evidence of myocardial dysfunction.[5]

In patients with cardiac hemosiderosis, certain areas of the heart contain heavier deposits than do other areas. The ventricular free walls and ventricular septa contain heavier deposits of iron than do the atrial walls. Of the various myocardial walls infiltrated by iron, the right atrial one—as so clearly demonstrated in the present patient—contains the least. The amount of iron in the various layers of ventricular myocardium also

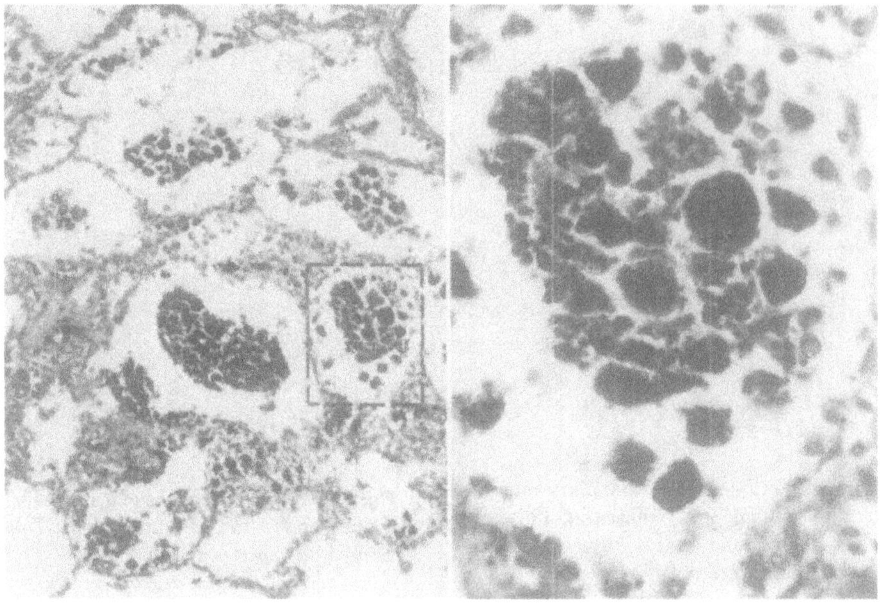

Fig. 13. Sections of lung disclosing heavy deposits of hemosiderin-laden macrophages in many alveoli. The right photomicrograph shows a single alveolus containing many iron-filled macrophages. (Hematoxylin and eosin stains; ×140 [left], ×560 [right].)

is variable: the epicardial third and the papillary muscles contain the most, the middle third the least, and the subendocardial third immediate between the two. The conduction tissue is relatively spared by iron deposits as compared to the contracting myocardial cells.[5] Serial sections of sinus node, A-V node and bundle, and proximal right and left bundle branches in the present patient and in those described previously from this laboratory[5] disclosed only small deposits of iron in the conducting tissues compared to heavy deposits in the contracting myocardial cells.

It would be difficult in the present patient with cardiac hemosiderosis to attribute the various atrial and ventricular arrhythmias to the presence of the few deposits of iron in the conducting tissues. The altered myocardial contracting cells more likely are the source of the arrhythmias. Support for this view also is provided by the His bundle electrogram which showed complete lack of impulse transmission through the His bundle prior to occurrence of ventricular ectopic beats.

The reason for the differences in the amounts of iron deposited in the various portions of heart is uncertain. Clearly, there is something different about the myocardial cells in the right atrium compared to those in the left atrium or in either ventricle.

The mechanism by which iron enters myocardial cells also is unknown. The deposits are most extensive in the perinuclear areas. Usually the myocardial contractile elements were fairly well preserved.

The occurrence of extensive foci of myocytolysis in the left ventricle of the present patient is probably more related to the occurrence of prolonged severe anemia than to the presence of iron deposits in the myocardial cells.

Dr. Neinhuis raised the issue as to how much of the myocardial dysfunction in the present patient resulted from the associated severe anemia and how much from the presence of myocardial hemosiderosis. The answer in the present patient is uncertain but other patients with similarly severe degrees of cardiac hemosiderosis and myocardial dysfunction have been observed in the absence of anemia.[5] The present patient was anemic his entire life, and evidence of cardiac dysfunction did not appear until about 6 months before death. Possibly chelation therapy during his last 6 months also had a deleterious effect on myocardial function.

The echocardiographic studies by Dr. Henry clearly show that dilatation of the cardiac ventricles is a late manifestation of cardiac hemosiderosis and that the ventricular cavities are of normal size before evidence of myocardial dysfunction appears.

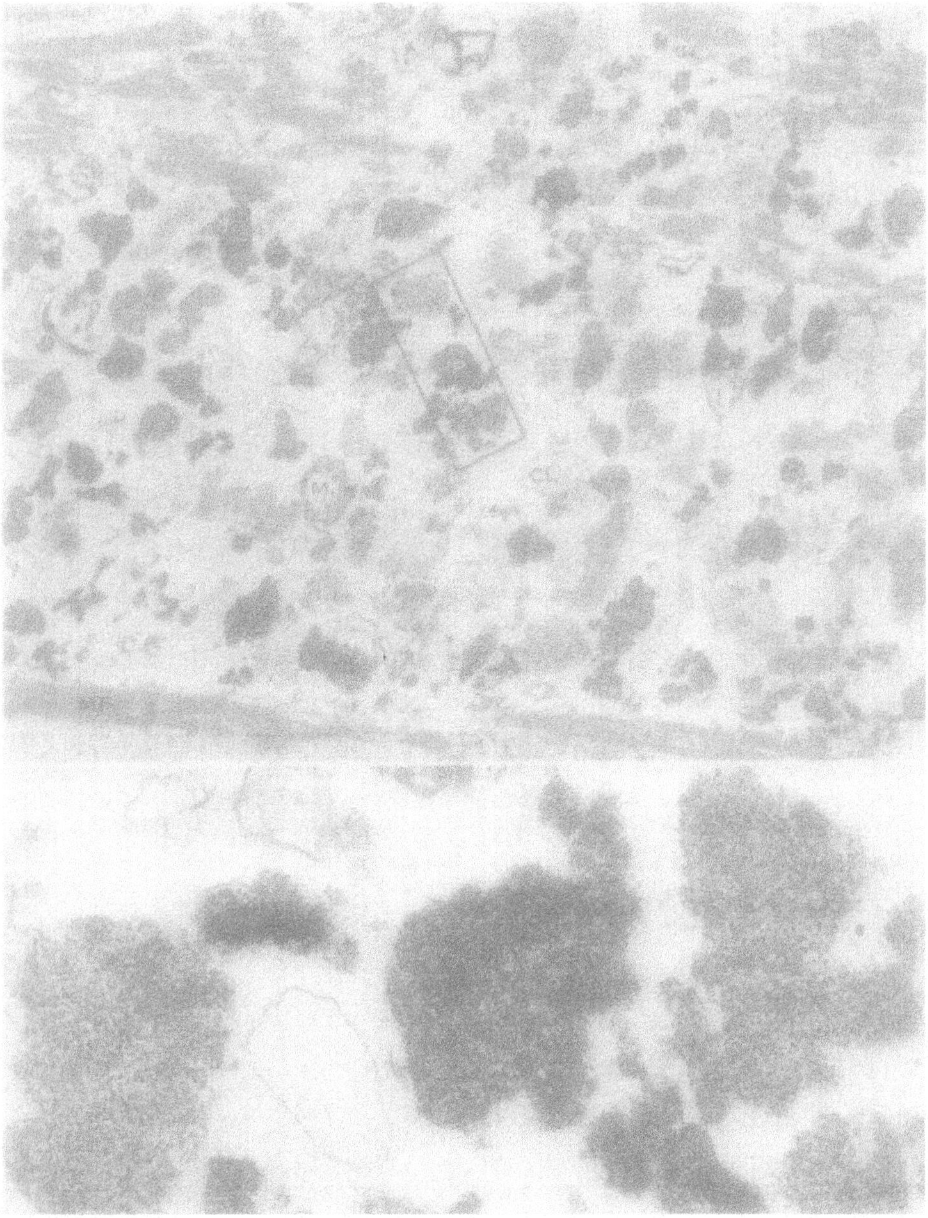

Fig. 14. Electron micrograph of part of left ventricular muscle cell (upper) shows large numbers of aggregates of iron particles (*IP*), decreased numbers of mitochondria (*M*) and myofibrils (*MF*), and scattered, concentric lamellae (*CL*) presumed to be derived from products of mitochondrial breakdown. Area within rectangle is shown at higher magnification below. The iron deposits in myocardium are composed of aggregates of electron-dense particles which measure from 90 to 100 A in diameter. (×11,750, upper; ×46,000, lower.)

Cardiac hemosiderosis is never an isolated occurrence. Iron deposits also are always present in most of the other body organs. In the present patient and in several others reported[5] the amount of iron in the heart is roughly proportional to that in the other body organs. Surprisingly, in contrast to its effect on the liver, for example, cardiac iron deposition does not produce a fibrous tissue reaction. Possibly the reason is due to its deposition nearly entirely *within* the myocardial cells and not within the interstitium as may occur in the liver.

In summary, extensive deposits of iron in the heart from whatever source–either endogenous or exogenous (as in the present patient > 500 blood transfusions)–may result in severe myocardial dysfunction. Thus, *the iron heart is not a strong heart, but a weak one.*

REFERENCES

1. Diamond, L. K., Allen, D. M., and Magill, F. B.: Congenital (erythroid) hypoplastic anemia, Am. J. Dis. Child **102**:403, 1961.
2. Allen, D. M., and Diamond, L. K.: Congenital (erythroid) hypoplastic anemia, cortisone treated, Am. J. Dis. Child **102**:416, 1961.
3. Hughes, D. W.: Hypoplastic anemia in infancy and childhood. Arch. Dis. Child. **36**:349, 1961.
4. Barry, M., Flynn, D. M., Lefsky, E. A., and Risdon, R. A.: Long-term chelation therapy in thalassemia major: Effect on liver iron concentration, liver histology and clinical progress, Br. Med. J. **2**:16-20, 1974.
5. Buja, L. M., and Roberts, W. C.: Iron in the heart. Etiology and clinical significance. Am. J. Med. **51**:209, 1971.

Sarcoidosis of the Heart

A Clinicopathologic Study of 35 Necropsy Patients (Group I) and Review of 78 Previously Described Necropsy Patients (Group II)

WILLIAM C. ROBERTS, M.D.
Bethesda, Maryland

HUGH A. McALLISTER, Jr., M.D.
Washington, D.C.

VICTOR J. FERRANS, M.D., Ph.D.
Bethesda, Maryland

Certain clinical and morphologic observations are described in 35 necropsy patients with cardiac sarcoidosis (group IA and IB), and similar observations are summarized in 78 previously described necropsy patients with cardiac sarcoidosis (group IIA and IIB). All patients had non-necrotic ("hard") granulomas in lymph nodes and either sarcoid granulomas in the heart (108 patients) or transmural myocardial scarring (five patients) unassociated with coronary arterial narrowing, i.e., healed granulomas. The 113 patients (groups I and II) whose data are analyzed also were divided into those in whom cardiac dysfunction clearly was the result of sarcoid granulomatous infiltration of the heart (89 patients) (groups IA and IIA), and those in whom cardiac dysfunction, if present, was clearly not the result of sarcoid involvement of the heart (24 patients) (groups IB and IIB).

Analysis of the 89 patients in groups IA and IIA disclosed that death was *sudden* (arrhythmia) in 60 (67 per cent), secondary to progressive *congestive cardiac failure* in 20 (23 per cent), from *recurring pericardial effusion* in three (3 per cent) and from other or unknown causes in six (7 per cent). Sudden death was the initial manifestation of sarcoidosis in 10 (17 per cent) of the 60 patients who died suddenly. Other than premature ventricular beats, *ventricular tachycardia* was the most common arrhythmia (17 patients), and *complete heart block* was the most common conduction disturbance (25 patients). *Complete bundle branch block* occurred in 21 patients. *Ventricular aneurysm* (eight patients) and *papillary muscle dysfunction* (possibly 16 patients) were other cardiac disturbances observed.

Although *corticosteroid therapy* tends to cause fibrous replacement of myocardial sarcoid granulomas, a possible consequence of this medication is the development of ventricular aneurysm.

Most patients with cardiac sarcoidosis causing dysfunction (groups IA and IIA) presented initially with manifestations related to the heart. Furthermore, most patients with cardiac sarcoidosis have little or no clinical evidence of dysfunction of an organ system other than the heart. Usually the course in patients with extensive cardiac sarcoidosis is not prolonged.

From the Pathology Branch, National Heart, Lung and Blood Institute, National Insitutes of Health, Bethesda, Maryland; and the Cardiovascular Department, Armed Forces Institute of Pathology, Washington, D.C. Requests for reprints should be addressed to Dr. William C. Roberts, Building 10A, Room 3E-30, National Institutes of Health, Bethesda, Maryland 20014. Manuscript accepted October 6, 1976.

Sarcoidosis, a systemic granulomatous disease of undetermined etiology and pathogenesis, most often involves lymph nodes, lungs, liver, spleen, skin, eyes, phalangeal bones and parotid glands, but other organs and tissues also may be affected. Cardiac involvement in patients with sarcoidosis has been reported on many occasions, but most reports are isolated case studies. The present study is a clinicopathologic analysis of a relatively large number of necropsy patients with cardiac sarcoidosis. It focuses on the varying types of functional and morphologic cardiac alterations in patients with cardiac sarcoidosis and, in addition, summarizes previous reports of this condition.

METHODS

The data on all the necropsy patients having cardiac sarcoidosis studied in the Pathology Branch, National Heart, Lung and Blood Institute, and in the Cardiovascular Registry of the Armed Forces Institute of Pathology are included in this analysis. A total of 35 patients was available for study (groups IA and IB). Prerequisites for inclusion in this study included (1) the presence of sarcoid-type, i.e., "hard" (non-necrotic) granulomas in lymph nodes, and (2) either the presence of sarcoid-type granulomas in the heart or the presence of transmural myocardial scarring unassociated with significant luminal narrowing of the extramural coronary arteries. The clinical and necropsy records, and the histologic sections from all body organs were reviewed. Excluding the one patient in whom the atrioventricular node and bundle were serially sectioned (sections cut a thickness of 6 μ and every fifth section was stained by hematoxylin and eosin), a total of 230 histologic sections of heart were examined, an average of six per patient (range one to 20). At least one histologic section of left ventricle was examined in every patient. Sections of other portions of the heart were available for reexamination in 31 patients: these included the ventricular septum (27 patients), the right ventricular free wall (25 patients), the right atrial wall (16 patients) and the left atrial wall (14 patients). The autopsy protocols also were examined for information regarding the presence or absence of granulomas in the various portions of the heart. Information was obtained regarding the presence or absence of sarcoid-type granulomas in lymph nodes (all patients) and lung, liver, and spleen (32 patients). Weights of the heart were available in 30 patients, and of the spleen, liver and both lungs in each of 20 patients. The available clinical information was examined in all 35 patients. Similar information was obtained on previously described cases of cardiac sarcoidosis. The classification used to group the 35 personally studied patients and the 78 previously described cases of cardiac sarcoidosis is outlined in Table I.

RESULTS

Certain clinical and morphologic observations in the 35 personally studied patients (groups IA and IB) are summarized in Tables II and III. For analysis of the cardiac disturbances, the 35 patients were subdivided into those in whom cardiac dysfunction clearly was the result of sarcoid granulomatous infiltration of the heart (26 patients, group IA, Table II), and those in whom cardiac dysfunction, if present, was clearly not the result of sarcoid granulomatous infiltration of the heart (nine patients, group IB, Table III).

At necropsy, 25 of these 26 patients (group IA) had grossly visible, usually large, granulomas in their hearts; the remaining patient had transmural myocardial scars unassociated with significant coronary arterial luminal narrowing. The other nine patients (group IB) were subdivided according to their predominant clinical features as shown in Table III. All nine of these patients had sarcoid granulomas in their hearts, but these granulomas were small; in eight patients they were visible only by histologic examination. This report focuses primarily on the 26 patients with cardiac dysfunction clearly secondary to sarcoid infiltration of the heart (group IA).

Observations in the Patients with Cardiac Dysfunction Secondary to Cardiac Sarcoidosis (Group IA). Cardiac dysfunction in the 26 patients in whom it was caused by cardiac sarcoidosis was variously manifested by arrhythmias and conduction disturbances, congestive cardiac failure and recurring pericardial effusions (Table II). These cardiac disturbances accounted for death in 25 of the 26 patients.

Arrhythmias or **conduction disturbances**, or both, were documented in 16 of these patients; electrocar-

TABLE I Cardiac Sarcoidosis: Necropsy Patients Analyzed

		Causing Cardiac Dysfunction (Subgroup A)		Not Causing Cardiac Dysfunction (Subgroup B)	
	Totals	No.	%	No.	%
Personally studied patients (group I)	35	26	74	9	26
Previously described patients (group II)	78	63	81	15	19
Totals	113	89	79	24	21

diograms were never recorded in six of the remaining 10 patients. Episodes of **ventricular tachycardia** were documented by electrocardiogram in five patients; 12 patients had ventricular premature beats. Four patients, two of whom also had episodes of ventricular tachycardia, had **atrial arrhythmias:** atrial fibrillation in two, atrial tachycardia in one and frequent atrial premature beats in one.

Heart block was confirmed by electrocardiogram in seven patients: prolongation of the P-R interval in one patient and complete heart block in six. In five of them the third degree heart block was present from two to six months; in the sixth patient it appeared about 2 hours before death. Three of the five patients with long-term complete heart block had syncope, which was the initial manifestation of sarcoidosis in each of them. Among the five patients with long-term complete heart block, the conduction disturbance, once it appeared, was persistent thereafter in four and periodic in one. In the latter patient, fibrous scarring associated with lymphocytic-cell infiltration was present at necropsy in the most cephalad portion of the muscular ventricular septum, whereas in the four patients with permanent complete heart block, large granulomas were still

TABLE II Cardiac Sarcoidosis Causing Cardiac Dysfunction: Clinical and Morphologic Observations in 26 Personally Studied Patients (Group IA)

	Mode of Death				
	Sudden	Congestive Heart Failure	Pericardial Effusion	Noncardiac	Totals
Patients (no.)	17	6	2	1	26
Age (yr)					
Range	21–74	26–73	35–47	34	21–74
Average	36	51	41	34	40
Race					
Black	9	3	2	0	14 (54)
White	7	2	0	1	10 (38)
Unknown or other	1	1	0	0	2 (8)
Sex					
Male	10	2	1	1	14 (54)
Female	7	4	1	0	12 (46)
Duration of symptoms (mo)					
Range	0–53	1–18	16, 18	48	0–53
Average	9*	7	17	48	11
Atrial arrhythmia	3	1	0	0	4 (15)
Ventricular premature beats	9	2	1	0	12 (46)
Ventricular tachycardia	5	0	1	0	6 (23)
Complete heart block	4	1	0	1	6 (23)
Syncope	3	0	0	0	3 (12)
Left bundle branch block	0	1	0	0	1 (12)
Right bundle branch block	1	1	0	0	2
Congestive heart failure	2	6	0	0	8 (31)
Diagnosis of sarcoid in life	5	0	2	1	8 (31)
Corticosteroid therapy	2	0	0	1	3 (12)
Heart weight (g)					
Range	300–550	300–660	350, 570	310	300–660
Average	430	536	460	310	428
Cardiac granulomas					
Left ventricle	17	6	2	0	25 (96)
Ventricular septum	15	4	0	0	19 (73)
Right ventricle	10	2	0	0	12 (46)
Papillary muscle	11	5	1	0	17 (65)
Atria	2	1	0	0	3 (12)
None	0	0	0	1	1 (4)
Ventricular aneurysm	2	0	0	0	2 (8)
Cardiac mural thrombi	0	0	0	1	1 (4)
Noncardiac granulomas					
Lymph node	17	6	2	1	26 (100)
Lung	15	4	1	0	20 (77)
Liver	11	4	2	1	18 (69)
Spleen	11	4	2	1	18 (69)
Other	6	2	2	1	11 (42)

NOTE: Figures in parentheses are per cents.

* This average includes six patients whose initial manifestation of sarcoidosis was sudden death.

present at necropsy in the most cephalad portion of the muscular ventricular septum. In addition to the six patients with complete heart block, three others had **complete bundle branch block** (right in two; left in one); one of these patients also had episodes of ventricular tachycardia, and another had atrial fibrillation.

It is presumed that an arrhythmia or a conduction disturbance was the cause of **sudden death,** which was the mode of death in 17 (65 per cent) of the 26 patients. Sudden death was the initial manifestation of sarcoidosis in six (35 per cent) of the 17 patients who died suddenly, and in each, death occurred during exertion. In none of these six patients was an electrocardiogram ever recorded. Of the remaining 11 patients who died suddenly, five had recurring episodes of ventricular tachycardia, and four others had complete heart block, three of whom had episodes of syncope (Stokes-Adams attacks). Of the remaining two patients who died suddenly, one was known to have ventricular premature beats, but he had always been asymptomatic and without any recognized features of sarcoidosis; the second patient, a 26 year old woman, began to lose weight about three years before her death, had a persistent cough, a right Horner's syndrome, and pulmonary lesions and hilar lymphadenopathy. Fatal rapid atrial fibrillation developed shortly after the patient underwent an open biopsy of lung.

Congestive cardiac failure occurred in eight of the

TABLE III Cardiac Sarcoidosis Not Causing Cardiac Dysfunction: Clinical and Morphologic Observations in Nine Personally Studied Patients (Group IB) and in 15 Previously Described Patients (Group IIB)

Data	Group IB (9 patients)			Group IIB (15 patients)			Totals
	Respiratory Failure	Nonsarcoid Cardiac Dysfunction	Noncardiac and Non-pulmonary	Respiratory Failure	Nonsarcoid Cardiac Dysfunction	Noncardiac and Non-pulmonary	
Patients	4	3	2	10	3	2	24*
References	...	...	...	[51–59, 61]	[22, 63, 64]	[60, 62]	[22, 51–64]
Ages (yr)							
Range	30–59	28–50	38–43	28–58	40–68	72, 83	28–83
Average	40	39	40	45	52	77	45
Race							
Black	3	2	1	3	0	0	9 (37)
White	1	1	1	4	2	1	10 (42)
Unknown	0	0	0	3	1	1	5 (21)
Sex							
Male	2	2	0	8	2	2	16 (67)
Female	2	1	2	2	1	0	8 (33)
Duration of symptoms (mo)							
Range	24–96	10–168	0–12	5–84	36–54	...	0–96
Average	72	71	6	36	45		46
Atrial arrhythmia	0	0	0	1	0	0	1 (4)
Ventricular premature beats	0	0	0	0	1	0	1 (4)
Bundle branch block	0	0	0	0	1	1	2 (8)
Congestive heart failure	...	3	0	...	3	0	6 (25)
Diagnosis of sarcoid during life	4	1	0	8	2	0	10 (42)
Corticosteroid therapy	2	0	0	0	1	0	3 (12)
Heart weight (g)							
Range	300–400	370–950	280–460	250–420	520–870	340	250–950
Average	345	623	370	336	670	340	440
Cardiac granulomas							
Left ventricle	4	3	2	3/3	...	2	14/14 (100)
Ventricular septum	1	1	0	2/3	...	1	5/14 (36)
Right ventricle	2	2	1	3/3	...	2	10/14 (71)
Papillary muscle	...	1	...	0/3	...	...	1/6 (17)
Atria	0	0	0	0/3	...	...	0
Noncardiac granulomas							
Lymph node	4	3	2	9/9	3	2	23/23 (100)
Lung	4	2	2	9/9	1	2	20/23 (87)
Liver	4	3	2	6/9	1	2	18/23 (78)
Spleen	4	2	2	7/9	1	2	18/23 (78)
Other	3	2	1	5/9	1	0	12/23 (52)

NOTE: Figures in parentheses are per cents.

* None of these 24 patients had ventricular tachycardia, complete heart block, syncope, cardiac aneurysm, intracardiac thrombi, or completely healed myocardial granulomas.

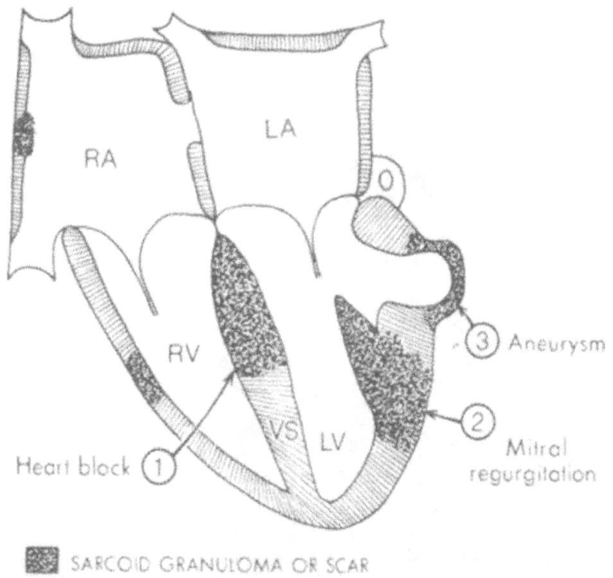

Figure 1. *Diagram showing the most common sites of sarcoid granulomas or scars in the heart and the most frequent functional consequences of these lesions.*

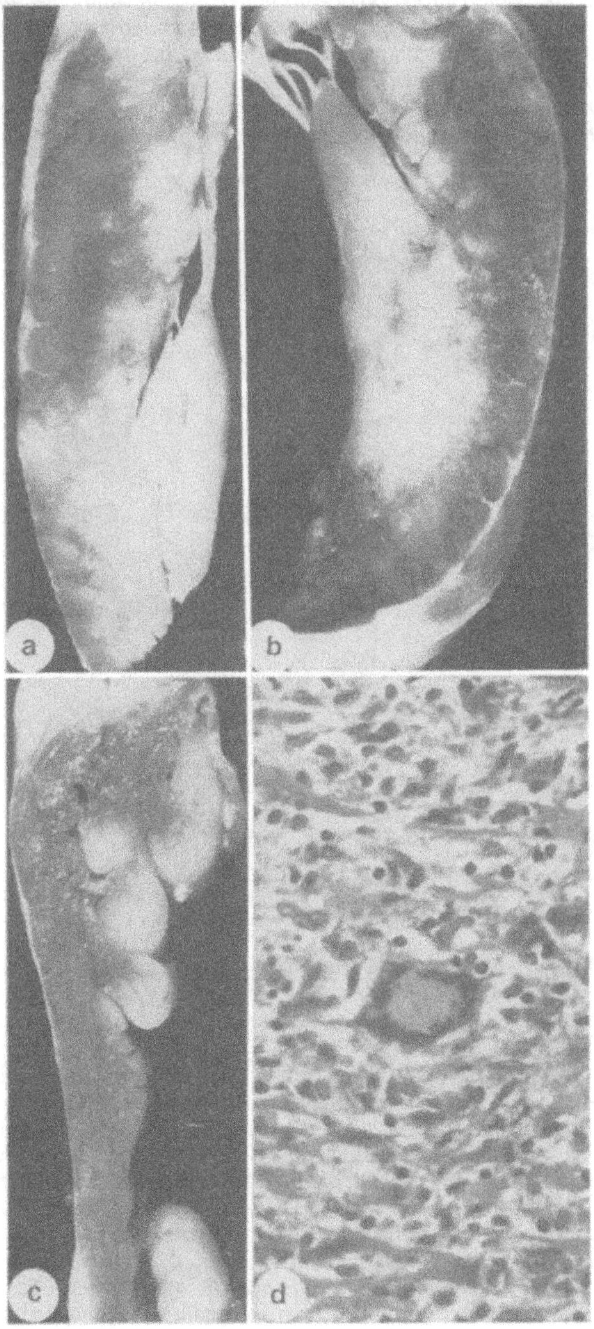

Figure 2. *The heart in a 26 year old black woman (A-70-541) who had been asymptomatic until 10 days before her death when dyspnea appeared. The dyspnea rapidly worsened, and when the patient was hospitalized on the day of death, she was in acute pulmonary edema. The blood pressure was 80/70 mm Hg, heart rate 160 beats/min and a grade 3-4/6 pansystolic blowing murmur, which radiated to the axilla, was audible. A chest roentgenogram showed congested lungs, cardiomegaly and prominent hilar adenopathy. Electrocardiogram showed nonspecific S-T segment and T-wave changes and atrial hypertrophy. Complete heart block developed and the patient died shortly thereafter.* ***a*** *and* ***b,*** *longitudinal sections of left ventricular free wall at sites of the papillary muscles. The latter are totally replaced by firm, white deposits, several of which also infiltrate the free wall.* ***c,*** *longitudinal section of right atrial wall showing similar white deposits.* ***d,*** *histologic section of a portion of a white deposit in the heart showing typical sarcoid granulomas. Similar hard granulomas were present in lymph nodes, liver, spleen and lung. Hematoxylin and eosin stain; original magnification X 400 (**d**), reduced by 12 per cent.*

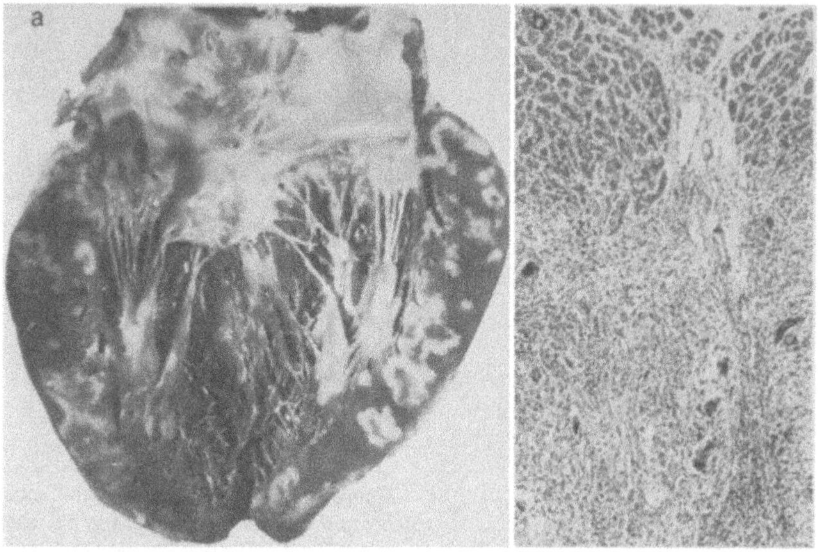

Figure 3. *Opened left atrium, mitral valve and left ventricle (**a**) and photomicrograph of a portion of the left ventricular wall (**b**) in a 28 year old black man (A-70-55) who died suddenly on his job as a construction worker. He had been well until two days earlier when he complained of "pain in his neck," but this had not prevented him from performing his usual activities. He had never sought medical care. At necropsy, sarcoid granulomas were found in the mediastinal lymph nodes, lung and heart. The heart weighed 420 g. Numerous sarcoid granulomas are present in the left ventricular free wall and in both papillary muscles. The posteromedial one is virtually replaced by the granulomas. Hematoxylin and eosin stain (**b**); original magnification × 100, reduced by 26 per cent.*

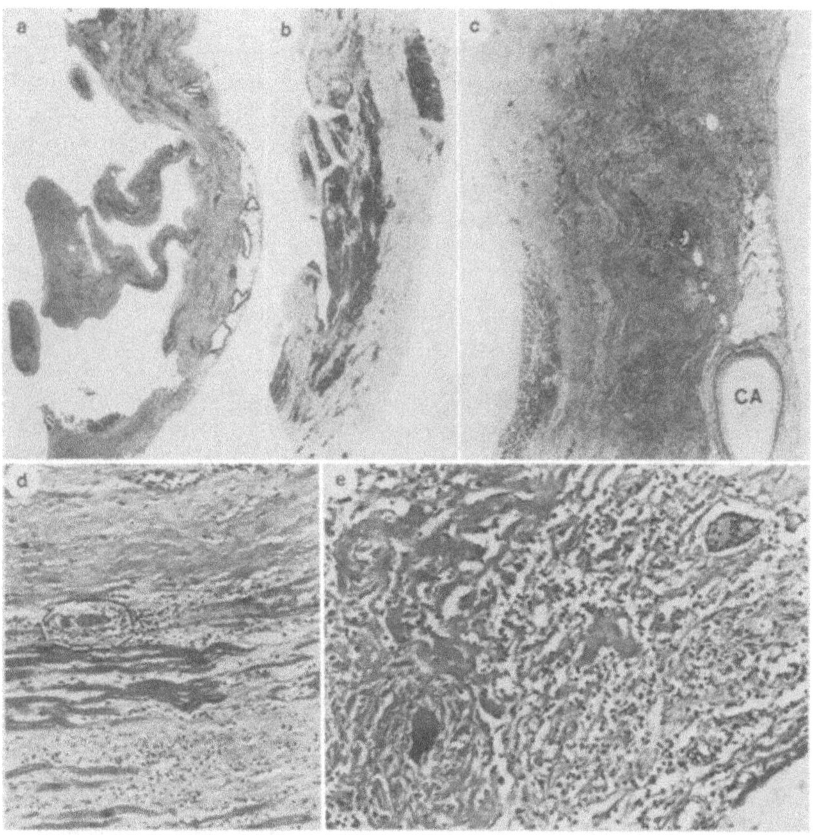

Figure 4. *Photomicrographs of the posterior left ventricular free wall in a 44 year old, extremely obese (260 pounds), white woman (A73-128) in whom evidence of congestive cardiac failure developed months before her death. A chest roentgenogram showed mild cardiomegaly and "pulmonary congestion." Several days before death, ventricular tachycardia developed suddenly. Episodes of this arrhythmia occurred until her death. Diagnosis of sarcoid was not suspected during life. **a, b, c,** longitudinal sections of left ventricular posterior wall at three different sites. In **a** and **c** there is complete transmural replacement of the wall primarily by fibrous tissue which contains occasional granuloma. The posteromedial papillary muscle is also completely replaced by sarcoid (**a**). Mainly the epicardial half of the portion shown in **b** is replaced. The coronary arteries (CA), one of which is shown in **c**, were wide open. In **d** only one granuloma (dashed circle) is present but the amount of fibrous tissue is extensive. In **e** more granulomas are seen. Far more granulomas were present in the lymph nodes than in the heart. Some also were found in the liver, spleen and lungs. Masson trichrome stain (**a** and **b**), hematoxylin and eosin stain (**c**, **d** and **e**); original magnification × 3 (**a** and **b**), × 15 (**c**), × 140 (**d**) and × 200 (**e**), reduced by 40 per cent.*

26 patients. Two of the eight patients had mild failure and died suddenly; the other six had progressive and eventually fatal failure. The left ventricular walls were extensively infiltrated by sarcoid granulomas in all eight patients with congestive cardiac failure. Of the six patients with severe, fatal heart failure, two had loud (grade 3–4/6) precordial, apical, systolic murmurs consistent with mitral regurgitation. At necropsy, both patients had extensive infiltration of their left ventricular papillary muscles by sarcoid granulomas; thus each had papillary muscle dysfunction as a result of myocardial sarcoidosis. Two patients had changes on the electrocardiogram that suggested recent myocardial infarction; one patient presented with acute failure, was symptomatic for only about one month and, during life, was considered to have the failure on the basis of acute myocardial infarction. Two patients, each of whom had had chronic failure for at least six months, had an acute exacerbation of the failure several days before death; at necropsy, each had large pulmonary emboli.

Recurring pericardial effusion was the cause of cardiac dysfunction in two of the 26 patients. The

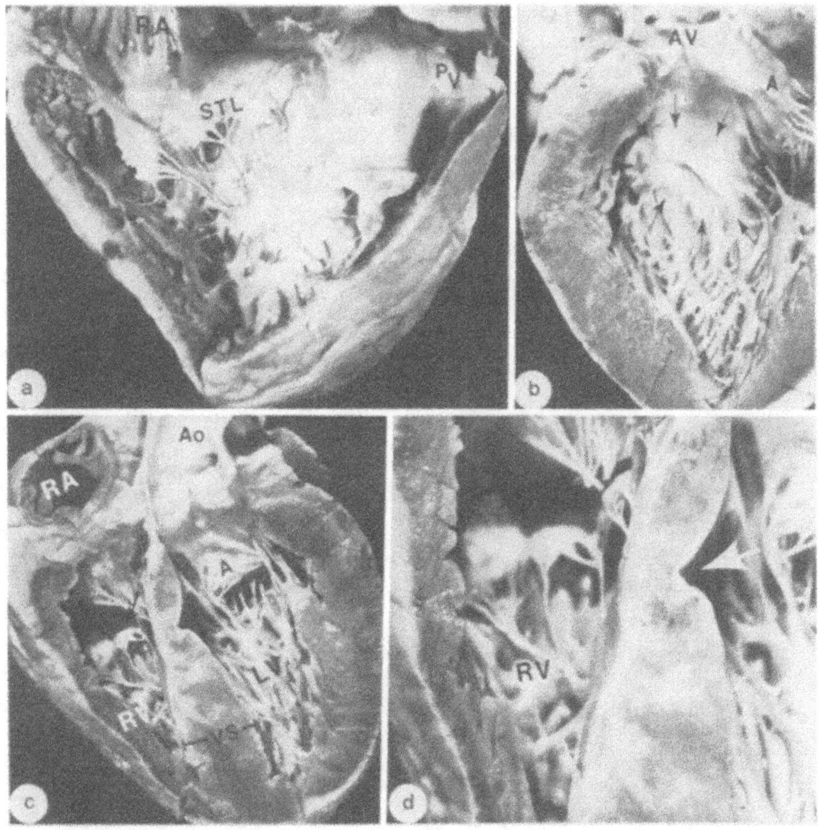

Figure 5. *Heart in a 30 year old black man (73-12-1146) who, three years before his death, was found to have bilateral pulmonary infiltrates. Open biopsy at that time disclosed sarcoidosis. He was asymptomatic until about 12 months before death when he noted occasional palpitations. Seven months before death he had the sudden onset of dyspnea, severe weakness and sweating, and he was found to have supraventricular tachycardia with a ventricular rate of 260 beats/min. Cardioversion restored his rhythm to sinus mechanism. An electrocardiogram shortly thereafter showed complete right bundle branch block, left ventricular hypertrophy and changes suggesting anteroseptal myocardial infarction of indeterminate age. A chest roentgenogram showed bilateral pulmonary infiltrates. Other electrocardiograms during this hospitalization showed atrial, nodal and ventricular premature beats, and periodic nodal tachycardia. Prednisone therapy was started at this time, initially 40 mg daily, and three months before death, 25 mg daily. The supraventricular tachycardia recurred thereafter about once a month until death despite prednisone, procainamide, diphenylhydantoin, and transiently, transvenous pacemaker, therapy. He was found dead in a hotel room while on a trip. At necropsy, the heart weighed 450 g. A small focus of fibrous pericardial adhesions was present posteriorly. The walls of both cardiac ventricles were hypertrophied. The endocardium of the right ventricular aspect of the ventricular septum was white and thick (**a**). RA = right atrium; PV = pulmonic valve; STL = septal tricuspid leaflet. A small indentation surrounded by white thick endocardium (**arrows**) was present on the left ventricular aspect of the ventricular septum (**b**). On longitudinal section (**c**) the cephalad portion of the ventricular septum (VS) was thinned and extensively infiltrated by firm white tissue which histologically was typical of sarcoid. LV = left ventricle; RV = right ventricle; A = anterior mitral leaflet; Ao = aorta. A close-up view of the sarcoid-infiltrated ventricular septum is shown in **d.** The indentation (**arrow**) of the ventricular septum is well shown.*

effusions had recurred over periods of 16 and 18 months, respectively, and both patients had huge cardiac silhouettes on chest roentgenogram. The diagnosis of sarcoidosis was established in each by biopsy of parietal pericardium one and two days, respectively, before death. At open biopsy, each patient had approximately 800 ml of serous pericardial effusion; at necropsy, each had sarcoid granulomas in the parietal pericardium, and both had left ventricular myocardial granulomas. Granulomas in one patient were small and in the second patient, huge.

Morphologic Observations. The weight of the heart in the 26 patients ranged from 310 to 700 g (average 461 g). The average weight among the 17 patients who died suddenly was less than that in the six patients with fatal congestive cardiac failure. Cardiac granulomas were observed grossly in 25 of the 26 hearts, and in the remaining one transmural myocardial scars were present. Sarcoid granulomas were present in the left ventricular free wall of all 25 patients, in the ventricular septum in at least 19 patients, in the right ventricular wall in 12 patients, in the right atrial wall in three patients and in the left atrial wall in two. The granulomas were most extensive in the left ventricular free wall and usually transmural (involving more than half of the thickness of the wall) (Figures 1 through 4). The deposits in the atrial wall were small (<1 cm) in all but one patient (Figure 2), in whom they were extensive in the right

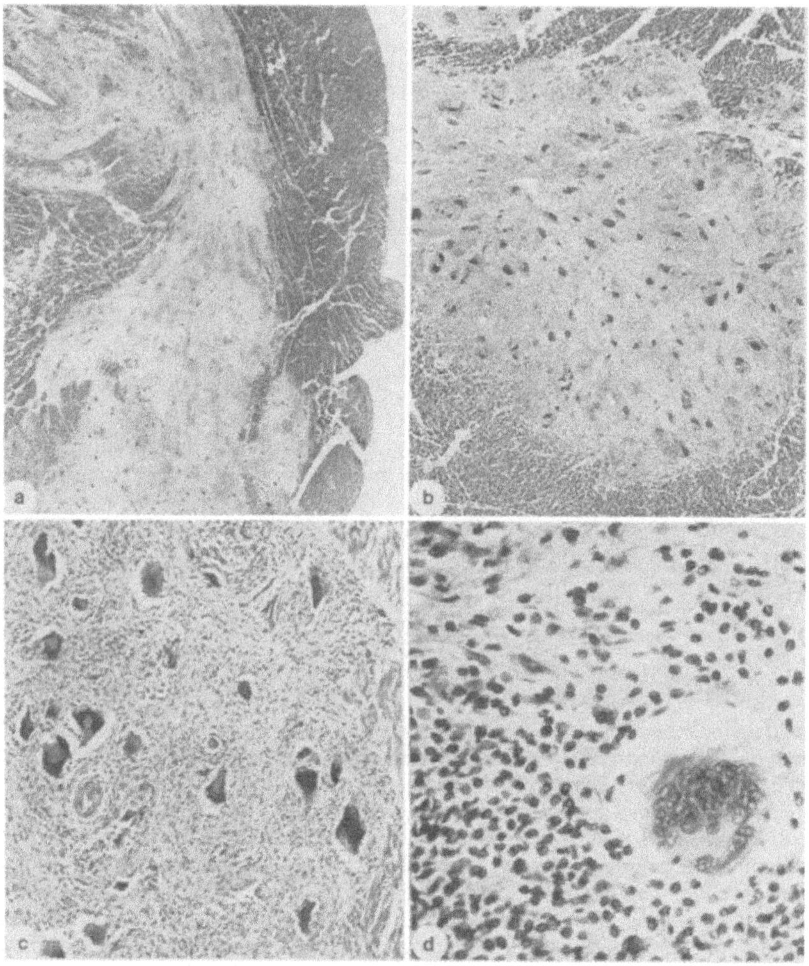

Figure 6. *Extensive, myocardial sarcoid in a 49 year old extremely obese (220 pounds) Indian woman (A-5559) who had been asymptomatic until two months before death when she fainted, and an electrocardiogram showed complete heart block with a ventricular rate of 32 beats/min. A chest roentgenogram disclosed mild cardiomegaly. Thereafter, she became quite dyspneic with only mild exertion. She collapsed while in the bathroom, and resuscitation was unsuccessful. Diagnosis of sarcoidosis was never suspected during life. At necropsy, the heart weighed 430 g. The entire cephalad portion of the ventricular septum, the entire anterolateral papillary muscle and several portions of left ventricular free wall were replaced by sarcoid granulomas.* ***a,*** *low power view of the ventricular septum showing extensive replacement of myocardium by sarcoid.* ***b, c*** *and* ***d,*** *progressive higher power views showing numerous giant cells, mononuclear cells and fibrous tissue. Hematoxylin and eosin stains; original magnification X 11 (**a**), X 35 (**b**), X 130 (**c**) and X 185 (**d**), reduced by 40 per cent.*

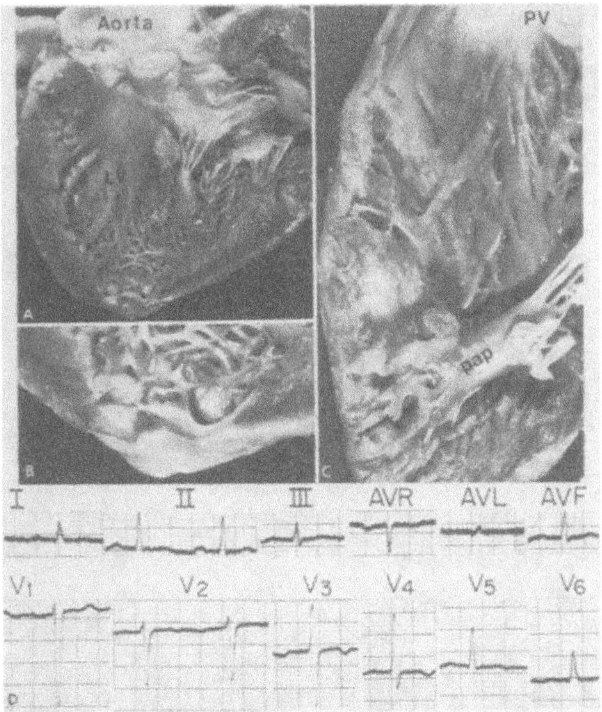

Figure 7. *Heart and electrocardiogram in a 34 year old man (A68-10) who noted swelling in his neck at age 29. Biopsy of the excised lump at age 30 disclosed that it consisted of lymph nodes infiltrated by hard granulomas. A diagnosis of sarcoidosis therefore was made. The liver was within normal limits on biopsy at age 31. A chest roentgenogram showed prominent bilateral hilar adenopathy, and prednisone therapy (10 to 20 mg daily) was begun and continued thereafter until his death. Five months later cryptococcal meningitis developed, but it was eradicated by amphotericin therapy. One year before death marked hypercalcemia developed. About one month before death a high degree of atrioventricular block developed, which at times progressed to complete heart block. The patient died of complications of peptic ulcer perforation. At necropsy the heart weighed 320 g. Both ventricular cavities were mildly dilated. Mural thrombi were present at the apices of both ventricles. The apical left ventricular wall beneath the thrombi was fibrotic; a small area of scarring was present in the basal anterior left ventricular wall, and the anterior right ventricular wall was focally scarred. Histologic study of the scarred areas disclosed some mononuclear cells but no giant cells. The area of the atrioventricular node and bundle was serially sectioned: considerable scarring with some mononuclear cells was present in the conduction tissue, but the node and bundle and proximal bundle branches were not interrupted at any point. Although no granulomas were observed in this patient's heart, it is nevertheless highly likely that the myocardial scars were the result of "healed" sarcoid granulomas. The myocardial scarring, for example, was similar to that observed in the lymph nodes, and the coronary arteries were normal. The healing appears to have been the result of steroid therapy given for three years.* ***A,*** *opened left ventricle (LV). At the apex is a thrombus, better seen in* ***B.*** *The myocardium beneath the thrombus is scarred.* ***C,*** *right ventricular wall shows severe focal scarring. Pap = papillary muscle.* ***D,*** *electrocardiograms recorded three days before death.*

atrium. The granulomas grossly were white and firm. In addition to the left ventricular free wall, granulomas often were observed in the left ventricular papillary muscles (at least 17 patients) (Figures 1, 2 and 3) and in the ventricular septum (at least 19 patients), primarily its cephalad portion (Figures 5 and 6). Of the six patients with complete heart block, five had granulomas in the most cephalad portion of the muscular ventricular septum (Figures 5 and 6), and one had scar tissue in this area (Figure 7). In the one patient in whom serial sections were studied (Figure 5), the atrioventricular bundle and the proximal portions of the right and left bundle branches were partially destroyed by granulomas. In a number of patients, large portions of the left ventricular free wall and ventricular septum were completely replaced by sarcoid granulomas (Figures 2 through 6). The white granulomas usually were visible on the endocardial surface of the left ventricle and, in several patients, they were grossly visible on the epicardial surface. Electron microscopic examination of a sarcoid granuloma in the myocardium was performed in one patient; ultrastructurally, the granulomas were similar to those present in the lungs (Figure 8). In several patients without grossly visible epicardial granulomas, histologic examination of the atrioventricular sulci and epicardium disclosed sarcoid granulomas. In each of the two patients with recurring pericardial effusions, sarcoid granulomas were present in both visceral and parietal pericardia (Figure 9).

Left ventricular aneurysm was present at necropsy in two patients, each of whom had myocardial granulomas. Sudden death was the initial manifestation of sarcoidosis in both patients.

In addition to occurring in the lymph nodes, granulomas consistent with sarcoidosis were present in the lung in 20 patients; in the liver in 18; in the spleen in 18 and in other organs or tissues in 11. The average weight of the liver and spleen was only slightly increased despite the presence of granulomas in these organs. The liver ranged in weight from 1,250 to 2,300 g (average 1,755 g) and the spleen, from 120 to 350 g (average 244 g). The weights of the lungs (together) were usually increased: they ranged from 800 to 1,600 g (average 1,132 g).

Observations in the Patients in Whom Cardiac Dysfunction, if Present, was Not Secondary to Cardiac Sarcoidosis (Group IB). In contrast to the 26 patients described, each of these nine patients had small (microscopic-sized in eight) myocardial sarcoid granulomas (Table III). Four had extensive pulmonary sarcoidosis resulting in cor pulmonale. Three had cardiac dysfunction on the basis of nonsarcoid cardiac conditions: valvular heart disease in two causing pure aortic regurgitation of uncertain etiology in one, and combined mitral and aortic regurgitation in one, presumably rheumatic in origin (this patient underwent mitral valve replacement three months before a fatal cerebral embolus); the third patient, a 50 year old man, had severe coronary atherosclerosis with a documented acute myocardial infarction nine years before his death and congestive cardiac failure probably on that basis. The myocardial granulomas in each of these three patients were minute and visible only by histologic examination. None of these nine patients had arrhythmias or conduction disturbances. None of the five patients without respiratory insufficiency had symptoms or signs definitely attributable to sarcoidosis. The diagnosis of

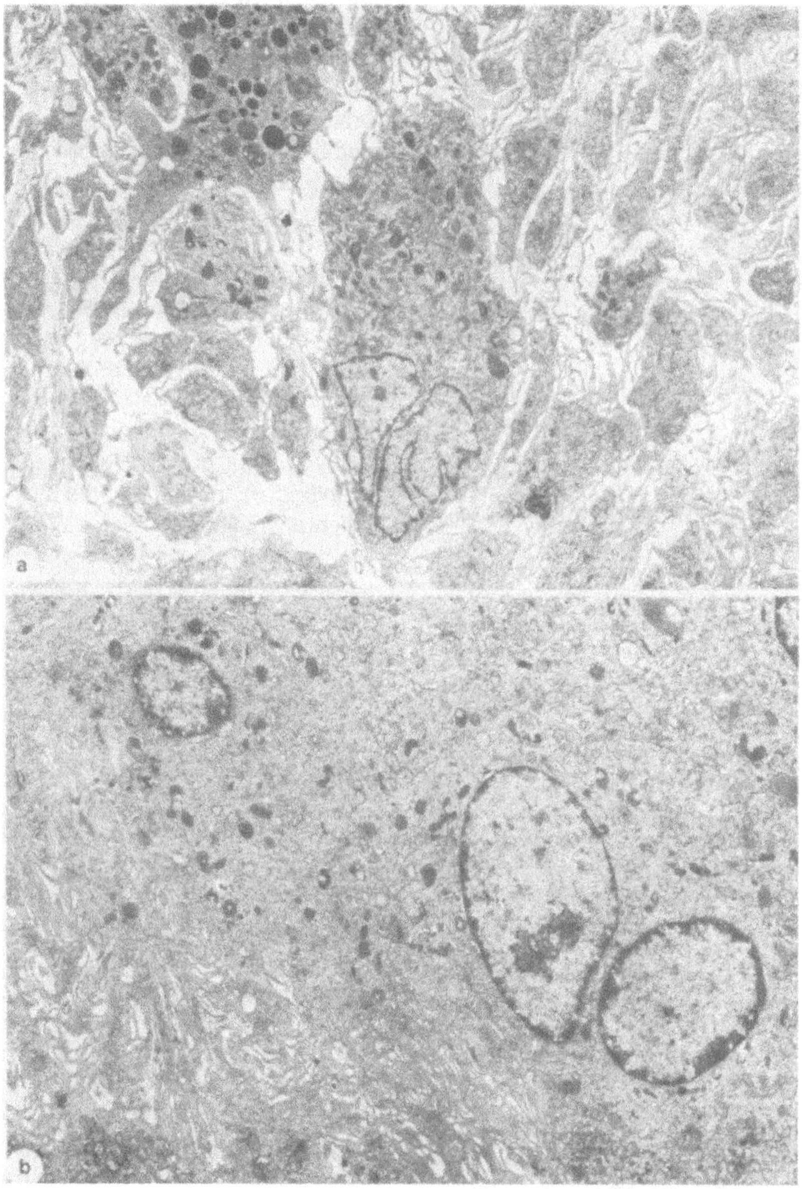

Figure 8. *Electron micrographs of portions of sarcoid granuloma from a biopsy specimen of lung tissue from a 24 year old white man. Similar granulomas were observed ultrastructurally in the myocardium in the one patient examined in the present study, but preservation of the myocardial tissue was not nearly as good as that of the lung biopsy specimen.* ***a,*** *in this electron micrograph an epithelioid cell is present in the central area; it has a multilobulated nucleus and numerous cytoplasmic dense bodies. The surface of this cell is highly irregular, with many flap- and pocket-like projections. Similar projections are present on the surfaces of adjacent cells. A macrophage-like cell is present at the upper left; it contains many large dense bodies.* ***b,*** *portion of multinucleated giant cell (same tissue as in* ***a****) showing parts of 4 nuclei and moderate numbers of dense bodies, mitochondria and cisterns of endoplasmic reticulum. The surface of this cell (lower left) is highly convoluted with complex, interdigitating folds. Original magnification × 6,000 (**a**) and × 7,500 (**b**), reduced by 38 per cent.*

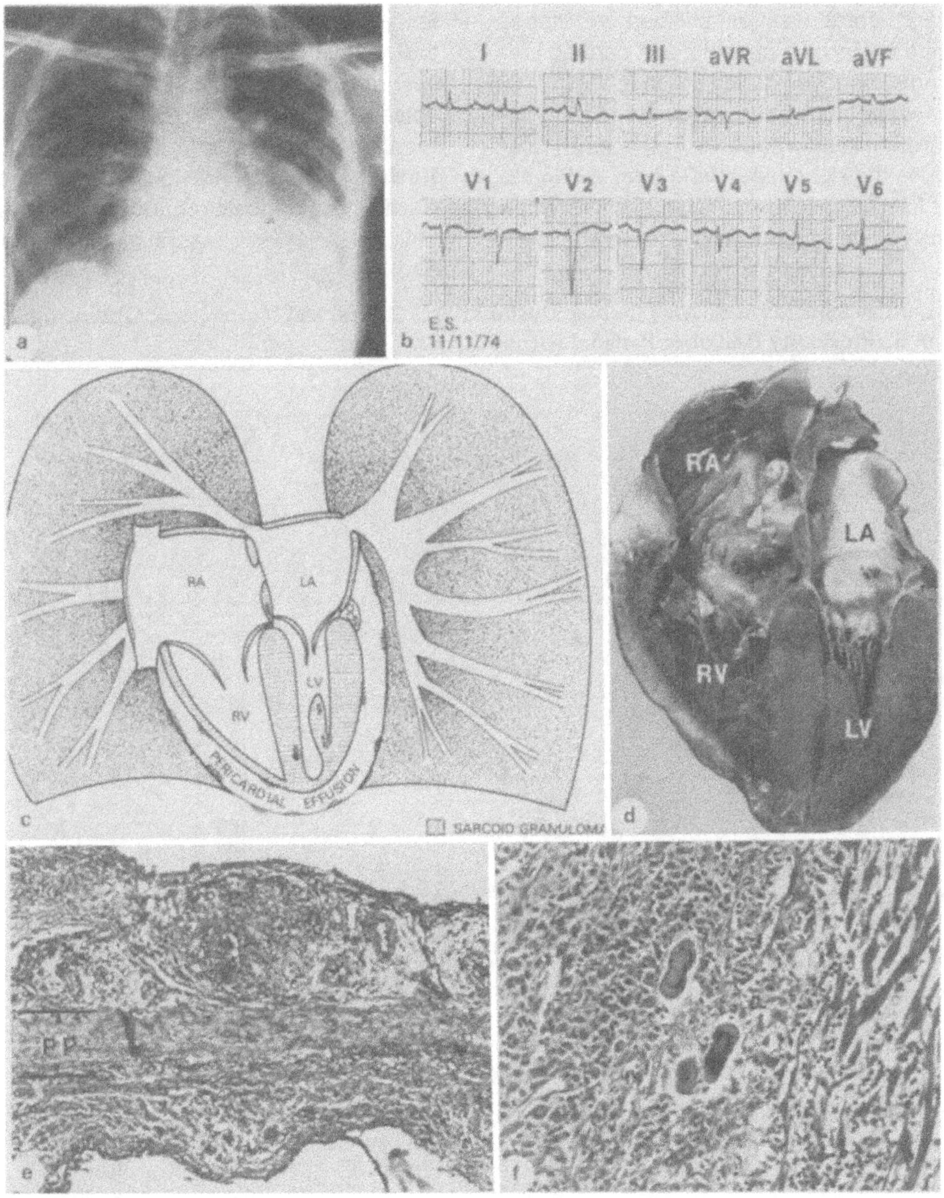

Figure 9. *Chest roentgenogram, electrocardiogram, diagram of heart and lungs, longitudinal cut of heart, and photomicrographs of parietal pericardium and left ventricular papillary muscle in a 47 year old black woman (74-A-223) who was well until 15 months before death when she noted exertional dyspnea, cough and retrosternal chest pain. Hospitalization a month later disclosed distended neck veins, a pericardial friction rub and bilateral pulmonary rales. A chest roentgenogram showed pulmonary "congestion" and mild cardiomegaly. A right-sided cardiac angiogram disclosed a large pericardial effusion. During her four month period in the hospital, infiltrates appeared in the lower lobes of both lungs, but a definite diagnosis was not made. During the next 10 months, she had only dyspnea on severe exertion and an occasional nonproductive cough. A week before death, she had the sudden appearance of severe dyspnea. Physical examination disclosed pulsus paradoxicus (12 mm Hg), distended neck veins and hepatosplenomegaly; roentgenography (**a**) disclosed bilateral pleural effusions, a large cardiac silhouette and interstitial pulmonary infiltrates. An electrocardiogram (**b**) showed low voltage and sinus tachycardia. An echocardiogram showed an echo-free space behind the posterior left ventricular wall. The pulmonary arterial pressure was 30/10 (mean 15) mm Hg. At open thoracotomy (for diagnostic purposes), 800 ml of straw-colored fluid was found in the pericardial sac (protein content = 2.5 g/100 ml; glucose = 105 mg/100 ml). The patient died three days later from progressive "respiratory insufficiency." At necropsy, many sarcoid granulomas were found in both lungs (**c**), hilar lymph nodes, liver and spleen. The parietal pericardium was thickened and contained many sarcoid granulomas (**e**). No lesions were noted on gross examination of the myocardium (**d**), but histologic study did disclose several sarcoid granulomas in the left ventricular free wall and papillary muscles. Granulomas also were present in the epicardium (**c**). The thickness of the normal parietal pericardium (PP) is shown in (**e**). Hematoxylin and eosin stains; original magnification × 85 (**e**) and × 220 (**f**), reduced by 38 per cent.*

noncardiac sarcoidosis was established by biopsy during life in five of the nine patients, and cardiac sarcoidosis was not diagnosed during life in any.

Granulomas were found at necropsy in the left ventricular myocardium in nine patients, in the ventricular septum in two, in the right ventricle in five, and in the atrium in none. In addition to their being present in lymph nodes in all nine patients, granulomas also were present in the lungs in eight, the liver in nine, the spleen in eight and in other organs or tissues in six. The weights of the liver ranged from 830 to 2,600 g (average 1,907 g); the spleen, from 70 to 400 g (average 211 g); and the lungs together, from 760 to 2,800 g (average 1,336 g).

Review of Data on Previously Described Patients with Cardiac Sarcoidosis (Group II). At least 78 necropsy patients have been described with sarcoid granulomas

TABLE IV Cardiac Sarcoidosis Causing Cardiac Dysfunction: Clinical and Morphologic Observations in 63 Previously Described Patients (Group IIA)

Data	Mode of Death: Sudden	Congestive Heart Failure	Pericardial Effusion	Non-cardiac	Uncertain	Totals
Patients (no.)	43	14	1	1	4	63
References	[1–34]	[10, 33, 35–44]	[47]	[2]	[48–54]	[1–51]
Age (yr)						
Range	18–76	24–67	27	42	18–38	18–76
Average	43	33	27	42	27	40
Race						
Black	13	10	1	1	2	27 (43)
White	14	2	0	0	1	17 (27)
Unknown or other	16	2	0	0	1	19 (30)
Sex						
Male	18*	9	0	1	2	30/62 (48)
Female	24*	5	1	0	2	32/62 (52)
Duration of symptoms (mo)						
Range	0–180	25–72	60	108	2–12	0–180
Average	27†	29§	60	108	7	28
Atrial arrhythmia	5	4	0	. . .	2	11 (17)
Ventricular premature beats	12	5	1	. . .	3	21 (33)
Ventricular tachycardia	8	4	0	. . .	1	13 (21)
Complete heart block	16	0	0	1	2	19 (30)
Syncope	14	1	0	1	1	17 (27)
Left bundle branch block	2	1	0	. . .	1	4 }
Right bundle branch block	8	2	0	. . .	1	11 } (32)
Indeterminate bundle block	3	1	0	. . .	1	5 }
Congestive heart failure	10	14	1	. . .	2	27 (43)
Diagnosis of sarcoid in life	10	5	0	. . .	1	16 (25)
Corticosteroid therapy	8	3	0	0	1	12 (19)
Heart weight (g)						
Range	225–640	320–660	745	. . .	300–450	225–745
Average	439‡	549§	745	. . .	385¶	476
Cardiac granulomas						
Left ventricle	28/30	9/9	1	0	2/2	40/41 (98)
Ventricular septum	27/30	4/9	1	0	1/2	33/41 (80)
Right ventricle	10/30	5/9	1	0	0/2	16/41 (39)
Papillary muscle	10/30	2/9	. . .	0	0/2	12/41 (29)
Atria	9/30	2/9	1	0	0/2	12/41 (29)
None	2	1	0	1	0	4 (6)
Ventricular aneurysm	4	2	0	0	0	6 (15)
Cardiac mural thrombi	0	4	0	0	0	4 (10)
Noncardiac granulomas						
Lymph node	41/41	12/12	1	1	4	59/59 (100)
Lung	35/41	9/12	1	0	4	49/59 (83)
Liver	22/41	8/12	1	0	4	35/59 (59)
Spleen	20/41	7/12	0	0	3	30/59 (51)
Other	9/41	6/12	1	0	1	17/59 (29)

* Sex not stated in one patient.

† Information from 30 patients; average includes four patients whose initial manifestation of sarcoidosis was sudden death. The average in the 26 patients with symptoms was 32 months.

‡ Eighteen patients.

§ Ten patients.

¶ Two patients.

(75 patients) or nonischemic myocardial scars, i.e., healed granulomas (three patients), in their hearts and sarcoid granulomas in at least one other body organ (Tables III and IV). The 78 patients were subdivided into two groups: (1) 63 patients with cardiac dysfunction resulting from extensive cardiac sarcoidosis (group IIA) [1–51] (Table IV) and (2) 15 patients with minute cardiac granulomas and either no (12 patients) cardiac dysfunction [51–62] or cardiac dysfunction (three patients) [22,63,64] not on the basis of cardiac sarcoidosis (group IIB) (Table III). Observations in these two groups of previously described cases are added to those in the personally studied patients and summarized in Table V.

Analysis of these 63 patients (group IIA, Table III) indicates that 43 died suddenly [1–34], 14 from progressive congestive cardiac failure [10,33,35–46], one from recurring pericardial effusion [47], one from noncardiac (suicide) [2] and four from unknown causes [48–51]. Sudden death was the initial manifestation of sarcoidosis in four of the 43 patients who died suddenly [4,6,12,27]; in the other 39 patients, symptoms were present from five days to 180 months (average 27 months). Electrocardiograms, obtained in 53 of the 63 patients, disclosed atrial **arrhythmias** in 11 [5,25–27,31,33,36,42,46,48,51], **ventricular premature beats** in 19 [7,12,16–18,20,27,28,31,34,35,37,40,45,46,49–51], **ventricular tachycardia** in 12 [10,17,27–29,32–35,37,39,40], **complete heart block** in 19 [2,7,11,13–16,20–24,30,31,49,50], second degree heart block in four [14,24,25,47], prolonged (>0.20 sec) P-R interval in five [18,27,36,40,46] and **complete bundle branch block** in 18 (left = three, right = 11, indeterminate = four) [5,7,11,14,16,18–20,25,26,31,33,36,41,46,51]. None of the 19 patients with complete heart block had ventricular tachycardia. Clinical evidence of **congestive cardiac failure** was present in 26 (50 per cent) [7,10,17,19,23,25–27,29,32,33,35–46,48,51] of the 52 patients in whom it was mentioned. The diagnosis of sarcoidosis was established during life in only 16 (25 per cent) of the 63 patients [3,10,14–16,22,27,29,31,34,37,38,40,44,46,51]. Twelve of the 63 patients received corticosteroid therapy at some time [15,19,20,22,27–29,34,44–46,51].

At necropsy, the **cardiac weight,** available in 31 of the 63 patients, ranged from 225 to 745 g (average 476 g). Although granulomas were present in "the heart" or "myocardium" of 60 patients, the **specific chambers involved** were mentioned in 44 patients: the left ventricle in 40 (91 per cent), the ventricular septum in 33 (75 per cent), the right ventricle in 16 (36 per cent) and

TABLE V Cardiac Sarcoidosis: Summary of Personally Studied and Previously Described Patients

Data	Causing Cardiac Dysfunction (Groups IA and IIA)	Not Causing Cardiac Dysfunction (Groups 1B and IIB)
Patients (no.)	89	24
Age (yr)		
Range	18–76	28–83
Average	40	45
Race		
Black	41	9
White	27	10
Unknown	0	3
Sex		
Male	45	16
Female	44	5
Unknown	0	3
Symptoms (mo)		
Range	0–180	0–96
Average	22	46
Syncope	20 (22)	0
Congestive heart failure	35 (39)	6 (25)
Atrial arrhythmia	15 (17)	1 (4)
Ventricular premature beats	33 (37)	1 (4)
Ventricular tachycardia	19 (21)	0
Complete heart block	25 (28)	0
Complete bundle branch block	23 (26)	2 (8)
Diagnosis of sarcoid in life	24 (27)	15 (62)
Corticosteroid treatment	15 (17)	3 (12)
Ventricular aneurysm	8 (9)	0
Intracardiac thrombi	5 (6)	0

NOTE: Figures in parentheses are per cents.

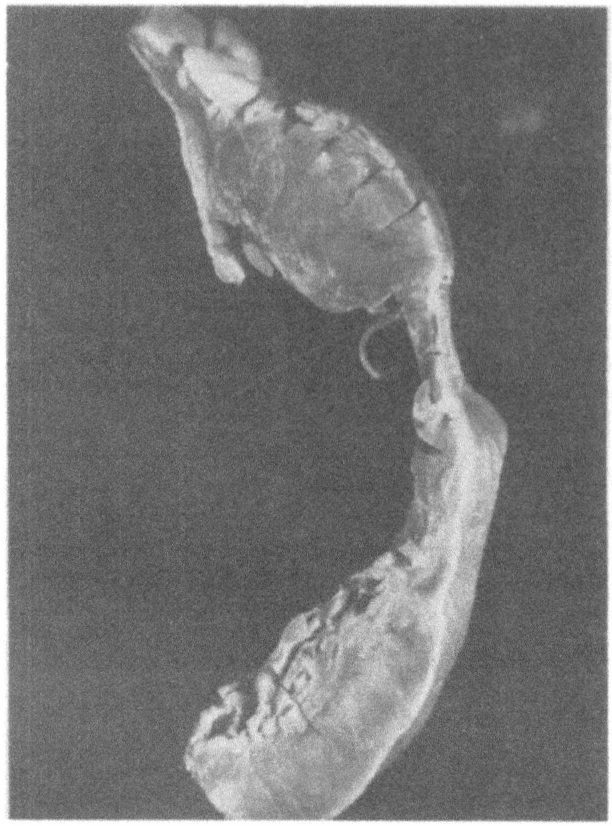

Figure 10. *Longitudinal section of left ventricular free wall showing an area of thinning which during life resulted in an aneurysm. This 49 year old black woman (A72-144), reported earlier by Chun and associates [34] and also examined by one of us (WCR), had 20 episodes of ventricular tachycardia during a 38-month period. She was treated with prednisone most of that time. She died suddenly. At necropsy, the wall of the left ventricular aneurysm consisted entirely of fibrous tissue and the coronary arteries were normal. No sarcoid granulomas were present in the heart but they were present in lymph nodes, spleen, liver and bone marrow. The heart weighed 470 g. It is believed that sarcoid granulomas were present in the heart at one time but that the prednisone therapy caused their healing with development of the above illustrated aneurysm.*

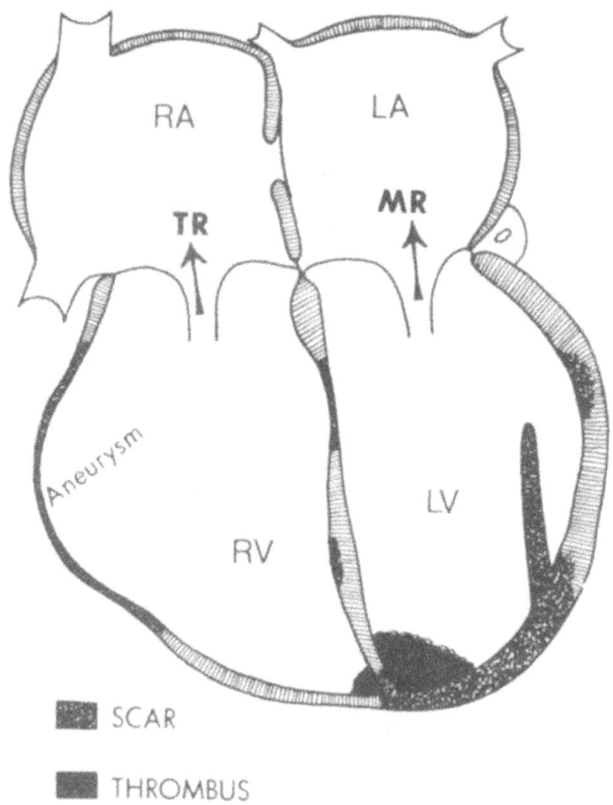

Figure 11. *Diagram of heart in a 37 year old white man (BIH A74-275) who was described in a New England Journal of Medicine CPC by Harthorne and Freiman [46]. (The heart was examined by one of us [WCR] through the courtesy of Walter H. Abelmann and David G. Freiman.) This case is of particular importance because the patient's course was eight years. During this period he had multiple arrhythmias, bilateral bundle branch block with prolongation of the P-R interval, systemic emboli, and progressive cardiomegaly, so that by necropsy both ventricles were enormously dilated and the right ventricular wall, so thinned that it was aneurysmal. Scars also were present in the left ventricular free wall and ventricular septum but no granulomas were present in the heart. Indeed, although sarcoid granulomas had been present in lymph nodes in an earlier biopsy, at necropsy no sarcoid granulomas were present in any organ. It is believed that corticosteroid therapy (two years) contributed to the disappearance of the granulomas. His heart at necropsy was very similar to the typical heart of idiopathic cardiomyopathy of the ventricular dilated type except for the presence of the healed granulomas (scars).*

the atrium in 12 (right atrium in eight, left atrium in seven and unspecified in one) (27 per cent). In at least 12 patients [1,3–6,10,12,14,18,32,40,43] sarcoid granulomas were stated to be present in one or more papillary muscles. The cardiac granulomas were visible grossly in all patients. One or more **ventricular aneurysms** were present in six patients [19,29,33,34,44,46] (Figures 10 and 11), and intracardiac thrombi in four patients [10,35,42,46] (Figure 11), all of whom had congestive cardiac failure. The specific location of sarcoid granulomas in organs other than the heart was described in 59 patients: lymph nodes in 59 (100 per cent); lung in 49 (83 per cent); liver in 35 (59 per cent); spleen in 31 (53 per cent) and other organs in 17 (29 per cent).

Observations in the previously described 15 patients in whom cardiac dysfunction, if present, was not secondary to cardiac sarcoidosis (group IIB) are summarized in Table II [22,51–64]. In contrast to the patients in group IIA, men were more numerous than women (12:3), the duration of symptoms was longer (average 38 months), arrhythmias and conduction defects were infrequent, the diagnosis of sarcoidosis was made in life in 10 of the 15 patients, and one patient died suddenly. The heart weights, available in 10 patients, were normal in seven and increased in the three patients with cardiac dysfunction from valvular disease of nonsarcoid origin. The cardiac sarcoid granulomas were minute in all 15 patients and usually visible only by histologic examination. Other body organs involved by sarcoid included the lymph nodes in all 15 patients, the lung in 12, the liver in nine, the spleen in 10 and other body organs or tissues in six.

COMMENTS

Study of our 35 patients (group I) and the 78 previously described necropsy patients (group II) allows certain general conclusions regarding cardiac sarcoidosis, and these items will be discussed in the following order: (1) the portions of the heart involved anatomically by sarcoid granulomas; (2) the determinants of whether or not cardiac sarcoidosis causes cardiac dysfunction; (3) the clinical types of cardiac dysfunction and their probable anatomic explanations; (4) the determinants of whether or not cardiac dysfunction from cardiac sarcoidosis is diagnosed clincally; (5) the modes of death and length of illness; (6) the effect of corticosteroid therapy on cardiac sarcoid granulomas and (7) the differences between cardiac sarcoidosis and idiopathic granulomatous (giant cell) myocarditis.

No portion of the heart is immune to infiltration by sarcoid granulomas. The granulomas may involve the pericardium, myocardium and endocardium, but of the three, the myocardium is, by far, the one most frequently involved. The portion of myocardium most frequently involved by sarcoid granulomas is the left ventricular free wall, followed by the ventricular septum, the right ventricle and, lastly, the atrial wall. Why the left ventricular free wall is the one most frequently involved and the atrial wall the one least frequently involved is uncertain, but the explanation may simply be that the largest fraction of the total myocardial mass is in the left ventricle, including the ventricular septum, and the smallest fraction is in the atrium. (Interestingly, the left ventricular wall also is the most frequent portion of myocardium invaded by secondary neoplasms of the heart [65–67].) Sarcoid granulomas within the left ventricle appear to be most common in the papillary muscles and in the free walls immediately beneath them. The cephalad half of the ventricular septum is more often involved than the caudal half. It is probable that the left ventricular papillary muscles and the cephalad portion of the ventricular septum are the preferential locations in the heart for sarcoid granulomas, but since these sites often are not incised at necropsy small granulomas in these locations may be missed. Thus, it is possible that the frequency of cardiac involvement by granulomas in patients with sarcoidosis may be higher than generally appreciated because of inadequate examination of these two structures.

Involvement of the epicardium (visceral pericardium) and mural endocardium by granulomas usually represents an extension of the myocardial involvement into these layers of the heart. None of our patients or those previously described had epicardial or mural endocardial involvement without concomitant myocardial sarcoid granulomas. The occurrence of sarcoid granulomas in the adipose tissue adjacent to the coronary arteries, particularly the atrioventricular sulci, however, is unusual, whereas this portion of the heart is the area most frequently invaded by metastatic neoplasm [65–67]. Although their occurrence on the mediastinal aspect of the parietal pericardium is common, the occurrence of sarcoid granulomas on the cardiac (serous) aspect of the parietal pericardium is unusual. Such an occurrence, however, was observed in each of our two patients with recurring pericardial effusions. Rarely, valvular endocardium may contain sarcoid granulomas: in one of our 35 patients these granulomas were present on the pulmonic valve cusps, but they were not of sufficient size to cause valvular malfunction. Sarcoid involvement of the tricuspid valve has also been reported [39].

Whether or not cardiac dysfunction occurs as a consequence of cardiac sarcoidosis is dependent on at least three factors: (1) the number of sarcoid granulomas in the heart, i.e., the amount of ventricular myocardium replaced by granulomas versus the amount of uninvolved ventricular myocardium; (2) the amount of ventricular wall scarring, i.e., the amount of ventricular myocardium replaced by scar versus the amount of uninvolved ventricular myocardium, and (3) the location of the granulomas or scars within the heart. Of our 26 patients in whom cardiac dysfunction resulted from cardiac sarcoid (Table I), 23 had large, granulomas or scars on the left ventricular wall: two had recurring pericardial effusions and sarcoid granulomas in the pericardium, and one had a scar in the most cephalad portion of ventricular septum resulting in complete heart block. The amount of myocardium replaced by sarcoid granulomas was minute in each of our nine patients who had cardiac sarcoidosis and no cardiac dysfunction as a result of the cardiac granulomas (Table II). Indeed, in eight of these nine patients the cardiac granulomas were observed only by histologic examination. This also was the situation in the 15 patients described by others as having cardiac sarcoidosis but no cardiac dysfunction as a result of that infiltration (Table II).

The types of cardiac dysfunction produced by cardiac sarcoidosis include: (1) arrhythmias, primarily ventricular ones; (2) high degrees of atrioventricular block and complete bundle branch block; (3) sudden death; (4) congestive cardiac failure; (5) papillary muscle dysfunction; (6) "acute myocardial infarction"; (7) ventricular aneurysm and (8) recurring pericardial effusion.

Other than premature ventricular beats, ventricular tachycardia was the most frequent major arrhythmia, occurring in at least six (23 per cent) of our 26 patients (group IA) and in at least 12 (19 per cent) of 63 previously described patients with cardiac dysfunction resulting from cardiac sarcoidosis (group IIA). The occurrence of ventricular tachycardia in these patients usually indicates extensive sarcoid granulomatous involvement of the heart or extensive scarring as a result of healing of the granulomas. Atrial arrhythmias, present in four (15 per cent) patients in group IA and in 11 (17 per cent) of the 63 patients in group IIA did not appear to be direct consequences of cardiac sarcoidosis because only two of the 15 patients with atrial arrhythmias had sarcoid granulomas in the atrial walls at necropsy. The atrial arrhythmias more likely were consequences of atrial dilatation arising as a result of the ventricular malfunction.

Severe conduction disturbances also were common. Complete heart block was documented in six (23 per cent) patients in group IA and in 19 (30 per cent) of the 63 patients in group IIA. Of the 25 patients with complete heart block, 17 (68 per cent) also had episodes of syncope (Stokes-Adams attacks). In each of our five patients and in most if not all of the 19 previously described patients with complete heart block, the cephalad portion of the muscular ventricular septum, and especially that portion in the vicinity of the atrioventricular bundle, was extensively infiltrated by sarcoid granulomas or, in one patient, by scar tissue. In our one patient with complete heart block in whom serial histologic sections of the atrioventricular node and bundle were examined, partial destruction of the atrioventricular bundle and complete disruption of the bundle branches from their origin were observed. Similar observations have been made by Morales and associates [33]. Thus, complete heart block in these patients appears to result from interruption of the conduction pathways by either sarcoid granuloma or scar or both.

Complete bundle branch block also was common. It occurred in three (12 per cent) of our patients (group IA) and in 20 (32 per cent) of the patients in group IIA. The bundle branch block was right in 13, left in five and indeterminate in five. The patients with bundle branch block also had either granulomas or scars in the cephalad portion of the ventricular septum, but the amount of granulomatous or scar tissue appeared to be less extensive than that in patients with complete heart block.

Sudden death is the most common cardiac manifestation of clinically significant cardiac sarcoidosis. It occurred in 17 (65 per cent) of the patients in group IA and in 43 (68 per cent) of the patients in group IIA. That the sudden death in these 60 patients was of cardiac origin cannot be unequivocally proved, but many had had preceding arrhythmias or complete heart block, and ventricular fibrillation was confirmed terminally in several of them. Thus, sarcoidosis is an important but neglected cause of sudden cardiac death. Sudden death may be the initial manifestation of sarcoidosis. This was the case in six (35 per cent) of our 17 patients who died suddenly and in four (9 per cent) of the 43 previously described patients who died suddenly. Among these 10 patients (age range, 18 to 53 years [average 31]), death occurred during exertion in eight, and, although none had had symptoms, one had had ventricular premature beats documented by electrocardiogram. Of the remaining 50 patients who died suddenly, complete heart block had been present in 20 (40 per cent), ventricular tachycardia in 12 (24 per cent), ventricular premature beats in 11 (22 per cent) and atrial arrhythmias in seven (14 per cent). Of the 50 patients who died suddenly (excluding the 10 in whom sudden death was the initial manifestation of sarcoidosis), either complete heart block or a ventricular arrhythmia had been documented by electrocardiogram in 38 (76 per cent); of the remaining 12 patients, four had atrial arrhythmias, one had complete right bundle branch block, and seven never had an electrocardiogram recorded. Thus, ventricular arrhythmias and complete heart block are bad omens in patients with sarcoidosis.

Congestive cardiac failure is another common form of cardiac dysfunction in patients with extensive cardiac

TABLE VI Cardiac Sarcoidosis: Cardiac Aneurysm

Case No.	Reference	Age (yr)	Sex	Precordial Murmur	CHF	CHB	VT	SD	Length of Illness (mo)	CS Rx	Length of CS Rx (mo)	Site of Aneurysm RV	Site of Aneurysm LV	Myocardial Granuloma	Myocardial Transmural Scarring	Heart Weight (g)
1	Hines, Sancetta [19]	44	F	+	+	0	0	+	17	+	3	+	+	0	+	465
2	Duvernoy, Garcia [29]	30	F	+	+	0	+	+	30	+	—	0	+	+	—	—
3	Morales et al. [33]	41	M	—	—	0	0	+	—	—	—	0	+	+	—	—
4	Chun et al. [34]	49	F	+	—	0	+	+	38	+	30	0	+	0	+	470
5	Clark, Blount [44]	28	M	+	+	0	0	0	12	+	—	+	0	+	+	650
6	Freiman [46]	37	M	+	+	0	0	0	96	+	24	+	0	0	+	700
7	Present study	21	M	—	0	—	—	+	0	0	—	0	+	+	0	400
8	Present study	41	F	—	0	—	—	+	0	0	—	0	+	+	0	300

NOTE: 0 = absent; + = present; — = no information available; CHB = complete heart block; CHF = congestive heart failure; CS Rx = corticosteroid treatment; LV = left ventricle; RV = right ventricle; SD = sudden death; VT = ventricular tachycardia.

sarcoidosis. It occurred in eight (31 per cent) (fatal in six) of the patients in group IA and in 27 (43 per cent) (fatal in 14) of the patients in group IIA. With rare exception these 35 patients with congestive cardiac failure had extensive granulomas or scars in the left ventricular free wall, with or without similar involvement of the ventricular septum. The patients with congestive failure, however, had varying clinical features. In some, consequences of complete heart block or ventricular tachycardia dominated the clinical course and the failure was episodic. Most patients, however, had chronic failure.

Precordial systolic murmurs may be consequences of cardiac sarcoidosis. They were noted in four (15 per cent) of the patients in group IA and in 12 (19 per cent) [10,16,17,19,29,32,34,37,43,46,50] of the patients in group IIA. The murmurs usually were apical in location and varied from grade 1 to 5 (on a scale of 6) in intensity. Cardiac catheterization was performed in five patients [19,29,34,43,46] with precordial murmurs; in each of the four patients [19,29,43,46] in whom pulmonary arterial pressures were recorded, mild to moderate pulmonary hypertension was present and in one [43] the pulmonary arterial wedge pressure was greatly increased (v waves to 66 mm Hg). The cause of the murmurs in most of the 16 patients is unclear, but papillary muscle dysfunction is the most likely explanation. Although sarcoid granulomas in papillary muscle were described at necropsy in 29 (33 per cent) of the 89 patients in group IIA (no mention of papillary muscle in at least 27 patients) with cardiac dysfunction from cardiac sarcoidosis, precordial murmurs had been recorded in only six of them. Conversely, of the 16 patients with precordial murmurs, in only six (38 per cent) were sarcoid granulomas noted in their left ventricular papillary muscles at necropsy. Thus, although sarcoid infiltration into one or both left ventricular papillary muscles and into the free walls beneath them may produce papillary muscle dysfunction with mitral regurgitation, more often, the presence of a precordial murmur in these patients is not indicative of sarcoid in these structures. More often, the murmurs appear to result from altered papillary muscle dynamics due to dilatation of the left ventricle.

Ventricular aneurysm may be a consequence of cardiac sarcoidosis. A ventricular aneurysm occurred in two (8 per cent) of the patients in group IA and in six (10 per cent) of the patients in group IIA (Table VI). The aneurysm may involve either or both ventricular walls; it may be discrete and relatively small in the left ventricle, as illustrated by the patient described by Chun and associates [34] (Figure 10), or it may be diffuse and involve a large portion of the right ventricular wall, as occurred in the patient described by Freiman [46] (Figure 11) and in the patient described by Clark and

Blount [44]. Scarring or thinning of the ventricular septum may be associated with protrusion of the septum toward the right ventricle, producing, in effect, an internal cardiac aneurysm. Such was the probable case in the patient described by Hines and Sancetta [19]. The aneurysmal wall may or may not contain sarcoid granulomas: of the eight patients with ventricular aneurysms from cardiac sarcoidosis whose data are summarized in Table III, five had residual granulomas in the heart and three had none. In each of the latter three patients, the aneurysmal wall consisted entirely of fibrous tissue. The dominant component of the aneurysmal wall, however, in the other five patients also appears to have been fibrous tissue. The myocardial scarring and aneurysmal formation in these patients may have been related in part to the administration of corticosteroids. Of the 89 patients in groups IA and IIA, only nine (seven previously described [15,19,22,27,29,34,46]) had received corticosteroid therapy for longer than one month, and five of these nine patients were among the eight with ventricular aneurysms. The eight patients with ventricular aneurysms were young (range 21 to 49 years [average 36 years]). In only one [29] was the presence of a ventricular aneurysm recognized during life (by left ventricular angiography). Six of the eight patients died suddenly, and in two sudden death was the initial manifestation of sarcoidosis; the other two patients died of progressive congestive cardiac failure, and it is likely that their ventricular aneurysms contributed to, or were responsible for, the congestive failure. None of the eight patients had significant coronary arterial luminal narrowing. The occurrence of either right or left ventricular aneurysm in the absence of significant coronary arterial luminal narrowing is quite suggestive of cardiac sarcoidosis (which may or may not have "healed").

Excision of a left ventricular aneurysm of sarcoid origin at times may be beneficial. Lull and associates [68] described such an aneurysm, "the size of a tennis ball," which was resected in a 22 year old man with evidence of sarcoidosis for five months. Preoperatively, the patient had had episodes of ventricular tachycardia unresponsive to therapy with corticosteroids or antiarrhythmic agents. After aneurysmectomy, the ventricular arrhythmia, at the time of the report, was "no longer a problem." Although histologic examination of the wall of the resected aneurysm disclosed mainly fibrous tissue, a few sarcoid-type granulomas were present.

Although an effusion into a body cavity is an unusual feature of sarcoidosis, recurring pericardial effusion on occasion may be a prominent clinical manifestation of cardiac sarcoidosis. Such was the case in two (8 per cent) of the patients in group IA and in one (2 per cent) [47] patient in group IIA. A living patient with recurrent pericardial effusion secondary to pericardial sarcoidosis also was described by Shiff and associates [69]. This patient, a 31 year old woman, had a 1,000 ml serous effusion and multiple sarcoid granulomas on the epicardium. A possibly similar patient was described by Bailey [70]. The three necropsy patients were 27, 35 and 47 years of age, respectively, and two were women. Each had huge cardiac silhouettes typical of pericardial effusion. Two underwent thoracotomy shortly before death because of cardiac tamponade from large (800 ml each) pericardial effusions. At necropsy two of the three patients also had severe pulmonary sarcoidosis with considerable right ventricular hypertrophy, but the third had no sarcoid granulomas in the lung. Pericardial adhesions were present in one patient. All three had epicardial sarcoid granulomas; in addition, two had large and one had minute myocardial granulomas. Marked dilatation of both ventricles secondary to active or healed myocardial sarcoidosis may produce a "water-bottle" configuration of the cardiac silhouette on chest roentgenogram and mimic a large pericardial effusion. This situation occurred in the patient described by Clark and Blount [44]. Their patient proved to have only a small pericardial effusion but aneurysmal dilatation of both cardiac ventricles.

Because of its ability to cause arrhythmias, conduction disturbances, precordial murmurs, huge cardiac silhouettes, ventricular aneurysm and electrocardiographic evidence of "myocardial damage," cardiac sarcoidosis may mimic other cardiac conditions. In at least eight (31 per cent) of the patients in group IA and in five (8 per cent) [9,18,19,25,36] of the patients in group IIA, the initial clinical diagnosis was "acute myocardial infarction." The myocardial damage evident on the electrocardiogram may be the consequence of a sudden arrhythmia or complete heart block, or it may result entirely from the replacement of myocardium by sarcoid granulomas. Chest pain simulating acute myocardial infarction also was described in a patient described by Stephen [9] and in another described by Forbes and Usher [18]. Electrocardiograms were not diagnostic of, but compatible with, acute myocardial infarction in both patients; if necropsy had not been performed, coronary heart disease would have remained their diagnosis. Papillary muscle dysfunction in cardiac sarcoidosis may mimic valvular heart disease. The presentation of features of congestive cardiac failure associated with a large cardiac silhouette obviously may mimic idiopathic dilated cardiomyopathy [71] as well as pericardial effusion. The occurrence of very dilated ventricular cavities, particularly when associated with intracardiac thrombi, may even suggest this diagnosis at necropsy. Five of the 89 analyzed patients with cardiac dysfunction from cardiac sarcoidosis (groups IA and IIA) had intracardiac thrombi at

TABLE VII Cardiac Sarcoidosis: Effect of Corticosteroid Therapy on the Cardiac Granulomas

Case No.	Reference	Age (yr)	Sex	VT	CHB	CHF	Length of Illness (mo)	Length of CS Rx (mo)	SD	Cardiac Granulomas LV	VS	RV	Atria	Heart Weight (g)	No. of Cardiac Granulomas	Cardiac Aneurysm RV	LV
1	Porter [15]	19	M	0	+	0	24	7	+	+	+	+	—	—	—	0	0
2	Hines, Sancetta [19]	44	F	0	0	+	17	3	+	0	0	0	0	465	Few	0	+
3	Johansen [22]	43	M	0	+	0	108	108	+	0	+*	0	0	500	Few	0	0
4	Bashour et al. [27]	48	F	+	0	+	10	9	+	+	+	—	—	500	Few	0	0
5	Duvernoy, Garcia [29]	30	F	+	0	+	31	7	+	+	—	—	—	—	Few	0	+
6	Chun et al. [34]	49	F	+	0	—	38	30	+	0	0	0	0	470	0	0	+
7	Freiman [46]	37	M	0	0	+	96	24	0	0	0	0	0	700	0	+	0
8	Present study	30	M	+	0	0	53	7	+	+	+	+	0	450	Few	0	0
9	Present study	34	M	0	+	0	48	36	0	0	0	0	0	310	0	0	0

NOTE: 0 = absent; + = present; — = no information available; * = microscopic-sized; CHB = complete heart block; CHF = congestive heart failure; CS Rx = corticosteroid treatment; LV = left ventricle; RV = right ventricle; SD = sudden death; VS = ventricular septum; VT = ventricular tachycardia.

necropsy; four of the five had had severe congestive cardiac failure.

Another type of cardiac involvement in some patients with sarcoidosis is calcification of the mitral anulus. Although ectopic and metastatic calcification is a well recognized occurrence in patients with sarcoidosis [72,73,83], calcification of the mitral anulus has not been described previously in this condition. Nevertheless, one of the conditions which predisposes to mitral anular calcification is hypercalcemia, irrespective of its cause [74,75]. Because hypercalcemia is a recognized manifestation of sarcoidosis, it therefore is reasonable to believe that mitral anular calcification should occur with increased frequency in this condition. We found minimal deposits of calcium in the mitral anulus in one of our 35 patients with cardiac sarcoidosis (group I). This man was only 34 years of age, but he had severe hypercalcemia [76]. We found heavy mitral anular calcific deposits in another patient (not included in this study) who also had severe hypercalcemia from sarcoidosis but no cardiac sarcoid granulomas or myocardial scars (Figure 12). Both of these patients also received corticosteroid therapy for several years, and this medication possibly might also predispose to mitral anular calcification.

The effect of corticosteroid therapy on patients with cardiac sarcoid granulomas has received little attention. Analysis of the data on our and previously described necropsy patients with cardiac sarcoidosis strongly suggests that this medication promotes healing of the cardiac granulomas. Only three of the patients in group IA and only 12 of the patients in group IIA received corticosteroid therapy at some time; only nine of these 15 patients received this medication for longer than one month. Certain clinical and morphologic observations in them are summarized in Table VII. Of these nine patients, four had no sarcoid granulomas in the heart—only myocardial scars at sites preferentially involved by sarcoid—and each of the remaining five patients had mainly myocardial scars with relatively few residual granulomas. The four patients without any cardiac granulomas were the only ones among the entire group of 113 patients (Tables II through IV) who had no cardiac granulomas, and three of the four also had one or more cardiac aneurysms at sites of myocardial scarring. Only one of the eight patients with a cardiac aneurysm had not received corticosteroid therapy. Thus, the evidence is substantial that corticosteroid therapy can cause healing of cardiac granulomas but that a possible consequence of this healing is the development of a cardiac aneurysm (Figure 13). The administration of corticosteroids over a period of several weeks during acute myocardial infarction resulting from severe coronary atherosclerosis also can lead rapidly to the development of a cardiac aneurysm [77].

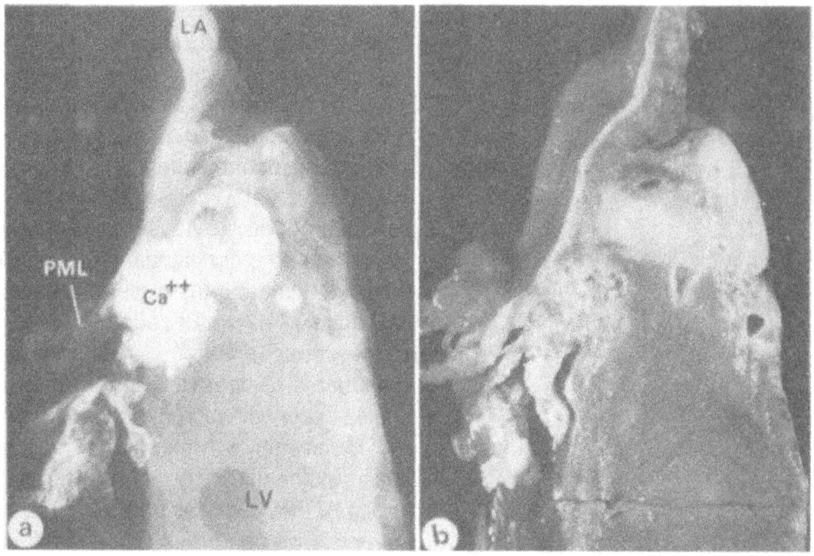

Figure 12. *Longitudinal cut of left atrium (LA), posterior mitral leaflet (PML) and left ventricle (LV) in a 44 year old black woman (A75-12) who had had evidence of noncardiac sarcoidosis for 18 years. Hypercalcemia developed and she died from rupture of a peptic ulcer, apparently a consequence of corticosteroid therapy. A surprise finding at necropsy was the presence of large calcific deposits (Ca++) in the mitral anular region as shown here. A tongue of calcium also protruded from the anular area into the space just behind the posterior mitral leaflet. Hypercalcemia, and possibly also prolonged corticosteroid therapy, are precursors to mitral anular calcification.* ***a,*** *roentgenogram.* ***b,*** *specimen itself.*

Indirect evidence that corticosteroid therapy causes "shrinkage" of the cardiac sarcoid granulomas is demonstrated by the reported diminution in the frequency of arrhythmias, conduction disturbances and electrocardiographic evidence of myocardial damage after initiation of this medication [78–81].

Sarcoid granulomas in the heart may be more responsive to corticosteroid therapy than are sarcoid granulomas located in other body organs. Of the four patients with no residual cardiac sarcoid granulomas, only one [46] had no residual granulomas in other body organs at necropsy. (Lymph node biopsy in the patient before he was given corticosteroid therapy had disclosed many sarcoid granulomas.) Of the other five patients with few cardiac sarcoid granulomas, all appeared to have relatively larger numbers of granulomas in other body organs. Obviously, a possible explanation for this observation is that the area for sarcoid granulomatous infiltration is larger in the liver or lung than in the heart; in other words, the area for granulomatous

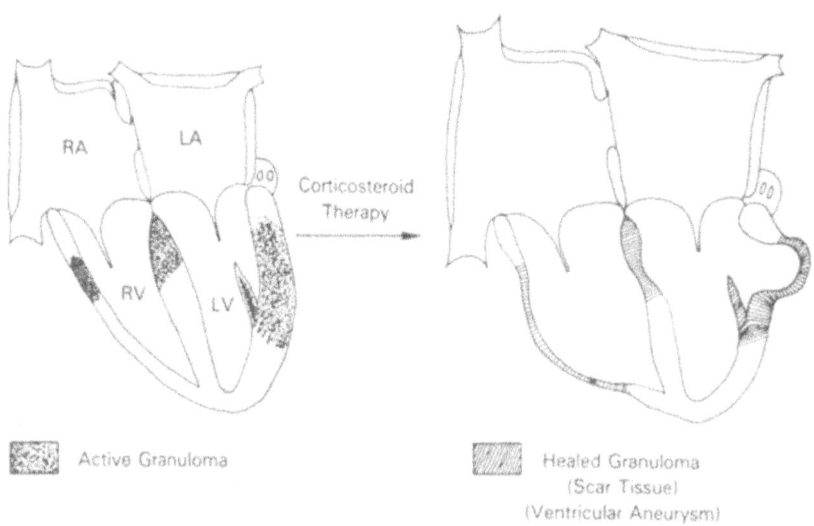

Figure 13. *Diagram showing the good and bad effects of corticosteroid therapy in patients with cardiac sarcoidosis.*

infiltration in the heart is smaller than that of some other body organs.

The majority of patients, in whom cardiac sarcoidosis causes cardiac dysfunction, present initially with manifestations related to the heart rather than to involvement of other body organs or systems. The initial manifestation of sarcoidosis in 23 (88 per cent) of the patients in group IA was related to the heart. Among the previously described 63 patients (group IIA), information regarding the initial manifestation was available in 38: in 28 (74 per cent) of them the initial manifestation was related to signs or symptoms of cardiac dysfunction. Furthermore, in the majority of these 89 patients (26 plus 63) there was never any clinical evidence of dysfunction of an organ system other than the heart. Indeed, the occurrence of symptomatic involvement of another body system by sarcoid generally indicates that symptom-producing cardiac involvement by sarcoid is unlikely to occur. Fleming [80], in search of patients with cardiac sarcoid, surveyed the chest, eye and skin clinics in his hospital in which patients with other forms of sarcoidosis were being followed and found this search unprofitable in revealing patients with cardiac sarcoid. Thus, cardiac sarcoidosis severe enough to cause cardiac dysfunction tends to be an all or none process: if it causes cardiac dysfunction, it tends not to cause dysfunction of another organ system; conversely, if it causes dysfunction of a noncardiac organ system, it infrequently causes cardiac dysfunction.

Although signs or symptoms of cardiac dysfunction from cardiac sarcoidosis may be present for many years, more often the course is not prolonged. The duration of symptoms of cardiac dysfunction from cardiac sarcoidosis was 12 months or less in 19 (73 per cent) of the patients in group IA and in 26 (58 per cent) of the 45 previously described patients (information not available in 18) in group IIA.

Although it appears to be the major cause of giant cell myocarditis, sarcoidosis is not the only condition in which giant cells unassociated with stainable organisms occur in the heart. Giant cells also have been observed in the hearts of patients with infective endocarditis [82], rheumatoid arthritis [83], Takayasu's arteritis [84], Wegener's granulomatosis [85] and, rarely, in patients with coronary heart disease with or without systemic hypertension [71]. "Idiopathic" granulomatous (giant cell) myocarditis has been reported by a number of investigators [86–94], but in many such reports the condition described may not have been "isolated" and, therefore, almost surely [86–90] or probably [91–94] was **cardiac sarcoidosis.** If the latter condition is defined as the presence of "hard" granulomas in at least one other body organ (always lymph node) in addition to the heart, then many patients described as having "isolated" giant cell or granulomatous myocarditis in actuality had cardiac sarcoidosis. It is probable that many patients reported to have isolated granulomatous (giant cell) myocarditis also had giant cells in lymph nodes but that these structures were not examined histologically. In several described patients and in a few of our patients with cardiac sarcoidosis, the lymph nodes were not enlarged grossly; if the nodes had not been studied histologically, sarcoidosis would not have been diagnosed. Thus, a diagnosis of "isolated granulomatous (giant cell) myocarditis" is justified only after thorough exclusion of extracardiac sarcoidosis. In contrast to Davies et al. [90], we believe that "idiopathic giant cell myocarditis" and "cardiac sarcoidosis" cannot be distinguished by histologic examination of the heart alone.

REFERENCES

1. Brosig W: Zur tuberkulösen Erkrankung des Herzmuskels. Zentralbl Allg Pathol 72: 161, 1939.
2. Longcope WT, Fisher AM: The effect of Schaumann's disease upon the heart and its mechanism. Acta Med Scand 108: 529, 1941.
3. Bates GS, Walsh JM: Boeck's sarcoid: observations on seven patients, one autopsy. Ann Intern Med 29: 306, 1948.
4. Scotti TM, McKeown CE: Sarcoidosis involving the heart. Report of case with sudden death. Arch Pathol 46: 289, 1948.
5. Vogt H: Morbus Besnier-Boeck-Schaumann. Klinische und pathologische-anatomie Studie. Helv Med Acta 16 (suppl 25): 1, 1949.
6. Kulka WE: Sarcoidosis of the heart. A cause of sudden and unexpected death. Circulation 1: 772, 1950.
7. Simkins S: Boeck's sarcoid with complete heart block mimicking carotid sinus syncope. Report of a case. JAMA 146: 794, 1951.
8. Oille WA, Ritchie RC, Barrie HJ: The age of lesions in a case of myocardial sarcoidosis. Can Med Assoc J 68: 277, 1953.
9. Stephen JD: Fatal myocardial sarcoidosis. A case of sudden death. Circulation 9: 886, 1954.
10. Powell LW Jr: Sarcoidosis of the myocardium. NC Med J 15: 28, 1954.
11. Gottfarb AG, Wahlgren F: Adams-Stokes syndrom framkallat av morbus Besnier-Boeck-Schaumann (sarcoidosis). Nord Med 52: 985, 1954.
12. Clinicopathologic conference. Cardiac arrhythmia. US Armed Forces Med J 8: 855, 1957.
13. Peacock RA, Lippschutz EJ, Lukas A: Myocardial sarcoidosis. Circulation 16: 67, 1957.
14. Poon TP, Forbus WD: Sudden death due to myocardial sarcoidosis, with a comment on the etiology of sarcoid. Arch Intern Med 104: 771, 1959.
15. Porter GH: Sarcoid heart disease. N Engl J Med 263: 1350, 1960.
16. Phinney AO Jr: Sarcoid of the myocardial septum with complete heart block. Report of two cases. Am Heart J 62: 270, 1961.
17. Chamovitz DL, Culley AW, Carlson KE: Cardiac sarcoidosis. Report of a case with paroxysmal ventricular tachycardia.

JAMA 182: 574, 1962.
18. Forbes G, Usher A: Fatal myocardial sarcoidosis. Br Med J 2: 771, 1962.
19. Hines JD, Sancetta SM: Myocardial sarcoidosis simulating healed myocardial infarction. Ohio State Med J 59: 689, 1963.
20. Smith WP: Primary sarcoid heart disease. Report of a case. J Fla Med Assoc 51: 652, 1964.
21. Chomette G, Auriol M, Daddi G, et al.: Localisations cardiaques massives d'une sarcoïdose de Besnier-Boeck-Schaumann. Ann Anat Pathol (Paris) 10: 177, 1965.
22. Johansen A: Isolated myocarditis versus myocardial sarcoidosis. A contribution to the discussion regarding points of resemblance between these and a report of three illustrative cases. Acta Pathol Microbiol Scand 67: 15, 1966.
23. Shimada N, Ishihara Y, Kojima A, et al.: Three cases of granulomatous myocarditis with giant cells. Acta Pathol Jap 17: 503, 1967.
24. Miyaji T, Ohara M, Funaki M, et al.: [A case of myocardial sarcoidosis with Adams-Stokes syndrome]. J Jap Soc Intern Med 56: 260, 1967.
25. Contreras R, Sánchez Torres G, Durán Rodríquez P: Sarcoidosis cardiaca. Arch Inst Cardiol Mex 37: 20, 1967.
26. Hishimoto Y, Takano Y, Tagaki M: Case of fatal myocardial sarcoidosis preceded by cardiac symptoms. Jap J Clin Med 26: 1244, 1968.
27. Bashour FA, McConnell T, Skinner W, et al.: Myocardial sarcoidosis. Dis Chest 53: 413, 1968.
28. Rajasenan V, Cooper ES: Myocardial sarcoidosis, bouts of ventricular tachycardia, psychiatric manifestations and sudden death. A case report. J Natl Med Assoc 61: 306, 1969.
29. Duvernoy WFC, Garcia R: Sarcoidosis of the heart presenting with ventricular tachycardia and atrioventricular block. Am J Cardiol 28: 348, 1971.
30. Rossi L: Sarcoid heart disease. Br Med J 1: 546, 1973.
31. Ghosh P, Fleming HA, Gresham GA, et al.: Myocardial sarcoidosis. Br Heart J 34: 769, 1972.
32. Zoneraich S, Gupta MP, Mehta J, et al.: Myocardial sarcoidosis presenting as acute mitral insufficiency. Chest 66: 452, 1974.
33. Morales AR, Levy S, Davis J, et al.: Sarcoidosis and the heart. Pathology Annual 1974 (Sommers SC, ed), New York, Appleton-Century-Crofts, 1974, p 139.
34. Chun SK, Andy JJ, Jilly P, et al.: Ventricular aneurysm in sarcoidosis. Chest 68: 392, 1975.
35. Johnson JB, Jason RS: Sarcoidosis of the heart. Report of a case and review of the literature. Am Heart J 27: 246, 1944.
36. Yesner R, Silver M: Fatal myocardial sarcoidosis. Am Heart J 41: 777, 1951.
37. Adickes GC, Zimmerman SL, Cardwell ES: Sarcoidosis with fatal cardiac involvement. Ann Intern Med 35: 898, 1951.
38. Arkless HA, Gokcebay TM, Mendell TH: Sarcoidosis of the heart. Am J Cardiol 1: 648, 1958.
39. Stein MH, Gross JM, Shulman H: A case of cardiac sarcoidosis manifested by uncontrollable ventricular tachycardia. Review of cardiac manifestations in sixteen cases of sarcoidosis. Am J Cardiol 10: 864, 1962.
40. Ferrans VJ, Hibbs RG, Black WC, et al.: Myocardial degeneration in cardiac sarcoidosis. Histochemical and electron microscopic studies. Am Heart J 68: 159, 1965.
41. Carvalhal S dos S, Rocha JC: Un caso de sarcoidose com comprometimento de coraçao. Rev Assoc Med Brasil 11: 89, 1965.
42. Deneberg M: Sarcoidosis of the myocardium and aorta. A case report. Am J Clin Pathol 43: 445, 1965.
43. Raftery EB, Oakley CM, Goodwin JF: Acute subvalvular mitral incompetence. Lancet 2: 360, 1966.
44. Clark EJ, Blount AW: A fatal case of myocardial sarcoidosis. Lancet 86: 568, 1966.
45. Bruno MS, Ober WB: Clinico-pathologic conference. Intractable heart failure with long-standing granulomatous disease. NY State J Med 68: 2790, 1968.
46. Case Records of the Massachusetts General Hospital. Case 46–1975. Harthorne JW, Freiman DG. N Engl J Med 293: 1138, 1975.
47. Gozo EG Jr, Cosnow I, Cohen HC, et al.: The heart in sarcoidosis. Chest 60: 379, 1971.
48. Cotter EF: Boeck's sarcoid. Autopsy in a case with visceral lesions. Arch Intern Med 64: 286, 1939.
49. Hirayama J: Ein Fall von diffuser spezifischer Myocarditis mit zahlreichen Riesenzellen. Trans Soc Pathol Jap 29: 261, 1939.
50. Botti RE, Young FE: Myocardial sarcoid, complete heart block and aortic stenosis. Ann Intern Med 51: 811, 1959.
51. Nissen AW, Berte JB: Cardiac arrhythmias in sarcoidosis. Arch Intern Med 113: 275, 1964.
52. Bernstein M, Konzlemann FW, Sidlick DM: Boeck's sarcoid. Report of a case with visceral involvement. Arch Intern Med 44: 721, 1929.
53. Nickerson DA: Boeck's sarcoid. Report of six cases in which autopsies were made. Arch Pathol 24: 19, 1937.
54. Spencer J, Warren S: Boeck's sarcoid. Report of a case, with clinical diagnosis confirmed at autopsy. Arch Intern Med 62: 285, 1938.
55. Granström KO, Gripwall E, Kristofferson CE, et al.: A case of uveoparotid fever (Heerfordt) with autopsy findings. Acta Med Scand 126: 307, 1946.
56. Skavlem JH, Ritterhoff RJ: Coexistent pulmonary asbestosis and sarcoidosis. Am J Pathol 22: 493, 1946.
57. Gendel BR, Young JM, Greiner DJ: Sarcoidosis. A review with twenty-four additional cases. Am J Med 12: 205, 1952.
58. Gilg I: Sarcoidosis involving the heart. Acta Derm Venereol 33: 318, 1953.
59. Brun J, Turiaf J, Perrin LF, et al.: Coeur et sarcoidose de Besnier-Boeck-Schaumann. Presse Med 63: 284, 1955.
60. Pascoe HR: Myocardial sarcoidosis. Report of a case with unexpected death. Arch Pathol 77: 299, 1964.
61. Peison B: Sarcoidosis of the heart associated with myocarditis: report of case. Ill Med J 130: 317, 1966.
62. Smith LH Jr: Case Records of the Massachusetts General Hospital. Weekly Clinicopathological Exercises. Case 8–1974. N Engl J Med 290: 504, 1974.
63. Laroche C, de Gennes J-L, Hazard J, et al.: Maladie de Besnier-Boeck-Schaumann avec manifestations polyarticulaires et localisations endo-myo-péricardiques mortelles. Bull Mém Soc Med Hôp Paris 71: 908, 1955.
64. Thorbjarnarson B, Glenn F: Sarcoidosis associated with sudden death during mitral valvulotomy. Arch Surg 73: 862, 1956.
65. Roberts WC, Bodey GP, Wertlake PT: The heart in acute leukemia. A study of 420 autopsy cases. Am J Cardiol 21: 388, 1968.
66. Glancy DL, Roberts WC: The heart in malignant melanoma. A study of 70 autopsy cases. Am J Cardiol 21: 555, 1968.
67. Roberts WC, Glancy DL, DeVita VT Jr: Heart in malignant lymphoma (Hodgkin's disease, lymphosarcoma, reticulum cell sarcoma and mycosis fungoides). A study of 196 autopsy cases. Am J Cardiol 22: 85, 1968.
68. Lull RJ, Dunn BE, Gregoratos G, et al.: Ventricular aneurysm due to cardiac sarcoidosis with surgical cure of refractory ventricular tachycardia. Am J Cardiol 30: 282, 1972.
69. Shiff AD, Blatt CJ, Colp C: Recurrent pericardial effusion secondary to sarcoidosis of the pericardium. A biopsy-proven case. N Engl J Med 281: 141, 1969.
70. Bailey RR: Systemic sarcoidosis with pericarditis and pericardial effusion. N Z Med J 65: 704, 1966.
71. Roberts WC, Ferrans VJ: Pathologic anatomy of the cardiomyopathies. Idiopathic dilated and hypertrophic types,

infiltrative types, and endomyocardial disease with and without eosinophilia. Hum Pathol 6: 287, 1975.
72. Lathan SR, Block RA, McLean RL: Sarcoidosis with metastatic calcification. Am J Med 44: 1000, 1968.
73. Fujita N, Torres A, Sharma OP: Ectopic calcification in sarcoidosis. JAMA 227: 556, 1974.
74. Roberts WC: Calcification of the mitral anulus: a study of 87 necropsy patients (abstract). Circulation 45 & 46 (Suppl II): 107, 1972.
75. Roberts WC, Perloff JK: Mitral valvular disease. A clinicopathologic survey of the conditions causing the mitral valve to function abnormally. Ann Intern Med 77: 939, 1972.
76. Bell NH, Bartter FC: Studies of ^{47}Ca metabolism in sarcoidosis: evidence for increased sensitivity of bone to vitamin D. Acta Endocrinol (Kbh) 54: 173, 1967.
77. Bulkley BH, Roberts WC: Steroid therapy during acute myocardial infarction. A cause of delayed healing and of ventricular aneurysm. Am J Med 56: 244, 1974.
78. Gold J, Cantor P: Sarcoid heart disease. A case with unusual electrocardiogram. Arch Intern Med 104: 101, 1959.
79. Unsigned Editorial. Myocardial sarcoidosis. Lancet 2: 1351, 1972.
80. Fleming HA: Sarcoid heart disease. Br Med J 1: 174, 1973.
81. Strauss GS, Lawton BR, Wenzel FJ, et al.: Detection of covert myocardial sarcoidosis by scalene node biopsy. Chest 69: 790, 1976.
82. Buchbinder NA, Roberts WC: Left-sided valvular active infective endocarditis. A study of forty-five necropsy patients. Am J Med 53: 20, 1972.
83. Roberts WC, Kehoe JA, Carpenter DF, et al.: Cardiac valvular lesions in rheumatoid arthritis. Arch Intern Med 122: 141, 1968.
84. Roberts WC, Wibin EA: Idiopathic panaortitis, supra-aortic arteritis, granulomatous myocarditis and pericarditis. A cause of pulseless disease and possibly left ventricular aneurysm in the African. Am J Med 41: 453, 1966.
85. Walton EW: Giant-cell granuloma of the respiratory tract (Wegener's granulomatosis). Br Med J 2: 265, 1958.
86. Jonas AF Jr: Granulomatous myocarditis. Bull Johns Hopkins Hosp 64: 45, 1939.
87. Kean BH, Koekenga MT: Giant cell myocarditis. Am J Pathol 28: 1095, 1952.
88. Tesluk H: Giant cell versus granulomatous myocarditis. Am J Clin Pathol 26: 1326, 1956.
89. Long WH: Granulomatous (Fiedler's) myocarditis with extracardiac involvement. A case report with sudden death. JAMA 177: 184, 1961.
90. Davies MJ, Pomerance A, Teare RD: Idiopathic giant cell myocarditis—a distinctive clinico-pathological entity. Br Heart J 37: 192, 1975.
91. Manger D: A case of fatal subacute myocarditis of unknown etiology. Am J Med Sci 198: 246, 1939.
92. Saphir O: Isolated myocarditis. Am Heart J 24: 167, 1942.
93. Dilling NV: Giant-cell myocarditis. J Pathol Bacteriol 71: 295, 1956.
94. Rab SM, Choudhury GM, Choudhury AR: Giant-cell myocarditis. Lancet 2: 172, 1963.

Cardiomyopathy and Myocarditis: Morphologic Features

WILLIAM C. ROBERTS

Pathology Branch, National Heart, Lung, and Blood Institute, National Institutes of Health, Bethesda, Md.

This report describes certain morphologic changes observed *at necropsy* in patients with various noniflammatory (cardiomyopathy) and inflammatory (myocarditis) heart muscle diseases. The disorders will be presented in the order shown in table I (fig. 1).

Noninflammatory Heart Muscle Diseases

Idiopathic Dilated Cardiomyopathy

An idiopathic cardiomyopathy may be defined as a disease of the myocardium not resulting from coronary, valvular, congenital, hypertensive or pulmonary heart disease [1]. Idiopathic cardiomyopathy is of two types: the ventricular dilated type and the hypertrophic (nonventricular dilated) type. Morphologic differences between these two types are summarized in table II.

Idiopathic cardiac enlargement, heart disease of unknown origin, primary myocardial disease, and *congestive cardiomyopathy* are other terms which have been used to describe what I prefer to call idiopathic dilated cardiomyopathy (DC). The reason for the latter term is that the major morphologic feature of this condition is dilation of both ventricular cavities. Although the degree of dilation of both ventricular cavities is usually similar, occasionally one ventricle is more dilated than the other one. The ventricular dilation is associated with poor ventricular contractions, which in turn produce low ejection fractions and high end-systolic volumes. The latter appear to limit atrial emptying, which in turn leads to high atrial end-diastolic volumes with resulting atrial dilatation.

The large end-systolic ventricular volumes lead to relative stasis of blood

Table I. Heart muscle diseases

Noninflammatory cardiomyopathy

- I. Idiopathic
  - A. Dilated type
  - B. Hypertrophic type
    - 1. With subaortic stenosis
    - 2. Without subaortic stenosis
- II. Endomyocardial disease
  - A. With eosinophilia (Löffler's fibroplastic parietal endocarditis)
  - B. Without eosinophilia (endomyocardial fibrosis of Davies)
- III. Infiltrative
  - A. Amyloid
  - B. Iron (hemosiderosis)
  - C. Glycogen
  - D. Lipids and mucopolysaccharides
  - E. Calcium

Inflammatory cardiomyopathy (myocarditis)

- I. Known infectious agent (bacteria, viruses, parasites, rickettsiae, spirochetes and treponemata, fungi)
  - A. Primary
  - B. Secondary
- II. Unknown agent (idiopathic)
- III. Associated with another known condition
  - A. Collagen disease
    - 1. Acute rheumatic fever
    - 2. Rheumatoid arthritis
    - 3. Systemic lupus erythematosus
    - 4. Other
  - B. Sarcoidosis

---

in the apical portions of the ventricular cavities and this results in intracavitary thrombosis. Thrombi also are frequent in one or both atrial appendages, presumably also the consequence of poor atrial emptying and relative stasis of blood in the appendages. The most frequent locations of thrombi in patients with DC are left ventricle, right ventricle, right atrial appendage and, lastly, left atrial appendage. About 75% of these patients have left ventricular thrombi at necropsy. I have never seen thrombus in the atria or right ventricle without thrombi being present also in the left ventricle. In addition to fibrin thrombi, focal endocardial thickenings often are present and they

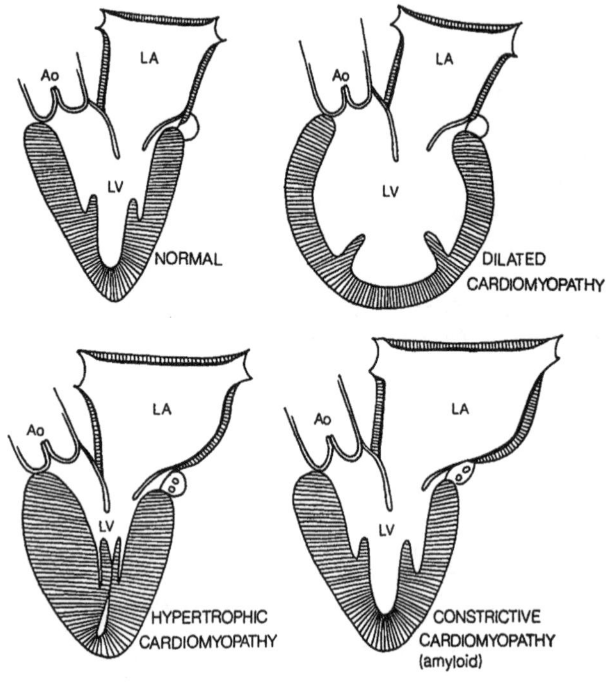

Fig. 1. Diagram illustrating the various types of cardiomyopathies, compared to the normal, to be discussed herein. In hypertrophic cardiomyopathy, the left ventricular cavity is small and in the constrictive variety, as illustrated by amyloidosis, the left ventricular cavity is of normal size. In the dilated type, the largest circumference of the left ventricle is not at its base but about midway between apex and base.

probably represent 'healed' or organized thrombi. The intracardiac thrombi obviously may give rise to pulmonary and systemic emboli.

The hearts are always increased in weight; the average in 100 personally studied necropsy patients is just under 600 g. Despite the increased weight, the maximal thickness of the left ventricular free wall and the ventricular septum is often < 1.5 cm.

Although interstitial myocardial fibrosis of varying degree usually is present by histologic examination, left ventricular free wall scarring is observed by gross inspection in only about 25% of the patients. Even when scarring is observed grossly, it is usually limited to papillary muscle and subendocardium (inner one-half of wall). Thus, the poor myocardial contractility cannot be explained by ventricular scarring.

The leaflets of the four cardiac valves are usually normal, but occasionally the margins of the mitral and tricuspid valve leaflets are focally thickened by fibrous tissue. The latter is most frequent in patients with atrioventricular valvular regurgitation for long periods. These valvular thickenings appear to be secondary to the regurgitation, and do not themselves cause valvular incompetence. The cause of valvular regurgitation in these patients appears to be papillary muscle dysfunction, because the tricuspid and mitral valvular anuli are usually only mildly dilated (< 25 % above normal) [2].

Histologic studies of the myocardial walls in these patients disclose nonspecific changes. Many myocardial cells appear hypertrophied; others, atrophied. The amount of fibrous tissue between myocardial cells usually is increased. Inflammatory cells are absent. The intramural coronary arteries are normal. Electronmicroscopy has confirmed these histologic observations and demonstrated other nonspecific changes icluding cellular edema; increased numbers of lipid droplets, lysosomes, and lipofuscin granules; dilatation of the tubules of the sarcoplasmic reticulum and the T system; mild myofibrillar damage, and the various mitochondrial alterations [3]. The mitochondria vary in size; many are smaller than normal. No virus particles have been observed in the myocardium of patients with fatal cardiomyopathy. The changes in myocardium in patients with histories of habitual alcoholism are indistinguishable from those in patients without positive histories. In general, the extent of the degenerative changes in the myocardial cells correlates with the duration and severity of cardiac dysfunction.

Although it is well recognized that DC may be confused clinically with coronary heart disease, separation of the two at necropsy may present problems if one adheres rigidly to a definition which includes 'absence of coronary arterial disease'. How much coronary arterial narrowing, in other words, is permissible to still allow the diagnosis of DC? Initially I included in a definition [1] of this entity 'less than 50 % cross-sectional area luminal narrowing', but this cut-off point prevented inclusion of patients who had typical clinical features of DC, including absence of chest pain, and in whom necropsy confirmed absence of myocardial scarring but showed up to 75 % cross-sectional area luminal narrowing of a major coronary artery. Because fatal coronary (atherosclerotic) heart disease is always associated with cross-sectional area luminal narrowing of > 75 % [4], a 75 % cut-off point appears more reasonable. Furthermore, there is apparently no reduction in flow through a tube (coronary artery) until more than 75 % of the cross-sectional area of the lumen is obliterated. Obviously, the associated coronary atherosclerosis presents no problem in the younger aged patients, but it might in the older ones.

Idiopathic Hypertrophic Cardiomyopathy

Hypertrophic cardiomyopathy (HC) is strikingly different both functionally and morphologically from DC (table II). The major problem is a *hyper*contracting left ventricle rather than a *hypo*contracting ventricle as in DC. The morphologic counterpart of this hypercontracting ventricle is a massive increase in ventricular muscle mass and small ventricular cavities. HC is the classic example of the 'muscle-bound heart'; DC, in contrast, is the classic example of the 'flabby heart', mostly cavity with comparatively little myocardial mass.

In his original description, Teare [6] applied the term *asymmetrical hypertrophy of the heart* to this condition. Subsequently, other terms including *functional subaortic stenosis, diffuse muscular subaortic stenosis, idiopathic hypertrophic subaortic stenosis, hypertrophic obstructive cardiomyopathy* and *asymmetric septal hypertrophy* have been applied. The terms which include the word stenosis or obstruction appear inappropriate because obstruction is more often absent than present [5]. The terms which emphasize asymmetry of the walls bordering the left ventricular cavity have served a useful purpose in emphasizing the characteristic morphologic feature of this condition, but it is now apparent that the ventricular septum may be thicker than the left ventricular free wall in some conditions (table III) other than HC, that a few patients with HC do not have asymmetric septal hypertrophy (i.e. septum thicker than free wall), and that the free wall on occasion in HC may not be hypertrophied.

Study at necropsy of 65 patients with HC has demonstrated the following characteristic features of this condition: (1) disproportional hypertrophy of the ventricular septum (95%); (2) disorientation of myocardial fibers in the ventricular septum (100%); (3) small or nomal-sized left and right ventricular cavities (90%); (4) mural endocardial plaque, left ventricular outflow tract (75%); (5) thickened mitral valve (75%); (6) dilated atria (100%); and (7) abnormal intramural coronary arteries (50%).

Disproportional septal hypertrophy was observed by Teare [6] in his initial description of HC. The thickest portion of the septum is not that portion immediately beneath the aortic valve, however, but that part located about midway between aortic valve and left ventricular apex. This level corresponds approximately to the apex of the right ventricle. The *maximal thickness of the ventricular septum* in our adult patients averaged 3.0 cm, and the *maximal thickness of the left ventricular free wall,* 1.8 cm.

When the echocardiogram measures what is believed to be the thickest portion of ventricular septum, the echo beam simultaneously delineates only

Table II. Morphologic differences between idiopathic DC and HC

		Dilated type	Hypertrophic type
1	Dilated ventricular cavities	+	0
2	Intracardiac thrombi	+	0
3	Asymmetric septal hypertrophy	0	+
4	Myocardial fiber disorientation	0	+
5	Endocardial plaque, left ventricular outflow tract	0	+
6	Thickened mitral valve	0	+
7	Abnormal intramural coronary arteries	0	+
8	Ventricular scarring	0–+	+
9	Thickened ventricular walls	0–+	+
10	Increased cardiac weight	+	+
11	Dilated atrial cavities	+	+

Table III. Causes of asymmetric septal hypertrophy

1. Hypertrophic cardiomyopathy
   A. With obstruction (IHSS)
   B. Without obstruction
2. Aortic stenosis
   A. Valvular
   B. Discrete subvalvular
   C. Supravalvular
   D. Tunnel
3. Systemic hypertension
4. Pulmonary hypertension
5. Basal myocardial infarct
6. Parachute mitral valve syndrome

that portion of left ventricular free wall which is located behind posterior mitral leaflet. In normal subjects and in patients with left ventricular hypertrophy from such causes as aortic valve stenosis and systemic hypertension, the thickest portion of the left ventricular free wall is located about 2 cm caudal to the base of the left ventricle, i.e., the area measured by echocardiography. In patients with the *obstructive type* of HC, this posterobasal portion

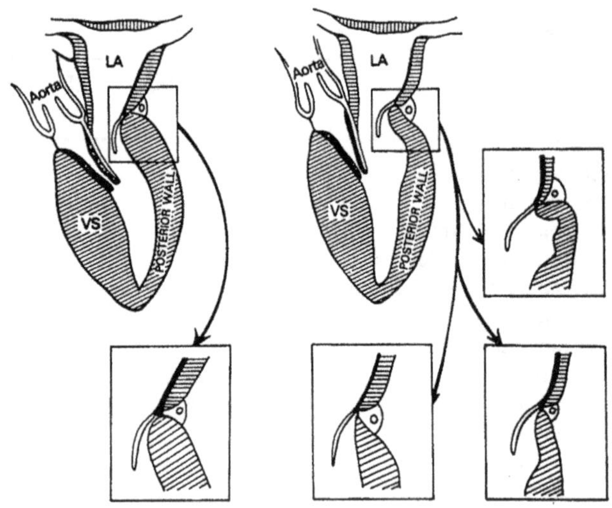

Fig. 2. Diagram illustrating the major differences between the obstructive and nonobstructive types of hypertrophic cardiomyopathy. In the obstructive type, the most basal portion of the posterior and lateral left ventricular free walls is rounded and thick. In the nonobstructive type, the left ventricular free wall beneath the posterior mitral leaflet is thinned and pointed.

of the left ventricular free wall represents the thickest portion of the free wall. In the patients with the *nonobstructive type* of HC, however, the portion of the left ventricular free wall directly behind the posterior mitral leaflet is not thickened and the thickest portion of the free wall is located more caudally, i.e., not measurable by echocardiogram. Differences in the configuration of the posterobasal left ventricular free wall between the obstructive and nonobstructive types are diagrammed in figure 2. Thus, by examination of the posterobasal portion of the left ventricular free wall, an accurate determination can be made as to whether the patient had the obstructive or the nonobstructive form of HC.

A second major anatomic feature of HC is focal disorganization of myocardial fibers in the ventricular septum. In TEARE's [6] original description he observed by histologic examination a 'bizarre arrangement of muscle bundles' and 'considerable variation in size' of the myocardial fibers in the ventricular septum. This myocardial fiber disarray in the septum occurs in patients of all ages (including infants) with HC of either the obstructive or nonobstructive variety [5]. The size and extent of the foci vary and between them are large areas of myocardium in which the muscle cells are hypertrophied but normally arranged (in parallel). The areas of disarray are composed of cells that are arranged in whorls or at random, the cells being wider (transverse diameters up to 80 μm, average 28 μm, normal 10–15 μm) and often shorter than normal. The abnormalities in cellular architecture are not unique to HC but they are clearly more severe and widespread in this condition than any other.

Not only does disorganization between *myocardial fibers* occur, but in addition, ultrastructural studies [7] have shown disarray of *myofibrilis* and *myofilaments* within individual cells. Again, the abnormalities of myofibrils and myofilaments are not absolutely specific for HC, but when disorganization of theses subcellular components is found in other cardiac conditions, the abnormal cells are in small numbers. The individual septal myocardial cells in HC also frequently show increased amounts of Z-band material and nonspecific changes of cellular hypertrophy and degeneration.

Myofiber disarray in the left and right ventricular free walls is more difficult to determine by light microscopy than that in the ventricular septum. Ultrastructural examination of the left and right ventricular free walls, however, discloses many bizarrely-shaped, disorganized cells in the ventricular free walls of patients *without obstruction,* whereas the bizarrely-shaped and disorganized myocardial fibers are virtually entirely absent from the ventricular free walls in the patients *with obstruction* [5]. Thus, the disorientation of groups of myocardial cells and the disarray of myofibrils and myofilaments within individual myocardial cells is not the result of left ventricular outflow obstruction or high intraventricular systolic pressures.

Another major anatomic characteristic of HC is lack of ventricular cavity dilatation. The left ventricular cavity usually has a flattened S-shape. The development of ventricular dilatation is rare (in 4 of our 65 necropsy patients) in HC and when it occurs transmural myocardial scars usually also are present. In contrast to the ventricular cavities, both atrial cavities at necropsy virtually always are dilated, more dilated than in DC.

In adults, the mural endocardium of the left ventricular outflow tract is usually thickened by fibrous tissue. This thickening is in direct apposition to the anterior mitral leaflet, which also is thickened by fibrous tissue. The caudal margin of the mural endocardial outflow plaque corresponds to the distal margin of the anterior mitral leaflet. This caudal margin probably represents the site of obstruction. If that is the case, then the fibrous thickening of the left ventricular outflow tract (includes both mural endocardium and anterior mitral leaflet) should be restricted to the patients with obstruction. This outflow thickening occurred in 95% of our necropsy patients with hemodynamically confirmed left ventricular outflow obstruction at rest and in only 50% of the patients without obstruction. Furthermore, the thickening was distinctly more severe in the patients with obstruction.

Not only is the anterior mitral leaflet thickened, but often (more frequently in the patients with obstruction) the posterior mitral leaflet is as well. The thickening of both leaflets is probably the consequence of the small left ventricular cavity in this condition. It is important to recall that the mitral valve resides in the left ventricle, which being small, causes abnormal contact of the leaflets with themselves and also causes the anterior one to contact the septum. In the patients without obstruction, the basal portion of the left ventricular cavity is larger than in the patients with obstruction because of the thinning of the basal portion of the free wall posteriorly and laterally. The local fibrous thickening of the posterior mitral leaflet probably results from abnormal contact during ventricular systole because there is not enough room in the ventricular cavity to easily accommodate the leaflets and chordae. The ventricle and mitral leaflets in this respect may be regarded as being similar to an accordion. The mitral leaflet thickening in HC is somewhat analogous to that which occurs normally as a consequence of aging. With aging, the left ventricular cavity becomes smaller, presumably in response to the lowered cardiac output; the mitral leaflets, thicker; the left ventricular muscle, less compliant, and the left atrium dilates in response to increased work required to fill the small left ventricle. Similar mechanisms appear to be accelerated in HC.

Most patients with HC have some degree of mitral regurgitation. It is not related to anular dilatation because the mitral anulus in this condition is smaller than normal. Furthermore, the leaflet thickening, in and of itself, is not extensive enough to cause valvular regurgitation. The most likely explanation appears to be abnormal bending of the papillary muscles, particularly the anterolateral one. These structures may be bent abnormally by the bulging ventricular septum with resulting excessive tension on the chordae tendineae preventing closure of the mitral orifice. Although they are usually present in the papillary muscles in HC, focal scars cannot account for the regurgitation. Although it is usually mild in HC, mitral regurgitation may be the predominant clinical feature of this condition. Mitral valve replacement in HC is hazardous because the small left ventricular cavity is rarely capable of freely accommodating a prosthesis [8].

Endomyocardial Disease with and without Eosinophilia

LÖFFLER in 1936 described 2 patients with 'fibroplastic parietal endocarditis with blood eosinophilia' [1]. In 1957, BOUSSER summarized reports of 13 patients with 'eosinophilic leukemia' and a number of reports subsequently described each of these two conditions [1]. In each, there is endocardial fibrosis of one or both ventricles and severe eosinophilia. Death is usually the result of congestive cardiac failure. From examination of previous reports and of our 8 necropsy patients [1], it appears that the clinical and morphologic features of eosinophilic leukemia and Löffler's endocarditis are similar and that these two conditions are indeed the same disease. Certain similarities also exist between endomyocardial fibrosis of the African (EMF) and EMF with eosinophilia, described by others as Löffler's endocarditis or eosinophilic leukemia. The mural endocardial thickening in the ventricles is seen in both conditions, and blood eosinophilia may occur in EMF.

The possibility that Löffler's fibroplastic parietal endocarditis, eosinophilic leukemia (without abnormal myelopoiesis), and EMF of the African are the same disease at different stages of development is an attractive hypothesis. Patients with eosinophilia associated with a transient, benign febrile illness, such as tropical eosinophilia or Löffler's pneumonia, may represent one end of the spectrum. Patients with severe EMF and no blood eosinophilia may represent the other end. Between these two extremes there may be patients who still have eosinophilia but less extensive endocardial scarring. The latter process is still active, and thus eosinophilia is still present, but as the inflammatory process dies down cardiac scar tissue remains and eosinophilia disappears.

Infiltrative Cardiomyopathies

These include various infiltrates into the walls of the cardiac chambers. The infiltrates may be localized to *myocardial interstitium* (amyloid) or within *myocardial cells* (iron, glycogen, lipids, calcium).

Amyloid

Amyloid may be deposited in any portion of the heart and the deposits may be large (grossly visible) or small (microscopic-sized) [9]. When cardiac dysfunction results from cardiac amyloidosis, the amyloid deposits are grossly visible and diffusely distributed throughout the ventricular walls which have firm, rubbery consistencies. Histologically, most ventricular myocardial cells are surrounded by amyloid fibrils. Thus, not only is ventricular motion restricted but most myofibers are constricted by the amyloid deposits. In addition to their being in the myocardial interstitium, amyloid is deposited in the walls and in the lumina of the intramural coronary arteries, in mural endocardium, particularly in the atria, in valvular endocardium, in epicardium and in both conduction tissue and cardiac nerves. The endocardial deposits usually are not large enough to produce valvular dysfunction. The deposits in the lumina of the small coronary arteries, however, may lead to focal myocardial ischemia with resulting necrosis and fibrosis. The amount of amyloid deposition in the conducting myocardium is minimal in comparison to that present in contracting myocardium. Nevertheless, conduction and rhythm disturbances are more common in these patients than in those of similar age and sex without cardiac amyloidosis. Amyloid may be viewed as an 'acellular cancer' in that the deposits infiltrate within and between normal tissues but no cells are present in the proliferating material.

Although the ventricular walls are made rigid by heavy amyloid deposits, the ventricular cavities are not dilated unless another cardiac condition also is present. Thus, cardiac amyloidosis joins hypertrophic cardiomyopathy and constrictive pericarditis as a cause of congestive cardiac failure in the absence of ventricular cavity dilatation. The atria, in contrast, usually are dilated. The enlargement of the cardiac silhouette on roentgenogram in this condition may well be related to the atrial dilatation. Most patients with symptomatic cardiac amyloidosis have electrocardiographic low voltage, conduction or rhythm disturbances, and congestive cardiac failure unresponsive to digitalis therapy. Diagnosis of clinically significant cardiac amyloidosis should be questioned in the absence of congestive cardiac failure and electrocardiographic low voltage [9].

Iron

For years it was debated whether or not iron deposition in the heart could cause cardiac dysfunction. It is now clear, just as with amyloid, that cardiac dysfunction will occur if the cardiac iron deposits are large enough [10], that cardiac dysfunction does not occur in patients with only microscopically visible iron deposits, and that cardiac dysfunction usually does occur when the deposits are grossly visible. In contrast to amyloid deposits which are between myocardial cells, the ironic deposits are within myofibers. The iron deposits are most extensive in ventricular myocardium, less in atrial myocardium, and least in conducting as contrasted to contracting myocardium. Most patients with large cardiac iron deposits have abnormal electrocardiograms, mainly arrhythmias and conduction disturbances, and congestive cardiac failure. In contrast to amyloid, the ventricular cavities typically are dilated. Thus, the iron heart is a weak heart, not a strong one.

Glycogen

A deficiency of one or more of the enzymes involved in the biosynthesis and degradation of glycogen produces glycogen storage disease, of which at least eight types have been described [1]. Cardiac involvement occurs in types II, III, and IV. Most patients with glycogen storage causing cardiomegaly belong to type II (Pompe's disease), caused by a deficiency of α-1,4-glucosidase, a lysosomal enzyme that hydrolyzes glycogen to glucose. As a result the heart enlarges, sometimes to a marked degree, and congestive cardiac failure supervenes. Survival rarely extends beyond infancy or early childhood. Microscopically, the muscle cells show a characteristic lacework pattern, with large, clear central spaces (which represent the sites of glycogen deposition) and a peripheral rim of compressed cytoplasm. Endocardial fibroelastosis of at least the left ventricle usually is present also. Although the deposits of glycogen usually involve all myocardial cells relatively uniformly, on occasion the fibers in the ventricular septum may contain disproportionately excessive quantities of glycogen and lead to subaortic stenosis. Myocardial involvement occurs to a variable extent in type III glycogenosis (glycogen debranching enzyme deficiency). In type IV glycogenosis (branching enzyme deficiency) deposits of abnormal glycogen are found free in the cytoplasm of cardiac muscle cells, hepatocytes and a variety of other cell types. These glycogen deposits are basophilic and are composed of nonbranching fibrils that measure 40–80 Å in diameter and resemble those in basophilic degeneration of the heart.

Lipids

Infiltration of cytoplasm of cardiac muscle cells by lipid droplets (fatty degeneration) is a nonspecific finding in many disorders, including hypoxia. *Fabry's disease* (angiokeratoma corporis diffusum universale) may be singled out among the lipid storage diseases as one in which extensive and clinically significant (cardiomegaly and congestive cardiac failure) accumulation occurs in cardiac muscle cells. In this condition, glycolipid deposits also are present in endothelium and vascular smooth muscle and in most other body tissues. The disease results from a deficiency of ceramide trihexosidase, an enzyme which hydrolyzes ceramide trihexoside. This glycolipid accumulates in the form of birefringent granules composed of concentric or parallel lamellae spaced 40–65 Å apart. In ordinary histologic preparations, the deposits are dissolved and the cardiac muscle cells resemble those in type II glycogenosis.

Calcium

Calcium is most commonly observed in the heart in the coronary arteries, mitral anulus, aortic and scarred mitral valve cusps, in large myocardial scars and in the pericardium. In these circumstances the calcific deposits are extracellular. Calcific deposits, however, also may occur within individual myocardial cells. This occurrence most commonly is observed in patients with fatal prolonged shock or renal failure. Its cause is uncertain, although severe hypoxia is the most likely explanation because the lesion may be produced experimentally by this means [1]. High serum levels of calcium also may be a factor. The myofibers infiltrated by calcium are always necrotic. Massive myocardial calcification may occur and produce cardiac dysfunction.

Inflammatory Heart Muscle Diseases

Known Infectious Agent

In contrast to noninflammatory ones, inflammatory heart diseases infrequently are observed today at necropsy. Acute myocarditis is now most commonly seen at necropsy only in patients with 'overwhelming' systemic acute infections, in those receiving immunosuppressive therapy, and those with infective endocarditis [11, 12].

Virtually every known bacterium, virus, parasite, rickettsia, spirochete and treponema, and fungus has been shown to produce myocarditis. The myocardial involvement is rarely primary but associated with involvement of other body organs and tissues.

Unknown Agent

An occasional patient at necropsy is observed to have foci of polymorphonuclear or mononuclear cell myocardial inflammation unassociated with stainable organisms or positive cultures. Most of these patients have received antibiotic therapy so that possibly the organisms, although not the inflammatory response, were eradicated.

Associated with Another Known Condition

Collagen Disease

Focal specific inflammatory infiltrates, namely Aschoff bodies and rheumatoid nodules, are recognized lesions in the heart in acute rheumatic fever and rheumatoid arthritis, respectively [13]. Fortunately, fatal acute rheumatic fever is infrequent today; when it does occur, the cardiac inflammatory response often has been altered by corticosteroid therapy. Rheumatoid nodules in the myocardium also may be affected by corticosteroid therapy. The latter occur in about 3% of patients with fatal rheumatoid arthritis. Aschoff bodies are found in most patients dying during the acute episode of rheumatic fever and at necropsy in about 5% of patients with mitral stenosis.

At one time, focal myocarditis was believed to be fairly common in systemic lupus erythematosus. In the corticosteroid era, however, myocarditis is extremely rare [14].

Sarcoidosis

A neglected cause of cardiac dysfunction is cardiac sarcoidosis, i.e., the replacement of portions of myocardial wall by sarcoid granulomas [15]. Hard granulomas are found in the heart in about 20% of patients with sarcoidosis studied at necropsy. Although sarcoid lesions are never limited to the heart, most patients with cardiac sarcoidosis have symptoms resulting primarily from cardiac dysfunction. In other words, a patient with sarcoidosis either has dominant cardiac involvement or the heart is spared [15]. The cardiac deposits preferentially involve the cephalad portion of the ventricular septum, producing severe conduction disturbances, particularly complete heart block; or the left ventricular papillary muscles and the adjacent free walls, producing papillary muscle dysfunction; or right or left ventricular free walls, which, after corticosteroid therapy, may scar and lead to ventricular aneurysm. Ventricular arrhythmias, particularly tachycardia, are frequent consequences. Sudden death is common and may be the initial manifestation of sarcoidosis.

References

1 ROBERTS, W. C. and FERRAS, V.J.: Pathologic anatomy of the cardiomyopathies. Idiopathic dilated and hypertrophic types, infiltrative types, and endomyocardial disease with and without eosinophilia. Hum. Path. *6:* 287–342 (1975).

2 Bulkley, B. H. and Roberts, W. C.: Dilatation of the mitral anulus. A rare cause of mitral regurgitation. Am. Heart J. *59:* 457–463 (1975).

3 Ferrans, V. J.; Massumi, R. A.; Shugoll, G. I.; Ali, N., and Roberts, W. C.: Ultrastructural studies of myocardial biopsies in 45 patients with obstructive or congestive cardiomyopathy; in Bajusz,, Rona, Brink and Lochner Recent advances in studies on cardiac structure and metabolism, vol. 2; Cardiomyopathies, pp. 231–272 (University Park Press, Baltimore 1972).

4 Roberts, W. C. and Buja, L. M.: The frequency and significance of coronary arterial thrombi and other observations in fatal acute myocardial infarction. A study of 107 necropsy patients. Am. J. Med. *52:* 425–443 (1972).

5 Epstein, S. E.; Clark, C. E.; Maron, B. J.; Redwood, D. R.; Henry, W. L.; Roberts, W. C.; Ferrans, V. J., and Morrow, A. G.: Asymmetric septal hypertrophy. Ann. intern. Med. *81:* 650–680 (1974).

6 Teare, D.: Asymmetrical hypertrophy of the heart in young adults. Br. Heart J. *20:* 1–18 (1958).

7 Ferrans, V. J.; Morrow, A. G., and Roberts, W. C.: Myocardial ultrastructure in idiopathic hypertrophic subaòrtic stenosis. A study of operatively excised left ventricular outflow tract muscle in 14 patients. Circulation *45:* 769–792 (1972).

8 Roberts, W. C.: Operative treatment of hypertrophic obstructive cardiomyopathy. The case against mitral valve replacement. Am. J. Cardiol. *32:* 377–381 (1973).

9 Buja, L. M.; Khoi, N. B., and Roberts, W. C.: Clinically significant cardiac amyloidosis. Clinicopathologic findings in 15 patients. Am. J. Cardiol. *26:* 394–405 (1970).

10 Buja, L. M. and Roberts, W. C.: Iron in the heart. Etiology and clinical significance. Am. J. Med. *51:* 209–221 (1971).

11 Roberts, W. C.; Bodey, G. P., and Wertlake, P. T.: The heart in acute leukemia. A study of 420 autopsy cases. Am. J. Cardiol. *21:* 388–413 (1968).

12 Buchbinder, N. A. and Roberts, W. C.: Left-sided valvular active infective endocarditis. A study of forty-five necropsy patients. Am. J. Med. *53:* 20–35 (1972).

13 Roberts, W. C.; Kehoe, J. A.; Carpenter, D. F., and Golden, A.: Cardiac valvular lesions in rheumatoid arthritis. Archs intern. Med. *122:* 141–146 (1968).

14 Bulkley, B. H. and Roberts, W. C.: The heart in systemic lupus erythematosus and the changes induced in it by corticosteroid therapy. A study of 36 necropsy patients. Am. J. Med. *58:* 243–264 (1975).

15 Roberts, W. C.; McAllister, H. A., jr., and Ferrans, V. J.: Sarcoidosis of the heart. A clinicopathologic study of 35 necropsy patients (group I) and review of 78 previously desribed necropsy patients (group II). Am. J. Med. *63:* 86–108 (1977).

W. C. Roberts, MD, Building 10A, Room 3E–30, National Institutes of Health, *Bethesda, MD 20014* (USA)

Myocardial Biopsy: A Useful Diagnostic Procedure or Only a Research Tool? *

VICTOR J. FERRANS, MD, PhD
WILLIAM C. ROBERTS, MD, FACC

Bethesda, Maryland

In 1962, Sakakibara and Konno[1] reported doing endomyocardial biopsies in patients using a catheter inserted into the right ventricle from a systemic vein. The right ventricular aspect of the ventricular septum was the portion of heart biopsied. Biopsy specimens of human left ventricular wall were obtained as early as 1956[2] with use of a transthoracic needle (using methods similar to those employed in a hepatic biopsy) and later by various modifications of the Konno catheter.[3–9] The report by Mason[10] in this issue of the Journal describes still another method of biopsy of the myocardium performed with a catheter and mentions that 1,300 cardiac biopsies have been performed in recent years by one or more catheter techniques in a single institution. It is now recognized that closed chest cardiac biopsy can be performed with a catheter at minimal risk and that several specimens can be obtained for examination during the same procedure. This editorial will attempt to summarize what has been learned to date from myocardial biopsies obtained by these closed chest catheter methods and to ask if the procedure is worth the risk, time and expense.

Since 1968, we have studied in our laboratory approximately 90 endomyocardial biopsy specimens, two thirds obtained with the Konno or the Olympus catheter from the right ventricle and one third with transthoracic Menghini needle biopsy of the left ventricular wall.[11] Most of these specimens were from patients who had some type of cardiomyopathy. The Konno catheter biopsies were performed by Drs. Rashid A. Massumi and Nayab Ali,[3,8] and the needle biopsies by Dr. Gerald I. Shugoll.[12] In addition, we have examined operatively obtained biopsy tissue from either the left or the right ventricle or the left atrium from more than 100 patients with various types of congenital and acquired heart diseases.[13–19] All biopsy samples were studied histologically; most were also studied with transmission electron microscopy and some were also studied histochemically. What was learned from these studies and from those of others?

1. Many details of the subcell pathology of human hearts were learned by study of the closed chest biopsy specimens. Similar observations were made, however, on cardiac biopsy tissue obtained from patients undergoing various types of cardiac operations, primarily open heart procedures. Thus, much of the "cell biology" type of information (as opposed to purely diagnostic information) derived from the closed chest biopsies also was obtained, often with fewer artifacts, at open chest biopsy.

2. The endomyocardial biopsies have had limited value from a diagnostic standpoint.

Idiopathic dilated cardiomyopathy: The biopsies provided the first opportunity to study ultrastructurally well preserved myocardium in patients with this condition.[20] Earlier ultrastructural studies[21] had been limited to tissues obtained at necropsy that showed considerable autolytic changes. The biopsies allowed documentation of the extent of the myocardial damage present but failed to disclose specific histologic or ultrastructural features that could be used as qualitative "markers" to establish the diagnosis of this condition. Thus, the diagnosis of idiopathic dilated cardiomyopathy cannot be made on the basis of myocardial biopsy, although there is generally a good correlation between the severity of the condition clinically and the extent of the morphologic changes.[11,22]

Especially disappointing have been the failures of biopsy studies to find viral particles or specific histochemical or immunohistochemical "markers" in the myocardium of patients with idiopathic dilated cardiomyopathy. Similarly, viral culture studies of myo-

From the Pathology Branch, National Heart, Lung, and Blood Institute, National Institutes of Health, Bethesda, Maryland 20014. Manuscript received January 16, 1978, accepted February 8, 1978.

cardial biopsy material from patients with idiopathic dilated cardiomyopathy appear to have met with little success. Although myocardial biopsies are potentially useful for biochemical studies, surprisingly little work has been published on this subject. The small size of the biopsy specimens severely limits the performance of many biochemical procedures, particularly those requiring extensive preparatory steps (such as cell fractionation). Nevertheless, a combined biochemical and ultrastructural study of tissue obtained by operative biopsy showed that cardiac muscle myosin from patients with hypertrophic cardiomyopathy does not differ from normal in its adenine triphosphatase activity, in its ability to form bipolar rods or in the morphologic features of such rods.[23]

Myocardial tissues from patients with idiopathic dilated cardiomyopathy appear to differ morphologically from those of patients with other types of heart disease quantitatively (that is, the extent of the hypertrophy and the damage) rather than qualitatively. Such differences must be evaluated in relation not only to the nature, but also to the severity and duration of the basic disease processes. Quantitative analysis (morphometry), including changes in surface/volume ratios and in the percent of cell volume occupied by myofibrils, mitochondria, nuclei and other organelles, presents a new approach to the study of cardiac ultrastructural alterations.[24,25] It is uncertain whether this methodology will have diagnostic applications, although it has become clear that morphometric analysis can detect various structural changes that are not recognizable from simple visual study of electron micrographs. Nevertheless, morphometric study presents formidable technical and statistical problems. It is only in the last few years that progress has been made in this area of cardiac pathology, and most of this progress has been in studies of relatively early and uncomplicated hypertrophy in small experimental animals.[24,25] The tissue fixation requirements considered necessary for such studies are extremely strict (including fixation by vascular perfusion) in order to minimize data scatter (that is, inhomogeneity in tissue structure) resulting from regional differences in the quality of the fixation. These requirements increase the practical difficulty of morphometric studies based on biopsy material, in which the tissue sample is small and often shows appreciable artifactual ultrastructural changes. These changes are due to tearing of tissue by the cutting edges of the biopsy instrument and to the unopposed contraction (leading to formation of hypercontraction bands and to translocation of cell organelles) of cells at the edges of the biopsy specimen. In fact, these changes can mimic true pathologic changes and can be the source of considerable difficulty in the qualitative evaluation of myocardial biopsy specimens.[11] An empirical answer has not yet been given to the complex question of how representative a biopsy sample (or two or three) is of the state of the whole heart. Obviously, the answer will depend not only on the exact site of the biopsy (right side of ventricular septum versus left ventricular free wall) but also on the focal or diffuse nature of the changes occurring in a given disease. Brooksby et al.[4] reported that the microscopic appearance of left and right ventricular biopsy specimens differed in 60 percent of their patients.

Idiopathic hypertrophic cardiomyopathy: The closed chest myocardial biopsy samples are of inadequate size to establish firmly the diagnosis of hypertrophic cardiomyopathy with this method. Nevertheless, the cardiac biopsy specimens obtained at open thoracotomy (at the time of the therapeutic cardiac operation) have provided much detailed ultrastructural information about myocardial cells in this condition.[26,27] The closed chest biopsy specimens are usually too small to evaluate disarray of groups of cells, but they have provided information about disarray of myofibrils and myofilaments within individual myocytes. A striking demonstration of these changes has been provided by a recent scanning electron microscopic study.[28] Most of the ultrastructural information on myocardium in patients with hypertrophic cardiomyopathy, however, has been obtained by study of either biopsy specimens or resected tissue obtained at open thoracotomy. Furthermore, it is now known that the foci of disarray of whole cells and of their contractile elements do not constitute a specific "marker" for the diagnosis of hypertrophic cardiomyopathy. Such changes also occur (although usually to a smaller extent than in hypertrophic cardiomyopathy) in certain patients with other types of heart diseases (see Ref 29 for review). Thus, additional ultrastructural information to be provided by closed chest endomyocardial biopsy in hypertrophic cardiomyopathy appears limited.

Infiltrative cardiomyopathies: Of the various types of cardiomyopathy, endomyocardial biopsy is most likely to be useful from a diagnostic standpoint in the infiltrative group. In the patient with cardiac dysfunction due to cardiac *amyloidosis*, the amyloid deposits are extensive throughout the ventricular wall and, therefore, myocardial biopsy studies are likely to be positive if the cardiac dysfunction is on the basis of cardiac amyloidosis. In amyloidosis involving the heart,[30] however, other organs usually contain amyloid deposits and, thus, biopsy studies of the tongue, liver, rectum, skin and other areas are also likely to be positive, and these tissues are more accessible to biopsy than is the heart. The same can be said for cardiac *hemosiderosis*.[31] When there is enough iron in the heart to cause it to function abnormally, iron deposits always are present in virtually every other body organ.[31] The same is true of the glycogen deposits in types II, III and IV *glycogen storage disease*.[32] *Granulomatous myocarditis*, which generally means *sarcoidosis*, is a focal process in the heart, in contrast to disease due to amyloid, iron or glycogen.[33] Thus, biopsy findings could be negative when many granulomas actually are present in the myocardium. Granulomas in sarcoidosis tend to involve preferentially the ventricular septum; therefore, biopsy may be worthwhile if this condition cannot be diagnosed by another means.[33]

Drug-induced cardiomyopathy: Endomyocardial biopsy studies in patients with *adriamycin cardiomy-*

opathy have proved informative by documenting damage to various myofiber organelles, but they have been less useful in predicting in which patients adriamycin cardiomyopathy will develop.[34]

Similarly, various myocardial changes have been documented by biopsy studies in patients with certain *congenital cardiomyopathies*,[35] but again the changes have not been useful diagnostically.

Cardiac transplants: In patients with cardiac transplantation the Stanford group[36] has demonstrated that endomyocardial biopsy is useful in diagnosing transplant rejection and in evaluating therapeutic intervention to counteract it. Thus, for this limited group of patients, endomyocardial biopsy appears useful from a diagnostic standpoint.

In summary, closed chest endomyocardial biopsy in the more common varieties of cardiomyopathy—the dilated and hypertrophic types—has been informative but rarely diagnostic. In the uncommon varieties of cardiomyopathy—amyloid, iron, glycogen, granuloma, neoplasm—this procedure is more useful from a diagnostic standpoint, but diagnosis of these disorders usually can be established more readily by biopsy of another more easily accessible tissue or organ.

References

1. **Sakakibara S, Konno S:** Endomyocardial biopsy. Jpn Heart J 3: 537–543, 1962
2. **Sutton DC, Sutton GC, Kent G:** Needle biopsy of the human ventricular myocardium. Q Bull Northwestern Univ Med Sch 30: 213–214, 1956
3. **Ali N, Ferrans VJ, Roberts WC, et al:** Clinical evaluation of transvenous catheter technique for endomyocardial biopsy. Chest 63:399–402, 1973
4. **Brooksby IAB, Jenkins BS, Coltart DJ, et al:** Left ventricular endomyocardial biopsy. Lancet 2:1222–1225, 1974
5. **Brooksby IAB, Swanton RH, Jenkins BS, et al:** Long sheath technique for introduction of catheter tip manometer or endomyocardial bioptome into left or right heart. Br Heart J 36:908–912, 1974
6. **Caves PK, Schulz WP, Dong E Jr, et al:** New instrument for transvenous cardiac biopsy. Am J Cardiol 33:264–267, 1974
7. **Richardson PJ:** King's endomyocardial bioptome. Lancet 1: 660–661, 1974
8. **Ali N:** Transvenous endomyocardial biopsy using the gastrointestinal biopsy (Olympus GFB) catheter. Am Heart J 87:294–297, 1974
9. **Kawai C, Kitaura Y:** New endomyocardial biopsy catheter for the left ventricle. Am J Cardiol 40:63–65, 1977
10. **Mason JW:** Techniques for right and left ventricular endomyocardial biopsy. Am J Cardiol 41:887–892, 1978
11. **Ferrans VJ, Massumi RA, Shugoll GI, et al:** Ultrastructural studies of myocardial biopsies in 45 patients with obstructive or congestive cardiomyopathy. In, Recent Advances in Studies on Cardiac Structure and Metabolism, Vol II, The Cardiomyopathies (Bajusz E, Rona G, Brink AJ, et al, ed). Baltimore, University Park Press, 1973, p 231–272
12. **Shugoll GI:** Percutaneous myocardial and pericardial biopsy with the Nenghini needle. Am Heart J 85:35–39, 1973
13. **Jones M, Ferrans VJ, Morrow AG, et al:** Ultrastructure of crista supraventricularis muscle in patients with congenital heart diseases associated with right ventricular outflow tract obstruction. Circulation 51:39–68, 1975
14. **Maron BJ, Ferrans VJ, Roberts WC:** Ultrastructural features of degenerated cardiac muscle cells in patients with cardiac hypertrophy. Am J Pathol 79:387–434, 1975
15. **Maron BJ, Ferrans VJ, Roberts WC:** Myocardial ultrastructure in patients with chronic aortic valve disease. Am J Cardiol 35: 725–739, 1975
16. **Jones M, Ferrans VJ:** Myocardial degeneration in congenital heart disease: a comparison of morphologic findings in young and old patients with congenital heart diseases associated with muscular obstruction to right ventricular outflow. Am J Cardiol 39:1051–1063, 1977
17. **Thiedemann K-U, Ferrans VJ:** Ultrastructure of sarcoplasmic reticulum in atrial myocardium of patients with mitral valvular disease. Am J Pathol 83:1–38, 1976
18. **Thiedemann K-U, Ferrans VJ:** Left atrial ultrastructure in mitral valvular disease. Am J Pathol 89:575–604, 1977
19. **Ferrans VJ, Thiedemann K-U, Maron BJ, et al:** Spherical microparticles in human myocardium. An ultrastructural study. Lab Invest 35:349–368, 1976
20. **Alexander CS:** Idiopathic heart disease. II. Electron microscopic examination of myocardial biopsy specimens in alcoholic heart disease. Am J Med 41:229–234, 1966
21. **Hibbs RG, Ferrans VJ, Black WC, et al:** Alcoholic cardiomyopathy: an electron microscopic study. Am Heart J 69:766–779, 1965
22. **Kunkel B, Kober G, Lapp H, et al:** Klinische, lichtund elektronenmikroskopische Befunde bei frühen und fortgeschrittenen Formen kongestiver Kardiomyopathien. Z Kardiol 68:198–202, 1977
23. **Maron BJ, Ferrans VJ, Adelstein RS:** Isolation and characterization of myosin from subjects with asymmetric septal hypertrophy. Circ Res 40:468–473, 1977
24. **Page E, Polimeni PI, Zak R, et al:** Myofibrillar mass in rat and rabbit heart muscle: correlation of microchemical with stereological measurements in normal and hypertrophied hearts. Circ Res 30: 430–439, 1972
25. **Page E, McCallister LP:** Quantitative electron microscopic description of heart muscle cells: application to normal, hypertrophied, and thyroxin-stimulated hearts. Am J Cardiol 31:172–181, 1973
26. **Ferrans VJ, Morrow AG, Roberts WC:** Myocardial ultrastructure in idiopathic hypertrophic subaortic stenosis. A study of operatively excised left ventricular outflow tract muscle in 14 patients. Circulation 45:769–792, 1972
27. **Maron BJ, Ferrans VJ, Henry WL, et al:** Differences in distribution of myocardial abnormalities in patients with obstructive and nonobstructive asymmetric septal hypertrophy (ASH): light and electron microscopic findings. Circulation 50:436–446, 1974
28. **Tulusan AH, Brandt G:** Morphologic differential diagnosis of idiopathic cardiomyopathies. Virchows Arch [Pathol Anat] 374:71–79, 1977
29. **Maron BJ, Ferrans VJ:** Ultrastructural features of hypertrophied human ventricular myocardium. Prog Cardiovasc Dis, in press
30. **Buja LM, Khoi NB, Roberts WC:** Clinically significant cardiac amyloidosis. Clinicopathologic findings in 15 patients. Am J Cardiol 26:394–405, 1970
31. **Buja LM, Roberts WC:** Iron in the heart. Etiology and clinical significance. Am J Med 51:209–221, 1971
32. **Howell RR:** The glycogen storage diseases. In, The Metabolic Basis of Inherited Disease, third edition (Stanbury JB, Wyngaarden JB, Fredrickson DS, ed). New York, McGraw-Hill, 1972, p 149–173
33. **Roberts WC, McAllister HA Jr, Ferrans VJ:** Sarcoidosis of the heart. A clincopathologic study of 35 necropsy patients (Group I) and review of 78 previously reported necropsy patients (Group II). Am J Med 63:86–108, 1977
34. **Bristow MR, Mason JW, Billingham ME, et al:** Endomyocardial biopsy and systolic time intervals in detection of adriamycin cardiotoxicity (abstr). Circulation 53, 54: Suppl II: II-80, 1976
35. **Hug G, Schubert WK:** Idiopathic cardiomyopathy. Mitochondrial and cytoplasmic alterations in heart and liver. Lab Invest 22: 541–552, 1970
36. **Caves PK, Stinson EB, Billingham ME, et al:** Percutaneous transvenous emdomyocardial biopsy in human heart recipients. Ann Thorac Surg 16:325–336, 1973

Clinical pathologic conference

Left and right ventricular myocardial infarction in idiopathic dilated cardiomyopathy

Jeffrey M. Isner, M.D.
Renu Virmani, M.D.
Samuel B. Itscoitz, M.D.
William C. Roberts, M.D.
Bethesda and Takoma Park, Md.

DR. ROBERTS: Dr. Isner will present the *patient's story* and *clinical findings.*

DR. ISNER: N. S. (Washington Adventist Hospital No. 14403-1), was a 62-year-old woman who died on September 23, 1978. Since age 53 years (1969), she had known of a "heart murmur" and a "large heart." She was asymptomatic until age 60 years when she developed exertional dyspnea and pedal edema. Examination then revealed distended neck veins, basilar pulmonary râles, a large heart, S_3 and S_4 sounds, an apical holosystolic murmur, and another systolic murmur, which increased with inspiration, at the left sternal border. The liver was palpable and both legs were edematous. Electrocardiogram disclosed sinus tachycardia with non-specific ST-T wave changes. The patient was started on digoxin and diuretics. She was hospitalized twice during the subsequent 2 years for overt congestive heart failure. Ten months before death an echocardiogram disclosed a dilated, poorly contracting left ventricle.

Because of increasing congestive cardiac failure she was hospitalized 5 days before death. She denied ever having chest pain. She had drunk alcohol infrequently and never had hypertension to her knowledge. Her blood pressure on admission was 110/90 mm. Hg with a pulsus paradoxus of 20 mm. Hg. Despite distention above the sternal angle of the neck veins, the lung fields were clear. The right ventricular impulse was more prominent than the left ventricular impulse. The remainder of the precordial examination was unchanged from the findings described 2 years earlier. The liver was enlarged and severe (4+/4+) subcutaneous edema was present in the lower legs. The hematocrit was 35 per cent; fasting serum glucose, 109 mg./dl.; serum total cholesterol, 170 mg./dl.; serum glutamic oxaloacetic transaminase, 61 mU./ml. (normal-7 to 40); lactic dehydrogenase, 302 mU./ml. (normal-100 to 225); creatinine phosphokinase, 208 mU./ml. (normal $<$145) with cardiac (MB) fraction, 1.9 (nl. $\leq$ 3 per cent). The electrocardiogram (Fig. 1) showed a vertical axis and inverted T waves in Leads III and aV_F, the chest radiograph (Fig. 2) showed marked cardiomegaly, and the echocardiogram (Fig. 3) was similar to the one recorded 10 months earlier. Her course worsened. On the day of death, her skin cooled and became moist, the blood pressure fell, and the electrocardiogram (Fig. 1) showed left bundle branch block. With ambu-bag pulmonary assistance, the arterial pO_2 was 69 mm. Hg; pCO_2, 55 mm. Hg, and pH 7.12. (On admission when breathing room air, the pO_2 had been 85 mm. Hg, pCO_2, 31 mm. Hg, and pH, 7.45.) The patient was intubated, and a Swan-Ganz catheter was inserted. Initial pressures (in mm. Hg) were: right atrial mean, 24; right ventricle, 55/24; pulmonary artery, 55/35; and mean pulmonary capillary wedge, 25. Despite intravenous administration of saline and dopamine, the systemic blood pressure continued to fall. Subxiphoid insertion of a needle ruled out cardiac tamponade. Shortly thereafter, fatal ventricular fibrillation occured.

From the Pathology Branch, National Heart, Lung, and Blood Institute, National Institutes of Health, Bethesda, Maryland, and the Department of Cardiology, Washington Adventist Hospital, Takoma Park, Maryland.

Received for publication Dec. 29, 1978.

Reprint requests: William C. Roberts, M.D., Building 10A, Room 3E30, National Institutes of Health, Bethesda, Md. 20014.

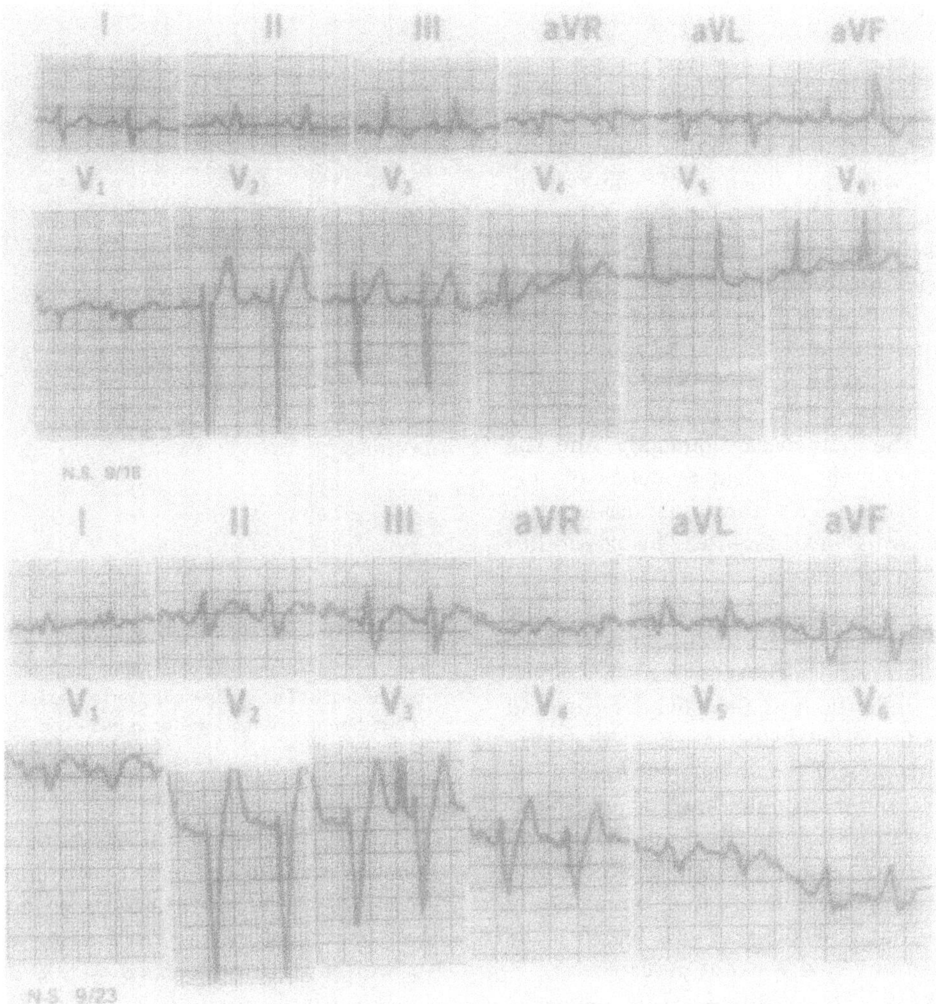

Fig. 1. Electrocardiograms. On admission (9/18), 5 days before death, the T-wave inversions in Leads III and aV_F are the only findings consistent with a scar in the posterior left ventricular free wall. Left bundle branch block appeared on the day of death (9/23).

Dr. Roberts: Dr. Virmani, would you decribe the *findings at necropsy.*

Dr. Virmani: At necropsy (WAH No. A7867), about 100 ml. of serous fluid was present in the pericardial sac. The heart weighed 580 grams. All four chambers were markedly dilated. There was transmural scarring of the posterior walls of both left and right ventricles and of the adjacent ventricular septum (Figs. 4 and 5). There were no foci of myocardial necrosis. Thrombi were present in both ventricles, and in the right atrial appendage. The major epicardial coronary arteries were wide open (Fig. 6). At no point were any portions of any epicardial coronary artery >25 per cent narrowed in cross-sectional area. The lungs together weighed 900 grams. Two hemorrhagic infarcts were present: one in the lower lobe of the left lung and the other in the upper lobe of the right lung. Some adjacent pulmonary arteries contained thromboemboli. Small healed infarcts were present in each kidney. The liver weighed 1,450 grams and was congested.

Dr. Roberts: Thus, we have a patient who was known to have cardiomegaly and an abnormal electrocardiogram for at least 10 years, evidence of chronic congestive heart failure for at least 2 years, never evidence of chest pain, and, at necropsy, very dilated ventricular cavities containing thrombi, large transmural scars involving the free walls of both left and right ventricles and the ventricular septum, and widely patent, virtually normal epicardial coronary arteries. Dr.

Itscoitz, what was your *clinical diagnosis* in this patient?

DR. ITSCOITZ: Three possibilities were considered. One was coronary heart disease, particularly in view of her age (62 years). Against this diagnosis, however, was the absence of chest pain, electrocardiographic absence of clear myocardial damage, and the absence of risk factors for atherosclerosis. Her total serum cholesterol was 170 mg./dl., she did not smoke, her blood pressure had always been normal, and her fasting blood sugar was normal. Idiopathic dilated cardiomyopathy was favored by the history of chronic congestive heart failure, the marked cardiomegaly, and the absence of chest pain, or clear evidence of "organic" valve disease. The third diagnosis considered was pericardial heart disease. This possibility was considered because of the extremely large cardiac silhouette by chest radiograph, the extreme prominence of features of right-sided congestive failure (the neck veins were enormously distended while the lung fields were clear, and she was able to lie flat in bed without distress), and the occurrence of diastolic pressures in the right ventricle and main pulmonary arteries similar to the mean pressures in the right atrium and pulmonary arterial wedge position. The possibility of cardiac tamponade was so high immediately before death that a needle was inserted into the pericardial sac but fluid was not detected.

DR. ROBERTS: Dr. Virmani, your necropsy observations in this patient are consistent with idiopathic dilated cardiomyopathy. What *morphologic criteria make this diagnosis at necropsy?*

DR. VIRMANI: To diagnose idiopathic dilated cardiomyopathy at necropsy, five criteria must be met: (1) both ventricular cavities must be dilated; (2) the heart weight must be increased (> 350 gms. in adult women and > 400 gms. in adult men); (3) the lumens of the major epicardial coronary arteries must be < 75 per cent narrowed in cross-sectional area by atherosclerotic plaque; (4) the four cardiac valves must be anatomically normal or have only minimal focal, small scars; and (5) no associated systemic or other known cardiovascular conditions can be present. In addition, intracardiac thrombi are usually present in one or more cardiac cavities, but this finding is not essential for diagnosis.

DR. ROBERTS: Dr. Itscoitz, although many clinical definitions of idiopathic dilated cardio-

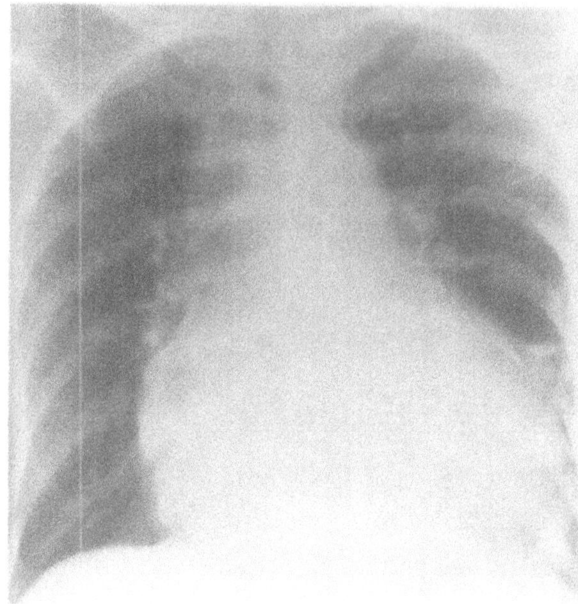

Fig. 2. Posteroanterior chest radiograph on admission 5 days before death The cardiac silhouette is markedly enlarged and the pulmonary vessels are prominent—i.e., "congested."

myopathy include the absence of systemic hypertension and the absence of valvular heart disease, many of these patients have systemic hypertension and most, before the end, have one or more precordial murmurs. *How do you diagnose idiopathic dilated cardiomyopathy in the presence of systemic hypertension or precordial murmurs or both?*

DR. ITSCOITZ: If systemic hypertension is present throughout the entire clinical course, I do not believe the diagnosis of idiopathic dilated cardiomyopathy would then be appropriate. If systemic hypertension were present, however, only at the beginning of the patient's course and was absent in the last few months, the diagnosis of idiopathic dilated cardiomyopathy could still be proper. In other words, if the blood pressure rises progressively and persists throughout the course, diagnosis of idiopathic dilated cardiomyopathy would not be appropriate.

In general, precordial murmurs appear relatively late in the course and the murmurs may get louder as the ventricular cavities get bigger. In the present patient, however, a precordial murmur preceded the presence of overt congestive heart failure, but that is unusual.

DR. ROBERTS: An unusual feature of this

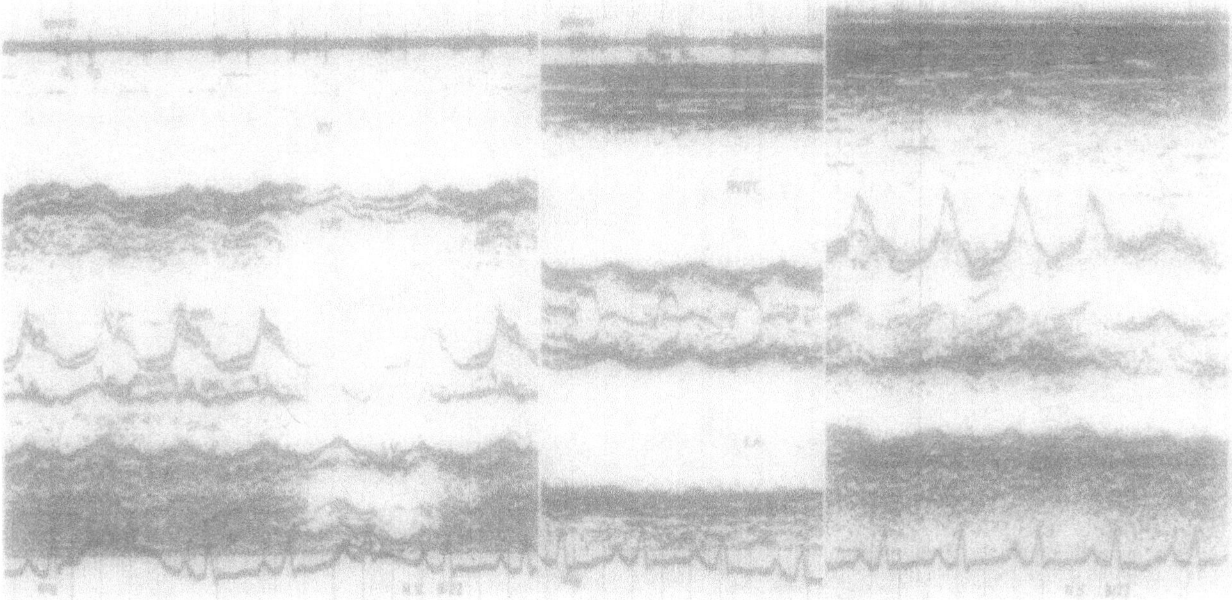

Fig. 3. Echophonocardiograms recorded one day before death. *Left*, ventricular dilatation with diminished excursion of both septum (*IVS*) and left ventricular (*LV*) free wall. There is no evidence of pericardial effusion. *RV* = right ventricle; *AML* and *PML* = anterior and posterior mitral leaflets, respectively. *Middle*, Severely dilated right ventricular outflow tract (*RVOT*). *Ao* = aortic valve within aorta; *LA* = left atrium; *SM* = systolic murmur. *Right*, Another view of the markedly dilated right ventricle at the level of the tricuspid valve (*TV*).

patient morphologically was the presence of a very large cardiac scar involving not only the left ventricular free wall and ventricular septum, but also the right ventricular free wall. I have studied the hearts of 153 necropsy patients with idiopathic dilated cariomyopathy and this patient had the largest ventricular scar of any. In addition, this is one of the few patients with idiopathic dilated cardiomyopathy seen personally at necropsy with extensive right ventricular scarring. Dr. Virmani, *could you enlighten us to the cause of ventricular scarring in patients with idiopathic dilated cardiomyopathy?*

DR. VIRMANI: The cause of cardiac ventricular scarring in patients with idiopathic dilated cardiomyopathy is unclear. By definition, the epicardial coronary arteries cannot be significantly narrowed in this condition, and, therefore, narrowing of these vessels is not a cause of the scarring. Embolism to the coronary arteries from thrombi located within the left side of the heart is a potential cause of left ventricular scarring. In patients with coronary embolism, however, whom we have studied at necropsy, there usually is evidence of occlusion of one or more of the intramural coronary arteries.[1] Multiple histologic sections of the ventricular walls in the present patient, however, disclosed no abnormality of the intramural coronary arteries and that observation is strong evidence aginst embolism as a cause of scarring. The extremely diminished cardiac output, which occurs in patients with idiopathic dilated cardiomyopathy, generally leads to a "global" myocardial ischemia and not so much to a focal myocardial ischemia. Ventricular scarring is always focal and, therefore, its explanation in these patients is uncertain.

DR. ROBERTS: Recently, Dr. Isner and I reviewed a large number of necropsy patients with coronary heart disease who had both right ventricular and left ventricular myocardial infarction.[2] The present patient, however, shows that right ventricular infarction may occur in the absence of coronary arterial luminal narrowing. Dr. Isner, *what features allow the clinical diagnosis of right ventricular infarction?*

DR. ISNER: From review of clinical and necropsy features of 33 patients with right ventricular myocardial infarction associated with left ventricular infarction, three findings suggest clinical-

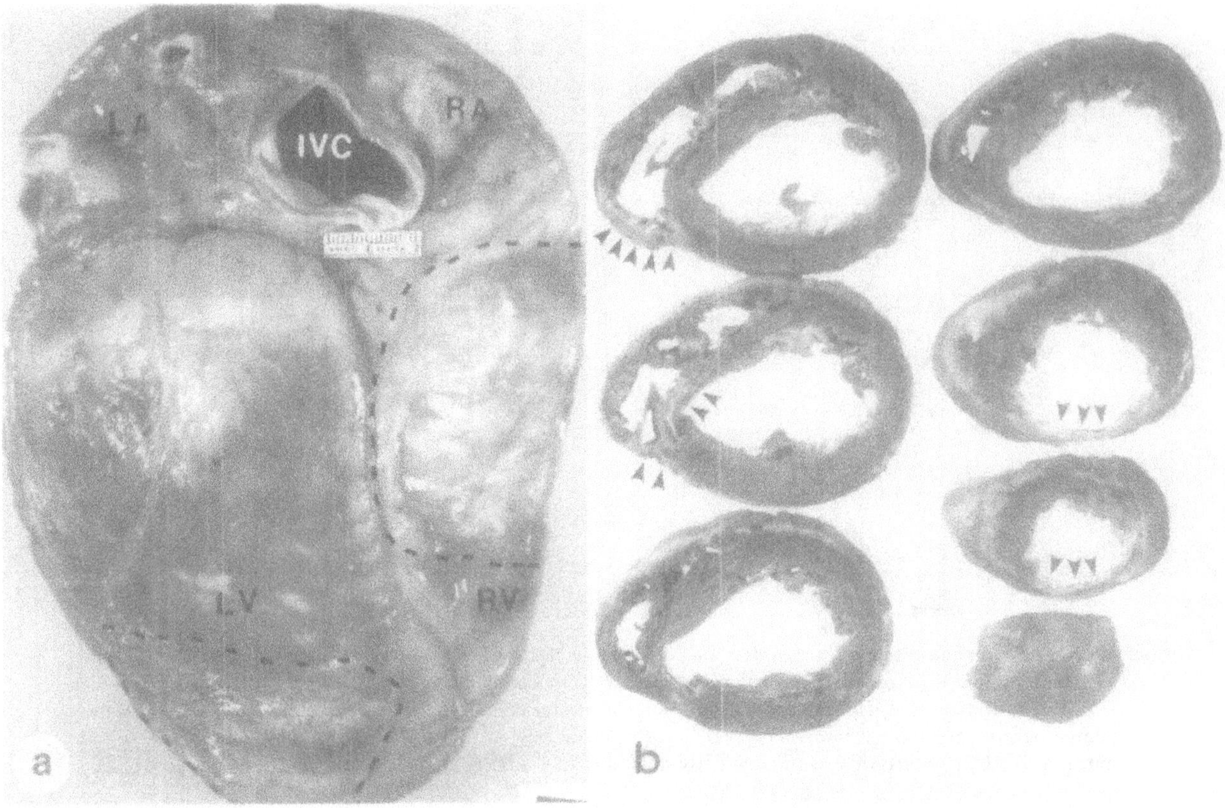

Fig. 4, a and b. Transmural ventricular scarring in the patient described. *a*, Posterior view of heart showing external appearance of left ventricular (*LV*) and right ventricular (*RV*) scars (*enclosed by dashed lines*). *b*, Transverse sections of ventricles from base (*upper left*) to apex (*lower right*). *The arrows* designate sites of transmural scarring. *LA* = left atrium; *RA* = right atrium; *IVC* = inferior vena cava.

ly the presence of right ventricular infarction[2]: (1) electrocardiographic evidence of an inferior or posterior left ventricular wall myocardial infarction, (2) evidence of right ventricular dilatation, and (3) a right ventricular filling pressure equal to or out of proportion to the left ventricular filling pressure. Of our 33 patients, all had an associated infarction of the posterior ("inferior") wall of the left ventricle. In contrast, of 97 patients with isolated anterior wall infarction of the left ventricle, none had associated right ventricular myocardial infraction. Furthermore, among the patients with posterior wall left ventricular infarcts, those with right ventricular myocardial infarcts had right ventricular dilatation observed at necropsy nearly three times more frequently than did the patients without right ventricular myocardial infarcts. Comparison of patients with right ventricular myocaridal infarction, however, disclosed no differences in the patient's age, sex, extent of coronary arterial luminal narrowing, presence of right ventricular hypertrophy, or right ventricular thrombi, or the length of symptoms of myocardial ischemia.

Dr. Roberts: Dr. Isner, *what clinical features in the present patient,* in retrospect, *might have suggested the presence of healed right ventricular infarction?*

Dr. Isner: First as Dr. Itscoitz pointed out, the signs of right ventricular failure were out of proportion to those of left ventricular failure. The neck veins were severely distended and yet the patient could lie flat in bed without respiratory distress. Secondly, echocardiograms done at 10 months and at one day before death both demonstrated severe right ventricular dilatation, a finding at least consistent with right ventricular myocardial infarction. Surprisingly, no electrocardiographic evidence of unequivocal infarction of the posterior wall of the left ventricle, however,

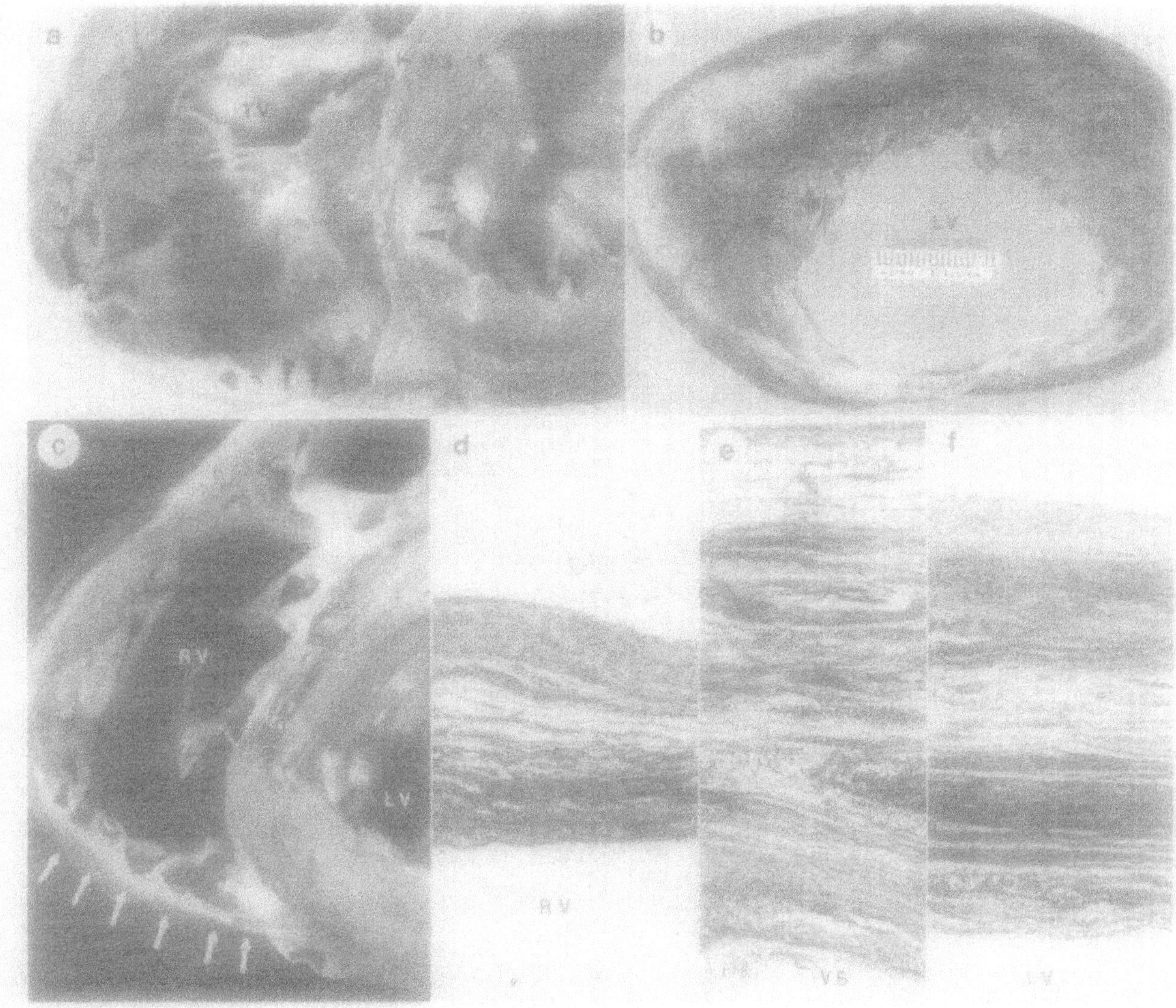

Fig. 5, a through f. Transmural ventricular scarring. *a, Arrows* designate thinning due to healed myocardial infarct of ventricular septum (*VS*) and posterior wall of ventricle (*RV*). *TV* = tricuspid valve. *b,* Posterior wall of left ventricle (*LV*) which is scarred and thinned. *c,* Posterior right ventricular scar (*arrows*) at level approximately 1 cm. caudad to *a*. *d, e, f,* Photomicrographs of healed transmural infarcts of RV, VS, and LV, respectively. (Movat stains; each original magnification ×36).

was present. The elevation of the pulmonary arterial diastolic pressure to a level of 9 mm. Hg greater than the mean pulmonary capillary "wedge" pressure was a reflection of pulmonary arterial hypertension, in this patient the result of pulmonary emboli. The elevation of right ventricular end-diastolic pressure, however, was out of proportion to both the elevated left ventricular end-diastolic pressure *and* the degree of pulmonary hypertension resulting from the pulmonary emboli. The degree of elevation of right ventricular end-diastolic pressure in this patient would be consistent with an associated right ventricular myocardial infarction.

Dr. Roberts: Dr. Isner, you[2] and others[3, 4] have mentioned that the signs of right ventricular infarction may mimic those of cardiac constriction or cardiac tamponade. How do you *distinguish the signs emanating from right ventricular infarction from those of pericardial heart disease?*

Dr. Isner: First, electrocardiographic or enzymatic evidence of myocardial infarction certainly would increase suspicion of an associated right

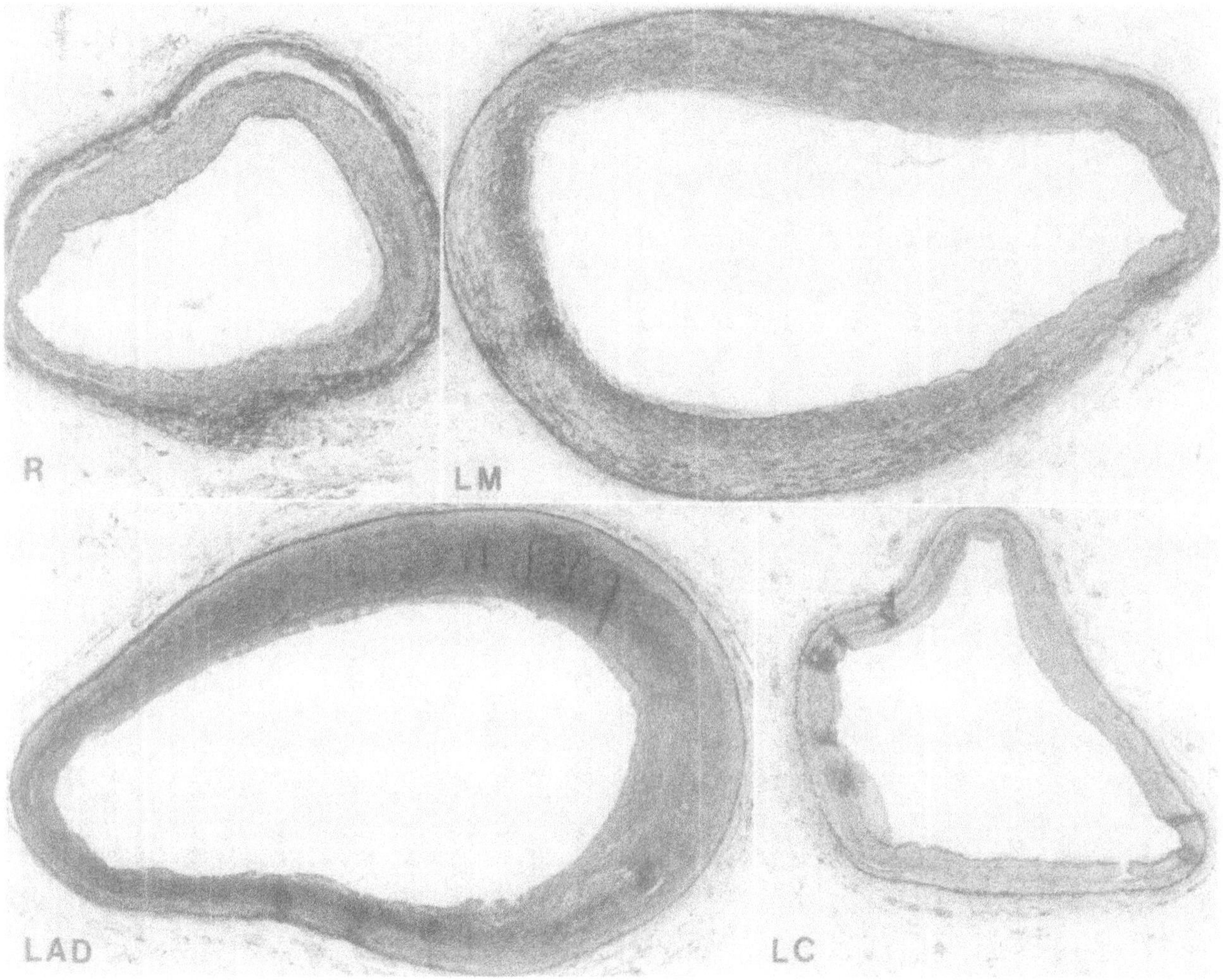

Fig. 6. Photomicrographs of each of the four major (right [*R*], left main [*LM*], left anterior descending [*LAD*], and left circumflex [*LC*]) coronary arteries at sites of maximal luminal narrowing. None of the coronary arteries were narrowed > 25 per cent in cross-sectional area. (Movat stain; each original magnification ×24).

ventricular infarction as opposed to primary pericardial disease. Secondly, right ventricular dilatation would be most unusual in a patient with impaired cardiac filling due to pericardial heart disease, whereas right ventricular dilatation is commonly present in patients with right ventricular myocardial infarcts. Finally, differentiation between pericardial heart disease and right ventricular myocardial infarction may not be possible on the basis of physical examination alone, and the use of noninvasive tools such as echocardiography and radionuclide angiography or invasive studies may be necessary to determine whether the clinical appearance of the patient is due to pericardial heart disease or to right ventricular myocardial infarction associated with left ventricular infarction.

DR. ROBERTS: The majority of patients with idiopathic dilated cardiomyopathy have mural thrombi in one or more ventricular cavities. The most frequent site is the left ventricle, next the right ventricle, third the right atrial appendage, and fourth, the left atrial appendage. The exact cause of these intracardiac thrombi is unclear, but it seems most reasonable to believe that they result simply from relative blood stasis or inadequate chamber emptying. The danger of intracardiac thrombi, obviously, is that they are sources of systemic and pulmonary emboli. In the present patient, emboli were observed at necropsy in both renal and pulmonary arteries with resulting infarcts of each organ. Dr. Isner, in retrospect, *what features suggested pulmonary embolism as the* terminal *event in our patient?*

DR. ISNER: The acute drop in blood pressure in spite of longstanding congestive heart failure, the drop in systemic arterial oxygen content, and the appearance of left bundle branch block suggested this possibility.[6]

REFERENCES

1. Roberts, W. C.: Coronary embolism: a review of causes, consequences, and diagnostic considerations, Cardiovasc. Med. **3**:699, 1978.
2. Isner, J. M., and Roberts, W. C.: Right ventricular infarction complicating left ventricular infarction secondary to coronary heart disease. Frequency, location, associated findings, and significance from analysis of 236 necropsy patients with acute or healed myocardial infarction, Am. J. Cardiol. **42**:885, 1978.
3. Lorell, B., Leinbach, R. C., Pohost, G. M., Gold, H. K., Dinsmore, R. E., Hutter, A. M., Pastore, J. O., and De Sanctis, R. W.: Right ventricular infarction. Clinical diagnosis and differentiation from cardiac tamponade and pericardial constriction, Am. J. Cardiol. **43**:465, 1979.
4. Jensen, D. P., Goolsby, J. P., and Oliva, P. B.: Hemodynamic pattern resembling pericardial constriction after acute inferior myocardial infarction with right ventricular infarction, Am. J. Cardiol. **42**:858, 1978.
5. Roberts, W. C., and Ferrans, V. J.: Pathologic anatomy of the cardiomyopathies. Idiopathic dilated and hypertrophic types, infiltrative types, and endomyocardial disease with and without eosinophilia, Hum. Pathol. **6**:287, 1975.
6. Lynch, R. E., Stein, P. D., and Bruce T. A.: Left-ward shift of frontal plane QRS axis as a frequent manifestation of acute pulmonary embolism, Chest **61**:443, 1972.

Cardiac Sarcoidosis*

A Major Cause of Sudden Death in Young Individuals

Renu Virmani, M.D.; J. Conrad Bures, M.D.; and William C. Roberts, M.D., F.C.C.P.

Dr. William C. Roberts: Herein we will discuss certain findings in a patient with cardiac sarcoidosis. Dr. Virmani will describe the patient.

Dr. Renu Virmani: A 35-year-old white man, a college philosophy professor who died Jan 9, 1979, was observed to have occasional ventricular premature beats during a medical check-up in March 1978 (ten months before death). No other abnormalities were found on examination. Specifically, he had no precordial murmur. He weighed 73.6 kg and was 175 cm tall. The ECG (Fig 1) showed low voltage, and chest roentgenogram (Fig 2) showed a normal sized heart and normal hilar and pulmonary shadows. In May 1978, he had an "upper respiratory infection," and in June 1978, he noted exertional dyspnea, two-pillow orthopnea, pedal edema, and severe fatigue. He was hospitalized in July 1978, his first and only hospitalization. The blood pressure was 110/70 mm Hg. The jugular veins were distended; rales were heard over both lungs; the heart was enlarged; a grade 2/6 holosystolic murmur now was heard at the lower left sternal border and it increased with inspiration; a third heart sound was present; and the feet were edematous. The blood hematocrit value was 45 percent; white blood cell count, 10,200/cu mm; blood urea nitrogen value, 38 mg/100 ml; serum creatinine level, 1.4 mg/100 ml; and serum total cholesterol value, 126 mg/100 ml. The IgG immunoglobulins were "low." The ECG was similar to the preceding one. The echocardiogram disclosed the maximal dimensions of the left ventricle to be 70 mm (normal, 40 to 52; left atrium, 45 mm (normal, 15 to 35); and the aorta, 30 mm (normal, 20 to 35). The walls of both the left ventricle and ventricular septum were 10 mm thick. Catheterization on July 25, 1979, disclosed the following pressures (mm Hg): pulmonary arterial wedge mean, 28; a-wave, 30, v-wave, 44; pulmonary trunk, 55/30 (mean 40);

*From the Pathology Branch, National Heart, Lung, and Blood Institute, National Institutes of Health, Bethesda, and the Department of Pathology, Montefiore Hospital, University of Pittsburgh Health Center, Pittsburgh.
Reprint requests: Dr. Roberts, NIH, Bldg 10A, Room 3E30, Bethesda 20205

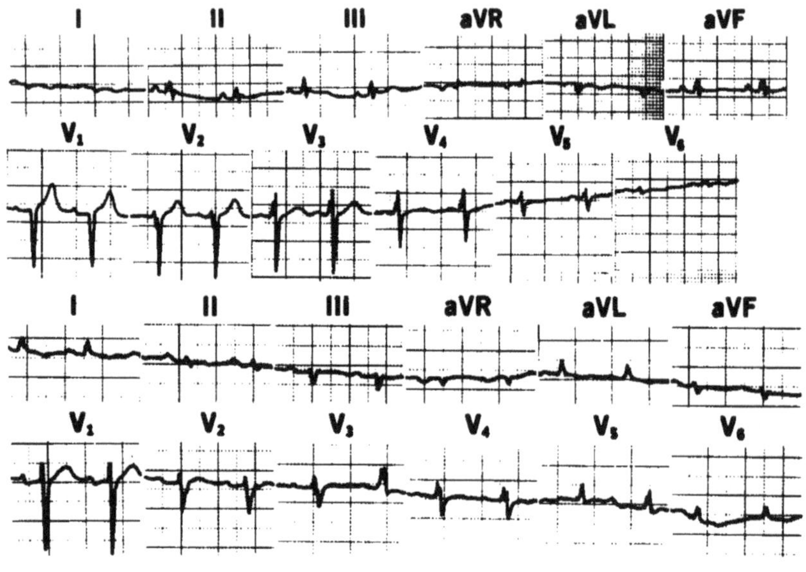

FIGURE 1. Electrocardiograms taken 3/6/78 (*upper*) and 9/6/78 (*lower*). Both show low voltage and nonspecific T-wave changes. One extrasystole is present in the lower electrocardiogram.

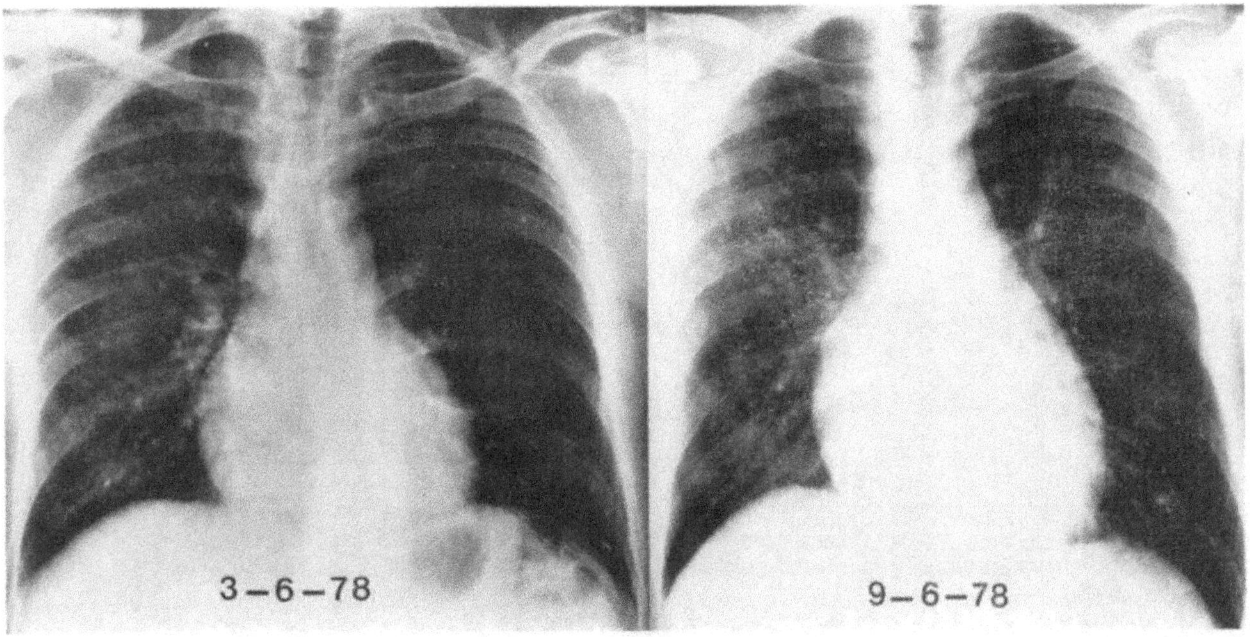

FIGURE 2. Chest roentgenograms taken 3/6/78 and 9/6/78. Cardiac silhouette has increased in size. Lung and hilar areas are normal.

right ventricle, 55/12; and right atrial mean, 10, a-wave 16. A diagnosis of idiopathic dilated cardiomyopathy was made and he was treated with digitalis, quinidine, chlorothiazide, and warfarin sodium. The dyspnea lessened considerably, the edema vanished, and he returned to his teaching duties. In September 1978, his weight was down to 146 pounds, his neck veins were flat, there was no edema, but a grade 3/6 murmur of tricuspid regurgitation persisted and a right ventricular lift was present. On Oct 13, 1978, he was started on a regimen of prednisone (10 mg daily), but during the next ten days, no subjective improvement was noted, and therefore, this medication was gradually discontinued over several more days. He remained asymptomatic until about Dec 20, 1978, when mild exertional dyspnea and orthopnea returned. His neck veins were distended, and the liver was both palpable and pulsatile. The weight had increased to 156 pounds, but he was not overtly edematous. He collapsed suddenly 19 days later while teaching and died.

Dr. Roberts: Dr. Bures, would you describe the findings at autopsy.

Dr. J. Conrad Bures: At necropsy (Montefiore Hospital, Pittsburgh), the heart weighed 460 g. All four cavities were dilated. The walls of both ventricles and both atria contained firm white deposits which histologically were typical sarcoid granulomas (Fig 3 to 6). The four cardiac valves and the coronary arteries were normal. Calcific deposits were present in a few myocardial fibers in the walls of all four cardiac chambers. The lungs together weighed 1,040 g; A 0.4-cm sized subpleural sarcoid granuloma was present in the right upper lobe. The tracheobronchial nodes measured up to 2 cm in diameter and they were nearly totally replaced by sarcoid granulomas (Fig 7). The liver (weight, 1,800 g) and spleen (weight, 300 g) were congested but free of granulomas. The rest of the organs were normal.

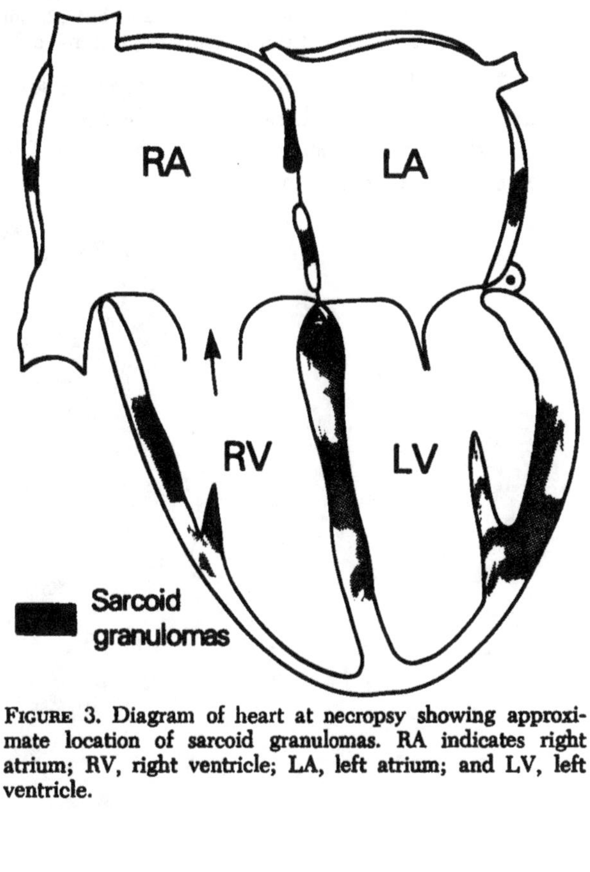

FIGURE 3. Diagram of heart at necropsy showing approximate location of sarcoid granulomas. RA indicates right atrium; RV, right ventricle; LA, left atrium; and LV, left ventricle.

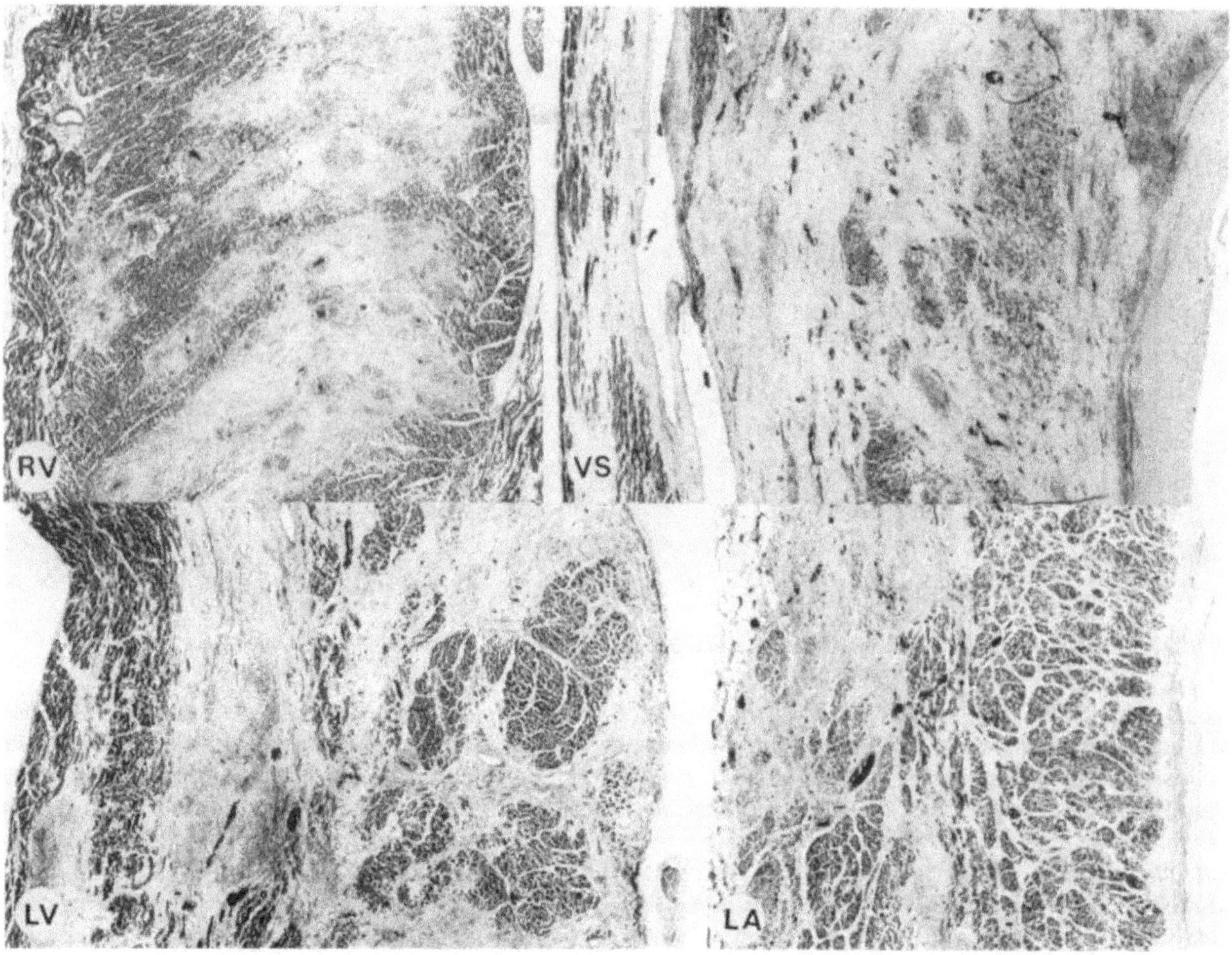

FIGURE 4. Sites of maximal involvement of walls of right ventricle (RV) ventricular septum (VS), left ventricle (LV), and left atrium (LA). There is extensive replacement by sarcoid granulomas (Movat stains, original magnification × 27), (RV, LV and LA) and × 21 (VS).

Dr. Roberts: The patient described exemplifies some of the diagnostic and therapeutic problems of patients with cardiac sarcoidosis. First, sarcoidosis was never diagnosed in life in our patient. Indeed, his clinical diagnosis was idiopathic dilated cardiomyopathy and this diagnosis seems, in retrospect, quite appropriate in view of the clinical findings. The patient was young (35 years old). His initial

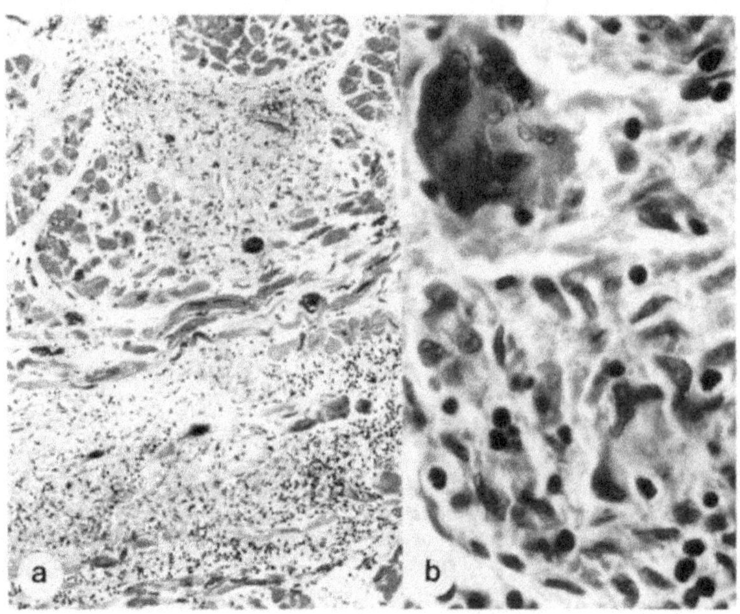

FIGURE 5. Extensive, sarcoid granulomatous involvement of left atrium. b (*right*), Close-up of giant cell, epitheloid cells and lymphocytes, a (*left*), Movat stain, original magnification × 130, and b (*right*), hematoxylin-eosin, original magnification × 880).

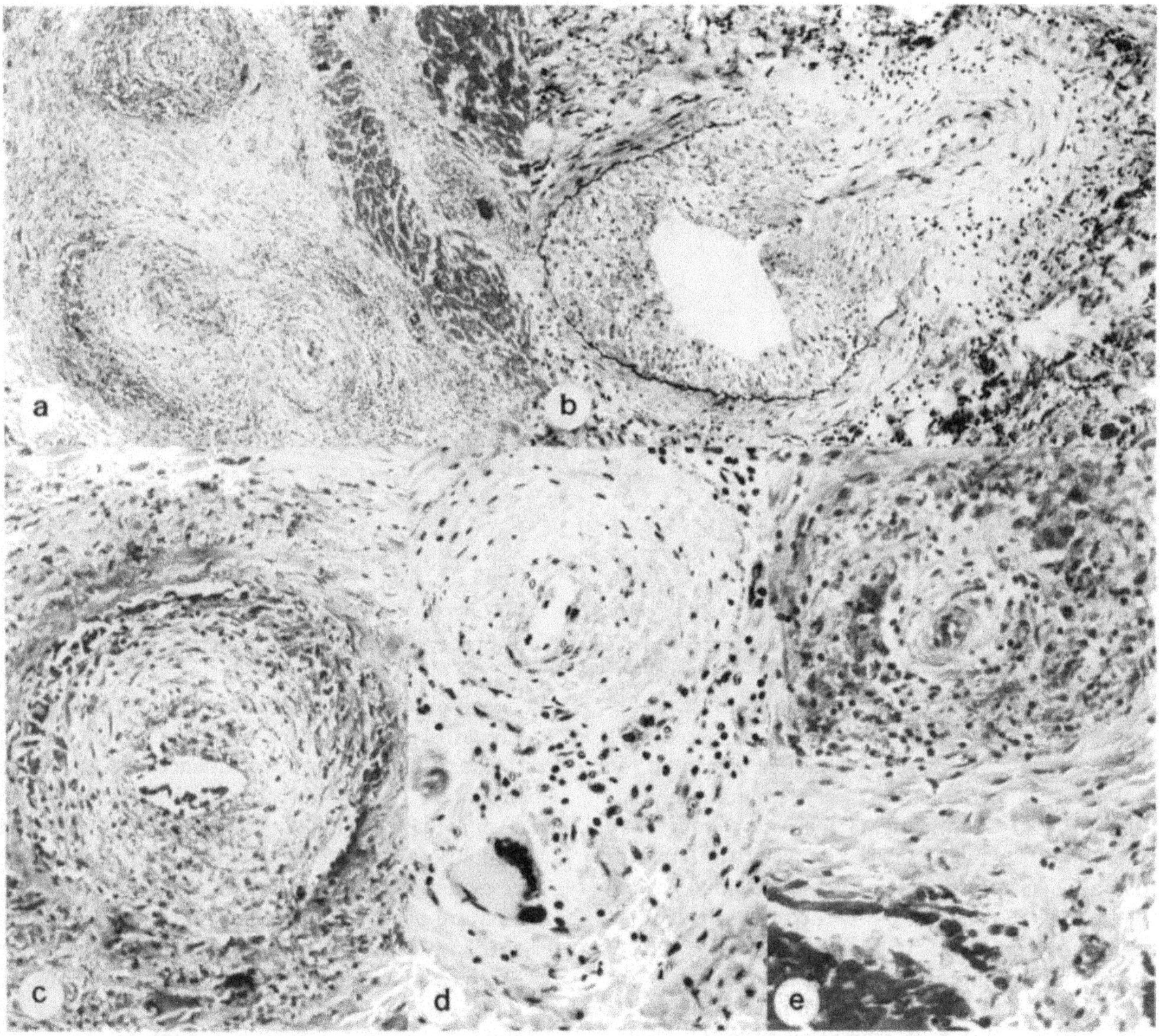

Figure 6. Intramural coronary arteries of ventricular septum, a, b, c, and d (*top figures* and *bottom, left* and *center*), and left ventricular free wall, e (*bottom right*) with surrounding sarcoid granulomas (sarcoid arteritis). Arteries or arterioles are surrounded by sarcoid granulomas and intima is thickened (Movat stains, original magnifications a [*top left*], × 80; b [*top right*], × 180; c [*bottom left*], × 220; d [*bottom center*], × 330; and e [*bottom right*, × 290]).

manifestation was ventricular premature beats which were noted on routine physical examination ten months before death, and he remained asymptomatic until six months before death when evidence of congestive heart failure appeared. He had cardiomegaly, a murmur of tricuspid regurgitation, and overt congestive heart failure which initially was quite responsive to medical therapy, but in his last month, reappeared. Because he was young and never had chest pain, coronary heart disease as a possibility never arose. The absence of a precordial murmur at the onset of his illness ruled out organic valvular heart disease as a reasonable diagnosis. During life, there were no signs suggesting the possibility of sarcoidosis. Chest roentgenogram showed normal lungs and no hilar adenopathy. Furthermore, lymph nodes were never palpated on physical examination. Moreover, there were no signs or symptoms of pulmonary disease. The mild hepatomegaly and splenomegaly were consistent with congestive heart failure and certainly did not suggest an infiltrative process, and at necropsy, no granulomas were present in either the liver or the spleen, and indeed, only one granuloma was observed in the lungs. There were no demonstrated ventricular arrhythmias other than an occasional ventricular premature beat during his illness. There were no cardiac conduction disturbances, heart block, syncope, or dizzy spells. Thus, clinically either retrospectively or prospectively, a diagnosis of sarcoidosis in the present patient would have been extremely difficult.

Approximately three months before death, the pa-

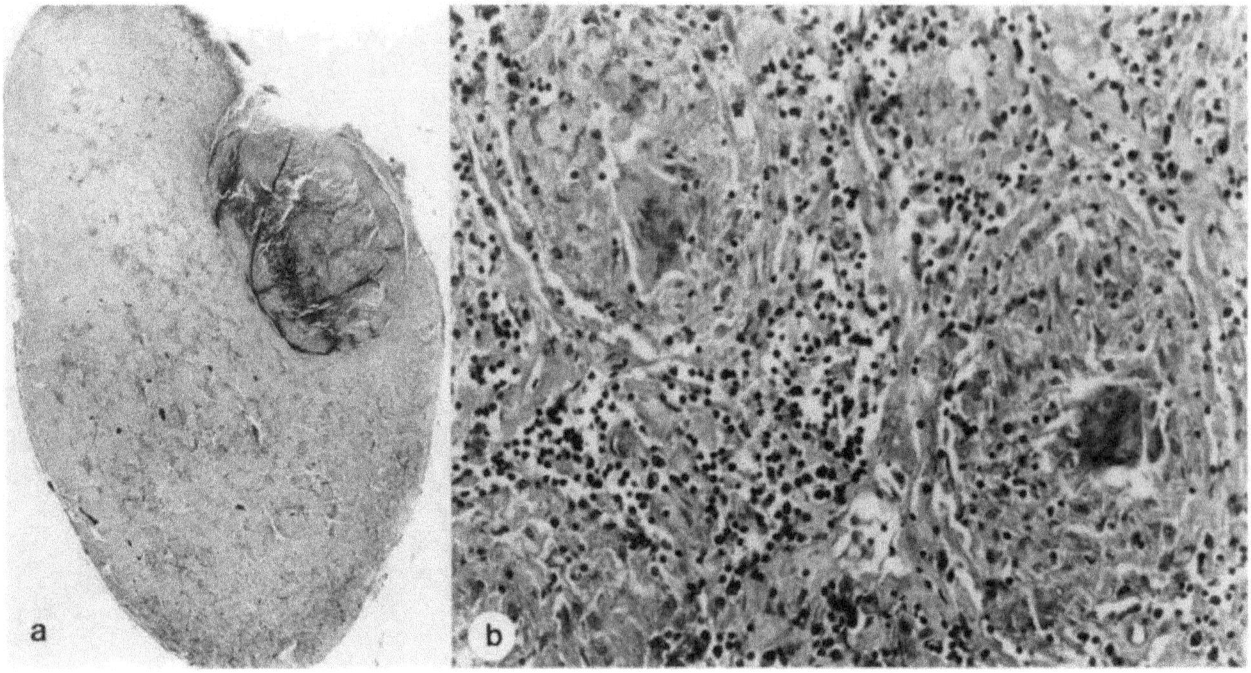

FIGURE 7. Tracheobronchial lymph node showing extensive replacement by sarcoid granulomas (hematoxylin-eosin, original magnificatoins a [*left*], × 8 and b [*right*], × 196]).

tient was given prednisone for about 15 days. Because no subjective improvement was noted, this medication was stopped. This patient brings up the possibility of a trial period of corticosteroid medication for all young patients who have congestive heart failure which is not secondary to valvular or coronary heart diseases or to hypertrophic cardiomyopathy. Possibly, if the corticosteroid treatment had been continued for a longer period and with higher doses, improvement may have occurred.

Sudden death is one of the well recognized modes of death in patients with cardiac sarcoidosis.[1] Indeed, it is the most common mode of death in patients with cardiac sarcoidosis extensive enough to cause cardiac dysfunction, and it is the first manifestation of sarcoidosis in about 20 percent of patients with cardiac sarcoidosis. It is relatively unusual, however, for a patient with cardiac sarcoidosis and evidence of chronic congestive heart failure to die suddenly. Most patients with sudden death from cardiac sarcoidosis have preceding evidence of ventricular arrhythmias (most commonly ventricular tachycardia) or evidence of high degrees of heart block (most commonly complete heart block). Our patient never had evidence of multifocal or runs of ventricular premature beats or ventricular tachycardia or complete heart block.

One of the unique features of cardiac sarcoidosis is that patients with infiltration of the heart by sarcoid granulomas extensive enough to cause cardiac dysfunction infrequently have evidence of dysfunction of another body organ.[1] Our patient only had evidence of cardiac dysfunction and no dysfunction of another body organ. At necropsy, only sites where sarcoid granulomas were observed were in the heart, mediastinal lymph nodes, and lung

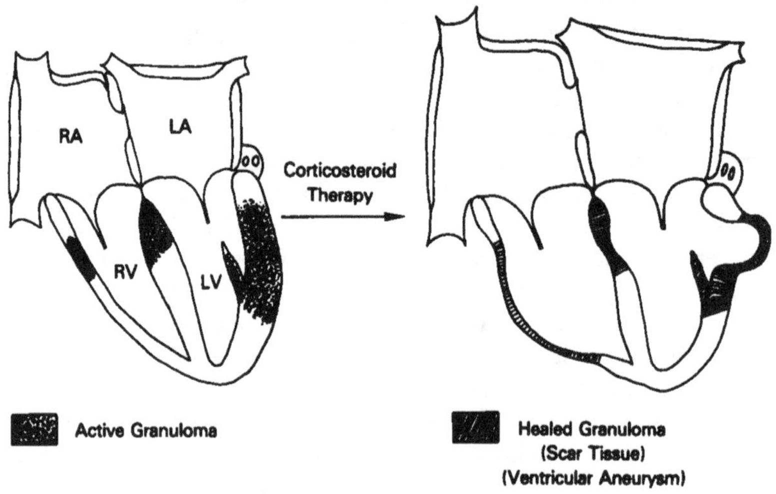

FIGURE 8. Good and bad effects of corticosteroid therapy in patients with cardiac sarcoidosis (reprinted with permission from Roberts WC, and the Yorke Medical Group[1]).

(one minute focus). A corollary to this is that the occurrence of symptomatic involvement of a noncardiac organ by sarcoid generally indicates that symptom-producing cardiac involvement by sarcoid is unlikely to occur. Flemming,[2] in search of patients with cardiac sarcoid, surveyed the chest, eye, and skin clinics in his hospital for patients with sarcoidosis and found this search unprofitable in revealing patients with cardiac sarcoid. Thus, cardiac sarcoidosis severe enough to cause cardiac dysfunction tends to be an all-or-none process: if it causes cardiac dysfunction, it tends not to cause dysfunction of another organ system; conversely, if it causes dysfunction of a noncardiac organ, it infrequently causes cardiac dysfunction. Although patients with fatal cardiac sarcoidosis may have sarcoid granulomas in other body organs, the extent of the sarcoid granulomas in the heart, in general, appears to be out of proportion to the extent in other body organs. Our patient had extensive granulomatous infiltrates in his myocardium, particularly the ventricles, but only one sarcoid granuloma was found in the lung and the only other body organ containing granuloma was lymph node.

One of the unusual histologic findings in sections of myocardium in our patient were granulomas around intramural coronary arteries. Dr. Virmani, can you summarize observations of others regarding cardiac sarcoid granulomas and their relationship to the coronary arteries?

Dr. Virmani: No one has reported sarcoid granulomas in extramural coronary arteries, but Morales and associates,[3] and more recently, James[4] pointed out that granulomas frequently surround the intramural coronary arteries of either cardiac atria or ventricles or both, and that the lumens of these arteries may be narrowed. The narrowing, in general, appears to result from intimal proliferation rather than from actual granulomatous invasion of the lumens. The medial and adventitial walls, however, have been observed to contain sarcoid granulomas. In our patient granulomas surrounded many intramural coronary arteries, particularly in the ventricles, and epithelioid cells were found to invade the wall of several intramural coronary arteries. Thus, sarcoidosis must be added to the list of causes of intramural coronary arterial disease. The functional significance of the involvement of the intramural coronary arteries, however, is uncertain. We suspect that it has little to no functional significance. Involvement of the small arteries in the lung by sarcoid granuloma has been noted in the past by others.[5] There is no surprise, therefore, that the small cardiac arteries may be involved by sarcoid granulomas.

Dr. Roberts: Dr. Virmani, the diagnosis of cardiac sarcoidosis clinically generally appears to be either simple or extremely difficult. Is this diagnosis easy at necropsy, and what morphologic criteria should be used to establish the diagnosis of cardiac sarcoidosis?

Dr. Virmani: To make the diagnosis of cardiac sarcoidosis at necropsy, we have required the presence of noncaseating granulomas in heart muscle and in lymph nodes.[1] The absence of noncaseating granulomas in lymph nodes, but their presence in the heart does not allow one to say, in our view, that sarcoidosis is the proper diagnosis. There have been a number of patients described with so-called "giant cell myocarditis." We believe that most of these patients in actuality had cardiac sarcoidosis. A problem here is that sarcoid may extensively involve the heart, and yet, although granulomas may be present in lymph nodes, the lymph nodes may not be enlarged. Because they are not enlarged at autopsy, histologic sections may not be prepared from them. If histologic sections are not prepared, certainly one cannot confirm or deny the presence of granulomas in these structures.

Dr. Roberts: One final comment regarding treatment. It seems reasonable to treat with corticosteroids any patient with documented cardiac sarcoidosis, be he (she) symptomatic or asymptomatic. As shown in the accompanying diagram (Fig 8), it appears that corticosteroid therapy causes shrinkage and conversion of the sarcoid granulomas into relatively dense scar tissue. In our patient, the cardiac sarcoid granulomas appeared quite active in that numerous lymphocytes surrounded the epithelioid and giant cell granulomas. In patients treated for long periods with corticosteroids, the cardiac sarcoid granulomas tend to be converted to scar tissue and the granulomas may disappear entirely. In our patient, relatively little myocardial scarring was observed.

References

1 Roberts WC, McAllister HA Jr, Ferrans VJ: Sarcoidosis of the heart; a clinicopathologic study of 35 necropsy patients (Group I) and review of 78 previously described necropsy patients (Group II). Am J Med 1977; 63:86

2 Flemming HA: Sarcoid heart disease. Br Med J 1973; 1:174

3 Morales AR, Levy S, Davis J, Fine G: Sarcoidosis and the heart. Pathol Ann 1974; 9:139

4 James TN: Sarcoid heart disease. Circulation 1977; 56:320

5 Carrington CB, Gaensler EA, Mikus JP, Schachter AW, Burke GW, Goff AM: Structure and function of sarcoidosis. Ann NY Acad Sci 1976; 278-265

Congenital Hypoplasia of Portions of Both Right and Left Ventricular Myocardial Walls

Clinical and Necropsy Observations in Two Patients With Parchment Heart Syndrome

BRUCE F. WALLER, MD*
ELDON R. SMITH, MD, FACC†
BRIAN D. BLACKBOURNE, MD‡
FELIX P. ARCE, MD†
NELLIE N. SARKAR, MD†
WILLIAM C. ROBERTS, MD, FACC*

Bethesda, Maryland
Halifax, Nova Scotia
Washington, D.C.

Clinical and morphologic findings are described in two patients with congenital hypoplasia of portions of both right and left ventricular free walls in the absence of associated coronary or valvular heart disease. One, a 61 year old man who had never had clinical evidence of cardiac dysfunction, died suddenly and unexpectedly. The second, a 55 year old woman, died of progressive, eventually intractable congestive heart failure of 29 months' duration. Although at least 22 necropsy patients have previously been reported to have "parchment-like" thinning of portions of the right ventricular free wall, only one patient has previously been described with such thinning of portions of both right and left ventricular free walls. The spectrum of right or right and left ventricular wall congenital hypoplasia is a broad one, with nearly half of described patients dying of congestive heart failure in the 1st year of life and the other half reaching adulthood with or without manifestations of cardiac dysfunction.

Partial to near complete absence of right ventricular myocardium ("parchment heart") with normal cardiac valves and normal or near normal coronary arteries has been reported in at least 22 necropsy patients (Table I),[1–22] only one of whom had associated thinning of the left ventricular free wall. In the report that follows, cardiac findings are described in two patients who had localized thinning of portions of both right and left ventricular free walls unassociated with coronary narrowing or abnormal cardiac valves. In addition, cardiac findings are summarized in previously described patients with the "parchment heart."

Description of Patients

Case 1

This was a 61 year old black man who died in August 1978. He had been well until the day of death when he complained of abdominal pain after consuming large quantities of alcohol the preceding day. While at home, he suddenly raised his arms, gasped for breath, collapsed and was dead. He had never had symptoms of cardiac dysfunction. A brief examination 5 years before death, at the time of a minor head injury, disclosed his blood pressure to be 130/70 mm Hg. No cardiac abnormalities were detected on precordial examination.

Necropsy findings: The heart weighed 350 g. A portion of the anterior wall of the right ventricular outflow tract was thin (Fig. 1) and histologic study revealed few myocardial fibers (Fig. 2). A similar area of thinning that bulged involved the apical portion of the left ventricle (Fig. 1). The wall of the thinned left ventricular apex contained a few myocardial fibers (Fig. 3). The four major epicardial coronary arteries (right, left main, left anterior descending and left circumflex) were virtually free of atherosclerotic plaque.

Case 2

This 55 year old white woman, who died in December 1979, had been well until July 1977 when she noted exertional epigastric distress, easy fatigability and,

From the Pathology Branch, National Heart, Lung, and Blood Institute, National Institutes of Health, Bethesda, Maryland*; the Departments of Medicine and Pathology, Dalhousie University, Halifax, Nova Scotia, Canada†; and the District of Columbia Medical Examiner's Office, Washington, D.C.‡ Manuscript received April 21, 1980; revised manuscript received June 3, 1980, accepted June 10, 1980.

Address for reprints: William C. Roberts, MD, National Heart, Lung, and Blood Institute, Building 10A, Room 3E30, 9000 Rockville Pike, Bethesda, Maryland 20205.

TABLE I

Clinical and Morphologic Observations in 22 Previously Described Necropsy Patients With Parchment Hearts

Reference													Location of Absent Ventricular Myocardium								
						Duration							RV					Thrombus		Defect of AS	
First Author	Year	Age at Death	Sex	CHF	P	Sy (mo)	C	M	CE (X-Ray)	Abnl ECG	Mode of Death	HW (g)	I	A	O	VS	LV	RV	LV	PFO	S
Patients Aged 5 Years or Less																					
Haworth[1]	1975	1 day	M	+	—	1 day	+	+	+	+	CHF	—	+	+	0	—	—	0	0	+	0
Diaz[2]	1973	4 mo	M	+	—	4	+	0	+	+	CHF	—	+	0	0	—	0	0	0	0	0
Novak[3]	1957	5 mo	M	+	—	5	+	0	+	+	CHF	—	+	+	0	—	0	0	0	+	0
Arcilla[4]	1961	6 mo	M	+	—	6	0	+	+	+	CHF	—	+	+	+	—	0	0	0	+	0
Uhl[5]	1952	7 mo	F	+	—	4	+	0	+	+	CHF	—	+	+	0	—	0	+	0	0	0
Cumming[6]	1965	7 mo	F	+	—	4	0	—	+	+	PO	48	0	+	0	—	0	0	0	+	0
Aherne[7]	1973	7 mo	F	+	—	3	0	—	+	+	CHF	—	+	+	+	—	0	0	0	0	0
Perrin[8]	1965	10 mo	M	+	—	7	+	+	+	+	CHF	—	0	+	0	—	0	—	—	0	0
Sherman[9]	1963	15 mo	F	+	—	12	+	0	+	+	CHF	—	+	+	+	—	0	—	—	0	0
Kinare[10]	1969	60 mo	F	+	0	60	+	0	+	+	CHF	130	+	+	+	—	0	0	0	0	0
Patients Aged More Than 15 Years																					
Abe[11]	1973	17 yr	F	+	0	48	0	0	+	+	PO	400	0	+	+	—	0	0	0	0	0
Murata[12]	1976	18 yr	F	+	0	12	0	0	+	+	CHF	400	0	+	+	—	0	+	0	0	0
Froment[13]	1968	19 yr	M	+	0	—	0	—	+	—	CHF	350	0	+	0	—	—	+	—	—	—
Vecht[14]	1979	19 yr	M	+	+	132	+	—	+	+	PO	435	+	0	0	—	—	0	0	0	+
Castleman[15]	1952	24 yr	F	+	0	12	0	+	+	+	CHF	300	+	+	+	—	0	+	0	0	0
Froment[13]	1968	26 yr	M	+	0	—	0	—	+	—	CHF	430	0	+	0	—	—	+	—	—	—
Bharati[16]	1978	29 yr	F	+	0	108	0	0	+	+	CHF +CHB	545	+	+	+	+	0	+	0	0	0
Osler[17] Segall[18]	1905 1950	"40's"	M	—	—	—	—	—	—	—	SD	168	+	+	+	—	+	0	0	0	0
Reeve[19]	1964	47 yr	F	+	+	432	+	+	+	+	CA	290	+	0	0	—	0	0	0	+	0
Forssman[20]	1972	47 yr	M	0	—	—	0	—	—	+	SD	—	0	+	0	0	—	—	—	—	—
Gould[21]	1967	66 yr	M	0	0	0	0	0	0	0	L	600	+	+	0	—	0	—	—	0	0
Sugiura[22]	1970	84 yr	F	0	0	0	0	0	0	0	AP	220	0	0	+	—	0	0	0	0	0

A = ventricular apex; Abnl = abnormal; AP = acute pneumonia; AS = atrial septum; C = cyanosis; CA = cerebrovascular accident; CE = cardiac enlargement; CHB = complete heart block; CHF = congestive heart failure; ECG = electrocardiogram; HW = heart weight; I = inflow tract; L = leukemia; LV = left ventricle; M = precordial murmur; O = outflow tract; P = chest pain; PFO = patent foramen ovale; PO = early postoperatively; RV = right ventricle; S = secundum; SD = sudden death; Sy = symptoms of cardiac dysfunction; VS = ventricular septum; — = no information available; + = present or positive; 0 = absent or negative.

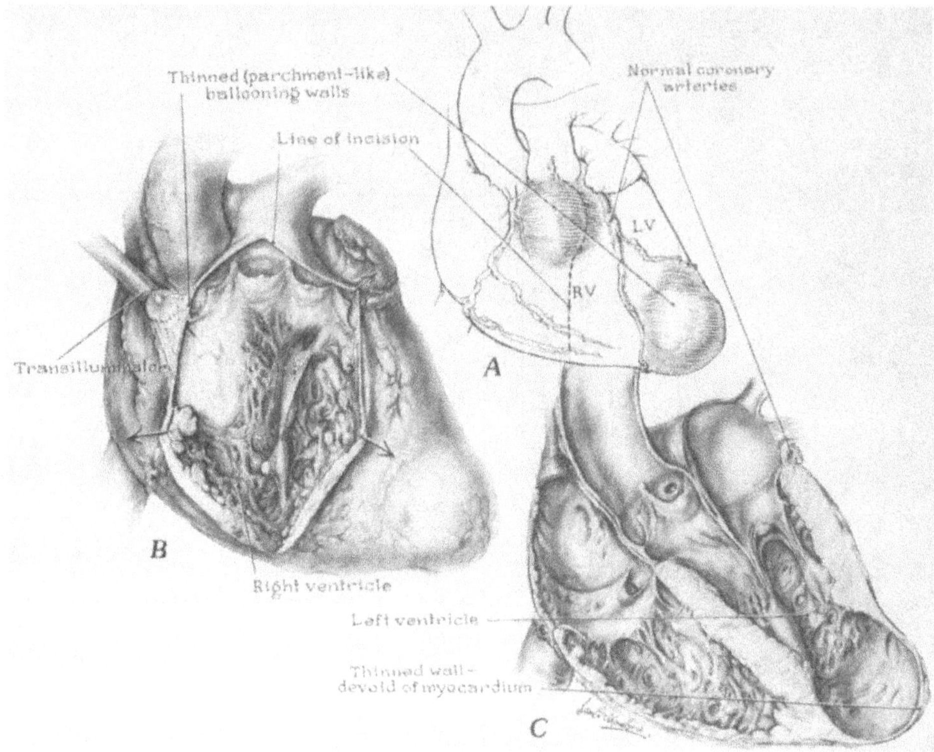

FIGURE 1. Case 1. Drawings of the heart showing the thinned portions of myocardium of the right ventricular outflow tract and left ventricular apex. LV = left ventricle; RV = right ventricle.

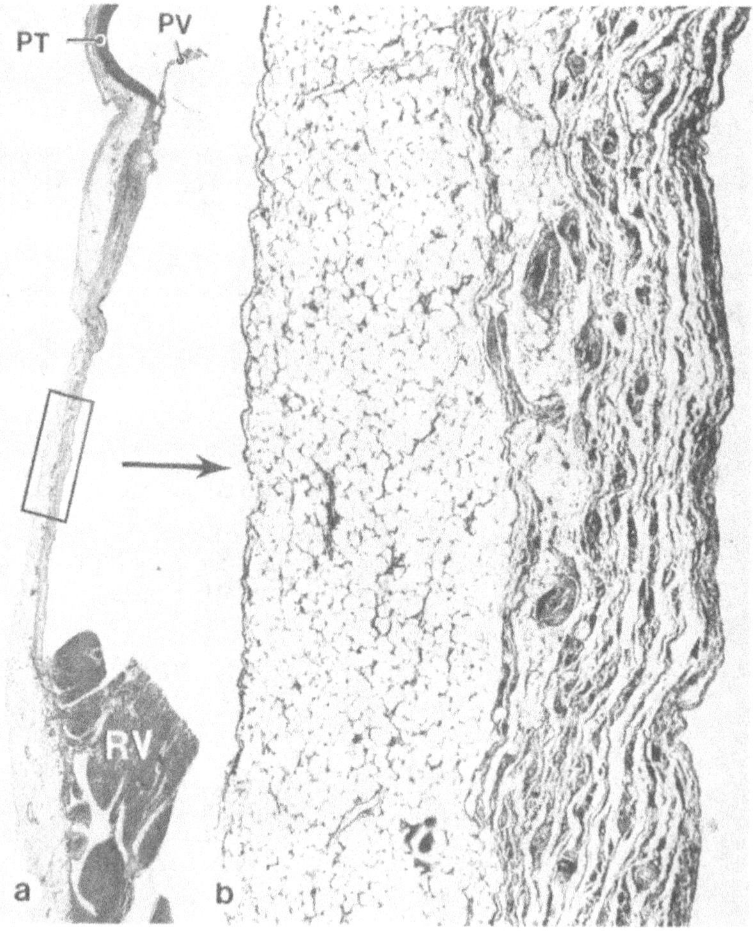

FIGURE 2. Case 1. Photomicrographs of the thinned right ventricular outflow tract. Lower power view (a) and higher magnification view (b) of the boxed area, showing a few myocardial fibers. PT = pulmonary trunk; PV = pulmonary valve; RV = right ventricle. (Movat stain X4 [a] and X55 [b], both reduced by 20 percent.)

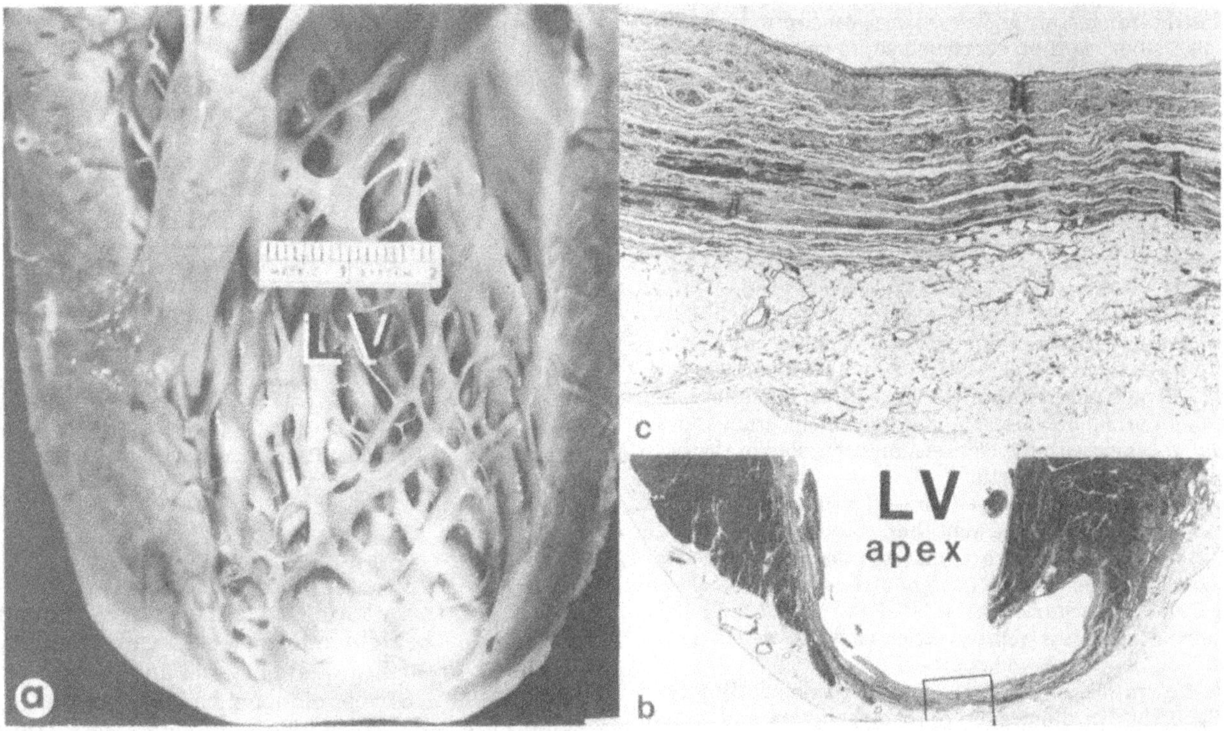

FIGURE 3. Case 1. Opened left ventricle (LV) showing the thinned apical portion (**a** and **b**). A close-up of the **boxed area** in **b** is shown in **c**. Relatively few myocardial fibers remain. (Movat stains ×10 [**b**], and ×55 [**c**], both reduced by 20 percent.)

subsequently, swelling of her abdomen and legs. She had exertional dyspnea but no orthopnea or nocturnal dyspnea. Diuretic therapy provided little improvement. On examination in February 1978, she was 157.5 cm tall, weighed 54 kg, and the blood pressure was 115/80 mm Hg without significant paradox. The venous pressure was markedly elevated with a rapid diastolic collapse. A right ventricular impulse was palpated and a third heart sound and soft pansystolic murmur of maximal intensity at the cardiac apex were audible. The liver and spleen were enlarged, tense ascites was evident and the legs were edematous. The chest was clear.

Laboratory findings: Hematologic and biochemical investigations were normal except for slight degrees of hypoalbuminemia and hyperbilirubinemia. A chest roentgenogram

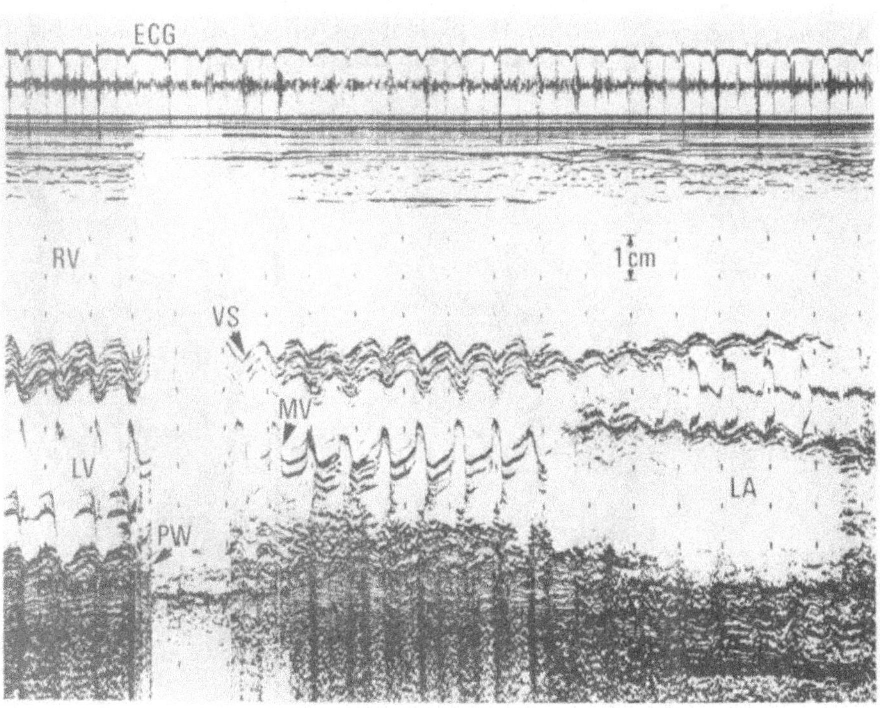

FIGURE 4. Case 2. Echocardiogram showing a scan from the aorta (**at right**) to the left ventricular (LV) cavity (**at left**). The right ventricle (RV) is dilated and the ventricular septum (VS) moves paradoxically (**arrow**). The posterobasal left ventricular free wall (PW) appears thinner than the septum and is hypokinetic. The left atrium (LA) is slightly dilated. MV = mitral valve.

disclosed cardiomegaly and clear lungs. An electrocardiogram revealed sinus rhythm, occasional supraventricular ectopic complexes, low voltage, incomplete right bundle branch block and changes compatible with old posterior myocardial infarct. An echocardiogram (Fig. 4) showed an enlarged right ventricle with paradoxical septal movement, a slightly enlarged left atrium and a thinned and hypokinetic posterobasal left ventricular free wall.

On cardiac catheterization, the cardiac pressures (in mm Hg) were: pulmonary artery, 28/20; right ventricle, 28/15 (mean 21); right atrial *a* wave, 22, v wave, 28 and mean, 22 (Fig. 5); left ventricle, 120/0 and aorta 120/65. The left ventriculogram disclosed a normal-sized chamber, an ejection fraction of 64 percent, akinesia of the posterobasal wall, and slight mitral regurgitation. Selective coronary arteriography revealed normal arteries. The right ventriculogram showed a dilated cavity with hypokinesia, most marked in the posterobasal and outflow portions.

Operative findings and course: To rule out pericardial disease, the patient underwent thoracotomy in March 1978. The pericardial layers were normal, and the sac contained 300 to 400 ml of serous fluid. The right atrial wall was hypertrophied; the right ventricle was dilated and contracted poorly. In several areas the right ventricular wall was extremely thin.

Postoperatively, the marked fatigue persisted. By August 1978, further cardiomegaly by roentgenogram and a right pleural effusion (transudate) were evident. In November 1979 she was rehospitalized with anasarca, oliguria and hypotension. She died in December 1979 from intractable heart failure complicated by atrial and ventricular arrhythmias.

Necropsy findings: The heart weighed 320 g. The wall of the right ventricular outflow tract and apex was "paper thin" and contained few myocardial fibers (Fig. 6). The posterobasal portions of both right and left ventricular free walls also were thinned, but more myocardial fibers surrounded by fibrous tissue were present in this portion of right ventricular free wall and a layer of myocardium was present beneath the endocardium in the thinned portion of left ventricular free wall. The right atrium, right ventricle and tricuspid valve anulus (12.5 cm in circumference) were dilated and the right atrial wall was hypertrophied. Several mural thrombi were present in the right ventricle and right atrium. All major coronary arteries were free of atherosclerotic plaques.

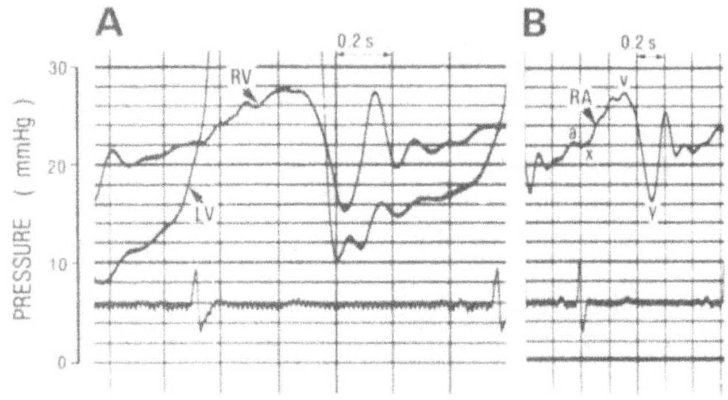

FIGURE 5. Case 2. **A,** simultaneous left ventricular (LV) and right ventricular (RV) pressures. The right ventricular end-diastolic pressure is elevated and the dip-end-plateau configuration in early diastole is present. **B,** high right atrial (RA) pressure with rapid y descent.

Comments

Each of these two patients had severe thinning of portions of the right and left ventricular free walls and each had normal coronary arteries and normal cardiac valves. One, a 61 year old man, had been asymptomatic all his life and died suddenly, and at necropsy the only abnormality was the localized deficiency of ventricular myocardium. The second patient, a 55 year old woman, had been asymptomatic until age 53 when congestive heart failure appeared; it became intractable and eventually fatal. The latter patient had a much larger loss of right ventricular myocardium than did the former patient; the amount of deficient left ventricular myocardium was roughly similar in each, although located at different sites.

Previously reported cases of thinning of the right ventricular wall: Osler[17] in 1905 was the first to describe a patient with "parchment-like" thinning of a ventricular wall in the absence of coronary or valve disease. His patient was believed to be a man in his 40s who died suddenly and unexpectedly while walking up

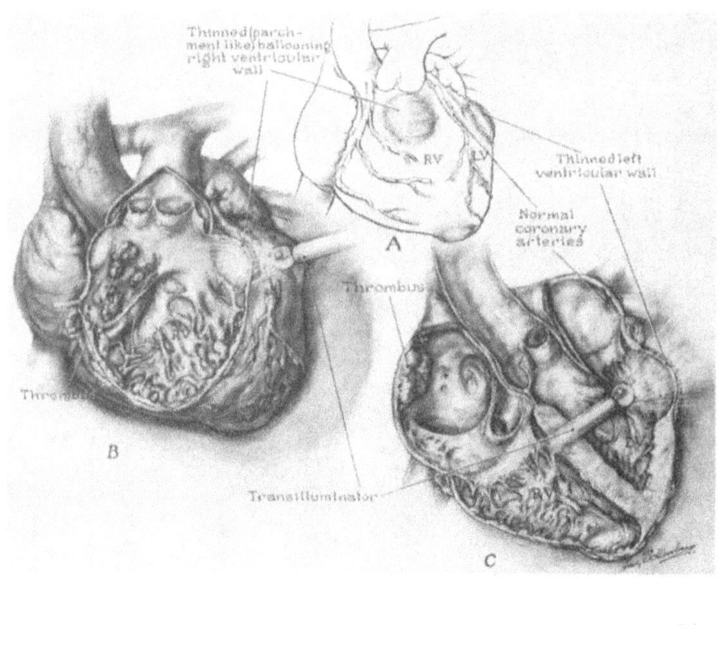

FIGURE 6. Case 2. Drawings of the heart showing thinned portions of right (RV) and left ventricular (LV) walls. Thrombi are present in the right atrial and right ventricular cavities.

a hill. At necropsy, the localized thinning involved portions of both ventricular walls as was the case in our two patients. Segall[18] in 1950 described in more detail the patient briefly referred to by Osler in the 1905 edition of his textbook. The second patient reported to have a parchment-like heart was a 23 year old woman who had chronic, eventually fatal congestive heart failure for nearly 1 year. This patient, reported on in May 15, 1952 in *The New England Journal of Medicine,*[15] was similar to our Patient 2. The third patient was described in 1952 by Uhl.[5] His patient was a 7 month old girl who had evidence of severe right-sided congestive heart failure and severe thinning of most of the right ventricular wall. Uhl's paper was entitled: "A previously undescribed congenital malformation of the heart: almost total absence of the myocardium of right ventricle." Since his report most authors describing patients with "parchment-like" thinning of the wall of right ventricle have referred to this condition as "Uhl's anomaly." It is true that Uhl was the first to describe a child with a parchment-like right ventricular wall, but he was preceded in describing this condition by Osler,[17] Segall,[18] and Castleman and Sprague[15] whose publications on this subject were overlooked by Uhl. Because Osler's description appeared only in a textbook, it is understandable how his description could have been missed. Overlooking Segall's report or possibly Castleman and Sprague's clinicopathologic conference in *The New England Journal of Medicine* is less understandable. We believe it best to eliminate the eponym for this condition, which we prefer to call "congenital hypoplasia of ventricular myocardium."

Clinical features: Since 1952, at least 21 additional patients with parchment-like thinning of portions of right ventricular free wall have been reported[1–22] (Table I). Surprisingly, the myocardial thinning in each was limited to the right ventricular wall and none had involvement of both ventricular free walls as did our two patients. One,[16] however, also had thinning of the ventricular septum. The described patients fall neatly into two age groups: those aged 5 years and younger[1–10] and those over age 15 years.[11–22] Of the 22 previously described patients, 8 were under age 1 year,[1–8] 1 was 15 months old,[9] 1 was 5 years old[10] and the remaining 12 patients were 17 to 84 years old.[11–22] In all 10 patients aged 5 years and under, congestive heart failure was clinically evident from birth and it became intractable and fatal. Of the 12 patients over age 15 years, 8 had chronic congestive heart failure, which was the cause of death in 5. Not all patients with parchment-like thinning of the right ventricular wall in the absence of coronary and valve disease have congestive heart failure or other clinical evidences of cardiac dysfunction. The 66 year old man reported on by Gould et al.[21] and the 84 year old woman reported on by Sugiura et al.[22] never had evidence of cardiac dysfunction and died from noncardiac conditions. Two of the older patients, as did our Patient 1, died suddenly.[17,18,20]

Hemodynamic and angiographic features: Hemodynamic studies have been reported in 6[4,6,11,12,14,16] of the 22 previously described patients and in 1 of our 2 patients. All seven had normal pulmonary arterial and right ventricular systolic pressures. However, the right ventricular end-diastolic pressure, (measured in six patients, was elevated in each (range 12 to 22 mm Hg). The right atrial pressure (measured in six patients)[4,6,11,12,14] was also elevated in each, with the mean pressure ranging from 8 to 28 mm Hg. In all but one patient,[16] the pulmonary arterial and right ventricular end-diastolic and right atrial mean pressures were the same or nearly the same. In our Patient 2, the similarity of these three pressures led to thoracotomy to rule out pericardial constriction. This patient was the only one of the seven patients who also had determination of left ventricular pressures, which were normal. Cardiac index (measured in three patients)[4,6,16] was severely depressed (1.3, 1.7, and 1.8 liters/min per m^2, respectively). Thus, parchment-like thinning of the right ventricular wall may cause equalization of pulmonary arterial, right ventricular end-diastolic and mean right atrial pressures and severe depression of cardiac output. Right ventricular angiography performed in five of the seven patients,[4,6,12,14] disclosed poor contractility of the ventricle in each, dilatation of this chamber in each with or without localized aneurysmal formation and focal or diffuse thinning of its wall, tricuspid valve regurgitation in one,[16] and right atrial dilatation in three patients.[4,6,12]

Differential diagnosis: Clinically, the differential diagnosis of congenital hypoplasia of the right ventricular myocardium includes Ebstein's anomaly of the tricuspid valve, idiopathic dilated cardiomyopathy and pulmonary or tricuspid valve atresia. The echocardiogram is useful in distinguishing congenital hypoplasia of the right ventricular myocardium from Ebstein's anomaly[20] by the presence of a dilated right ventricular cavity (as in our Case 2), delayed tricuspid valve closure, and diastolic opening of the pulmonary valve in patients with the former.[23] Angiographically, dilatation of the right ventricular cavity may not be useful in differentiating idiopathic dilated cardiomyopathy from congenital hypoplasia of the right ventricular myocardium, but the presence of left ventricular dilatation obviously favors the diagnosis of cardiomyopathy.

References

1. **Haworth SG, Shinebourne EA, Miller GAH.** Right to left interatrial shunting with normal right ventricular pressure. Br Heart J 1975; 37:386–91.
2. **Diaz LP, Jimenez MQ, Granados FM, Martinez VP, Batres GM.** Congenital absence of myocardium of right ventricle: Uhl's anomaly. Br Heart J 1973;35:570–2.
3. **Novak G, Szanto PB, Gasul B, Dillon E.** Congenital aplasia of the myocardium of the right ventricle. Proc Inst Med Chic 1957;21: 334–9.
4. **Arcilla RA, Gasul BM.** Congenital aplasia or marked hypoplasia of the myocardium. J Pediatr 1961;58:381–8.
5. **Uhl HS.** A previously undescribed congenital malformation of the

heart: almost total absence of the myocardium of the right ventricle. Bull Johns Hopkins Hosp 1952;91:197–209.
6. **Cumming GR, Bowman JM, Whytehead L.** Congenital aplasia of the myocardium of the right ventricle (Uhl's anomaly). Am Heart J 1965;70:671–6.
7. **Aherne WA.** Uhl's anomaly (abstr). Arch Dis Child 1973;48:160.
8. **Perrin EV, Mehrizi A.** Isolated free-wall hypoplasia of the right ventricle. Am J Dis Child 1965;109:558–66.
9. **Sherman FE.** An Atlas of Congenital Heart Disease. Philadelphia: Lea & Febiger, 1963:270, 290–1.
10. **Kinare SG, Panday SR, Deshmukh SM.** Congenital aplasia of the right ventricular myocardium (Uhl's anomaly). Chest 1969;55: 429–31.
11. **Abe T, Kuribayashi R, Sato M, Nieda S, Abe S.** Congenital hypoplasia of the right ventricular myocardium (Uhl's anomaly). A case report and review of literature. J Cardiovasc Surg 1973;14: 431–8.
12. **Murata K, Matsuo H, Yoshitake Y, Ishizawa Y, Shigiya R, Okamato K.** Functionally atrialized parchment-like right ventricle with extensive myocardial fibrosis of left ventricle. Jpn Heart J 1976; 17:428–35.
13. **Froment R, Perrin A, Loire R, Dalloz CJ.** Ventricule droit papyrace du jeune adultre par dystrophie congenitale. Arch Mal Coeur 1968;61:477–503.
14. **Vecht RJ, Carmichael JS, Gopal R, Philip G.** Uhl's anomaly. Br Heart J 1979;41:676–82.
15. **Castleman B, Sprague HB.** Case records of the Massachusetts General Hospital. Weekly clinicopathological exercises. N Engl J Med 1952;246:785–90.
16. **Bharati S, Ciraulo DA, Bilitch M, Rosen KM, Lev M.** Inexcitable right ventricle and bilateral bundle branch block in Uhl's disease. Circulation 1978;57:636–44.
17. **Osler W.** The Principles and Practice of Medicine. 6th ed. New York: Appleton-Century-Crofts 1905:820.
18. **Segall HN.** Parchment heart (Osler). Am Heart J 1950;40:948–50.
19. **Reeve R, MacDonald D.** Partial absence of the right ventricular musculature—partial parchment heart. Am J Cardiol 1964;14: 415–9.
20. **Forssman O, Bjorkman G.** Absence of the solid part of the right ventricular musculature. Acta Pathol Microbiol Scand[A] 1972; 80:263–70.
21. **Gould K, Guttman AB, Carrasco J, Lyon AF.** Partial absence of the right ventricular musculature. A congenital lesion. Am J Med 1967;42:636–41.
22. **Sugiura M, Hayashi T, Ueno K.** Partial absence of the right ventricular muscle in an aged. Jpn Heart J 1970;11:582–5.
23. **French JW, Baum D, Popp RL.** Echocardiographic findings in Uhl's anomaly. Demonstration of diastolic pulmonary valve opening. Am J Cardiol 1975;36:349–53.

Hemochromatosis Heart Disease: An Unemphasized Cause of Potentially Reversible Restrictive Cardiomyopathy

D. JOSHUA CUTLER, M.D.*
JEFFREY M. ISNER, M.D.†
ARTHUR W. BRACEY, M.D.
CHARLES A. HUFNAGEL, M.D.
PETER W. CONRAD, M.D.
WILLIAM C. ROBERTS, M.D.
DONALD M. KERWIN, M.D.
ALAN M. WEINTRAUB, M.D.
Washington, D.C.

Cardiac involvement in hemochromatosis typically results in congestive cardiomyopathy; a restrictive cardiomyopathy due to hemochromatosis is distinctly rare. A restrictive cardiomyopathy, which developed in the patient described in this report, was due to hemochromatosis which mimicked constrictive pericarditis clinically, echocardiographically and hemodynamically, and resulted in a thoracotomy for attempted surgical therapy. The fact that hemochromatosis represents the only cause of a restrictive cardiomyopathy that is potentially reversible by medical therapy makes early recognition of hemochromatosis heart disease important.

Distinguishing restrictive cardiomyopathy from constrictive pericardial disease is often difficult. Even invasively-obtained hemodynamic data may not be diagnostic [1,2]. The fact that hemochromatosis may present initially as a restrictive cardiomyopathy mimicking constrictive pericarditis is not well appreciated. We describe such a patient and stress the importance of early recognition of this potentially, medically-reversible disorder.

CASE REPORT

A 61 year old white woman (CT 381808) was transferred to Georgetown University Hospital with the diagnosis of constrictive pericarditis. She had been asymptomatic until four weeks before death when exertional dyspnea, lethargy and episodes of mental confusion developed. Two years before death the serum glutamic oxaloacetic transaminase (SGOT) level had been elevated, and two months before death, the serum glucose level was found to be elevated. The patient had never received blood transfusions or other known sources of excess exogenous iron. Her family denied that she had consumed alcohol.

On physical examination the patient responded sluggishly to painful stimuli. The systolic blood pressure was 110 mm Hg with a pulsus paradoxus of 10 mm Hg. The skin over the trunk was slate gray. The jugular veins were distended above the mandible with the patient at 45 degrees with prominent x and y descents. The carotid pulse was normal in contour but small in volume. The lungs were clear. The cardiac apex was not palpable. The first and second heart sounds were normal. A "pericardial knock" sound was present in early diastole. There were no precordial murmurs or rubs. Neither the liver nor the spleen was enlarged, and there was no evidence of ascites. There was 2+ pretibial and presacral pitting edema.

The hematocrit value was 39 percent; serum glucose, 333 mg/dl; blood urea nitrogen, 62 mg/dl; creatinine, 1.4 mg/dl; sodium, 125 meq/liter; potassium, 5.4 meq/liter; chloride, 92 meq/liter; carbon dioxide, 22 meq/liter; SGOT, 170 Karmen units (normal <40 Karmen units); alkaline phosphatase, 1.5 Bessey-

From the Cardiology Division, Department of Medicine, the Cardiovascular Surgery Division, Department of Surgery, and the Department of Pathology, Georgetown University Hospital, Washington, D.C.; and the Pathology Branch, National Heart, Lung, and Blood Institute, National Institutes of Health, Bethesda, Maryland. Requests for reprints should be addressed to Dr. Alan M. Weintraub, Cardiology Division, Georgetown University Hospital, 3800 Reservoir Road, N.W., Washington, D.C. 20007. Manuscript accepted December 10, 1979.

* Present address: Division of Cardiology, Veterans Administration Hospital, 50 Irving Street, N.W., Washington, D.C. 20422.
† Present address: Division of Cardiology, Tufts University School of Medicine, The New England Medical Center Hospital, Boston, MA 02153.

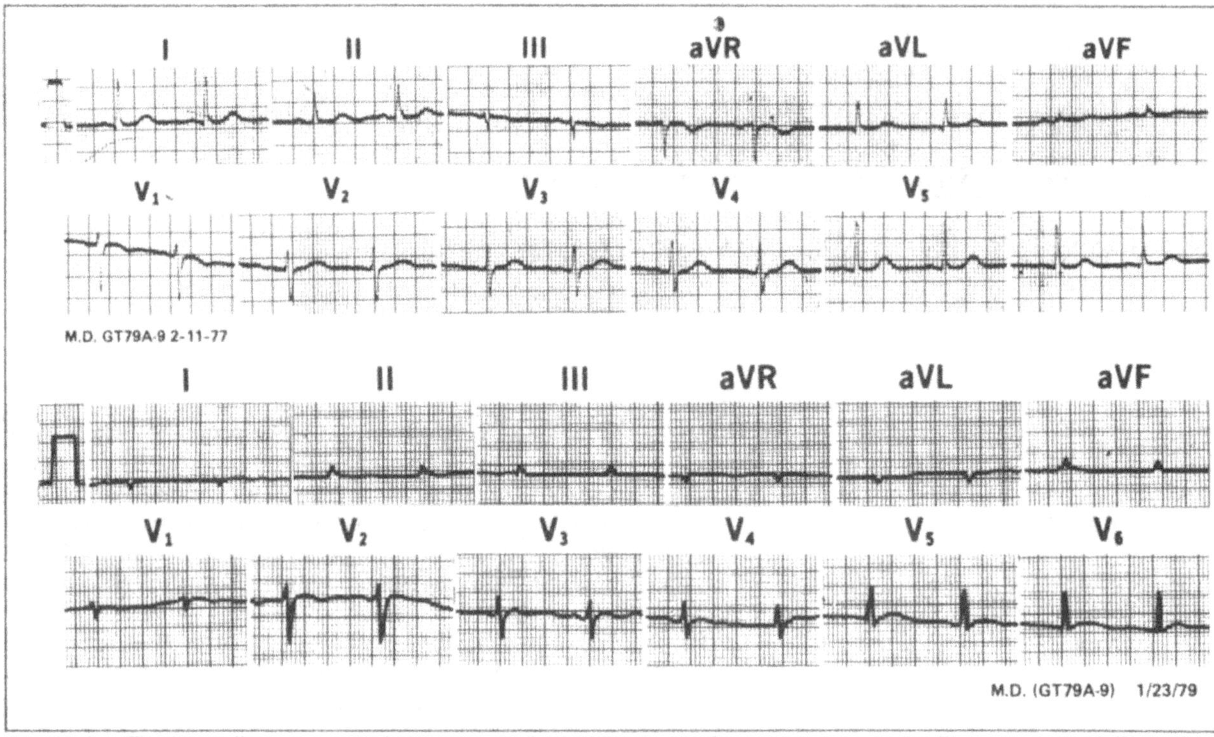

Figure 1. Electrocardiograms recorded two years (**top**) and one day (**bottom**) before death. There is marked diminution in the QRS voltage in both the standard and precordial leads of the later tracing.

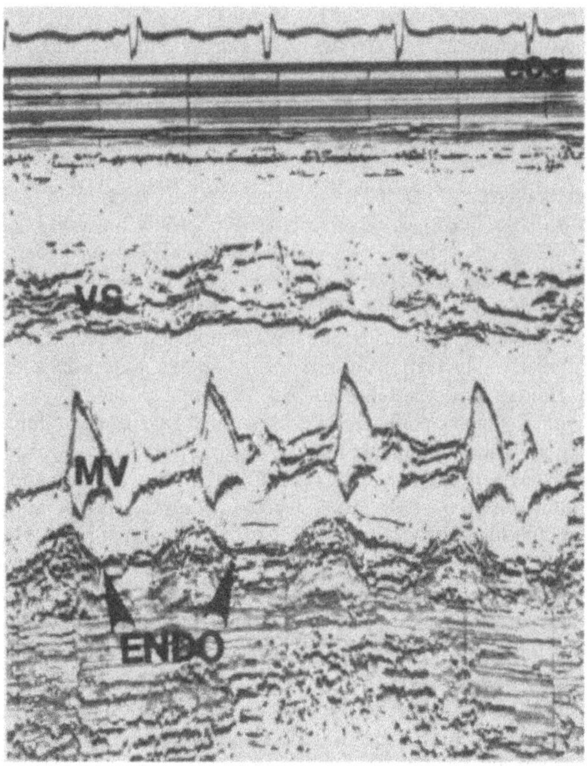

Figure 2. Echocardiogram at the level of the mitral valve (MV) recorded 10 days before death. The normal posteriorward diastolic motion of the left ventricular endocardium (ENDO) is absent; it is severely flattened. (VS = ventricular septum.)

Lowry units (normal = 0.8 to 2.3 Bessey-Lowry units); total bilirubin, 1.4 mg/dl with direct bilirubin, 0.8 mg/dl; and lactic dehydrogenase (LDH), 146 Wroblerwski units (normal = 42 to 120 Wroblerwski units). The blood ammonia level was 274 μg/dl (normal <65 μg/dl). The serum iron was 104 mg/dl (normal 30 to 130 mg/dl) and total iron-binding capacity, 175 mg/dl (normal = 250 to 400 mg/dl). The prothrombin time was 16 seconds (control 11 seconds). Chest roentgenogram showed bilateral pleural effusions and pulmonary vascular congestion. The electrocardiogram (**Figure 1**) showed severe diminution of the QRS amplitude and nonspecific changes in the S-T segment compared to a previous tracing. Echocardiography (**Figure 2**) disclosed a flattened slope of the left ventricular free wall during diastole. Cardiac catheterization on the right side of the heart disclosed the following pressures: mean right atrium, 18 mm Hg; right ventricle, 35/22 mm Hg; pulmonary artery, 35/22 mm Hg and mean pulmonary capillary wedge, 22 mm Hg (**Figure 3**). The cardiac output was 3.4 liters/min. Diabetes mellitus, hepatic encephalopathy and cardiac disease, either constrictive pericarditis or a restrictive cardiomyopathy due to hemochromatosis, were diagnosed. Hepatic biopsy was deferred because of the patient's unstable clinical status. Effusive-constrictive pericardial disease remained suspect and the patient underwent thoracotomy. At surgery, the amount and composition of the pericardial fluid was normal as were the visceral and parietal pericardia. The patient died five days later with evidence of progressively diminishing cardiac output.

At necropsy the heart weighed 305 g. The parietal and visceral pericardia were normal. Both ventricles were mildly dilated and both atria were of normal size. Thrombi were present in both the right atrial appendage and the right ven-

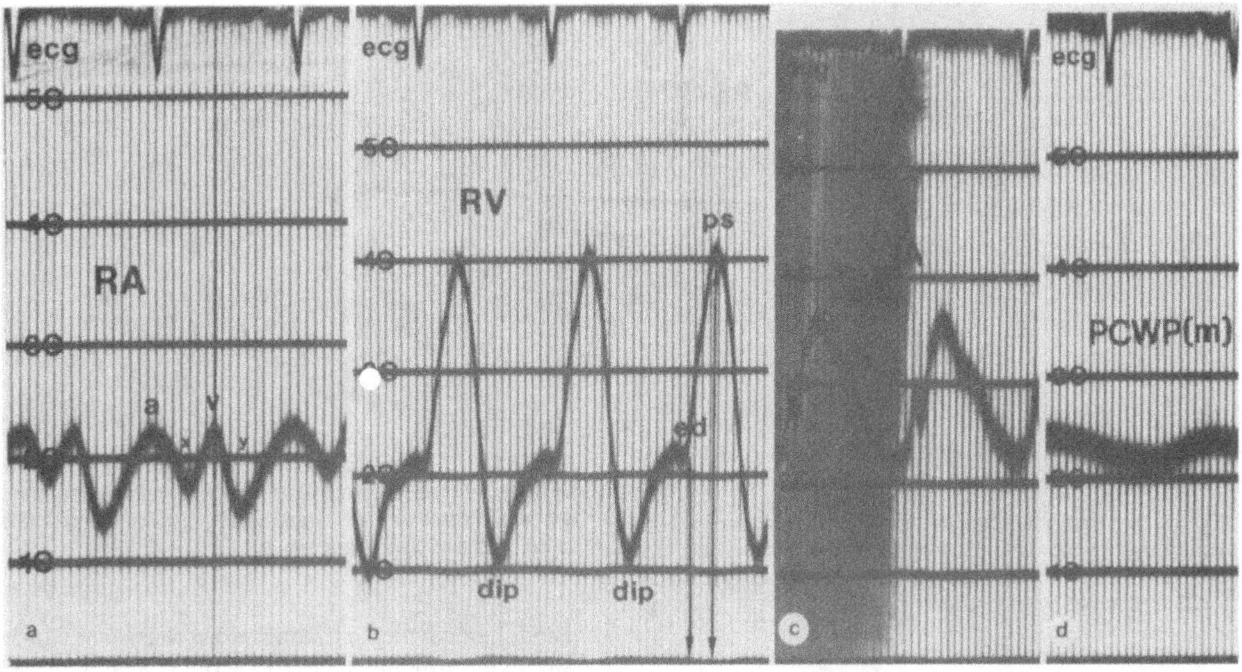

Figure 3. Intracardiac pressure recordings obtained six days before death. **a,** the right atrial (RA) pressure is "M-shaped" with equal a and v waves and a prominent y trough. **b,** the right ventricular (RV) pressure contour displays an early diastolic dip; the right ventricular end-diastolic (ed) pressure is greater than one third of right ventricular peak systolic (PS) pressure. There is approximation of mean right atrial pressure, right ventricular end-diastolic pressure; **c,** pulmonary arterial (PA) diastolic pressure, and **d,** mean pulmonary capillary wedge pressure (PCWP).

tricle. Myocardial foci of fibrosis and necrosis were absent. The myocardium, liver, pancreas, spleen, lymph nodes and bone marrow, when immersed in potassium ferricyanide, stained intensely blue (**Figure 4**). Histologic sections disclosed extensive deposits of iron within the myocardial cells (**Figure 5**). Ashed tissue sections of myocardium from the wall of each of the four cardiac chambers were quantitatively analyzed for iron content by mass photospectrometry. The results were compared to those obtained in analogous specimens obtained from an age and sex-matched control subject who had neither heart disease nor a disorder of iron metabolism (**Table I**). The iron content of the heart was markedly increased, more in the ventricles than in the atria.

The liver (weight, 1,290 g) was brown, firm, and there was micronodular cirrhosis. Histologic examination revealed grade 4 iron staining (classification of Scheuer et al. [3]). The iron deposits were located in the hepatocytes, the biliary ductular epithelium, the macrophages in the fibrous portal bands and in the Kupfer cells (**Figure 6**). The pancreas was brown. Iron deposits were observed in the islet cells of Langerhans' acinar cells and in the ductular epithelium. The number of islet cells did not appear to be diminished. Extensive iron deposits were present in the spleen, bone marrow and lymph nodes, and less extensive deposits were present in the kidneys (proximal tubules), thyroid, adrenal, parathyroid and anterior pituitary glands.

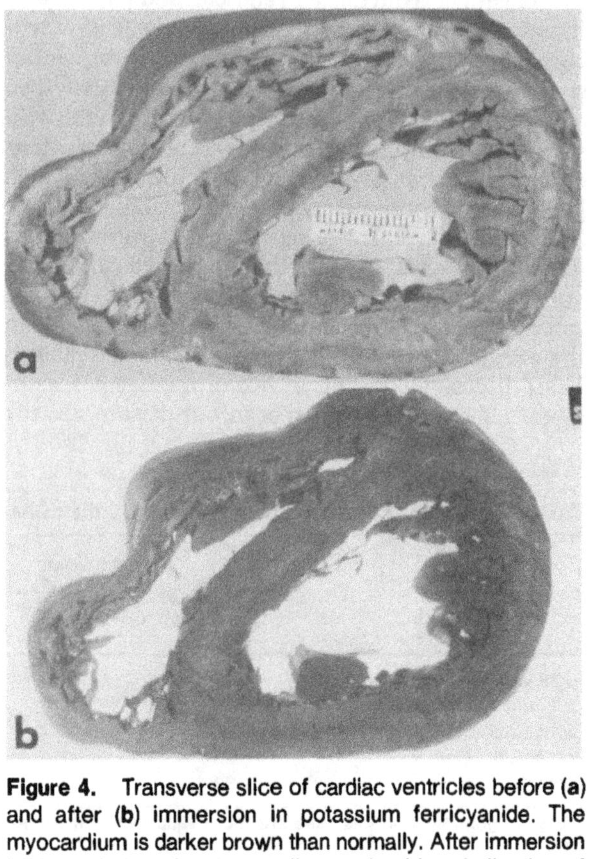

Figure 4. Transverse slice of cardiac ventricles before (**a**) and after (**b**) immersion in potassium ferricyanide. The myocardium is darker brown than normally. After immersion in the solution, the myocardium stains blue, indicative of heavy iron deposits.

COMMENTS

The differential diagnosis of restrictive cardiomyopathy is usually limited to amyloidosis, endomyocardial fibrosis with or without eosinophilia and an idiopathic

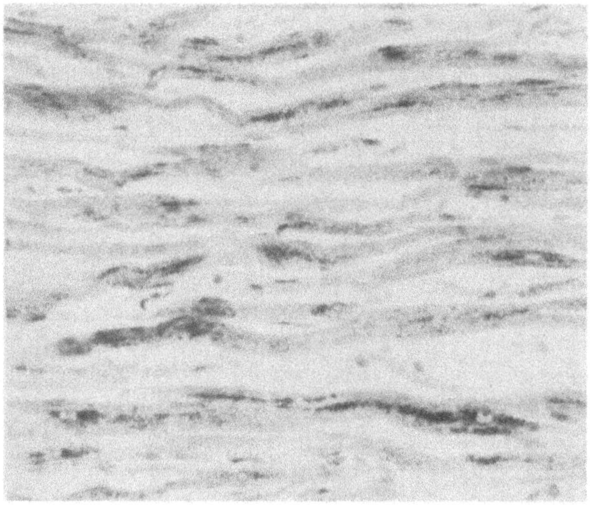

Figure 5. Photomicrograph of histologic section of left ventricular myocardium showing extensive intracellular iron deposits. Potassium ferricyanide stain; original magnification × 330, reduced by 21 percent.

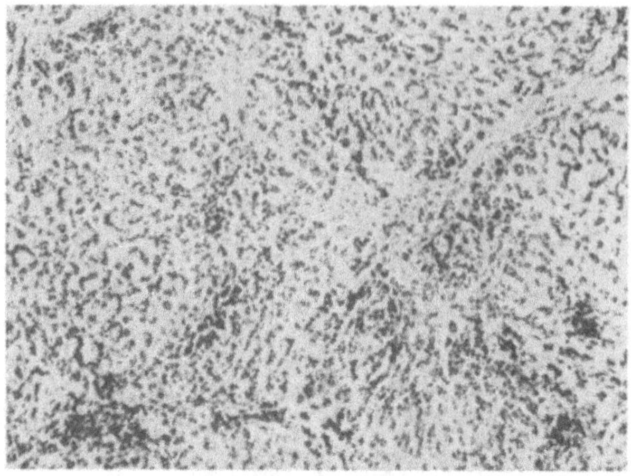

Figure 6. Photomicrograph of histologic section of liver showing increased fibrous tissue and extensive hepatic iron deposits. Potassium ferricyanide stain; original magnification × 80, reduced by 28 percent.

form. Although cardiac involvement in hemochromatosis is common (heart failure was the cause of death in nearly one half of the largest series of cases reported to date [4]), heart failure secondary to hemochromatosis (or exogenous iron overload) has usually been described as "congestive" with dilated ventricles and poor systolic function [4–12]. That cardiac involvement in hemochromatosis may be manifested by a restrictive cardiomyopathy is not well appreciated. Indeed, only two cases have been reported, to our knowledge, with a restrictive cardiomyopathy secondary to hemochromatosis or exogenous iron overload [13,14], only one of which [13] included confirmatory pressure tracings. Evidence contained in several other reports of iron overload heart disease, however, suggests that restrictive cardiac involvement may have gone unrecognized. Cardiac catheterization, for example, has been performed and the results reported in five cases of hemochromatosis heart disease [13,15–18]. In two of the five cases (including the patient with recognized disease already cited) hemodynamic findings were consistent with restrictive cardiomyopathy. Descriptions of markedly dilated, pulsatile neck veins in the absence of clinical or necropsy evidence of cardiac dilatation in three other cases [6–7] suggests restriction of ventricular diastolic filling. Furthermore, Finch and Finch [4] in their review of idiopathic hemochromatosis noted that "One of the most striking features in this type (i.e., hemochromatosis) of failure is the predominance of right-sided signs of congestive failure." Such a predominance of right-sided signs might be the result of a restraint on ventricular diastolic filling. Finally, it is conceivable that some patients who have been diagnosed as having "idiopathic" restrictive cardiomyopathy may, in fact, have had hemochromatosis. Our patient, for example, would have been classified as such had a necropsy not been performed.

Our patient's condition is remarkably similar to that in two other cases, one reported by Wasserman [13] and the other by Nody and co-workers [14], as examples of restrictive cardiomyopathy secondary to hemochromatosis. All three patients were asymptomatic until the

TABLE I Iron (Fe) Content of Liver and Cardiac Chambers

Tissue Assayed	Dry Weight* (µg Fe/100 µg dry weight) Patient	Dry Weight* Control Subject	Wet Weight (µg Fe/mg wet weight) Patient	Wet Weight Control Subject
Right ventricle	0.51	0.04	1.06	0.07
Left ventricle	0.47	0.04	0.99	0.09
Right atrium	0.12	0.03	0.48	0.05
Left atrium	0.07	0.05	0.47	0.08
Liver	3.84	0.07	7.87	0.20

* Dry weight values in this case are more valid than wet weight values since all specimens were formalin-fixed and therefore not truly wet.

onset of rapidly progressive cardiac decompensation culminating in death within one to three weeks. In none of the three patients was the diagnosis of hemochromatosis made during life. Failure to establish the diagnosis was, to a large degree, the result of the manner in which the restrictive cardiomyopathy simulated the clinical and hemodynamic signs of constrictive pericarditis. In the present case, diagnosis of hemochromatosis was considered because of the constellation of hepatic disease, diabetes mellitus and cardiac disease. Serum iron and iron-binding studies, however, revealed no abnormalities. Deterioration of the patient's hemodynamic status in the face of an abnormal prothrombin time prompted a decision to defer hepatic biopsy and, as was described in the patients of Wasserman [13] and Nody [14], to proceed to thoracotomy because of the suspicion of constrictive pericarditis.

The hemodynamic criteria considered as helpful in differentiating restrictive cardiomyopathy from constrictive pericarditis [1,2] supported the latter in this patient. These findings serve to emphasize the caveat that these criteria are not specific for the etiology of impaired diastolic filling.

The finding in our case also demonstrate that the difficulties which often obscure the clinical and hemodynamic distinctions between restrictive cardiomyopathy and constrictive pericarditis extend to the echocardiographic examination. Diastolic "flattening" of the left ventricular endocardial motion, described as the most consistent echocardiographic finding of constrictive pericarditis [19], was clearly and consistently observed in our patient with restrictive cardiomyopathy. Furthermore, there are presently no other recognized echocardiographic findings which can be used to reliably distinguish constrictive disease from restrictive disease [20-22]. In addition, echocardiographic findings observed by others [23] in patients with myocardial iron overload secondary to chronic transfusion or idiopathic hemochromatosis (increased left ventricular wall thickness, left ventricular transverse diastolic dimension and left ventricular mass) were absent in our patient (both by echocardiography and necropsy).

Although the mechanism by which cardiac iron deposition leads to cardiac dysfunction (systolic and/or diastolic) is not understood, the degree of dysfunction tends to parallel the amount of iron deposited in the myocardial cells [24,25]. It has been suggested that replacement fibrosis following degeneration of iron-laden myocytes may be the basis for cardiac dysfunction in hemosiderosis, but there was no increase in fibrous connective tissue in the myocardium of our patient.

The importance of our case and the two previously documented cases is (1) that restrictive cardiomyopathy due to hemochromatosis may be clinically indistinguishable from constrictive pericarditis, and (2) that hemochromatosis may represent the only potentially reversible cause of restrictive cardiomyopathy. Clinical [17] and hemodynamic [16] improvement of cardiac systolic function had been described in patients with hemochromatosis following repeated venesection. Although the patients with documented hemodynamic improvement had the "congestive" type of cardiomyopathy, it is reasonable to believe that the beneficial effect achieved in those patients with impaired systolic function might be duplicated in the treatment of patients with impaired diastolic function.

ACKNOWLEDGMENT

We gratefully acknowledge the assistance of Dr. Joseph Graziano, Department of Hematology, Columbia-Presbyterian Hospital, who performed the analyses of hepatic and myocardial iron content in our patient, and Dr. Frank A. Carroll, Alexandria, Virginia, who referred this patient to Georgetown University Hospital.

REFERENCES

1. Shabetai R, Fowler NO, Fenton JC: Restrictive cardiac disease, pericarditis and the myocardiopathies. Am Heart J 1965; 69: 271.
2. Conti CR, Friesinger GC: Chronic constrictive pericarditis. Clinical and laboratory findings in 11 cases. Johns Hopkins Med J 1967; 120: 262.
3. Scheuer PJ, Williams R, Muir AR: Hepatic pathology in relatives of patients with haemochromatosis. J Pathol 1962; 84: 53.
4. Finch SC, Finch CA: Idiopathic hemochromatosis, an iron storage disease. Medicine (Baltimore) 1955; 34: 381.
5. Tucker HS, Moss LF, Williams JP: Hemochromatosis with death from heart failure. Am Heart J 1948; 35: 993.
6. Horns HL: Hemochromatosis: Cardiac failure associated with extensive hemosiderosis of the myocardium. Am J Med 1949; 6: 272.
7. Bothwell TH, Van Lingen B, Alper T, Dupreeze, ML: The cardiac complications of hemochromatosis. Am Heart J 1952; 43: 333.
8. Swan WGA, Dewar HA: The heart in hemochromatosis. Br Heart J 1952; 14: 117.
9. Levin EB, Galum A: The heart in hemochromatosis. Am Heart J 1953; 45: 277.
10. Lewis HP: Cardiac involvement in hemochromatosis. Am J Med Sci 1954; 277: 554.
11. Castleman B, ed: Case records of the Massachusetts General Hospital. Discussion: Field RA, Pathology: Castleman B. N Engl J Med 1960; 263: 88.
12. Grosberg SJ: Hemochromatosis and heart failure. Ann Intern Med 1961; 54: 550.
13. Wasserman AJ, Richardson DW, Baird CL, Wyso EM: Cardiac hemochromatosis simulating constrictive pericarditis. Am J Med 1962; 32: 316.
14. Nody AC, Bruno MS, DePasquale NP, Bienstock PA: Fulminating idiopathic hemochromatosis presenting as constrictive pericarditis. Ann Intern Med 1975; 83: 373.
15. Schreiber AW: Hemochromatosis and the heart. Ann Intern Med 1957; 47: 1015.
16. Aronow WS, Melster L, Kent JR: Atrioventricular block in familial hemochromatosis treated by permanent synchronous pacemaker. Arch Intern Med 1969; 123: 433.
17. Easley RM, Schreiner BF, Yu PN: Reversible cardiomyopathy associated with hemochromatosis. N Engl J Med 1972; 287: 866.

18. Skinner C, Kenmure ACF: Haemochromatosis presenting as congestive heart failure and responding to venesection. Br Heart J 1973; 35: 466.
19. Voelkel AG, Pietro DA, Folland ED, Fisher ML, and Parisi AF: Echocardiographic features of constrictive pericarditis. Circulation 1978; 58: 871.
20. Candell-Riera J, Garcia Del Castillo H, Permanyer-Miralda G, Soler-Soler J: Echocardiographic features of the interventricular septum in chronic constrictive pericarditis. Circulation 1978; 57: 1154.
21. Candell-Riera J, Garcia Del Castillo H, Permanyer-Miralda C, Soler-Soler J: Interventricular septum in chronic constrictive pericarditis. Circulation 1979; 59: 847.
22. Acquatella H, Puigbo JJ, Suaree C, Mendoza J: Sudden early diastolic anterior movement of the septum in chronic constrictive pericarditis. Circulation 1979; 59: 847.
23. Henry WL, Nienhuis AW, Wiener M, Miller DR, Canale VC, Piomelli S: Echocardiographic abnormalities in patients with transfusion-dependent anemia and secondary myocardial iron deposition. Am J Med 1978; 64: 547.
24. Buja LM, Roberts WC: Iron in the heart: etiology and clinical significance. Am J Med 1971; 51: 209.
25. Arnett EN, Nienhuis AW, Henry WL, Ferrans VJ, Redwood DR, Roberts WC: Massive myocardial hemosiderosis: a structure-function conference at the National Heart and Lung Institute. Am Heart J 1975; 90: 777.

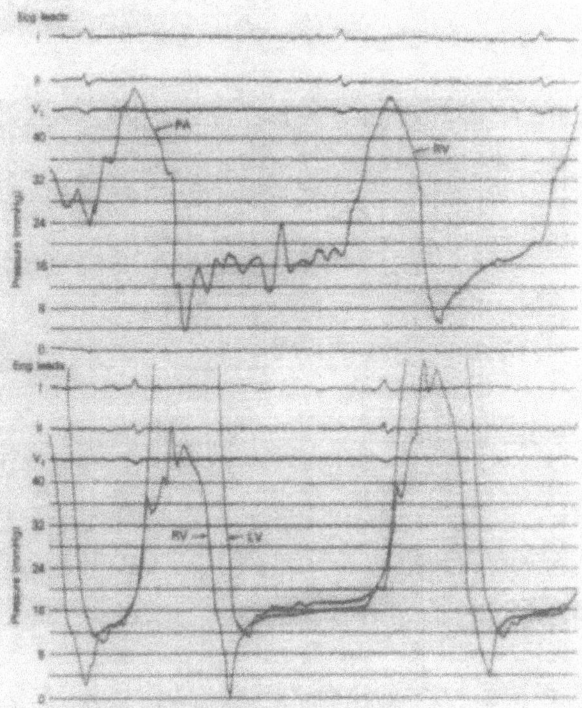

F.G. Age 62 Recorded 9/17/79 Died 9/4/80

Fig. 1. Pressure tracings recorded approximately 1 year before death which occurred on September 4, 1980. *Top panel,* Pullback from pulmonary trunk to RV showing similarly elevated diastolic pressures. *Bottom panel,* Simultaneous RV and LV pressures showing similarly elevated diastolic pressures, and RV early diastolic dip with plateau.

Hemodynamic cardiac constriction without anatomic myocardial restriction or pericardial constriction

Bruce M. McManus, M.D., Ph.D.,
George B. Bren, M.D., E. Arthur Robertson, M.D.,
Richard J. Katz, M.D., Allan M. Ross, M.D., and
William C. Roberts, M.D. *Bethesda, Md., and Washington, D.C.*

Most patients with hemodynamic evidence of right (RV) and left (LV) ventricular myocardial constriction have distinct anatomic conditions such as amyloidosis,[1] endomyocardial fibrosis,[2] hemosiderosis,[3] and the pericardial diseases,[4] responsible for the hemodynamic alterations. Recently, Benotti et al.[5] described nine patients with typical hemodynamic evidence of ventricular myocardial constriction, but the specific causes of the constriction were not delineated despite extensive studies.

Recently, we studied a 63-year-old woman with evidence of mixed connective tissue disease for at least 13 years and clinical and hemodynamic features of myocardial constriction for about 2 years. At cardiac catheterization 1 year before death, the right atrial mean, RV and LV end-diastolic, pulmonary arterial (PA) diastolic and PA wedge mean pressures were identical (18 mm Hg) with late diastolic plateau and "square root" configuration of the RV tracings (Fig. 1). Examination at that time disclosed 15 mm Hg pulsus paradoxus, distended neck veins, subcutaneous edema, and a murmur typical of tricuspid valve regurgitation. Both one- and two-dimensional echocardiograms were normal except for a dilated RV.

Pericardiotomy and partial pericardiectomy at that time disclosed normal parietal and visceral pericardia. She developed multiple arrhythmias (Fig. 2) for undetermined reasons and died a year later of progressive congestive heart failure (Fig. 3). At necropsy, the heart weighed 360 gm, the coronary arteries, the pericardium, and the valvular and mural endocardium and myocardium were normal except for a small posterobasal LV scar. Thus, classic clinical and hemodynamic features of cardiac constriction may not always have a demonstrable anatomic cause at necropsy.

From the Pathology Branch, National Heart, Lung, and Blood Institute, National Institutes of Health; and the Departments of Medicine and Pathology, George Washington University Hospital.

Received for publication March 13, 1981; accepted March 20, 1981.

0002-8703/81/070134 + 03$00.30/0 © 1981 The C. V. Mosby Co.

REFERENCES

1. Buja LM, Khoi NB, Roberts WC: Clinically significant cardiac amyloidosis: Clinicopathologic findings in 15 patients. Am J Cardiol **26**:394, 1970.

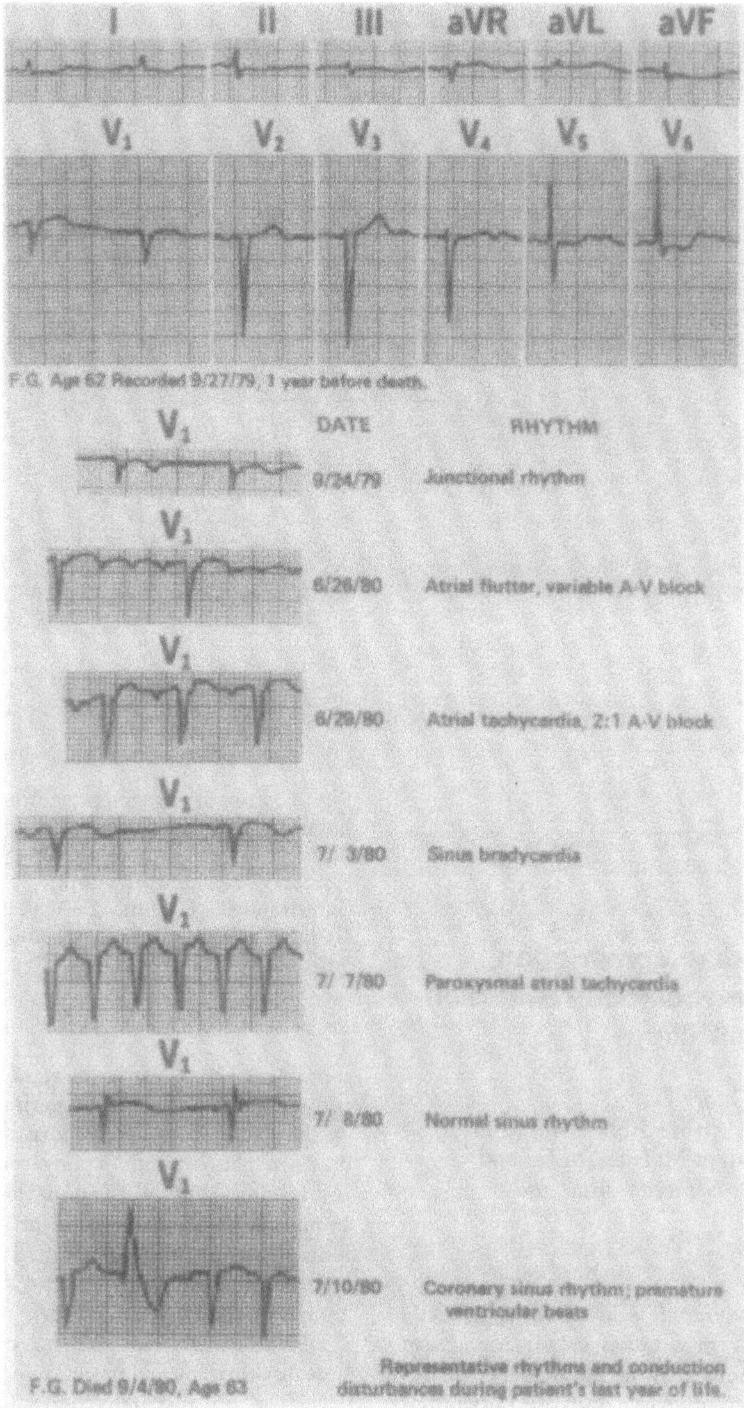

Fig. 2. Electrocardiograms showed a variety of arrhythmias and low voltage.

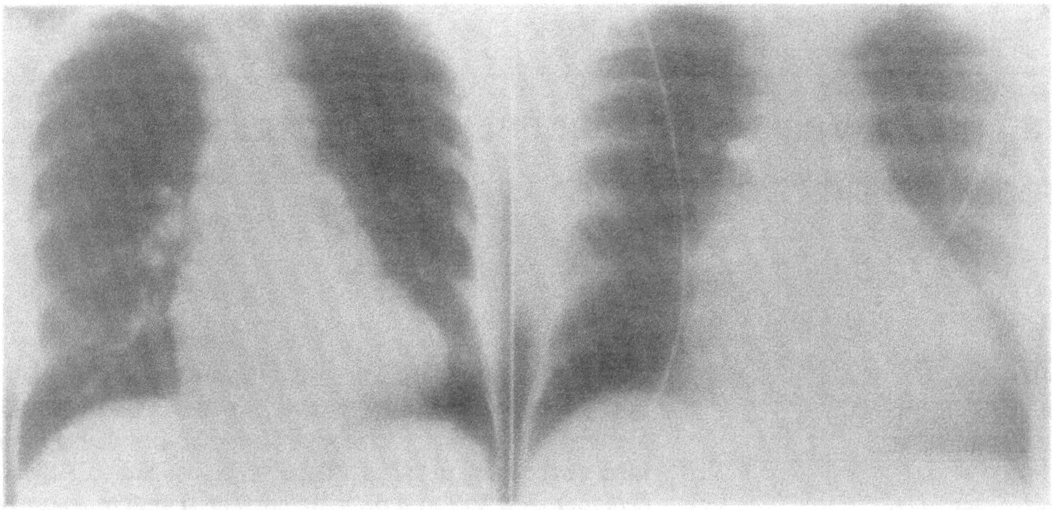

Fig. 3. Chest roentgenograms. *Left,* 1 year before death. *Right,* 3 months before death.

2. Somers K, Brenton DP, D'Arbela PG, Fowler JM, Kanyerezi BR, Sood NK: Haemodynamic features of severe endomyocardial fibrosis of right ventricle, including comparison with constrictive pericarditis. Br Heart J **30**:322, 1968.
3. Cutler DJ, Isner JM, Bracey AW, Hufnagel CAA, Conrad PW, Roberts WC, Kerwin DM, Weintraub AM: Hemochromatosis heart disease: An unemphasized cause of potentially reversible restrictive cardiomyopathy. Am J Med **69**:923, 1980.
4. Wood P: Chronic constrictive pericarditis. Am J Cardiol **7**:48, 1961.
5. Benotti JR, Grossman W, Cohn PF: Clinical profile of restrictive cardiomyopathy. Circulation **61**:1207, 1980.

Atrioventricular Valve Replacement in the Idiopathic Hypereosinophilic Syndrome

JOHN B. HARLEY, M.D., Ph.D.*
CHARLES L. McINTOSH, M.D.
JOHN J. W. KIRKLIN, M.D.
BARRY J. MARON, M.D.
JOHN GOTTDIENER, M.D.
WILLIAM C. ROBERTS, M.D.
ANTHONY S. FAUCI, M.D.
Bethesda, Maryland

Three patients with the idiopathic hypereosinophilic syndrome and the associated endocardiopathy are described who underwent atrioventricular valve replacement after intractable congestive heart failure secondary to valvular dysfunction developed. Following valve replacement, all three patients sustained striking improvement in exercise tolerance and control of congestive heart failure. Thus, atrioventricular valve replacement may be beneficial to selected patients with congestive heart failure associated with the endocardial process of the idiopathic hypereosinophilic syndrome.

Patients with the idiopathic hypereosinophilic syndrome (HES) present a variety of serious clinical problems. One is the progressive and often acute deterioration of cardiac function associated with severe thickening of the mural ventricular endocardium of one or both ventricles [1,2]. Clinically detectable heart disease eventually occurs in most patients with HES, and cardiac involvement is the most common cause of morbidity and mortality [1,2]. Mural endocardial thickening and superimposed thrombus, the characteristic anatomic features of HES, often lead to a restrictive cardiomyopathy which may be accompanied by atrioventricular (A-V) valve regurgitation [2]. In addition to the A-V valve regurgitation and endocardial fibrosis, many patients with HES have other complications which may include a poorly understood myeloproliferative component; therefore, there has been reluctance on the part of physicians to perform valve replacement. However, since hematologic complications can generally be controlled using chemotherapy with an improved prognosis [3], and since the major source of morbidity and mortality in these patients is the condition of cardiac function [2], we have recently replaced the mitral and/or tricuspid valves in three patients with HES and intractable congestive heart failure. Our findings and the results of surgery in these patients are the subject of this report.

PATIENTS AND METHODS

Three male patients from the group of 48 patients with HES followed at the National Institute of Allergy and Infectious Diseases [4] have undergone valve replacement. The preoperative clinical data from these patients are summarized in **Table I**. All three patients were initially treated with prednisone (up to 1 mg/kg per day) and subsequently received hydroxyurea (1 to 1.5 g/day) in accordance with the results of previous studies [3,4]. This therapy decreased, but did not eliminate their eosinophilia. After two years of hydroxyurea therapy, the eosinophilia in Patient 3 completely resolved. Clinical heart disease was first appreciated in these patients between 10 and 12 months after their original presentation with eosinophilia. In each patient, HES-related heart disease with a valvular component was relentlessly pro-

From the Laboratory of Immunoregulation, National Institute of Allergy and Infectious Diseases, and the Surgery, Cardiology and Pathology Branches, National Heart, Lung, and Blood Institute, National Institutes of Health, Bethesda, Maryland and the Department of Surgery, University of Alabama, Birmingham, Alabama. Requests for reprints should be addressed to Dr. John B. Harley, National Institutes of Health, NIAID, LIR, Building 10, Room 11B–13, Bethesda, Maryland 20205. Manuscript accepted December 21, 1981.

*Present address: Department of Medicine, University of Oklahoma and Oklahoma Medical Research Foundation, Oklahoma City, Oklahoma 73104.

TABLE I **Summary of Preoperative Clinical Data in Three Patients with HES**

	Patient 1	Patient 2	Patient 3
Age at onset (years)	24	32	29
Organ involvement*	Heart Spleen Liver Brain Eye	Lung Skin Spleen Heart Eye	Lung Spleen Liver Skin Heart
Range of eosinophilia/mm^3	6,000 to 30,000	5,000 to 19,500	250 to 9,000
Years from onset of symptoms to valve replacement	4.5	2.0	6.5
Physical examination			
Abnormal S_3	+	+	+
Peripheral edema	+	+	+
Pulmonary edema	+	+	+
Mitral regurgitation†	+	+	+
Tricuspid regurgitation†	+	0	0‡
Multiple emboli	+	+	0
Electrocardiogram			
Rhythm§	ST	NSR	NSR → AF
Nonspecific T-wave changes	+	+	+

+ = present; ST = resting sinus tachycardia; NSR = normal sinus rhythm; AF = atrial fibrillation.
* Involved organs listed in the order of clinical appearance.
† The clinical presence of mitral and tricuspid regurgitation was determined by the appropriate bedside maneuvers.
‡ At surgery this patient was found to have severe tricuspid regurgitation.
§ Rhythms are indicated by ST (sinus tachycardia at rest), NSR (normal sinus rhythm and AF (atrial fibrillation).

gressive and led to intractable congestive heart failure. Digoxin and diuretics were administered to all three patients for their congestive heart failure. Trials of hydralazine and nitrates, to reduce afterload, were not clearly beneficial. A-V valve replacements were performed between two and six and a half years after onset of disease when all other alternatives of available medical management had been exhausted. Surgery was performed as indicated using cardiopulmonary bypass and previously described surgical techniques [5].

RESULTS

All three patients who underwent A-V valve replacement sustained substantial improvement in most measures of cardiac performance. New York Heart Association functional class improved from IV to I or II in each patient, which was maintained throughout the period of postoperative follow-up in Patients 2 and 3 (28 and 21 months, respectively) or until fatal prosthetic valve endocarditis supervened in Patient 1 (eight months). In addition to severe A-V valve regurgitation, Patient 3 also had poor ventricular contractility, atrial fibrillation, and a filling defect at the apex of the left ventricle, which had been first appreciated two years before A-V valve replacement. In this patient, the benefit of valve replacement and apical thrombus removal was striking.

Left ventricular end diastolic and end systolic dimensions returned to or toward the normal range in each patient after operation. The end diastolic dimension decreased from an average of 67 mm to 48 mm (normal, 40 to 52 mm) whereas the end systolic dimension decreased from an average of 46 mm to 31 mm (normal, 25 to 35 mm).

In Patients 2 and 3, cardiac catheterization data were obtained at the sixth postoperative month. Pulmonary artery pressures decreased in both patients, although pulmonary hypertension persisted in Patient 3. The improved clinical state of these two patients was reflected by the marked decrease in their mean pulmonary artery wedge pressures, from a level compatible with intractable congestive heart failure to one that was only mildly abnormal (**Table II**). On the other hand, valve replacement did not improve cardiac output or ejection fraction. Indeed, the decrease in ejection fraction after surgery seen in Patient 2 appears to be a common consequence of mitral valve replacement [6].

At the first valve replacement, Patient 1 had mural thrombus adherent to both native A-V valves (**Figure 1**) and in the apex of the left ventricle. Initially Björk-Shiley prostheses were chosen for him. However, recurrent thrombotic involvement of the valves, despite systemic anticoagulation with warfarin sodium and heparin, led to a second valve replacement within four months where Hancock porcine heterografts were used. This patient died eight months after the second valve re-

TABLE II **Cardiac Catheterization Data Before (B) and After (A) Valve Replacement in Three Patients with HES**

	Patient 1	Patient 2		Patient 3	
	B	B	A	B	A
Pulmonary artery pressures (normal, 15/3 to 30/12 mm Hg)	60/28	52/20	25/13	62/30	50/25
Pulmonary artery mean wedge pressures (normal, 1 to 10 mm Hg)	30	24	14	33	14
Cardiac index (liters/min/m^2) (normal, 2.5 to 4.2 liters/min/m^2)	2.3	3.3	3.3	2.1	2.6
Left ventriculogram					
Ejection fraction (normal, >0.60)	0.66	0.51	0.26	0.17*	0.18
Apical filling defect	0	0	0	+	0
Posterobasal filling defects	0	+	+	0	0

+ = present.
* Gated blood pool scan (normal, 0.45 to 0.72) performed immediately before valve replacement while in atrial fibrillation.

placement with Straphylococcus aureus septicemia and acute bioprosthesis endocarditis. At necropsy, mural thrombi were absent from both ventricular cavities (**Figure 2**); however, small thrombi were present on both Hancock bioprostheses, despite long-term treatment with warfarin sodium. Microscopically, organisms were present in the bioprosthetic valves, but valve function had not been compromised.

The A-V native valves in Patients 2 and 3 were focally thickened by fibrous tissue. In both patients, these valves were devoid of thrombus whereas mural thrombi were present in the left ventricle. The large (approximately 30 g) calcified thrombus found in the ventricular apex of Patient 3 was successfully excised at operation.

COMMENTS

This study demonstrates the A-V valve replacement is beneficial for selected patients with idiopathic HES and severe A-V valve regurgitation in association with the characteristic endocardial heart disease. In each of our three patients, A-V valve replacement led to substantial improvement in exercise tolerance, reduction in left ventricular cavity dimension, as determined by echocardiography, and improved hemodynamics (Tables I and II).

The past surgical experience with valvular heart disease in patients with persistent eosinophilia appears to be limited to two patients. Bell et al. [7] described a patient in whom mitral anuloplasty was successfully performed and Weyman et al. [8] described a patient with mitral and tricuspid stenosis who underwent successful mitral valve replacement (porcine bioprostheses) and tricuspid commissurotomy. Both patients were alive six months after operation.

Some degree of cardiac involvement develops in from 40 to 95 percent of the patients with idiopathic HES [2,4]. This involvement ranges from T-wave inversion on electrocardiogram [2] to congestive heart failure, with endocardial fibrosis and mural thrombi at autopsy. Mitral regurgitation is the most common valvular lesion detected clinically [2], although valvular lesions have generally been considered to be a minor aspect of the cardiac abnormalities encountered in HES [1,2,9]. Decreased motion of the posterior mitral leaflet and thickening of the posterobasal left ventricular free wall are characteristic two-dimensional echocardiographic findings in patients with HES and mitral regurgitation [10].

The choice of a valve prosthesis for patients with HES is especially difficult. There are almost no data to evaluate the thrombotic potential and long-term structural integrity of the available valve prostheses in this disease. Of the patients reported by Hess et al. [11] who underwent A-V valve replacement and decortication of the concomitant endomyocardial fibrosis, one had an associated eosinophilia (46 percent). This patient's condition was stable at one-year follow-up, and no thrombotic difficulties were described despite the use of a Björk-Shiley prosthesis in the mitral position. Our unfortunate experience with Björk-Shiley prostheses in Patient 1, in addition to the knowledge that these valves are thrombogenic and that mural thrombi are characteristic of the HES-associated heart disease [3,4,12–15], has led us to prefer porcine heterograft prostheses in patients with this disease when prostheses are required and to administer anticoagulant therapy to those patients who have undergone A-V valve replacement.

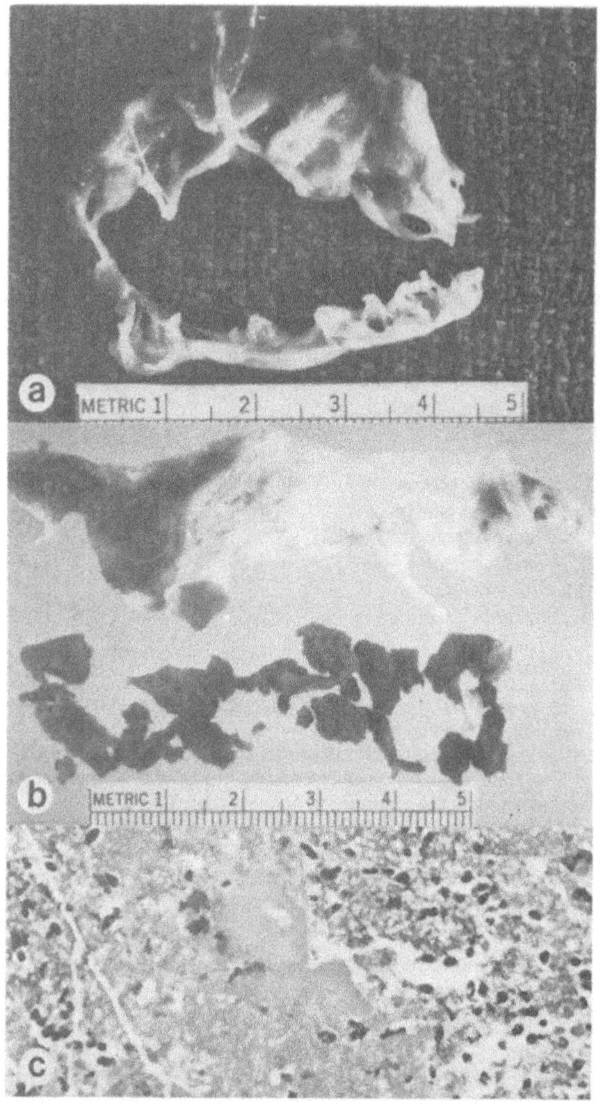

Figure 1. *Patient 1. Operatively excised tricuspid valve (**a**) and mitral valve (**b**). On the undersurface, i.e., ventricular surface of one tricuspid valve leaflet (**a**) and of one posterior mitral leaflet (**b**), large fibrous deposits containing some inflammatory cells (**c**) are present. Additionally, some mural endocardial thrombus was removed from left ventricle. H and E; magnification × 330, reduced by 24 percent.*

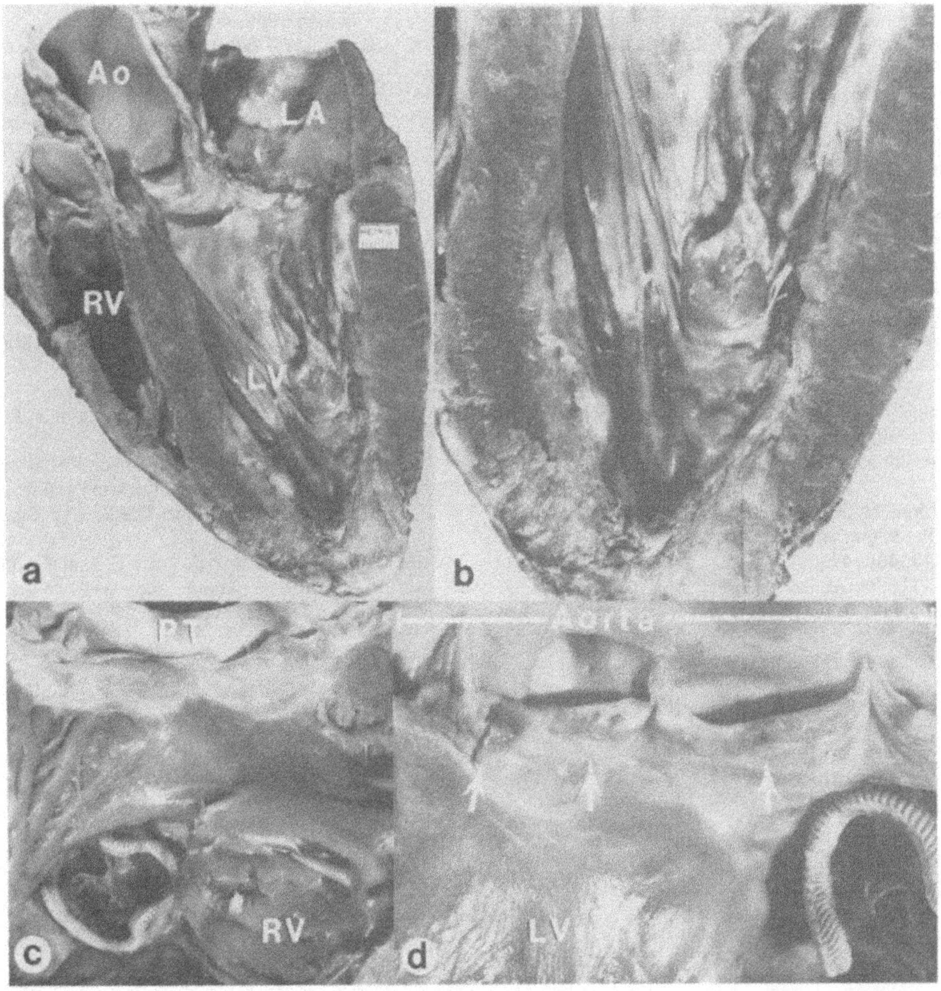

Figure 2. *Patient 1.* ***a,*** *Anterior-posterior cut of heart showing left ventricular (LV) mural endocardial thickening limited to its inflow tract. Ao = aorta; LA = left atrium; RV = right ventricle.* ***b,*** *close-up of left ventricular endocardial thickening.* ***c,*** *opened right ventricle with thrombus on the porcine bioprosthesis in the tricuspid valve position.* ***d,*** *opened aortic valve and left ventricular outflow tract showing fibrous thrombus (arrows) on each of the three aortic valve cusps. The porcine bioprosthesis in the mitral position is also visible.*

Several patients have been described with endocardial fibrosis without eosinophilia in whom A-V valve incompetence has also developed, and subsequently, they have undergone A-V valve replacement with successful decortication of the associated endocardial fibrosis [11,16–19]. It is unclear whether an antecedent eosinophilia was associated with the development of their heart disease. However, the cardiac pathology of certain patients with endocardial fibrosis without eosinophilia (such as Davies endomyocardial fibrosis) cannot be grossly or histopathologically differentiated from the endomyocardial pathology of HES [12–15].

In summary, this study demonstrates the feasibility of prosthetic valve replacement and its potential for dramatic benefit in patients who have severe valvular heart disease associated with the endocardial fibrosis of HES.

REFERENCES

1. Chusid MJ, Dale DC, West BC, et al.: The hypereosinophilic syndrome: analysis of fourteen cases with review of the literature. Medicine (Baltimore) 1975; 54: 1–27.
2. Parrillo JE, Borer JS, Henry WL, et al.: The cardiovascular manifestations of the hyperosinophilic syndrome: prospective study of 26 patients with review of the literature. Am J Med 1979; 67: 572–582.
3. Parrillo JE, Fauci AS, Wolff SM: Therapy of the hypereosinophilic syndrome. Ann Intern Med 1978; 89: 167–172.
4. Fauci AS (moderator): The idiopathic hypereosinophilic syn-

drome. Ann Intern Med (in press).
5. McIntosh CL, Michaelis LL, Morrow AG, et al.: Atrioventricular valve replacement with the Hancock porcine zenograft. Surgery 1975; 78: 768–775.
6. Schuler G, Peterson KL, Johnson A, et al.: Temporal response of left ventricular performance to mitral valve surgery. Circulation 1979; 59: 1218–1231.
7. Bell JA, Jenkins BS, Webbe-Reploe MM: Clinical, hemodynamic and angiographic findings in Löfflers eosinophilic endocarditis. Br Heart J 1976; 38: 541–548.
8. Weyman AE, Rankin R, King H: Loefflers endocarditis presenting as mitral and tricuspid stenosis. Am J Cardiol 1977; 40: 438–444.
9. Brink AJ, Weber HW: Fibroplastic parietal endocarditis with eosinophilia. Am J Med 1973; 34: 52–70.
10. Gottdiener JS, Schooley RS, Maron BS, Fauci AS: Cardiac abnormality in the hypereosinophilic syndrome—identification of a unique mechanism for mitral regurgitation by two-dimensional echocardiography. Circulation 1979; 65: II–19.
11. Hess OM, Turina M, Senning A, et al.: Pre- and postoperative findings in patients with endomyocardial fibrosis. Br Heart J 1978; 40: 406–415.
12. Roberts WC, Leigler DG, Carbone PP: Endomyocardial disease and eosinophilia. A clinical and pathologic spectrum. Am J Med 1969; 46: 28–32.
13. Roberts WC, Buja LM, Ferrans VJ: Löffler's fibroplastic parietal endocarditis, eosinophilic leukemia, and Davies' endomyocardial fibrosis: the same disease at different stages. Pathologica Microbiol 1970; 35: 90–95.
14. Brockington IF, Olsen EGJ: Löffler's endocarditis and Davies' endomyocardial fibrosis. Am Heart J 1973; 85: 308–322.
15. Roberts WC, Ferrans VJ: Pathologic anatomy of the cardiomyopathies: idiopathic dilated and hypertrophic types, infiltrative types, and endomyocardial disease with and without eosinophilia. Hum Pathol 1975; 6: 287–342.
16. Lepley DA, Aris A, Korns ME, et al.: Endomyocardial fibrosis: a surgical approach. Ann Thorac Surg 1974; 18: 626–633.
17. Dubost C, Maurice P, Gerbaux A, et al.: The surgical treatment of constrictive fibrosis endocarditis. Ann Surg 1976; 184: 303–307.
18. Laing HC, Sharratt GP, Johnson AM, et al.: Endomyocardial fibrosis in a European woman and its successful surgical treatment. J Thorac Cardiovasc Surg 1977; 74: 803–807.
19. Moraes CR, Buffalo E, Victor E, et al.: Endomyocardial fibrosis: report of 6 patients and review of the surgical literature. Ann Thorac Surg 1979; 29: 243–248.

The Idiopathic Hypereosinophilic Syndrome

Clinical, Pathophysiologic, and Therapeutic Considerations

Moderator: ANTHONY S. FAUCI, M.D. *Discussants:* JOHN B. HARLEY, M.D., Ph.D.; WILLIAM C. ROBERTS, M.D.; VICTOR J. FERRANS, M.D., Ph.D.; HARVEY R. GRALNICK, M.D.; and BARBARA H. BJORNSON, M.D.; Bethesda, Maryland

The idiopathic hypereosinophilic syndrome (HES) represents a heterogeneous group of disorders with the common features of prolonged eosinophilia of an undetectable cause and organ system dysfunction. Fifty patients with the idiopathic HES were studied over 11 years at the National Institutes of Health. Multiple organ systems were involved; bone marrow hypereosinophilia was common to all patients, but the most severe clinicopathologic involvement was of the heart and nervous system. Postmortem gross pathologic examination of the hearts of patients with idiopathic and nonidiopathic HES suggested that the common mechanism of cardiac disease is the eosinophilia. Endomyocardial biopsy findings showed that the endothelial cells in the endocardium and of the microvasculature were the primary targets of the tissue damage. This damage initiates thrombosis; endocardial fibrosis and restrictive endomyocardopathy may follow. In-vitro culture of circulating eosinophil colony-forming units showed some normal studies, some studies showing increased progenitor cells committed to eosinophil development, and others showing an excess production of eosinophil colony-stimulating factor. Chemotherapy to lower the eosinophil counts has resulted in marked improvement of HES prognosis, as have agressive medical and surgical approaches to cardiovascular complications.

DR. ANTHONY S. FAUCI (Chief, Laboratory of Immunoregulation, National Institute of Allergy and Infectious Diseases): Since the discovery of the eosinophil was announced by Paul Ehrlich at the meeting of the Physiological Society of Berlin on 17 January 1879 in his paper "Contribution of Granulated Connective Tissue Cells and of Eosinophil Leukocytes" (1), investigators have been both fascinated and perplexed by this cell whose precise function eludes us even today. The presence of circulating and tissue eosinophils in allergic and parasitic diseases is a universally recognized phenomenon. However, the beneficial or detrimental role of the eosinophil in these disease states is unclear. During the past 10 years, there has been a surge of interest in delineating the precise functional capabilities and the purpose of this cell (2, 3). There are several potential roles for the eosinophil in normal and abnormal physiologic responses.

▶ An edited transcription of a Clinical Staff Conference at the Clinical Center, Bethesda, Maryland, 12 February 1981, sponsored by the National Institute of Allergy and Infectious Diseases, National Institute of Health, U.S. Department of Health and Human Services.

▶ Authors who wish to cite a section of this conference and specifically indicate its author can use this example for the form of reference:

HARLEY JB. Clinical manifestations of patients with hypereosinophilic syndrome, pp. 82-4. In: FAUCI AS, moderator. The idiopathic hypereosinophilic syndrome: clinical, pathophysiologic, and therapeutic considerations. *Ann Intern Med.* 1982;**97**:78-92.

Characteristics of the Syndrome

ROLE OF THE EOSINOPHIL

The presence of eosinophilia in certain parasitic infections, particularly those helminthic infections that invade tissue, has been recognized practically from the time the eosinophil was discovered. Yet, its role in parasitic diseases is still disputed (4).

Because of the presence of eosinophils in abundance in the skin and mucosal surfaces of the respiratory and gastrointestinal tracts, it has been suggested that the cells have a major role in protecting the host from the initial invasion by organisms from the external environment. Although eosinophils are capable of phagocytosing bacteria and other microorganisms (5-9), their efficiency in this regard is felt to be far inferior to the neutrophil (10). Therefore, it was felt that their protection was predominantly against parasites. In this regard, several investigators have found mechanisms whereby the eosinophil can actually kill various forms of certain parasites after tissue invasion (11, 12). The most predominant of these mechanisms are antibody-dependent cellular cytotoxicity or complement-dependent cellular killing of the parasite. In this process, it has been suggested that the eosinophil binds firmly to the parasite by the above mentioned mechanisms and subsequently releases its intracytoplasmic enzymes, particularly major basic protein, onto and into the parasite, which results in the death of the organism (12-14).

Although many eosinophils are involved in the cytotoxic effect on one multicellular nematode or helminth, a word of caution should be introduced: as yet there is no convincing evidence that the eosinophil plays a direct role in vivo in the killing of parasites. However, substantial data exist to show that, if eosinophils are depleted from parasite-infected animals by treatment of the animal with an anti-eosinophil serum, mortality is higher than in control groups and greater numbers of parasites as well as eggs are recovered from the treated groups (11, 15).

In the United States and Europe, the commonest causes of eosinophilia are allergic reactions, particularly immediate hypersensitivity responses. Yet, the precise role of the eosinophil in these reactions is not entirely clear. However, substantial evidence is accumulating that enzymes present in the eosinophil can markedly modulate immediate hypersensitivity responses by inactivating various mediators that have a role in the initiation or perpetuation of these responses (13).

Finally, the presence of eosinophilia in certain diseases

characterized by circulating immune complexes has been well recognized. Eosinophils accumulate in response to immune complexes (16) and have been shown to be capable of phagocytosing immune complexes (17, 18), and so it has been postulated that a potential in-vivo role for these cells is in the clearance of deposited immune complexes in normal states and in pathologic conditions of immune complex deposition.

FACTORS INFLUENCING BLOOD AND TISSUE EOSINOPHILIA

Perhaps more is known of the mechanisms resulting in eosinophilia than is known of the functions of the eosinophils themselves. A number of mechanisms of eosinophilia have been proposed, and it is likely that several of these combine under any given circumstances to result in the net effect of increased numbers of eosinophils in the blood and tissues.

An elegant series of in-vitro studies have clearly established that, on triggering and degranulating of mast cells and basophils, peptides are released that are strongly chemotactic for eosinophils (19). The most studied of these is eosinophil chemotactic factor of anaphylaxis (20, 21). In addition, at appropriate concentrations, histamine has been shown to be chemotactic for eosinophils (22). Because IgE-mediated immune reactions are the hallmark of immediate hypersensitivity responses (23), and because IgE is directly involved in the triggering of mast cells with subsequent degranulation (24), the association of eosinophilia and such reactions can be easily and feasibly explained by such chemotactic mechanisms.

A number of experiments have firmly established a major role of the T lymphocyte in the development of eosinophilia (25). Under conditions of depletion of T lymphocytes, the eosinophilia normally seen in response to infestation and challenge of certain parasites in animal models is obviated (26). In this regard, it has been shown that a number of factors are derived from lymphocytes that are responsible for the proliferation and chemotaxis of eosinophils (27). It is surprising that eosinophilia is not seen more frequently in immune responses in animal models and humans, given the large body of evidence that eosinophilic chemotactic factors are elaborated in a wide variety of immunologic reactions.

Another potentially important mechanism operable in the production of eosinophilia is a direct increase in bone marrow production of eosinophils either in response to stimulatory factors such as eosinophilopoietin (28) or in primary myeloproliferative states that involve eosinophils primarily or secondarily. Lastly, there may be a prolongation of the eosinophil half-life, as has been shown in the idiopathic hypereosinophilic syndrome (HES) (29).

DISEASES CHARACTERIZED BY HYPEREOSINOPHILIA

Eosinophilia is found in different degrees in a wide variety of diseases, and this subject has been reviewed extensively (10). Table 1 contains a partial list of diseases in which circulating and tissue eosinophilia is not uncommonly found. Clearly, the two commonest groups are the allergic, or immediate hypersensitivity reactions, and parasitic diseases. The potential eosinophilotactic mechanisms associated with several of the allergic disorders, noted above, can easily explain this finding. It is important to point out that the mere presence of a parasitic infestation in the host is not necessarily associated with an eosinophilia. Within the spectrum of parasitic diseases, eosinophilia is almost exclusively found in those metazoan parasitic diseases in which the parasite actually invades that host tissue as opposed to merely residing on a surface such as the gut lumen (10). Diseases where eosinophilia is commonly encountered are strongyloidiasis, trichinosis, schistosomiasis, filariasis, toxocara, and other tissue-invasive helminths.

Table 1. Disorders Associated with a Secondary Eosinophilia

- Allergic or hypersensitivity diseases (predominantly respiratory)
  - Asthma
  - Seasonal rhinitis
  - Pulmonary aspergillosis
  - Certain drug reactions
- Parasitic diseases
  - Strongyloidiasis
  - Trichinosis
  - Schistosomiasis
  - Filariasis
  - Toxocara
  - Other tissue invasive helminths
- Cutaneous diseases
  - Known allergic cause (such as drug reactions, atopic dermatitis)
  - Suspected allergic cause (such as dermatitis herpetiformis)
  - Unknown cause
- Connective tissue diseases
  - Systemic necrotizing vasculitis—particularly allergic angiitis and granulomatosis (Churg-Strauss syndrome)
  - Eosinophilia with fasciitis
  - Rheumatoid arthritis, systemic lupus erythematosus scleroderma (rarely)
- Neoplastic diseases
  - Lymphoma—Hodgkin's disease, T cell lymphomas (mycosis fungoides)
  - Certain leukemias—acute lymphoblastic leukemia, Sezary syndrome (T-cell leukemia)
  - Solid tumors—particularly metastatic carcinoma of mucin-secreting epithelial origin
- Immunodeficiency states
  - Wiscott-Aldrich syndrome
  - Hyper-IgE with infections
  - Selective IgA deficiency

Under certain circumstances, even after a thorough diagnostic evaluation, no underlying cause can be found for an observed eosinophilia. Hence, the eosinophilia would have to be categorized as "idiopathic." Idiopathic hypereosinophilia is of no special clinical relevance except as a curiosity and diagnostic dilemma. However, when the eosinophilia is associated with organ system dysfunction that cannot be explained by another mechanism apart from the presence of eosinophils, and the probability exists (for lack of another explanation) that the tissue damage causing the organ system dysfunction is directly or indirectly related to the eosinophil itself, then a frustrating and serious clinical problem arises. Over the past 11 years we have had prospective experience with 50 patients with the idiopathic HES (30, 31).

Table 2. Potential Mechanisms of Tissue Damage in Hypereosinophilic Syndromes

Tissue infiltration with eosinophils (space occupying)
Damage relating to an eosinophil function
  Direct cytotoxicity
  Antibody dependent cellular cytotoxicity
Damage related to eosinophil products
  Secretion or release by cell death of intracytoplasmic contents into tissues.
  Secretion or release by cell death of intracytoplasmic contents into the circulation with subsequent damage to selective tissues.
Thromboembolic phenomena
  Related to thombi associated with endomyocardial disease
  Related to hypercoagulable state (no direct evidence)
Damage related to mechanisms apart from eosinophils themselves
  Related to the underlying cause of the eosinophilia
  Unrelated to the underlying cause of the eosinophilia

THE IDIOPATHIC HYPEREOSINOPHILIC SYNDROME

Empiric threefold criteria have been established for idiopathic HES (30, 31): persistent eosinophilia of 1500 eosinophils/mm^3 for at least 6 months or death before 6 months with signs and symptoms of HES disease; lack of evidence for parasitic, allergic, or other recognized causes of eosinophilia (Table 1) despite careful evaluation; and signs and symptoms of organ system involvement or dysfunction either directly related to eosinophilia or unexplained in the given clinical setting. Although unexplained eosinophilia of 1500 eosinophils/mm^3 is not clinically uncommon and often resolves unexplained, it is the persistence of the eosinophilia that is the hallmark of the syndrome along with the enigmatic organ system dysfunction.

Patients who have entered the HES protocol of the National Institute of Allergy and Infectious Diseases (NIAID) have undergone a thorough diagnostic evaluation for the usual causes of eosinophilia (Table 1). All patients had a careful history taking and a complete physical examination. Laboratory data included serial complete blood counts, urinalysis, liver and renal function tests, multiple serologic tests for infectious and connective tissue diseases, chest roentgenograms, electrocardiograms, pulmonary function tests, roentgenograms of any involved organ where appropriate, bone marrow aspirate, and biopsy with chromosomal analysis. Markers for certain leukemias, such as serum vitamin B12 levels and leukocyte alkaline phosphatase, were also determined. Where indicated and appropriate, other involved organs were biopsied to document the presence or absence of eosinophils and the type of histopathologic findings present. Multiple stool samples were examined for ova and parasites, and duodenal aspirates were obtained to exclude specific parasites such as Strongyloides. Extensive cultures for bacteria, fungi, and mycobacteria were obtained on all patients. These thorough evaluations were usually repeated at 3- to 6-month follow-up visits (31). Extensive immunologic evaluation of these patients has shown various nonspecific abnormalities such as the presence of circulating immune complexes in 32% of patients, elevated IgE levels in 38% of patients, and mild decreases in proportions of circulating T cells in certain patients (32). No apparent correlation with these observed abnormalities and patterns of disease could be found, except in patients with indications of a hypersensitivity phenomenon (albeit of unknown cause), such as elevated serum IgE levels. These patients were usually more responsive to corticosteroid therapy and, although they did have organ system dysfunction, it generally was milder than that in patients without such manifestations. If such attempts at delineating an underlying cause of the eosinophilia were unsuccessful, the patient was designated as having the idiopathic HES.

The most significant component of this designation is the fact that this syndrome is distinct, with a range of organ system dysfunctions from minor skin involvement to serious and often life-threatening cardiovascular, hematologic, and neurologic manifestations (30, 31, 33). There is no question that HES is a heterogeneous group of disorders whose common denominator is persistent eosinophilia with organ system involvement, dysfunction, or both, related either to infiltration of eosinophils or secondary to an eosinophil-associated damage to tissue (30, 31).

Of particular interest is the fact that organ system dysfunction, which is likely related directly or indirectly to the eosinophils themselves, may be seen in certain patients with eosinophilia of a known cause. Specifically, cardiac lesions similar to those seen in HES have been reported in patients with eosinophilic responses secondary to drug reactions (35) and parasitic disease (36). In fact, we have seen patients who presented with unexplained eosinophilia that either spontaneously resolved or resolved after empiric treatment with an antihelminthic agent and in whom clear-cut endomyocardopathy developed.

MECHANISMS OF TISSUE DAMAGE

In addition to the frustrating fact of the idiopathic nature of the HES is the realization that we lack the knowledge of the precise mechanisms whereby eosinophils exert their tissue damaging effects. In the past few years, however, as we have become more aware of certain of the functional capabilities of the eosinophil (1, 2, 13), potential mechanisms of eosinophil-related tissue damage in the syndrome have been appreciated (Table 2).

Clearly, eosinophils can infiltrate virtually any organ system that is involved in the HES. Infiltration of large amounts of eosinophils in the lungs and the skin can explain certain of the manifestations in those organs. Also, a large amount of eosinophilic infiltration in the bone marrow can clearly result in a myelophthisic effect. Of particular note, however, is the fact that the two organ systems most severely involved in the syndrome, namely the heart and the nervous system, have degrees of tissue damage, functional impairment, or both that cannot be explained on the basis of the mere infiltration of eosinophils into the tissues themselves (30, 31). Thus, other alternative mechanisms must be involved. Although these mechanisms are still at the stage of hypothesis, experimental data and clinicopathologic observations suggest a real potential for certain pathophysiologic mechanisms.

Of particular interest concerning the tissue-damaging potential of the eosinophil has been the recent description of the intracellular contents of the eosinophil, particularly its granule contents (19). The ability of the eosinophil or its contents to cause tissue damage was noted inadvertently as far back as 1933, when Gordon found that the intracerebral injection of lymph node homogenates from patients with Hodgkin's disease into laboratory animals led to a neurotoxic effect (37). This has subsequently been referred to as the "Gordon phenomenon." It was not realized until 1938 that this neurotoxic reaction was dependent on the presence of eosinophils in the lymph nodes (38, 39). Most recently, a neurotoxic fraction has been isolated from human eosinophils and not from human neutrophils (40). The clinical significance and relationship of the Gordon phenomenon to the neurologic manifestations of the HES are uncertain at present.

Further information on the potential tissue-damaging effects of the eosinophil has emerged from recent precise delineation of the broad range of intracytoplasmic contents of the eosinophil, some of which are exclusively found in the eosinophil or are more concentrated in that cell than in other leukocytes (19, 41). Of these, the eosinophil major basic protein (42, 43) and the eosinphil cationic protein (44) deserve special comment. Of particular interest and potentially great importance in our understanding of the pathogenesis of the endothelial damage in the syndrome is the fact that concentrations of major basic protein shown in the serum of several of our patients with the HES (45) are capable of causing severe damage to tracheal epithelial cells (46); these levels exceed those needed for direct cytoxicity in vitro and are much higher than levels needed to inhibit growth of aortic endothelial cells (45). Some of the highest serum levels of major basic protein were seen in certain of our patients with the most severe organ system involvement with HES. However, there was not a direct relation between severity of disease and serum level of major basic protein in every patient. This raises the interesting possibility of factors other than the mere presence of large numbers of eosinophils, particularly major basic protein, that may be involved in the discharge of eosinophil contents either directly into tissue or into the circulation. Thus, factors that may be responsible for the degranulation of eosinophils may be influential in the ultimate tissue damage in the HES.

The other eosinophil protein that is felt to have a potential role in the tissue damage seen in HES is eosinophil cationic protein (44). This protein has been found in high levels in the sera of patients with HES and has been reported to have profound effects on the coagulation system in vitro (44). Eosinophil cationic protein may be partially responsible for the thromboembolic phenomena (particularly mural thrombi and consequent embolizations) characteristic of the HES (which will be discussed later).

With regard to the cardopathy of the HES, it is highly

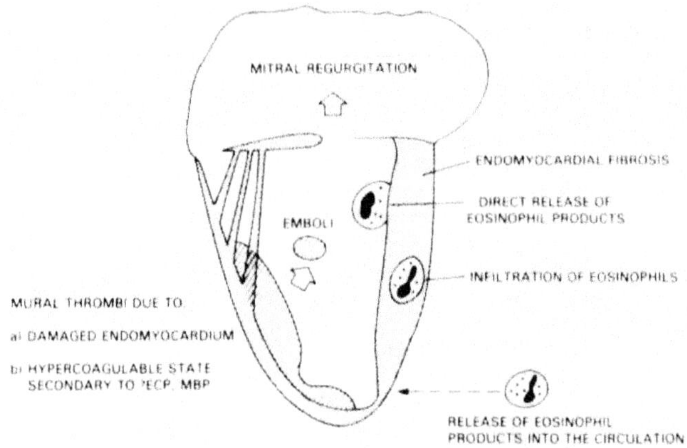

Figure 1. Schematic diagram of the various potential mechanisms of cardiovascular disease in the hypereosinophilic syndrome. The initial damage is to the endocardium with subsequent thrombus formation. Thrombi may involve the atrioventricular valves resulting in impaired function and valvular incompetence. Also, thrombi may dislodge and result in pulmonary or peripheral embolization. Fibrosis of the damaged endocardium may lead to a secondary restrictive endomyocardopathy.

likely that the initial and primary lesion is damage to the endocardium. Subsequent to this, platelet thrombi form over the injured or denuded endocardium and a mural thrombus is propagated. Such thrombi often involve the posterior leaflet of the mitral or tricuspid valves leading to the atrioventricular valvular insufficiency that we have clearly documented as being characteristic of the endocardopathy of the HES (33). Peripheral embolization would readily follow the deposition of mural thrombi. Furthermore, high serum levels of eosinophil cationic protein with its potential hypercoagulable effects (44) may contribute to the thromboembolic phenomena. Lastly, it is possible (although no evidence exists in this regard) that mechanisms unrelated to the eosinophils themselves are responsible for the tissue damage, particularly the endomyocardial disease. The multiple potential mechanisms of the cardiac damage in the HES are schematically diagrammed in Figure 1.

THERAPY

Historically, HES has carried an extremely poor prognosis. Multiple reviews of the literature showed an extremely high morbidity and mortality of patients with the syndrome (30, 47, 48).

In a recent review of 57 cases in the literature (31), we found an average survival of 9 months and a 3-year survivial of 12%. On this basis, we instituted a vigorous treatment regimen directed at lowering the eosinophil count in patients with the syndrome, because this was the only consistently abnormal laboratory variable. We also aggressively treated the organ system complications of the syndrome where possible (31). Given the recent information of the potential tissue-damaging capabilities of eosinophils, attempts at lowering the eosinophil counts have assumed a renewed rational basis.

Our treatment regimen for patients with the syndrome has been previously described in detail (31, 49, 50). Patients without progressive organ system dysfunction are not treated and are followed closely at 3-to 6-month in-

Table 3. Presenting Signs and Symptoms in Patients with the Idiopathic Hypereosinophilic Syndrome

	Patients (n = 50)
	n(%)
Weakness and fatigue	13 (26)
Cough	12 (24)
Dyspnea	8 (16)
Myalgias	7 (14)
Angioedema	7 (14)
Rash	6 (12)
Fever	6 (12)
Incidental discovery of eosinophilia	6 (12)
Rhinitis	5 (10)

tervals. If patients show organ system dysfunction, they are treated initially with prednisone, 1 mg/kg body weight·d on a daily basis followed by conversion to an alternate day regimen. Again they are followed on a 3-month basis with careful evaluation particularly with regard to cardiovascular complications. If the disease stabilizes or improves, the corticosteroid is continued and ultimately tapered to the lowest possible dosage that will control the disease. If the disease progresses despite corticosteroid therapy, a cytotoxic agent, specifically hydroxyurea (0.5 to 1.5 g/d), is added to the regimen with the aim of maintaining the leukocyte count at less than 10 000/mm^3. Rarely, a patient is treated with leukopheresis when extremely high levels of eosinophils (100 000/mm^3 or greater) are acutely encountered during the induction period with hydroxyurea. The most recent follow-up on our total of 50 patients managed with this regimen will be discussed below.

Clinical Manifestations

Dr. John B. Harley (Clinical Associate, Laboratory of Immunoregulation, National Institute of Allergy and Infectious Diseases): Over the past 11 years patients with unexplained eosinophilia have been evaluated and treated at the National Institutes of Health (NIH). Fifty-five patients were referred to NIH as apparently satisfying the diagnostic criteria for idiopathic HES. Alternative diagnoses were established for five patients who were shown to have polyarteritis nodosa, allergic angiitis, and granulomatosis of Churg and Strauss; rheumatoid arthritis with vasculitis; allergic eosinophilic gastroenteritis; or *Strongyloides* infestation. The remaining 50 patients were considered to have the idiopathic HES because they all satisfied the criteria for diagnosis as has been described above, and the subsequent discussion will be limited to this group of patients.

PATIENTS

In this population the mean age of disease onset was 33 years. The mean duration of disease has been 4.8 years (range, 1 to 24 years). This group has been followed at the NIH between 0.1 to 11 years with a mean of 3.2 years. The age distribution by decade shows that although the disease can occur at any age, 70% of the patients had their onset of disease between 20 and 50 years of age.

The patients originally presented with various nonspecific symptoms (Table 3) that in no way revealed their underlying diagnosis. In fact, in 12% of the patients, the eosinophilia was discovered incidentally at routine medical check-up or was noted during the management of an apparently unrelated medical problem.

Virtually any organ system can be involved in the idiopathic HES and, by definition, all patients have had hematologic involvement (Table 4). In addition to eosinophilia, hematologic problems included anemia, thrombocytopenia, venous thrombosis, and elevated serum B12 levels. Abnormal leukocyte alkaline phosphatase was found in most patients but, as has been noted previously (30), the results of this test are highly variable in patients with the syndrome. Karyotype abnormalities, when present, are usually nonspecific. However, one of our patients had a Philadelphia chromosome and another was a male Turner's syndrome mosaic. Eight of the 33 patients studied had some chromosomal abnormality with the commonest finding being aneuploidy in a minority of the mitoses. One patient in our series died in blast crisis.

Peripheral blood smear and bone marrow may also show abnormalities beyond eosinophilia. Eosinophil hypogranulation and vacuolization is frequently found in the peripheral blood, but is uncommon in the bone marrow. Patients may also show evidence of myeloid dyspoiesis in the peripheral blood with immature cells present. In the marrow, findings ranged from benign eosinophilia to blast crisis with a range of intermediate findings found in most patients.

Neurologic manifestations of the syndrome included three major categories of neurologic dysfunction. A diffuse central nervous system abnormality was found, characterized by altered behavior and cognitive function, spasticity, and occasionally ataxia. A peripheral neuropathy was particularly common, usually in the distribution of a symmetrical polyneuropathy. Focal central nervous system deficits from cardiac emboli or hematologic disturbances were also noted (Moore PM, Harley J, Fauci AS. In preparation).

Most of the patients had cutaneous disease; 28% had dermatographism and 10% had angioedema. Also, a wide variety of different rashes have been seen in our

Table 4. The Relative Frequency of Organ System Involvement in the Idiopathic Hypereosinophilic Syndrome

	Patients (n = 50)
	n (%)
Hematologic	50 (100)
Neurologic	32 (64)
Skin	28 (56)
Cardiovascular	27 (54)
Spleen	23 (46)
Pulmonary	20 (40)
Liver	16 (32)
Nose and sinuses	13 (26)
Ocular	9 (18)
Gastrointestinal	7 (14)
Lymph nodes	6 (12)
Muscles	6 (12)

patients, none of which could be considered typical. Skin biopsies from these rashes almost invariably showed inflammatory changes with the pathologic findings rangings from eosinophilic vasculitis to nonspecific inflammatory infiltrates (51).

Cardiac disease is the major source of morbidity and mortality in patients with the syndrome (30, 31, 33). These patients are at risk to develop the characteristic endocardial fibrosis with overlying thrombus. Progressive pump failure, which in some cases cannot be completely explained by the endocardial fibrosis and restrictive endomyocardopathy, may be relentlessly progressive, its course ranging from days to years. In our series, 8% of the patients had otherwise unexplained progressive pump failure. The supporting structures of the atrioventricular valves are especially affected by the processes of fibrosis and thrombus that often result in clinical valvular incompetence; 30% of the patients have had progressive mitral regurgitation. Tricuspid regurgitation was manifest as well in a few patients. Multiple emboli were seen in 18% of our patients and this finding was viewed as evidence for HES-related cardiac involvement. Finally, two of our patients have developed bacterial endocarditis.

Pulmonary disease with unexplained eosinophilia comprises a heterogeneous spectrum of disorders with various manifestations and clinical courses. A subgroup of such patients may have transient pulmonary infiltrates with eosinophilia, with or without bronchospasm that may resolve spontaneously. Several of our patients presented with this illness and, had they not later gone on to develop more extensive and severe organ system involvement, could rightfully have been considered to have had Löffler's syndrome or the pulmonary infiltration with eosinophilia syndrome and not the idiopathic HES. In fact, a short benign clinical course with spontaneous resolution actually precludes the diagnosis of the idiopathic HES. However, our patients with this type of initial pulmonary manifestations went on to a more persistent form of pulmonary disease almost always associated with other organ system dysfunction. Some of these patients have progressed from inflammatory pulmonary disease to substantial pulmonary fibrosis, most commonly with the development of HES-related heart disease (30, 31, 33). Unfortunately, the ultimate clinical course of patients with initially benign and self-limiting pulmonary involvement cannot be accurately predicted at the time of presentation. This observation emphasizes the need for comprehensive evaluation even in those patients in whom the more benign forms of pulmonary disease are considered more likely.

Patients with HES and pulmonary disease may pose certain difficult diagnostic and management problems. Cough, bronchospasm, dyspnea, infiltrates, and effusions may be manifestations of pulmonary infection, embolus, or infarction, as well as HES-related pulmonary or cardiac involvement. Because therapy for each of these possibilities may be quite different, careful diagnostic evaluation is needed in each instance. Hepatic involvement was typified by hepatomegaly and minor abnormalities of liver function tests. The spectrum of pathologic findings included congested sinusoids, chronic hepatitis without cirrhosis, and periportal inflammation.

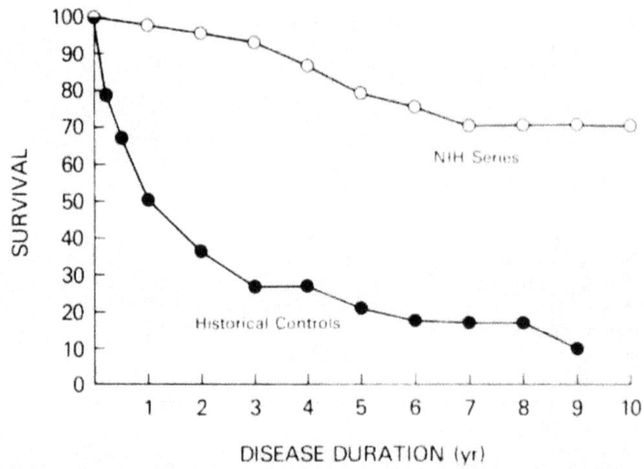

Figure 2. Survival in the idiopathic hypereosinophilic syndrome of 58 cases from the literature (-●-) taken from the study by Parrillo and associates (5) and of the 50 patients in the updated National Institutes of Health series (-o-).

Ocular manifestations, when present, generally reflected the effects of embolic events. Also, two patients had findings consistent with retinal vein thrombosis: one showed changes consistent with hyperviscosity, and the other had nodular episcleritis.

Gastrointestinal involvement was manifestd clinically by diarrhea, nausea, and abdominal cramps. In most of these patients, Charcot-Leyden crystals were found in stools. Eosinophilic infiltrates of the gastrointestinal mucosa were found in all but one biopsy; the exception showed flattened villi.

In patients with muscular involvement, swelling or wasting was generally seen, but such involvement was unusual. Pathologically, diverse inflammatory infiltrates were found with different degrees of tissue destruction.

Renal disease as a primary consequence of the idiopathic HES was also rare. Pathologically there were inflammatory infiltrates with eosinophilic predominance that primarily involved the interstitial areas, but also, to a lesser extent, involved the glomeruli. Proliferative glomerular lesions in the absence of inflammatory infiltrates have also been described (34).

Abnormalities of the immune system were seen in certain patients and were quite different. Although only a few patients were shown to have lymphadenopathy or anergy, almost half of the patient population had circulating immune complexes, elevated IgE, or hyperimmunoglobulinemia involving IgM, IgG, or IgA. Thus, the syndrome may involve multiple organ systems with various pathologic findings and a broad range of clinical findings and disease courses.

THERAPY

Because the precise pathophysiologic mechanisms of tissue damage in patients with HES are not entirely clear (Table 2), the major thrust of therapy has been aimed at lowering the eosinophil counts and alleviating the clinical manifestations of cardiac involvement. The chemotherapeutic approach to these patients has been outlined

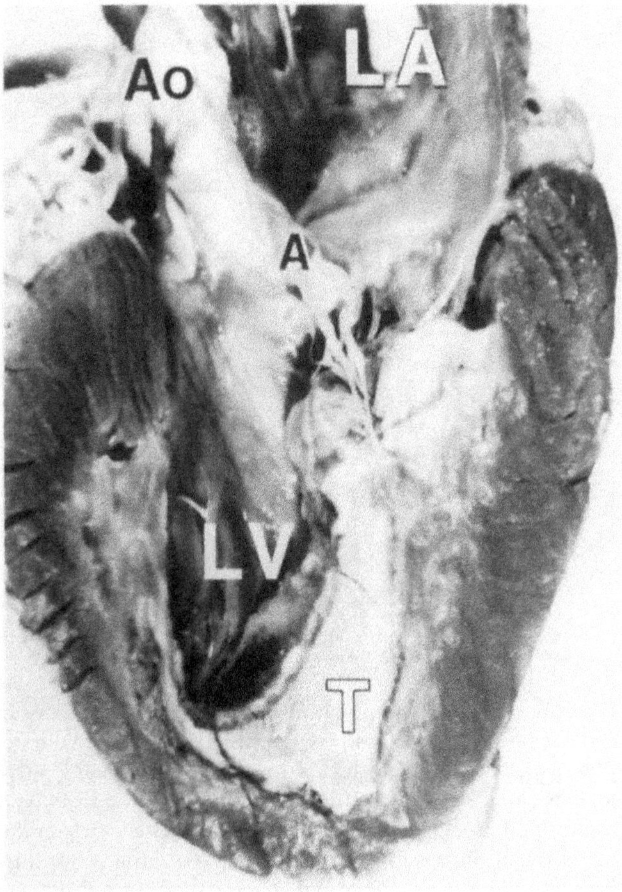

Figure 3. Longitudinal cuts of left ventricle (LV) in a 47-year-old man with chronic myelogenous leukemia showing a large thrombus (T) in the in-flow portion. A = anterior mitral leaflet; Ao = aorta; LA = left atrium.

above. Using such an approach over the past 11 years, our patients have shown remarkable improvement in survival and prognosis as compared with those of controls taken from the literature (5) (Figure 2). Because the cardiovascular manifestations of the syndrome are clearly the most important clinical factor because they, more than any other organ system involved, dictate the ultimate prognosis (30, 31, 33), a particularly aggressive medical and surgical approach to the cardiovascular manifestations of the disease has been assumed in our patient population. We believe this approach has been a major factor in the improved survival.

In brief, our approach was to treat patients with a medical regimen of digitalis and diuretics, if needed. In some cases, afterload reduction was attempted. Patients with evidence of thromboembolic phenomena of cardiac origin have been treated with additional surgical and medical therapies including thrombectomy and systemic anticoagulation with heparin. Finally, despite continued activity of the underlying disease, we have done atrioventricular valve replacement in three patients who had relentless and progressive valvular heart disease related to the syndrome. Two patients had mitral and tricuspid valves replaced, and the third needed only mitral valve replacement. Also, an old organized thrombus was surgically removed in one patient. Substantial improvement in functional class was realized in each patient. One patient died in staphylococcal sepsis with prosthetic valve endocarditis 8 months after surgery but the other two patients are doing well 7 and 13 months after surgery, respectively. An aggressive cardiovascular surgical approach to this group of patients with an underlying disease of previously poor prognosis has contributed to the improved ultimate survival of the patients, because the severity of their cardiovascular functional impairment would have almost invariably led to a rapid deterioration in their clinical course (33).

Cardiopathy

Dr. William C. Roberts (Chief, Pathology Branch, National Heart, Lung, and Blood Institute): As mentioned before, the clinical cardiovascular manifestations in patients with the idiopathic HES are striking and in many cases dominate the clinical picture. However, pathologic findings in the hearts of patients with eosinophilia associated with another recognized and well-defined underlying disease can be strikingly similar, if not identical, to the pathologic findings in patients with the idiopathic HES. In fact, it is interesting and informative to review the historic evolution of the concept of severe cardiovascular disease associated with various types of eosinophilic syndromes.

In 1936, Löffler (52) in Zurich described two patients seen 20 years apart: a 37-year-old man with a 21-month illness and a 45-year-old woman with a 12-month illness; each had severe blood eosinophilia (to 70%), mild leukocytosis (12 000 to 18 000/mm^3), severe chronic congestive heart failure, hepatomegaly, splenomegaly, precordial murmurs of mitral regurgitation, and at autopsy, extensive fibrous thickening of the mural endocardium of both the right and left ventricles with superimposed thrombus in the left ventricles. Löffler called the condition "fibroplastic parietal endocarditis with blood eosinophilia." In his first patient the eosinophilia vanished before death, and in his second patient, it remained near its maximal level. Löffler considered the eosinophilia to be an expression of an allergic reaction, but it was a "phasic sign," present only as long as the allergic condition was present. He ascribed the chronic congestive heart failure in both his patients to the fibrous thickening of the mural endocardium of both ventricles that "prevented normal diastolic relaxation" and to the thrombotic masses that "decreased the capacity of the ventricles." He believed the clinical consequences of the mural endocardial thickening produced clinical features indistinguishable from those resulting from chronic constrictive pericarditis.

After Löffler's report, many single case descriptions of similar patients appeared. By 1957 Weiss-Carmine (53), working in Löffler's department, collected 26 additional cases, including two from the United States, and thereafter many more reports followed (48, 54).

Patients described under various other designations have had clinical and morphologic features similar to those described in patients with Löffler's fibroplastic parietal endocarditis. Bousser (55) and, later, Odebery (56) noted from the study of autopsy findings of 25 pa-

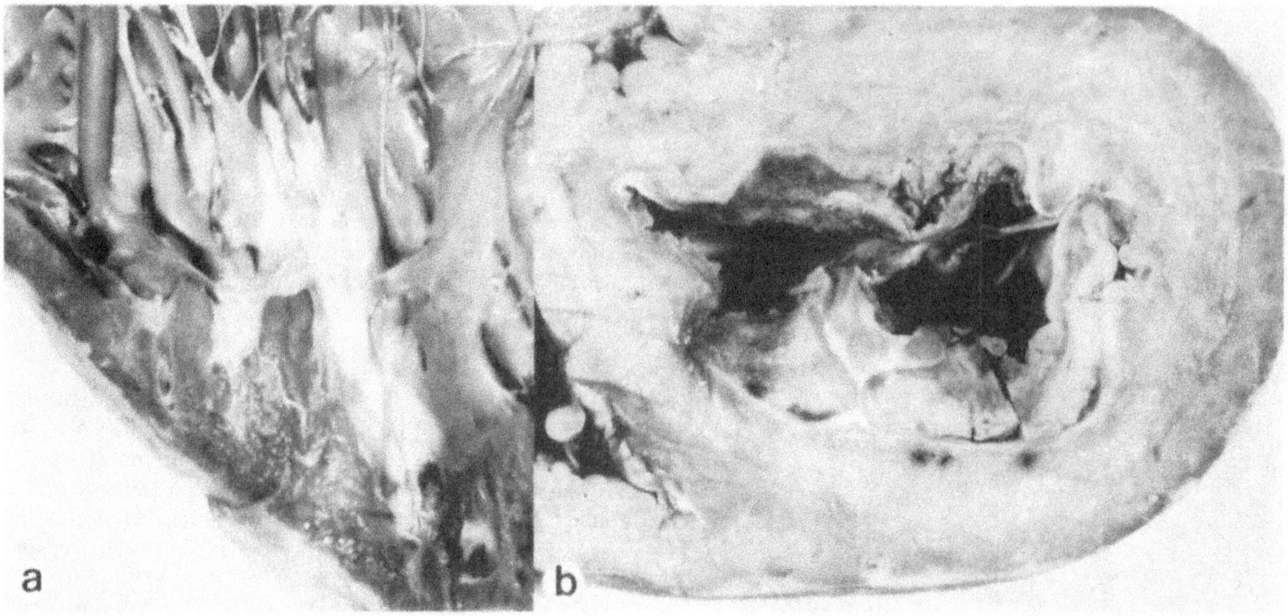

Figure 4. Right ventricle (*a*) showing endocardial fibrous thickening and transverse cut of left ventricle (*b*) showing considerable thrombus with underlying fibrous tissue in a 30-year-old man with idiopathic hypereosinophilic syndrome of 24-months duration.

tients with "eosinophilic leukemia" that over half of the patients had extensive endocardial fibrosis with superimposed thrombosis, that most died within 2 years after onset of symptoms, and that death usually resulted from chronic congestive cardiac failure. Although most patients reported as having "eosinophilic leukemia" did not appear to have neoplastic proliferation of malignant eosinophils or myeloblastic precursors, abnormal myelopoiesis and eosinophilia with or without the Philadelphia chromosome was present in a few patients (48, 57-59).

The heart in the condition described in 1948 in West Africa by Davies (60), originally called "endocardial fibrosis" and later "endomyocardial fibrosis" (61-64), is indistinguishable from the heart of patients with Löffler's "fibroplastic parietal endocarditis" and the heart of patients with "eosinophilic leukemia." Davies was the first to point out that the mural endocardial fibrosis and thrombosis was virtually limited to the inflow tracts of the cardiac ventricles and frequently involved the ventricular aspects of the posterior mitral and tricuspid valve leaflets, making each at times immobile. Although Davies mentioned in his initial report that patients with endomyocardial fibrosis ". . . sometimes show an eosinophilia for which none of the usual causes of eosinophilia account," Ive and associates (64) later documented eosinophilia (absolute count greater than $1000/mm^3$, or differential count greater than 20% of the total leukocyte count) in 17 of 40 patients autopsied who had proven endomyocardial fibrosis. In 1956, Gerbaux and associates (65) were the first to suggest that endomyocardial fibrosis and Löffler's endocarditis were essentially the same disease, and this viewpoint has been supported (66, 67).

That Löffler's endocarditis, eosinophilic leukemia with or without abnormal myelopoiesis, endomyocardial fibro-

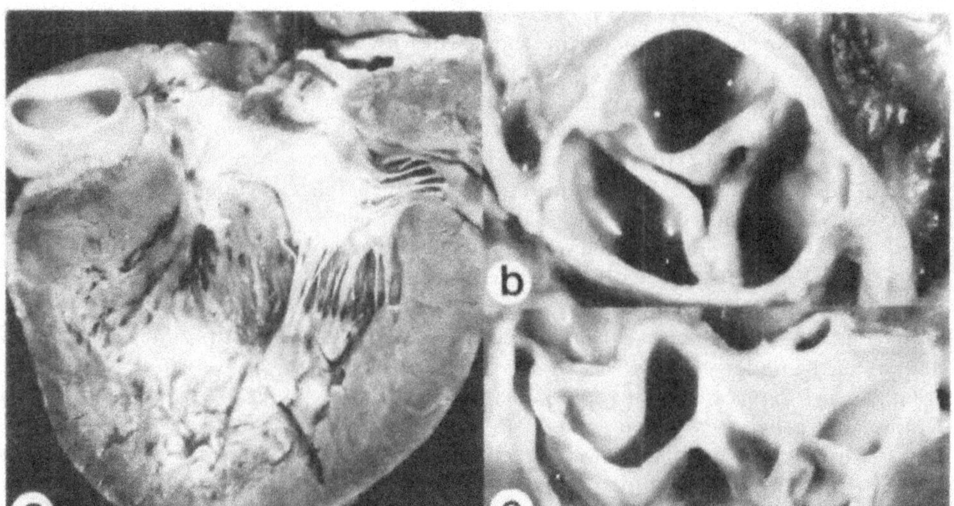

Figure 5. Opened left ventricle and aortic valve (*a*) showing marked fibrous thickening of the mural endocardium of the apical portion; aortic valve from above (*b*) showing fibrous thickening of all cusps with fusion of two of three commissures; and opened aortic valve (*c*) showing superimposed thrombus (fibrin) on the fibrotic cusps in a 46-year-old man with idiopathic hypereosinophilic syndrome. It is likely that the involvement of the aortic valvular endocardium is by the same process that involved the mural endocardium.

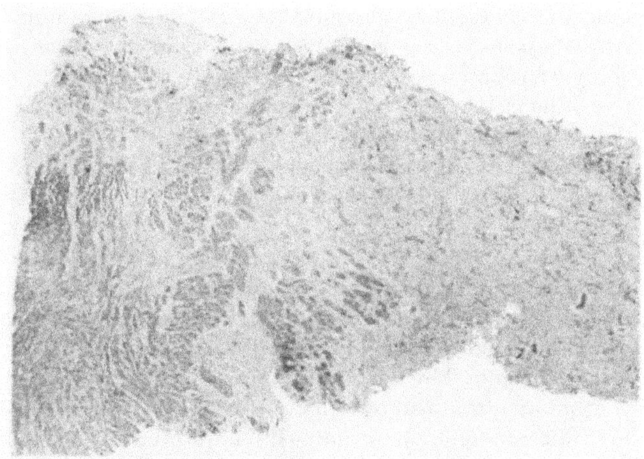

Figure 6. Histologic section of endomyocardial biopsy from a patient with hypereosinophilic syndrome and cardiac involvement, showing marked fibrosis in endocardium and immediately adjacent layers of myocardium. (Hematoxylin and eosin; original magnification, × 50.)

sis of Davies, and endocardial fibrosis (68-71) are the same disease simply seen at different stages of development is a most reasonable supposition (67). At one end of the spectrum may be patients with eosinophilia associated with a transient benign febrile illness, such as tropical eosinophilia or Löffler's pneumonia or trichinosis (72), and at the other end of the gamut may be patients with endomyocardial fibrosis with only mild or absent eosinophilia. Between these two extremes may be patients who still have eosinophilia, but less extensive ventricular endocardial scarring and more extensive mural thrombosis. The latter process may be considered active and eosinophilia is still present, but as the inflammatory process vanishes the endocardial ventricular scar tissue remains and eosinophilia disappears.

From 1958 through 1980, I autopsied 16 patients with hypereosinophilic syndromes who were admitted to NIH or referred from a number of institutions. Representative findings in the hearts in three of these patients are illustrated in Figures 3 to 5. The 16 patients ranged in age from 5 to 52 years (14 patients were 18 years or older); 14 were white and two were black; four were women and 12 were men or boys. The length of the symptomatic illnesses ranged from 7 to 72 months (mean, 30 months). The maximal eosinophils in the peripheral blood differential ranged from 19% to 90%. Chronic congestive heart failure was present in 13 of the 16 patients. The HES was idiopathic or primary in eight patients and associated with another condition in eight (leukemia in five, lymphoma in two, and polyarteritis nodosa in one). At autopsy, the heart in 14 adults ranged in weight from 26 to 550 g, and it was increased in size in 11. The mural endocardium of the right ventricle was thickened in 13, with superimposed thrombi in four; on the other hand, the mural endocardium of the left ventricle was thickened in 15, with superimposed thrombi in seven. The spleen (11 patients) ranged in weight from 1400 to 2800 g and was increased in 11. Enlargement of the spleen or liver or both was as frequent in the patients with idiopathic HES as in those with another condition (nonidiopathic).

Thus, it is clear that the gross pathologic findings in certain patients with the idiopathic HES and HES associated with well-defined underlying diseases can be strikingly similar. Because the cause of the eosinophilia is different in several of these disorders, it is thus likely that the common denominator of the cardiac disease is the eosinophilia itself and not an unrecognized underlying factor found in all patients. Hence, the cardiac dysfunction seen in our patients with the idiopathic HES appears to reflect an eosinophil-related pathophysiologic mechanism as opposed to an unidentified underlying cause.

Ultrastructural Studies of Cardiac Biopsies

Dr. Victor J. Ferrans (Head, Ultrastructure Section, Pathology Branch, National Heart, Lung, and Blood Institute): Before summarizing our experience with ultrastructural studies of cardiac biopsies from patients with HES and cardiac involvement, it may be helpful to review the histologic features of the endomyocardial disease associated with HES that have been reported in the literature (67, 73-76) thus far:

1. Fibrotic thickening of endocardium by collagen-rich connective tissue, which has a layered appearance, is variably cellular, and can measure up to several millimeters in thickness. This fibrous tissue can extend into the innermost layers of ventricular muscle cells, and can also involve the cardiac valves, binding them to mural endocardium; this change can cause considerable restriction in the mobility of the leaflets, particularly the posterior mitral leaflet, with resulting valvular regurgitation. The deeper layers of the areas of fibrous thickening may contain granulation tissue with numerous growing blood vessels. More superficial areas may contain significant amounts of fibrin-like material. Calcific deposits may be present in areas of endocardial thickening.

2. Mural thrombosis, which affects mural endocardium and is thought to be the factor that initiates endocardial thickening. The latter change is regarded as a consequence of organization of mural thrombi. These thrombi can be present in thickened as well as in nonthickened areas of endocardium, and they can contain large numbers of eosinophils.

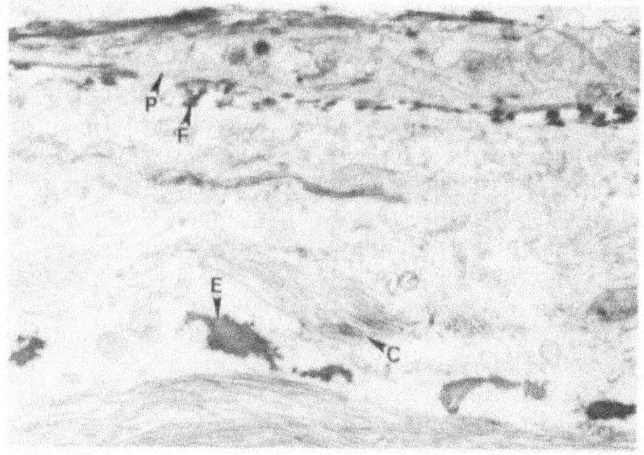

Figure 7. Surface of endocardium showing thin layer of thrombus composed of platelets (*P*) and strands of fibrin (*F*); overlying layer composed of collagen (*C*) and elastic fibers (*E*). (Original magnification, × 23 500.)

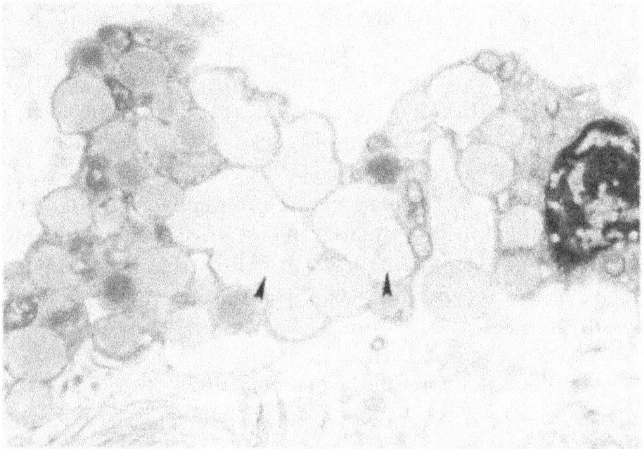

Figure 8. Mast cell in subendocardium shows loss of normal density of its specific granules as well as labyrinth formation, characterized by coalescence of several specific granules (*arrows*). (Original magnification, × 21 750.)

3. Thrombosis, fibrinoid change, and inflammatory cell reaction involving small intramural coronary vessels.

4. Infiltration of eosinophils into myocardium and endocardium may be present, but is not a consistent finding.

The extent to which these four changes are present is a function of the stage and degree of activity of the cardiac involvement. Several investigators (67, 76, 77) have postulated that the release of products derived from eosinophils produces endocardial damage, that this damage is manifested by mural thrombosis, and that organization of the mural thrombi leads to the severe endocardial thickening that is a hallmark of the disease. However, most of the anatomic information on the heart in the HES has been obtained from autopsy studies (76), and little is known of the cardiac morphologic changes that occur in the early stages of the disease. Cardiac biopsies done on patients with advanced stages of the syndrome have shown severe fibrotic changes (73, 75), but have not provided clues as to the pathogenesis of the disorder.

We have recently studied transvenous endomyocardial biopsies from 12 patients (nine men and three women) with the syndrome, who ranged in age from 20 to 62 years. The duration of symptoms in these patients had clinical or echocardiographic evidence of cardiac involvement. Only one of these patients had evidence of right ventricular disease, manifested as an apical filling defect on angiographic study. At the time of biopsy, 10 patients had hypereosinophilia, and all had received treatment with either corticosteroids or cytotoxic agents. Eosinophilia in the other two patients had resolved at the time of biopsy. Each patient underwent biopsy of the right side of the ventricular septum with a catheter bioptome. Tissues were fixed with formalin for light microscopic study and with gluteraldehyde for electron microscopic study. For the latter, tissues were postfixed with OsO_4 and embedded in Maraglas resin.

The endocardial layer was of normal thickness in six patients, and slightly to moderately thickened with increased amounts of fibrous tissue (Figure 6) in four patients, all of whom also had myocardial interstitial fibrosis. The endocardial layer was not seen in histologic sections in the other two patients, but a mild degree of interstitial fibrosis was present. Microscopic evidence of cardiac hypertrophy was found in only two of the biopsies. In the other 10 patients, the cardiac muscle cells showed only alterations that could be attributed to interstitial fibrosis, such as partial dissociation of intercellular junctions and subsarcolemmal accumulations of Z-band-like material.

Endocardial mural thrombi composed of fibrin, platelets, and erythrocytes were found in three biopsies (Figure 7). In one of these, the thrombus showed evidence of extensive organization. Eosinophils were present in each of the thrombi, but were more numerous in the two recent unorganized thrombi than in the one that was organized. Eosinophils in thrombi often showed changes of degranulation, and Charcot-Leyden crystals were found within the thrombus in one biopsy. Eosinophils also were identified within the lumina of myocardial capillaries in seven patients, but were found in myocardial interstitium in only two patients. However, eosinophils were found only infrequently in the interstitial space in the biopsies from these two patients. These cells did not show consistent structural abnormalities, although they occasionally showed some reversal of the normal staining pattern of their specific granules.

Macrophages and mast cells were found frequently in fibrous connective tissue in eight patients. Many of the granules in the mast cells showed labyrinth formation (Figure 8). This change was characterized by the coalescence of granules and by disorganization and partial loss of granule content. Capillary endothelial cells in eight biopsy specimens showed edematous swelling and formation of blebs, which often caused some degree of luminal obstruction. Other endothelial cells in these biopsy specimens had markedly pyknotic cytoplasm (Figure 9), and others showed evidence of regeneration, manifested by increases in the thickness of their cytoplasm and in their numbers of ribosomes (Figure 10). These changes were seen in areas not involved in the formation of granulation tissue.

The observations just described suggest that the endo-

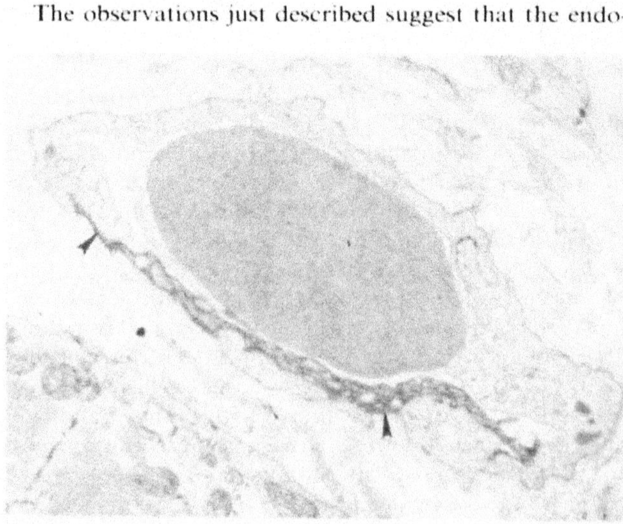

Figure 9. Markedly pyknotic endothelial cell (*arrows*) forms part of the wall of a capillary adjacent to a cardiac muscle cell. (Original magnification, × 25 000.)

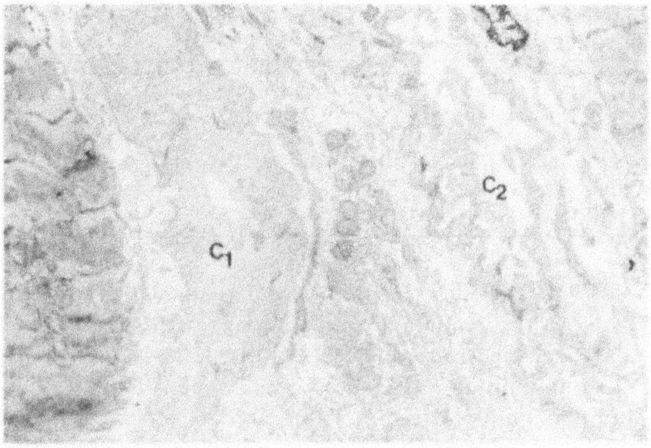

Figure 10. Two capillaries are present in fibrotic interstitium between the cardiac muscle cells. One of these capillaries (C_1) had an endothelial cell with thick, dense cytoplasm; the other capillary (C_2) has numerous cytoplasmic projections extending into its lumen. (Original magnification, × 15 000.)

thelial cells in the endocardium and of the microvasculature, and not the cardiac muscle cells, are the primary tissue targets of the disease process by which cardiac lesions develop in patients with HES. The muscle cell alterations appeared to be relatively minimal and to be a consequence of proliferation of fibrous tissue, with subsequent separation of the muscle cells. Fibrosis was associated with alterations in endothelial cells, which showed evidence of damage as well as regeneration. It is important to point out that we have not found these endothelial cell alterations in myocardial biopsy specimens from patients with other types of heart disease, including rheumatic and nonrheumatic valvular disease, hypertrophic cardiomyopathy, and various congenital heart diseases. Furthermore, it is noteworthy that endothelial cell alterations were seen in myocardial biopsies of the three patients who had no clinical evidence of cardiac involvement. Thus, it may be concluded that these are early alterations. The alterations indicative of degranulation of mast cells are of interest because they provide evidence suggesting that release of mast cell products may mediate some of the pathologic changes observed in the study. It remains to be ascertained whether such mediation is dependent on interactions between mast cells and eosinophils.

Thus, this evidence suggests that endothelial damage serves as the initiator of thrombosis in HES, as it does in other disease processes, and that repeated episodes of damage, thrombosis, and organization of thrombi lead to eventual fibrous thickening of the endocardial lining.

Hematologic Factors

Dr. Harvey R. Gralnick (Chief, Hematology Service, Clinical Pathology Department, National Institute of Health Clinical Center): Although the pathogenesis of HES is unknown, it has been suggested that this may represent a hematologic disorder. This is based primarily on the findings of increased numbers of eosinophils in the peripheral blood and bone marrow, as well as the various names previously given to this syndrome, such as eosinophilic leukemia, and eosinophilic myelosis (47, 48, 52, 57, 59, 66, 78, 79). Obviously, this does not indicate that the syndrome is a primary hematologic disorder; however, my discussion will focus on certain of the hematologic variables of this syndrome.

It has been suggested that persons with eosinophilia and cardiovascular disease have abnormalities of their eosinophils (76, 77). These abnormalities have usually been described as vacuolated or hypogranulated eosinophils. Similar findings have been described in patients with asthma or allergies as well as in those with tropical pulmonary eosinophilia (18, 80-82). We have examined bone marrow smears and peripheral blood smears prepared from patients with the syndrome. This material was examined in a blind manner for vacuolization and hypogranularity of bone marrow and peripheral blood eosinophils at the time of the first NIH admission. The criteria for vacuolization were related to the presence of 10 or more distinct vacuoles in the cytoplasm of 50% of the eosinophils or 30% or more of the eosinophils had to be hypogranular where 50% of the visible cytoplasm was devoid of granules. The studies indicated that bone marrow material cannot be used for studies of vacuolization or hypogranularity because very few of the bone marrow cells appear to be affected. However, using fingerstick peripheral blood samples from these patients, we were able to correctly identify 12 of 13 patients with the syndrome who had cardiovascular disease, by the presence of either hypogranular or vacuolated eosinophils, and eight of 10 patients who did not have cardiovascular disease by the relative absence of these cells. Using these criteria, we were able to specifically separate the patients with cardiovascular disease from those who had no clinical or laboratory evidence of heart disease. As there is a high incidence of thrombotic episodes, mural thrombi, and endocardial fibrosis in patients with HES, attempts have been made to implicate the eosinophil in coagulation and thrombosis. Lisiewicz and Okulski (83) described increased tissue factor activity of leukemic eosinophils, whereas Barnhart and Riddle (84, 85) indicated that eosinophils are the site of storage or synthesis of plasminogen. Venge and associates (86) showed that the eosinophil cationic protein caused enhancement of factor-XII-dependent reactions and also enhanced urokinase-induced plasminogen activation (87).

Despite these numerous laboratory findings indicating eosinophil augmentation of coagulation and fibrinolysis, clinical studies have shown very few abnormalities. One study has indicated intravascular coagulation in HES (88), whereas other studies have described normal hemostasis except for thrombocytopenia, platelet dysfunction, or both (89, 90).

Studies in our laboratory of peripheral blood eosinophils collected from four patients with HES showed reduced fibrinolytic or proteolytic activity compared with normal granulocytes. When the eosinophils were incubated with streptokinase, an activator of plasminogen, no enhancement of the eosinophil proteolytic or fibrinolytic activity was observed, although the fibrinolytic activity of normal granulocytes increased 25%. This suggests that if plasminogen is present in the eosinophils, it is not in a state that is functionally competent; alternatively in the syndrome, eosinophil plasminogen may be deficient or consumed. Studies of the clot-promoting activity of eosinophils using a two-stage assay for tissue factor activity also showed minimal amounts of tissue factor activity in the eosinophils compared with normal granulocytes or other cell lines. Thus, the role of the circulating eosinophil in pathogenesis of the thrombotic lesions is not clear.

We recently initiated a study of platelets and blood coagulation in HES. Such studies may show significant changes in blood coagulation, fibrinolysis, or platelet secretion in the HES that may shed some light on the cardiovascular and thromboembolic complications. To date, our studies of coagulation and fibrinolysis have not shown any characteristic abnormality of HES.

Is the syndrome a malignant proliferation of eosinophils? Unfortunately, this question cannot be directly answered because no specific markers are available to indicate whether the eosinophils in HES are really a clonal proliferation of cells. Despite this lack of markers, there are similarities between some patients with HES and those with myeloproliferative or myelodysplastic syndromes. In the latter syndromes, eosinophils have been shown to be part of the clonal proliferation by the presence of the Philadelphia chromosome (58) and the presence of one G6PD variant in the eosinophils of a patient heterozygous for the common electrophoretic variant of the G6PD gene and chronic granulocytic leukemia (91). Also, there are other similarities in the idiopathic HES, both clinically and hematologically, to these disorders. Many of these similarities have been used in the hematologic scoring system. Various chromosome abnormalities have been described, in our patients and other patients, that are suggestive of possible clonal proliferation of eosinophils (92-99). Studies by Mahmoud and associates (100) indicate that the patients with HES and high levels of circulating eosinophils do not have eosinophilopoietin in their blood, similar to the finding in polycythemia vera, where patients with elevated erythrocyte masses do not have elevated erythropoietin levels, suggesting that the proliferation itself may be autonomous rather than under physiologic control. One of our patients who presented with HES has had intermittent polycythemia (elevated erythrocyte mass) needing phlebotomy and met the criteria for polycythemia vera.

The argument that infiltration of eosinophils into tissue be used as evidence for a malignant state is refuted by the fact that the presence of eosinophils in tissue other than bone marrow or peripheral blood may be reactive because it is seen in many nonmalignant conditions. The question of the relation between HES and eosinophilic leukemia remains in doubt despite many reports in the literature (56, 58, 88-90, 92-99, 101-106). We have seen one of our patients develop blast formation similar to that seen in chronic granulocytic leukemia; a second patient developed histiocytic medullary reticulosis and a T-cell lymphoma; and a third patient, who was lost to follow-up, developed a similar clinical picture. This latter association has been previously described (107, 108).

Table 5. Characteristics of Lymphoproliferative Disease Associated with Hypereosinophilia

Primarily in men
Hypereosinophilia—responsive to chemotherapy
Hypereosinophilia—heralds relapse
Eosinophils—hypogranular, vacuolated, or both
High incidence of cardiovascular disease
High incidence of T-cell malignancies

We have seen three additional patients with HES associated with lymphoma or acute leukemia, an association also previously reported (109-120). The characteristics of lymphoproliferative disease associated with hypereosinophilia are outlined in Table 5.

In-Vitro Culture of Circulating Eosinophil Cells

Dr Barbara H. Bjornson (Fellow in Hematology, Department of Medicine, Tufts-New England Medical Center): Stem cell studies were done to examine some of the factors that control eosinophilopoiesis in patients with the HES. Because the group of patients was heterogenous, probably various causes are involved. For example, some patients clinically have a disease resembling a myeloproliferative disorder, whereas others probably have eosinophilia secondary to an unidentified antigen. Through the in-vitro culture of peripheral blood progenitor cells, we studied circulating stem cells committed to eosinophil differentiation in these patients. Also, the production of eosinophil colony-stimulating factor by mononuclear cells from these patients was examined (Bjornson BH, Harley JB, Andre-Schwartz J, Fauci AS, Des Forges J. Unpublished observations).

The method is a modification of the double-layer soft agar technique originally described by Pike and Robinson (121). Whole mononuclear cells were separated from heparinized blood by Ficoll hypaque centrifugation. This preparation contained lymphocytes and monocytes and, because monocytes are a source of colony-stimulating factor, a portion of cells was put aside to provide this material in the feeder layer of the culture (122). The remaining whole mononuclear cells were incubated in petri dishes to remove adherent monocytes. Nonadherent cells, which include the progenitor cells, were collected from the supernatant.

With autologous whole mononuclear cells in the feeder layer, 20 samples from normal male subjects produced from 43% to 57% pure eosinophil colonies with a mean of 49.6 ± 3.5%. The range for the 13 patients with HES studied was much greater (from 31% to 79%). Five of the patients produced 63% or greater colonies. There was no correlation between percent eosinophil colonies and total eosinophil count, but all five patients clearly had a myeloproliferative syndrome. One patient died from a blast crisis 6 weeks after the study. Another patient also had polycythemia vera that developed 8 years after HES was diagnosed. In this particular patient, in addition to the high percent of eosinophil colonies, many trilinear colonies containing neutrophils, eosinophils and normoblasts were noted. The presence of normoblastic proliferation, which was confirmed by electron microscopy, was distinctly abnormal because erythroid precursors do not usually grow in culture without added erythropoietin (123). However, this finding is characteristic of patients with polycythemia vera (123) and lends support to the diagnosis of myeloproliferative disease in this patient. Such trilinear colonies were noted in an additional patient with clinically proliferative disease but no evidence of polycythemia vera. All of the patients whose results were within the normal range had splenomegaly and needed cytotoxic therapy. Thus, of the 13 patients with HES studied, seven did not differ from controls. One sample contained fewer eosinophil colonies than normals and five had an increased percentage of eosinophil colonies. The increased growth of eosinophil colonies correlated with more aggressive clinical disease.

To distinguish an increase in circulating stem cells committed to eosinophil development from an increased production of eosinophil colony-stimulating factors, normal nonadherent cells were grown over feeder layers from patients with HES. When normal progenitor cells were incubated over HES whole mononuclear cells, feeder layers from three of the five patients with myeloproliferative disease stimulated the normal nonadherent cells to produce more than 70% eosinophil colonies. This suggested that the whole mononuclear cell feeder layer from these particular patients produced increased amounts of eosinophil colony-stimulating factor.

The response of progenitor cells from patients with HES to a normal feeder layer was then examined. Samples from two of the patients with myeloproliferative disease grew an increased percent of eosinophil colonies with a normal source of colony-stimulating factor. This is consistent with an increased number of circulating eosinophil progenitor cells in these patients. Samples from the remaining patients produced a normal percent of eosinophil colonies.

Of the five patients with proliferative disease clinically and an abnormal pattern of growth in culture, two patients had an increased number of circulating eosinophil committed stem cells as evidenced by an increase in eosinophil colonies both in their own feeder layer and a normal feeder layer. Two patients showed an excess production of eosinophil colony-stimulating factor in that their feeder layer stimulated their own progenitor cells as well as those from a normal donor to produce an increased number of eosinophil colonies. Finally, an increased number of eosinophil colonies were grown from nonadherent cells of one patient only when autologous whole mononuclear cells were used in the feeder layer. Thus, there appears to be a component of defective regulatory control as well as abnormalities in proportion of eosinophil stem cells in this myeloproliferative disease.

In-vitro culture of circulating eosinophil colony-forming units has shown that patients with HES are a heterogenous group. Some cells do not differ from normal cells; others have an abnormal pattern of growth. There may be an increased number of circulating progenitor cells committed to eosinophil development, or there may be an excess production of eosinophil colony-stimulating factor. Abnormal behavior in culture seems to correlate with clinically more serious diseases and may provide a key to the cause of the syndrome in individual patients.

▶ Requests for reprints should be addressed to Dr. Anthony S. Fauci; Building 10, Room 11B09, National Institutes of Health, Bethesda, MD 20205

References

1. Hirsch JG, Hirsch BI. Paul Erhlich and the discovery of the eosinophil. In: Mahmoud AAF, Austen KF, eds. *The Eosinophil in Health and Disease.* New York: Grune & Stratton; 1980:3-23.
2. Beeson PB, Bass DA. *The Eosinophil.* Philadelphia: W.B. Saunders; 1977.
3. Mahmoud AAF, Austen KF. *The Eosinophil in Health and Disease.* New York: Grune & Stratton; 1980.
4. Beeson PB. The clinical significance of eosinophilia. In: Mahmoud AAF, Austen KF, eds. *The Eosinophil in Health and Disease.* New York: Grune & Stratton; 1980:313-21.
5. Cohen SD, Sapp TM. Phagocytosis of bacteria by eosinophils in infectious-related asthma. *J Allergy.* 1969;**44**:113-17.
6. Michenberg ID, Root RK, Wolff SM. Bactericidal and metabolic properties of human eosinophils. *Blood.* 1972;**39**:67-80.
7. Cline MJ, Hanafin J, Lehrer RI. Phagocytosis by human eosinophils. *Blood.* 1968;**32**:922-34.
8. Ishikawa T, Dalton AC, Arbesman CE. Phagocytosis of Candida albicans by eosinophilic leukocytes. *J Allergy Clin Immunol.* 1972;**49**:311-5.
9. Zucker-Franklin D, Davidson M, Thomas L. The interactions of mycoplasmas with mammalian cells. I. Hela cells, neutrophils and eosinophils. *J Exp Med.* 1966;**124**:521-31.
10. Ottesen EA, Cohen SG. The eosinophil, eosinophilia, and eosinophil-related disorders. In: Middleton JRE, Reed CE, Ellis EF, eds. *Allergy, Principles and Practice.* St. Louis: CV Mosby Co; 1978:584-632.
11. Kazura JW. Protective role of eosinophils. In: Mahmoud AAF, Austen KF, eds. *The Eosinophil in Health and Disease.* New York: Grune & Stratton; 1980:321-51.
12. Butterworth AE, Vadas MA, David JR. Mechanism of eosinophil mediated helminthotoxicity. In: Mahmoud AAF, Austen KF, eds. *The Eosinophil in Health and Disease.* New York: Grune & Stratton; 1980:253-73.
13. Butterworth AE, David JR. Eosinophil function. *N Engl J Med.* 1981;**304**:154-6.
14. Butterworth AE, Wassom DL, Gleich GL, Loegering DA, David JR. Damage to schistosomula of *Schistosoma mansoni* induced directly by eosinophil major basic protein. *J Immunol.* 1979;**122**:221-9.
15. Grove DI, Mahmoud AAF, Warren KS. Eosinophils and resistance to *Trichenella spiralis.* *J Exp Med.* 1977;**145**:755-9.
16. Cohen SG, Sapp TM, Gallia AR. Experimental eosinophilia. V. Specificity of regional lymph node responses to antigen-antibody systems. *Proc Soc Exp Biol Med.* 1963;**113**:29-32.
17. Sabesin SM. A function of the eosinophil: Phagocytosis of antigen-antibody complexes. *Proc Soc Exp Biol Med.* 1963;**112**:667-70.
18. Litt M. Studies in experimental eosinophilia: VI. Uptake of immune complexes by eosinophils. *J Cell Biol.* 1964;**23**:355-61.
19. Goetzl EJ, Austen KF. Natural eosinophilotactic peptides: Evidence of heterogeneity and studies of structure and function. In: Mahmoud AAF, Austen KF, eds. *The Eosinophil in Health and Disease.* New York: Grune & Stratton; 1980:149-65.
20. Kay AB, Stechschulte DJ, Austen KF. An eosinophil leukocyte chemotactic factor of anaphylaxis. *J Exp Med.* 1971;**133**:602-19.
21. Goetzl EJ, Austen KF. Purification and synthesis of eosinophilotactic tetrapeptides of human lung tissues: Identification as eosinophil chemotactic factor of anaphylaxis. *Proc Natl Acad Sci (USA).* 1975;**72**:4123-7.
22. Clark RAF, Gallin JI, Kaplan AP. The selective eosinophil chemotactic activity of histamine. *J Exp Med.* 1975;**142**:1462-76.
23. Ishizaka T, Ishizaka K. Biology of immunoglobulin E. Molecular basis of reaginic hypersensitivity. *Prog Allergy.* 1975;**19**:60-121.
24. Sullivan TH, Kulczycki A. Immediate hypersensitivity responses. In: Parker CW, ed. *Clinical Immunology.* Philadelphia: WB Saunders Co.; 1980:115-42.
25. Colley DG. Lymphocyte products. In: Mahmoud AAF, Austen KF, eds. *The Eosinophil in Health and Disease.* New York: Grune & Stratton; 1980:293-309.
26. Basten A, Beeson PB. Mechanism of eosinophilia. II. Role of the lymphocyte. *J Exp Med.* 1970;**131**:1288-305.
27. Colley DG. Lymphokine-related eosinophil responses. *Lymphokine Rep.* 1980;**1**:133-55.
28. Mahmoud AAF, Stone MK, Kellermeyer RW. Eosinophilopoietin: A circulating low molecular weight peptide-like substance which stimulates the production of eosinophils in mice. *J Clin Invest.*

1977;**60:**675-82.

29. Dale DC, Hubert TR, Fauci A. Eosinophil kinetics in the hypereosinophilic syndrome. *J Lab Clin Med.* 1976;**87:**487-95.
30. Chusid MJ, Dale DC, West BC, Wolff SM. The hypereosinophilic syndrome: Analysis of fourteen cases with review of the literature. *Medicine.* 1975;**54:**1-27.
31. Parrillo JE, Fauci AS, Wolff SM. Therapy of the hypereosinophilic syndrome. *Ann Intern Med.* 1978;**89:**167-72.
32. Parrillo JE, Lawley TJ, Frank MM, Kaplan AP, Fauci AS. Immunologic reactivity in the hypereosinophilic syndrome. *J Allergy Clin Immunol.* 1979;**64:**113-21.
33. Parrillo JE, Borer JS, Henry WL, Wolff SM, Fauci AS. The cardiovascular manifestations of the hypereosinophilic syndrome. Prospective study of 26 patients, with review of the literature. *Am J Med.* 1979;**67:**572-82.
34. Hardy WR, Anderson RE. The hypereosinophilic syndromes. *Ann Intern Med.* 1968;**68:**1220-9.
35. Edge JR. Myocardial fibrosis following arsenical therapy: report of a case. *Lancet.* 1946;**2:**675-7.
36. Sternon J, Parmentier R, Kenis J. Filariose et endocarditi fibroplastique. *Ann Soc Belge Med Trop.* 1962;**3:**351-66.
37. Gordon MH. Remarks on Hodgkin's disease. A pathogenic agent in the glands, and its application in diagnosis. *Br Med J.* 1933;**1:**641-7.
38. McNaught JB. The Gordon test for Hodgkin's disease. A reaction to eosinophils. *JAMA.* 1938;**111:**1280-4.
39. Turner JC, Jackson H Jr, Parker F Jr. The etiologic relation of the eosinophil to the Gordon phenomenon in Hodgkin's disease. *Am J Med Sci.* 1979;**76:**1443-7.
40. Durack DT, Sumi SM, Klebanoff SJ. Neurotoxicity of human eosinophils. *Proc Natl Acad Sci (USA).* 1979;**76:**1443-7.
41. Weller PF, Wasserman SI, Austen KF. Selected enzymes preferentially present in the eosinophil. In: Mahmoud AAF, Austen KF, eds. *The Eosinophil in Health and Disease.* New York: Grune & Stratton; **1980:**115-30.
42. Gleich GJ, Loegering DA, Maldonado JE. Identification of a major basic protein in guinea pig eosinophil granules. *J Exp Med.* 1973;**137:**1459-71.
43. Gleich GJ, Loegering DA, Frigas E, Wassom DL, Solley GO, Mann KG. The major basic protein of the eosinophil granule: Physiochemical properties, localization, and function. In: Mahmoud AAF, Austen KF, eds. *The Eosinophil in Health and Disease.* New York: Grune & Stratton; 1980: 79-97.
44. Venge P, Dahl R, Hallgren R, Olsson I. Cationic proteins of human eosinophils and their role in the inflammatory reaction. In: Mahmoud AAF, Austen KF, eds. *The Eosinophil in Health and Disease.* New York: Grune & Stratton; 1980: 131-44.
45. Wassom DL, Loegering DA, Solley GO, et al. Elevated serum levels of the eosinophil granule major basic protein in patients with eosinophilia. *J Clin Invest.* 1981;**67:**651-61.
46. Gleich GJ, Frigas E, Loegering DA, Wassom DL, Steinmuller L. Cytotoxic properties of the eosinophil major basic protein. *J Immunol.* 1979;**123:**2925-7.
47. Brink AJ, Weber HW. Fibroplastic parietal endocarditis with eosinophilia. Löffler's endocarditis. *Am J Med.* 1963;**34:**52-70.
48. Roberts WC, Liegler DG, Carbone PP. Endomyocardial disease and eosinophilia. A clinical and pathologic spectrum. *Am J Med.* 1969;**46:**28-42.
49. Parrillo JE, Fauci AS, Wolff SM. The hypereosinophilic syndrome: Dramatic response to therapeutic intervention. *Trans Assoc Am Physicians.* 1977;**90:**135-44.
50. Schooley RT, Parrillo JE, Wolff SM, Fauci AS. Management of the idiopathic hypereosinophilic syndrome. In: Mahmoud AAF, Austen KF, eds. *The Eosinophil in Health and Disease.* New York: Grune & Stratton; 1980: 323-43.
51. Kazmierowski JA, Chusid MJ, Parrillo JE, Fauci AS, Wolff SM. Dermatologic manifestations of the hypereosinophilic syndrome. *Arch Dermatol.* 1978;**114:**531-5.
52. Löffler W. Endocarditis parietalis fibroplastica mit bluteosinophilie. Ein eigenartiges Krankheitsbild. *Schweiz Med Wochenschr.* 1936;**66:**817-20.
53. Weiss-Carmine S. Die endocarditis parietalis fibroplastica mit bluteosinophilie (Löffler) und ihre stellung im rahmender parietalendokardifibrosen. *Schweiz Med Wochenschr.* 1957;**87:**890-8.
54. Roberts WC, Ferrans VJ. Pathologic anatomy of the cardiomyopathies: Idiopathic dilated and hypertrophic types, infiltrative types, and endomyocardial disease with and without eosinophilia. *Hum Pathol.* 1975;**6:**287-342.
55. Bousser J. Eosinophilie et Leucémie. *Sang.* 1957;**28:**553-80.
56. Odeberg B. Eosinophilic leukemia and disseminated eosinophilic collagen disease—a disease entity. *Acta Med Scand.* 1965;**177:**129-44.
57. Benvenisti DS, Ultmann JE. Eosinophilic leukemia. Report of five cases and review of literature. *Ann Intern Med.* 1969;**71:**731-45.
58. Gruenwald H, Kiossoglou KA, Mitus WJ, Dameshek W. Philadelphia chromosome in eosinophilic leukemia. *Am J Med.* 1965;**39:**1003-10.
59. Bentley HP Jr, Reardon AE, Knoedler JP, Krivit W. Eosinophilic leukemia. Report of a case, with review and classification. *Am J Med.* 1961;**30:**310-22.
60. Davies JNP. Endocardial fibrosis in Africans. *East Afr Med J.* 1948;**25:**10-4.
61. Ball JD, Williams AW, Davies JNP. Endomyocardial fibrosis. *Lancet.* 1954;**1:**1049-54.
62. Edington GM, Jackson JG. The pathology of heart muscle disease and endomyocardial fibrosis in Nigeria. *J Pathol Bacteriol.* 1963;**86:**333-44.
63. Parry EHO, Abrahams DG. The natural history of endomyocardial fibrosis. *Q J Med.* 1965;**34:**383-08.
64. Ive FA, Willis AJP, Ikeme AC, Brockington IF. Endomyocardial fibrosis and filariasis. *Q J Med.* 1967;**36:**495-516.
65. Gerbaux A, deBrux J, Bennaceur M, Lenegre J. L'endocardite pariétale fibroplastique avec éosinophile sanguine endocardite de Löeffler. *Bull et Mem Soc Med Hôp Paris.* 1956;**72:**456-65.
66. Engfeldt B, Zetterström R. Disseminated eosinophilic "collagen disease." A clinical and pathological study of a clinical entity related to Löffler's syndromes. *Acta Med Scand.* 1956;**153:**337-53.
67. Roberts WC, Buja LM, Ferrans VJ. Löffler's fibroplastic parietal endocarditis, eosinophilic leukemia, and Davies' endomyocardial fibrosis: the same disease at different stages. *Pathol Microbiol.* 1970;**35:**90-5.
68. Gray IR. Endocardial fibrosis. *Br Heart J.* 1951;**13:**387-96.
69. McKusick VA, Cochran TH. Constrictive endocarditis. Report of a case. *Bull Johns Hopkins Hos.* 1952;**90:**90-7.
70. McNicol C, MacMahon HE, Benenson AS, Winship T. Recurrent parietal thromboendocarditis. *Circulation.* 1953;**7:**497-502.
71. Clark GM, Valentine E, Blount SG Jr. Endocardial fibrosis simulating constrictive pericarditis. Report of a case with determinations of pressure in the right side of the heart and eosinophilia. *N Engl J Med.* 1956;**254:**349-55.
72. Andy JJ, O'Connell JP, Daddario RC, Roberts WC. Trichinosis causing extensive ventricular mural endocarditis with superimposed thrombosis. Evidence that severe eosinophilia damages endocardium. *Am J Med.* 1977;**63:**825-9.
73. Somers K, Hutt MSR, Patel AK, D'Arbela PG. Endomyocardial biopsy in diagnosis of cardiomyopathies. *Br Heart J.* 1971;**33:**822-32.
74. Brockington IF, Olsen EGJ. Löffler's endocarditis and Davies' endomyocardial fibrosis. *Am Heart J.* 1973;**85:**308-22.
75. Grosgogeat Y, Nicolas G. La biopsie endomyocardique: son interet en pathologie tropicale. A propos de 3 nouveaux cas. *Arch Mal Coeur.* 1977;**70:**179-83.
76. Olsen EGJ, Spry CJF. The pathogenesis of Löffler's endomyocardial disease, and its relationship to endomyocardial fibrosis. *Prog Cardiol.* 1979;**8:**281-303.
77. Spry CJF, Tai PC. Studies on blood eosinophils. II. Patients with Löffler's cardiomyopathy. *Clin Exp Immunol.* 1976;**24:**423-34.
78. Stillman RG. A case of myeloid leukemia with predominance of eosinophil cells. *Med Records.* 1912;**81:**594-5.
79. Evans TS, Nesbitt RR. Eosinophilic leukemia. Report of a case with autopsy confirmation; review of the literature. *Blood.* 1949;**4:**603-13.
80. Connell JT. Morphological changes in eosinophils in allergic disease. *J Allergy.* 1968;**41:**1-9.
81. Saran R. Cytoplasmic vacuoles of eosinophils in tropical pulmonary eosinophilia. *Am Rev Respir Dis.* 1973;**108:**1283-5.
82. Tai PC, Spry CJF. Studies on blood eosinophils. I. Patients with a transient eosinophilia. *Clin Exp Immunol.* 1976;**24:**415-22.
83. Lisiewicz J, Okulski J. Thromboplastic activity of leukemic eosinophils. *Haematologica (Budapest).* 1970;**4:**213-20.
84. Barnhart MI, Riddle JM. Cellular localization of profibrinolysin (plasminogen). *Blood.* 1963;**21:**306-21.
85. Riddle JM, Barnhart MI. The eosinophil as a source of profibrinolysin in acute inflammation. *Blood.* 1965;**25:**776-94.
86. Venge P, Dahl R, Hallgren R. Enhancement of factor XII dependent reactions by eosinophil cationic protein. *Thromb Res.* 1979;**14:**641-9.
87. Dahl R, Venge P. Enhancement of urokinase-induced plasminogen activation by the cationic protein of human eosinophil granulocytes. *Thromb Res.* 1979;**14:**599-608.
88. Lamotte-Barrillon S, Carbon C, Bernard JF, Gaudin H, Teillet F, Barge J. Leucemie A esonophiles et coagulation intra-vasculaire disseminée. *Sem Hop Paris.* 1976;**52:**987-98.
89. Zoller VH. Blutgerinnungsstorung bei einer chronischen eosinophilen-leukamie. *Munch Med Wochenschr.* 1973;**115:**1036-8.
90. Wautier JL, Souchon H, Dupuis D, Caen JP, Nurden AT. A platelet defect in a patient with eosinophilic leukaemia: absent ristocetin-induced platelet aggregation associated with a reduced platelet sialic acid content. *Scand J Haematol.* 1979;**22:**267-76.
91. Koeffler HP, Levine AM, Sparkes M, Sparkes RS. Chronic myelocytic leukemia: Eosinophils involved in the malignant clone. *Blood.*

1980;**55:**1063-5.

92. Goh K, Swisher SN, Rosenberg CA. Cytogenetic studies in eosinophilic leukemia. The relationship of eosinophilic leukemia and chronic myelocytic leukemia. *Ann Intern Med.* 1965;**62:**80-6.
93. Flannery EP, Dillon DE, Freeman MVR, Levy JD, D'Ambrosio U, Bedynek JL. Eosinophilic leukemia with fibrosing endocarditis and short y chromosome. *Ann Intern Med.* 1972;**77:**223-8.
94. Goldman JM, Najfeld V, Th'ng KH. Agar culture and chromosome analysis of eosinophilic leukaemia. *J Clin Pathol.* 1975;**28:**956-61.
95. Weinfeld A, Westin J, Swolin B. Ph[1]-negative eosinophilic leukaemia with trisomy 8. Case report and review of cytogenetic studies. *Scand J Haematol.* 1977;**18:**413-20.
96. Cabrol C. Chromosomal anomaly in eosinophilic leukemia [Letter]. *N Engl J Med.* 1979;**301:**439.
97. Ellman L, Hammond D, Atkins L. Eosinophilia, chloromas and a chromosome abnormality in a patient with a myeloproliferative syndrome. *Cancer.* 1979;**43:**2410-3.
98. Lonnqvist B, Gahrton G, Ericksson P, Friberg K, Zech L. Isochromosome 17 in a patient with a myeloproliferative disorder terminating in eosinophilic leukemia. *Acta Med Scand.* 1979;**206:**321-5.
99. Huang CS, Gomez GA, Kohno S, Sokal JE, Sandberg AA. Chromosomes and causation of human cancer and leukemia. XXXIV. A case of "hypereosinophilic syndrome" with unusual cytogenetic findings in a chloroma, terminating in blastic transformation and CNS leukemia. *Cancer.* 1979;**44:**1284-9.
100. Mahmoud AAF, Billings FT III, Stone MK, Kellermeyer RW. Human eosinophilopoietin [Abstract]. *Clin Res.* 1978;**26:**555A.
101. Rickles FR, Miller DR. Eosinophilic leukemoid reaction. Report of a case, its relationship to eosinophilic leukemia and review of the pediatric literature. *J Pediatr.* 1972;**80:**418-28.
102. Yam LT, Li CY, Necheles TF, Katayama I. Pseudoeosinophilia, eosinophilic endocarditis and eosinophilic leukemia. *Am J Med.* 1972;**53:** 193-202.
103. Miller RR, Lewis JP, Knapp W. Acute eosinophilic leukemia associated with neutropenia. *West J Med.* 1975;**123:**399-404.
104. Dvilansky A, Alkan ML, Ho W, Kaplan H, Tiberin P, Rachmilewitz B. Chronic eosinophilic leukemia complicated by epidural myeloblastoma. *Acta Haematol.* 1975;**53:**356-61.
105. Presentey B, Jerushalmy Z, Mintz U. Eosinophilic leukaemia: Morphological, cytochemical and electron microscopic studies. *J Clin Pathol.* 1979;**32:**261-71.
106. Sjogren J. Bone marrow morphology in acute eosinophilic-monocytic leukaemia. *Acta Haematol.* 1979;**62:**17-9.
107. Henderson DW, Sage RE. Malignant histiocytosis with eosinophilia. *Cancer.* 1973;**32:**1421-8.
108. Liao KT, Rosai J, Daneshbod K. Malignant histiocytosis with cutaneous involvement and eosinophilia. *Am J Clin Pathol.* 1972;**57:**438-48.
109. Spitzer G, Garson OM. Lymphoblastic leukemia with marked eosinophilia: A report of two cases. *Blood.* 1973;**42:**377-84.
110. Blatt PM, Rothstein G, Miller HL, Cathey WJ. Löffler's endomyocardial fibrosis with eosinophilia in association with acute lymphoblastic leukemia. *Blood.* 1974;**44:**489-93.
111. Kaufmann U, Lampert F. Eosinophilie bei akuter lymphoblastischer leukamie and lymphosarkom: Indikator fur immunologische vorgange? *Klin Paediatr.* 1974;**186:**492-9.
112. Weinger RS, Andre-Schwartz J, Desforges JF, Baker M. Acute leukaemia with eosinophilia or acute eosinophilic leukaemia: A dilemma. *Br J Haematol.* 1975;**30:**65-70.
113. Nelken RP, Stockman JA III. The hypereosinophilic syndrome in association with acute lymphoblastic leukemia. *J Pediatr.* 1976;**89:**771-3.
114. Manthorpe R, Egeberg J, Hesselvik M, Videbaek AA. Unique eosinophil granules in a case of T-cell lymphoma. *Scand J Haematol.* 1977;**19:**129-44.
115. Pereira F, Hernan M, Crist W, Ermocilla R. Loffler's endomyocardial fibrosis, eosinophilia and acute lymphoblastic leukemia. *J Pediatr.* 1977;**59:**950-1.
116. Wimmer RS, Raney RB Jr, Naiman JL. Hypereosinophilia with acute lymphocytic and acute myelocytic leukemia in childhood. *J Pediatr.* 1978;**92:**244-6.
117. Hamilton PJ, Dawson AA. Successful treatment of apparent eosinophilic leukaemia. *Br Med J.* 1977;**1:**1195.
118. Geltner D, Friedman G, Naparstek E, Granot H, Polliack A. Acute lymphoblastic leukemia. Its occurrence with 'Hypereosinophilic syndrome' and bilateral spontaneous pneumothorax. *Arch Intern Med.* 1978;**138:**292-3.
119. Youinou P, Andrieu JM, Casassus P. Leucemie aigue lymphoblastique accompagnee d'une eosinophilie sanguine et meningee. *Nouv Presse Med.* 1979;**8:**527.
120. Catovsky D, Bernasconi C, Verdonck PJ, et al. The association of eosinophilia with lymphoblastic leukaemia or lymphoma: a study of seven patients. *Br J Haematol.* 1980;**45:**523-34.
121. Pike BL, Robinson WA. Human bone marrow colony growth in agar gel. *J Cell Physiol.* 1970;**76:**77-84.
122. Burgess AW, Metcalf D. The nature and action of granulocyte-macrophage colony stimulating factors. *Blood.* 1980;**56:**947-58.
123. Lacombe C, Casadevall N, Varet B. Polycythaemia vera: in vitro studies of circulating erythroid progenitors. *Br J Haematol.* 1980;**44:**189-99.

Two-dimensional Echocardiographic Assessment of the Idiopathic Hypereosinophilic Syndrome

Anatomic Basis of Mitral Regurgitation and Peripheral Embolization

John S. Gottdiener, M.D., Barry J. Maron, M.D., Robert T. Schooley, M.D., John B. Harley, M.D., Ph.D., William C. Roberts, M.D., and Anthony S. Fauci, M.D.

SUMMARY Important cardiac manifestations in the idiopathic hypereosinophilic syndrome include mitral regurgitation and peripheral embolization. To determine the anatomic basis of these abnormalities, real-time, wide-angle, two-dimensional echocardiography (2-D echo) was performed in 21 patients with the hypereosinophilic syndrome. Nine patients (43%) had clinical evidence of mitral regurgitation, and each had localized thickening of the posterobasal left ventricular wall behind the posterior mitral leaflet and absent (seven patients) or diminished (two patients) motion of the posterior leaflet. Anatomic observations at operation or necropsy in four patients with mitral regurgitation demonstrated that the echocardiographic abnormalities resulted from posterior mitral leaflet thickening and adherence of the leaflet to the underlying mural endocardium of the posterobasal wall. On 2-D echo, each of the six patients with peripheral emboli had either apical left ventricular echo-dense targets consistent with thrombus or thickening of the posterobasal wall of the left ventricle, and these findings were validated at autopsy or operation in three patients.

Hence, in patients with the hypereosinophilic syndrome, 2-D echo is useful in identifying the probable etiology of two important cardiac manifestations. Thickening of the posterobasal wall is usually associated with impairment of posterior mitral leaflet function, resulting in mitral regurgitation. Because the hypereosinophilic syndrome is associated with peripheral embolization, thrombus formation and subsequent endocardial scarring, the noninvasive identification of intracavitary ventricular thrombi may be important.

CARDIAC INVOLVEMENT is a major cause of death in the idiopathic hypereosinophilic syndrome, a systemic illness characterized by a persistently elevated blood eosinophil count without an identifiable etiology for the eosinophilia.[1, 2] Although almost any organ may be affected, cardiovascular abnormalities have been identified in most patients.[3] Roberts et al.[4] suggested that intracavitary thrombi and extensive endocardial fibrosis are causally related to the occurrence of restrictive cardiomyopathy, atrioventricular valve abnormalities (particularly mitral regurgitation) and peripheral embolism. To determine the morphologic cause of the mitral regurgitation and peripheral embolization, wide-angle two-dimensional echocardiography (2-D echo) was performed in 21 patients with the hypereosinophilic syndrome, and the findings were compared with other clinical features.

Methods

Patients

Twenty-one consecutive patients with the idiopathic hypereosinophilic syndrome who had been identified prospectively at the National Institutes of Health constitute the study group (table 1). All patients had been admitted to the clinical center and extensively evaluated to exclude other causes of peripheral blood eosinophilia. The details of this diagnostic evaluation have been described.[5]

The criteria for diagnosis of the idiopathic hypereosinophilic syndrome included a persistent, total eosinophil count of more than 1500 cells/mm^3; an extensive evaluation that excluded other known causes of hypereosinophilia, such as parasitic infection, allergy or neoplasm; and clinical or biopsy evidence of organ system involvement. All patients except 1, 3, 6, 7, 9 and 16 (table 1) were being treated with prednisone or hydroxyurea or both at the time of the echocardiographic recording.

Clinical Evaluation

The diagnosis of mitral regurgitation was based on the identification of an apical holosystolic murmur that responded appropriately to bedside physiologic maneuvers. The murmur decreased in intensity with the Valsalva maneuver and with the administration of amyl nitrate, and increased in intensity with squatting. In patients 5, 8 and 10, left ventriculography confirmed the presence of marked mitral regurgitation; each patient subsequently underwent mitral valve replacement. A history of transient ischemic attacks (three patients), or cerebrovascular accident (three patients) was considered evidence of previous peripheral embolism.

Echocardiographic Evaluation

Two-dimensional echocardiograms were obtained with a commercially available, real-time, phased-ar-

From the Cardiology and Pathology Branches, National Heart, Lung, and Blood Institute, and the Laboratory of Immunoregulation, National Institute of Allergy and Infectious Diseases, National Institutes of Health, Bethesda, Maryland.

Address for correspondence: John S. Gottdiener, M.D., Cardiology Section (151D), Veterans Administration Medical Center, 50 Irving Street N.W., Washington, D.C. 20422.

Received July 1, 1982; accepted September 3, 1982.

Circulation 67, No. 3, 1983.

TABLE 1. *Clinical Features in 21 Patients with Hypereosinophilic Syndrome*

Pt	Age (years)	Sex	Highest eosinophil count (mm^3)	Duration of illness (years)	First organ system involved‡	MR	PE	2-D echo: Apical LV cavity density	2-D echo: Abnormal PML motion	2-D echo: Thickened P-B LV wall
1	16	M	83,000	11	Skin	0	0	0	0	0
2	21	F	11,000	2	Heart	0	0	0	0	0
3	23	M	7,600	1	GI	0	0	0	0	0
4	27	M	350,000	3	Spleen	+	0	0	+	+
5	28	M	30,000	4	Heart	+	0	+	+	+
6	30	M	72,000	1	Heart	0	0	0	0	0
7	33	M	48,000	1	Liver	0	0	+	0	0
8*	33	M	19,000	2	Lung	+	0	0	+	+
9	33	F	8,000	3	Skin	0	0	0	0	0
10	35	M	8,500	5	Lung	+	0	+	+	+
11	36	F	16,400	3	Spleen	+	0	0	+	+
12	38	M	12,000	2	Heart	0	+	+	0	0
13†	44	M	3,000	13	Heart	+	+	+	+	+
14	45	M	11,000	4	GI	+	+	+	+	+
15	47	M	200,000	7	Spleen	0	0	0	0	+
16	51	M	39,000	1	Skin	0	0	0	0	0
17	51	M	26,000	10	Heart/kidney	+	+	0	+	+
18	51	F	6,100	1	Lung	0	0	0	0	+
19	53	M	70,000	12	GI	0	0	0	0	0
20	58	M	52,000	4	Spleen	+	+	0	+	+
21	61	M	8,500	6	Lung	0	+	+	0	0

*Evaluation 11 months previously showed no 2-D echocardiographic abnormalities or clinical evidence of either mitral regurgitation or peripheral emboli.

†Evaluation 3 months previously showed no 2-D echocardiographic abnormalities or clinical evidence of peripheral embolization; mitral regurgitation, however, was present.

‡Exclusive of bone marrow.

Abbreviations: GI = gastrointestinal; LV = left ventricular; MR = mitral regurgitation; P-B = posterobasal; PE = peripheral emboli; PML = posterior mitral leaflet; 2-D echo = two-dimensional echocardiography.

ray, 80° ultrasonic sector scanner (V3000 or 3400) using a hand-held 2.25-MHz transducer. Echocardiograms were recorded on either one-half-inch cassette videotape, 1-inch reel-to-reel videotape, or a rhodium-plated chromium disc for subsequent review in real-time, slow-motion or stop-action mode. Single-frame photographs were made from the television monitor using a 35-mm camera.

Two-dimensional echocardiographic examination included the imaging of a number of cross-sectional planes through the heart.[6–8] Serial short-axis views of the left ventricle were obtained by orienting the sector plane perpendicular to the long axis of the left ventricle from a standard transducer placement on the chest. The short-axis sweep was performed by maintaining the transducer in a fixed location on the chest wall and slowly angling the image plane from aorta (cephalad) to apex (caudad). Care was taken to assure proper transducer angulation so that the left ventricle appeared circular rather than oval or elliptical.

The long-axis view was obtained by orienting the sector plan parallel to the longitudinal axis of the left ventricle, taking care to avoid improper angulation of the scan plane tangentially through the ventricle. The apical four-chamber view was obtained with the transducer placed at the cardiac apex and the tomographic plane directed perpendicular to the ventricular and atrial septa and through the plane of the mitral and tricuspid valve orifices to permit simultaneous display of both atria and ventricles, atrioventricular valves and cardiac septa.

Two-dimensional echocardiograms were reviewed independently by two of the authors, one of whom was unaware of the clinical findings. Increased posterobasal wall thickness was identified in the parasternal long-axis view as an abrupt displacement of the endocardial contour at the level of the posterior mitral leaflet, so that the posterobasal region was substantially thicker than was the ventricular free wall distal to the mitral leaflets. This "thickening" of the posterobasal wall was considered to represent either recent thrombus formation, organizing thrombus, or scarring superimposed on the posterobasal left ventricular wall (which itself was of normal or slightly increased thickness).[4, 9, 10]

Echocardiograms were interpreted as showing absent or markedly limited posterior mitral leaflet motion if no leaflet motion, or only a barely perceptible sug-

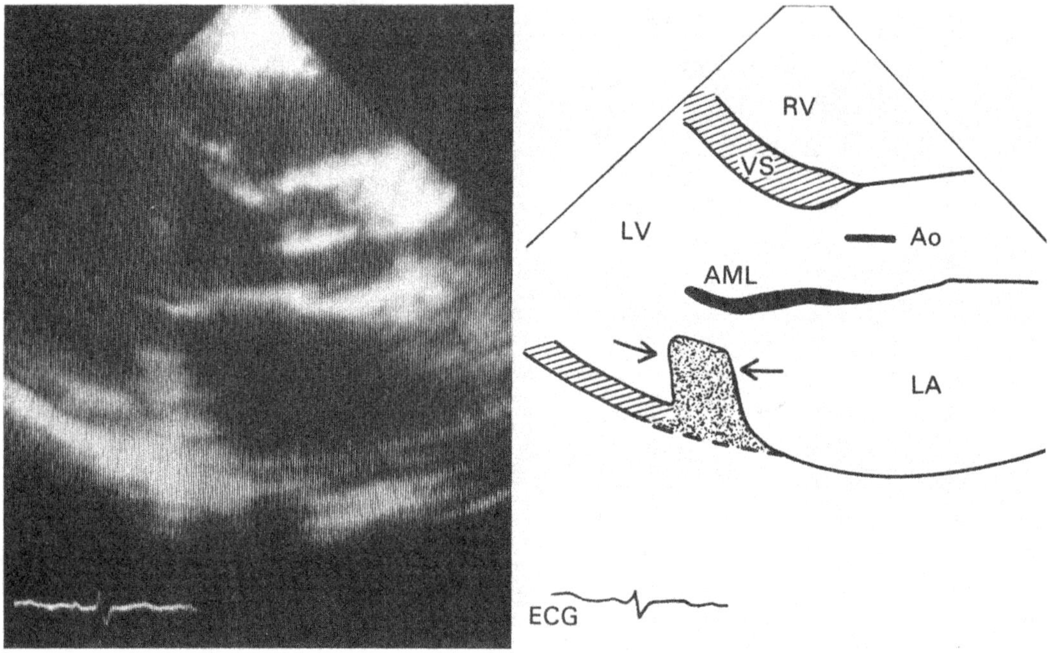

FIGURE 1. *Two-dimensional echocardiogram during diastole in parasternal long-axis view from patient 5 shows localized thickening (arrows) of the posterobasal wall. AML = anterior mitral leaflet; Ao = aorta; RV = right ventricle; LV = left ventricle; LA = left atrium; VS = ventricular septum.*

gestion of motion, was evident in all three echocardiographic image planes. Left ventricular thrombus was considered present if an echo density with distinct margins was present within the ventricular cavity in continuity with the endocardium, but unassociated with the papillary muscles.[11-13]

Pathologic Studies

Material for pathologic examinations was available in four patients. In three, the mitral valve had been excised at operation[14] 2–4 weeks after the echocardiographic study; one patient was studied at necropsy 6 months after the echocardiographic studies.

Results

Mitral Regurgitation

Mitral regurgitation was identified in nine patients (table 1). In each, the 2-D echo showed increased thickness (range 15–26 mm) of the portion of posterobasal left ventricular wall behind the posterior mitral leaflet (fig. 1). The M-mode echocardiogram (fig. 2), recorded simultaneously and under direct visualization with the 2-D echo, confirmed that the posterobasal wall at the level of the mitral valve was markedly thickened compared with the left ventricular free wall distal to the mitral valve. Each patient with mitral regurgitation and posterobasal wall thickening had ab-

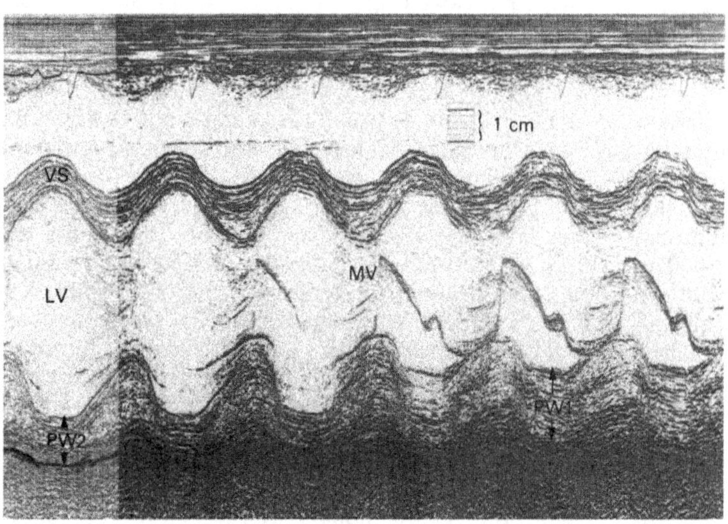

FIGURE 2. *M-mode echocardiogram recorded under direct visualization with two-dimensional echocardiography in same patient as in figure 1. The posterior left ventricular (LV) wall at the level of the mitral leaflets (PW1) is markedly thickened compared with the segment of posterior wall distal to the mitral leaflet (PW2). MV = mitral valve; VS = ventricular septum.*

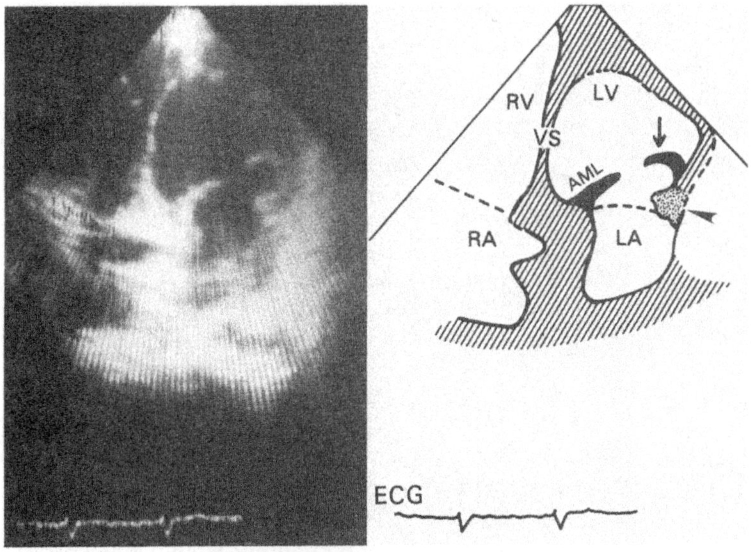

FIGURE 3. *Two-dimensional echocardiogram during diastole in apical four-chamber view from patient 5. Note the apically displaced structure (arrow), which showed motion characteristic of mitral valve on real-time display. The proximal (basilar) portion of this leaflet is not visible because of incorporation within echo-dense material (arrowhead), representing organized thrombus, extending from left ventricular inflow tract. AML = anterior mitral leaflet; LA = left atrium; LV = left ventricle; RA = right atrium; RV = right ventricle; VS = ventricular septum.*

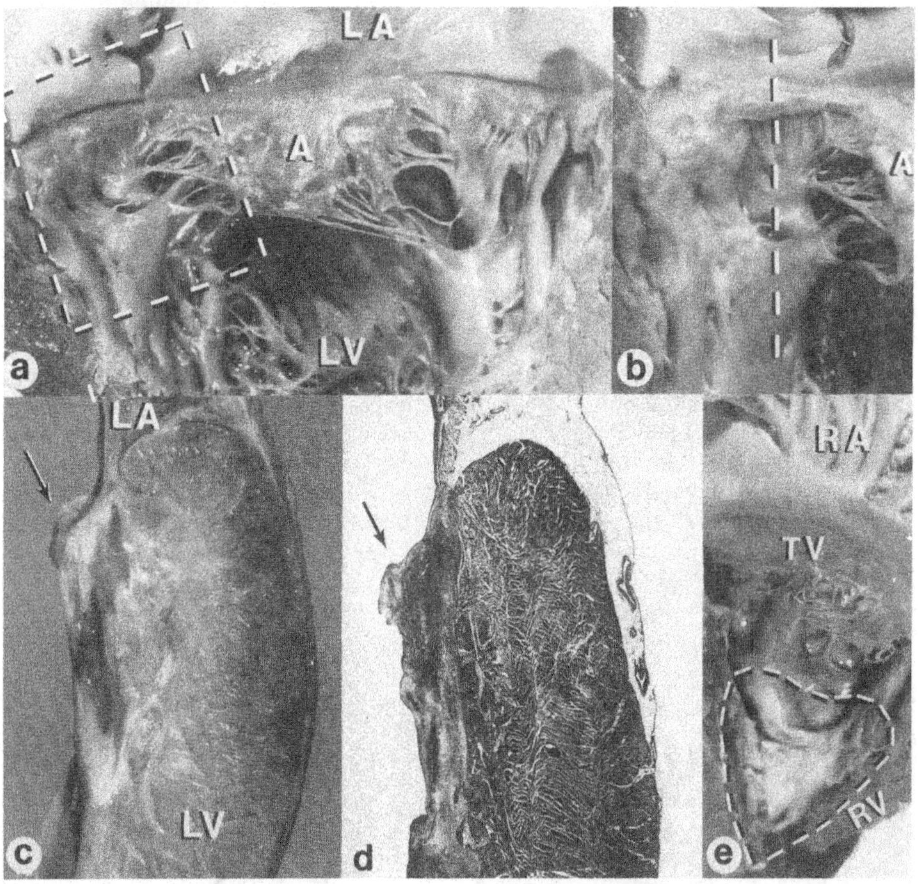

FIGURE 4. *Gross anatomic findings in patient 4, who had severe mitral regurgitation. (A) View of left ventricular inflow tract showing the anterior (A) and posterior (within box) leaflets and their chordal attachments to the papillary muscles. The anterior leaflet is normal, but the posterior leaflet is scarred and adheres to the posterior left ventricular wall. (B) Closer view of the fixed posterior leaflet shown within the box in panel A. Broken line indicates the plane of section producing the view of the left ventricular inflow tract seen in panel C. (C) Posterobasal left ventricular free wall showing substantial endocardial scarring which has obliterated the posterior mitral leaflet except for the area indicated by the arrow. (D) Photomicrograph of histologic section taken from panel C, stained with hematoxylin-eosin. (E) Inflow tract of right ventricle (RV) shows endocardial scarring (within broken line). LA = left atrium; LV = left ventricle; RA = right atrium; TV = tricuspid valve.*

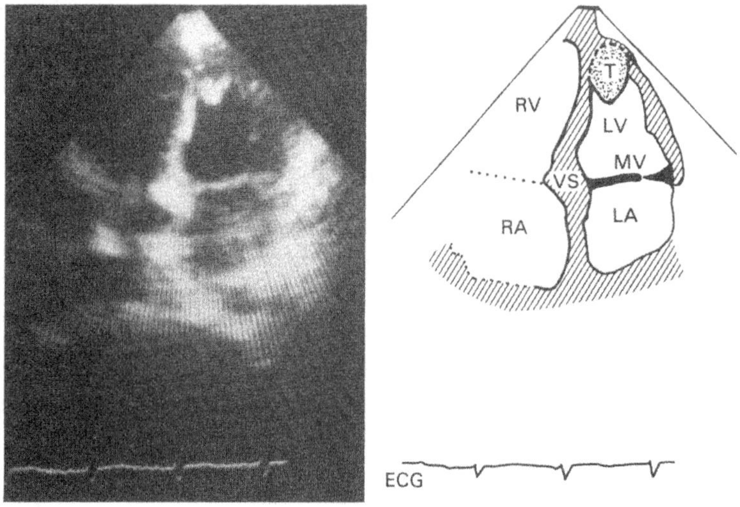

FIGURE 5. *Stop-frame two-dimensional echocardiogram during systole in the apical four-chamber view from patient 5, with the transducer angulated more posteriorly than in figure 3. The apical left ventricular echo density was confirmed as thrombus at operation. LA = left atrium; LV = left ventricle; RA = right atrium; RV = right ventricle; T = thrombus; VS = ventricular septum.*

sent (seven patients) or diminished (two patients) motion of the posterior mitral leaflet. In the two patients with diminished motion, no posterior leaflet motion could be visualized in the parasternal long- or short-axis views; however, the apical four-chamber view demonstrated that only the most distal "apical" portion of the posterior mitral leaflet was mobile (fig. 3). Leaflet motion was not evident in the proximal portion of the posterior leaflet, presumably because it adhered to the posterobasal wall. This alteration of mitral valve anatomy also appeared to prevent normal systolic coaptation between the posterior and anterior mitral leaflets. Patients 15 and 18, without evidence of mitral regurgitation, had increased posterobasal wall thickness, but both had normal mitral leaflet motion.

Anatomic confirmation of the mitral valve abnormality identified by 2-D echo (figs. 1 and 3) was available in four patients. In each, the posterior mitral leaflet was thickened and adherent to the underlying endocardium of the posterobasal wall (fig. 4), by virtue of its incorporation within accumulations of calcified and fibrotic material attached to the mural endocardial surface. In addition, in patient 5, thrombus also was present on the tricuspid valve leaflets and the anterior mitral leaflet, which were partially destroyed.

Peripheral Embolization

Each of the six patients with clinical events suggestive of peripheral emboli had evidence by 2-D echo of thrombus formation in either the left ventricular apex (two patients) or left ventricular inflow tract (two patients) or both (two patients) (figs. 5 and 6). Of the 15 other patients who did not have clinical events compatible with peripheral embolization, 10 had evidence of intraventricular thrombus, three in the left ventricular apex and seven in the inflow tract.

Supporting evidence or anatomic confirmation for the 2-D echo finding of apical left ventricular thrombus was available in five patients; an apical thrombus was observed at operation in patients 5, 8 and 10 and at

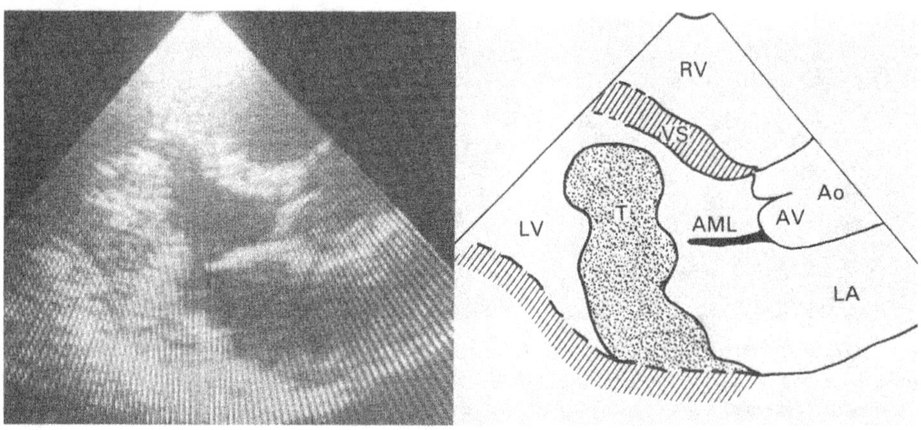

FIGURE 6. *Two-dimensional echocardiogram during diastole from patient 13 in the parasternal long-axis view. A massive intracavitary echo-dense structure extends from the left ventricular inflow tract to the apex, shown at operation to represent thrombus and scar. Posterior mitral leaflet, absent on echocardiogram, was incorporated within the echo-dense mass, resulting in severe mitral regurgitation. AML = anterior mitral leaflet; Ao = aorta; AV = aortic valve; LA = left atrium; T = thrombus; VS = ventricular septum.*

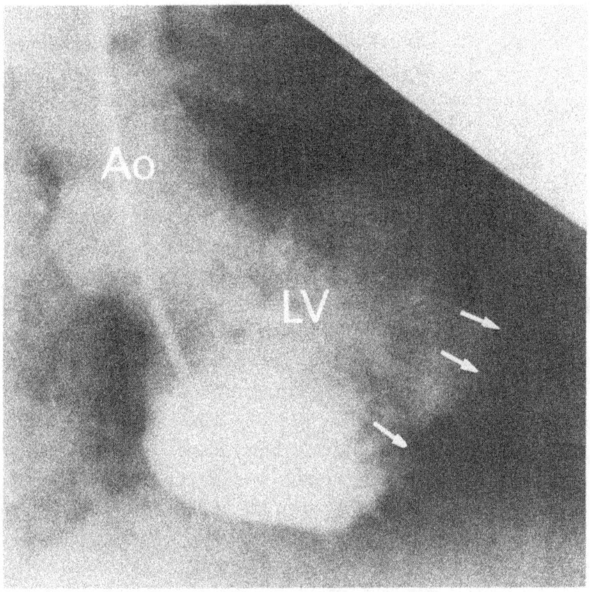

FIGURE 7. *Contrast left ventriculogram in right anterior oblique position from patient 21. The large apical filling defect (arrows) is consistent with thrombus. Ao = aorta; LV = left ventricle.*

necropsy in patient 4; contrast ventriculography (fig. 7) showed a left ventricular apical filling defect in patient 21.

Discussion

The echocardiographic findings demonstrate a probable mechanism for mitral regurgitation in patients with idiopathic hypereosinophilic syndrome. The patients with mitral regurgitation had thickened posterobasal left ventricular walls and impaired or absent posterior mitral leaflet motion. Morphologic observations at operation or necropsy in four patients with mitral regurgitation showed that the posterobasal left ventricular wall thickening, identified by 2-D echo, was due to the accumulation of thrombofibrotic material between the ventricular aspect of the posterior mitral leaflet and the mural endocardium of left ventricular free wall behind this leaflet and this material in the submitral angle adhered these two structures together.

Our findings regarding the mechanism of mitral regurgitation in hypereosinophilic syndrome support the observations of Davies[9] and Brockington and Olsen.[10] Davies,[9] in a necropsy study of patients with this disease, reported thickening of the posterior mitral leaflet and noted that the leaflet in some patients adhered to organized, fibrotic thrombus on the surface of the posterior left ventricular wall. Brockington and Olsen[10] reported three patients with this disease in whom the posterior mitral leaflet was incorporated within the fibrotic tissue.

We hypothesize that turbulence of blood flow in the left ventricular inflow tract and apex make these sites on the endocardial surface of the left ventricular wall particularly susceptible to eosinophilic injury and subsequent thrombus formation. Thereafter, clot organization, scarring and new thrombus formation occurs. Eventually, the posterior mitral leaflet motion is impaired or abolished as the leaflet becomes adherent to, and ultimately incorporated in, the scar and thrombus. The extension of thrombus to adjacent endocardial surfaces followed by thrombus organization and subsequent scarring may result in a restrictive-type ventricle.

Two-dimensional echocardiography was of value in identifying left ventricular thrombi in our patients and also was a sensitive method of identifying patients with hypereosinophilic syndrome who were at risk for peripheral embolization. Each of the six patients with peripheral emboli had evidence of intracavitary thrombi by 2-D echo, including four with thrombi in the apex of the left ventricle. Ten other patients without peripheral embolization also had echocardiographic evidence of thrombus formation, however, either in the left ventricular inflow tract or apex. Nevertheless, because of the relatively high incidence of peripheral emboli in patients with the hypereosinophilic syndrome, patients with evidence of intraventricular thrombi should be considered at risk for peripheral emboli, and hence are candidates for chronic anticoagulation therapy. Patients with thrombus in the left ventricular inflow tract alone may also be at risk for peripheral embolization, of course, since such posterobasal wall "thickening" may represent fresh thrombus. In contrast, patients with the hypereosinophilic syndrome who do not have either posterobasal wall thickening or apical thrombi by 2-D echo do not appear to be at substantial risk of embolization. Anticoagulation therapy may modify the development of the restrictive ventricle in the hypereosinophilic syndrome, which appears to be the consequence of organization of intraventricular thrombi and subsequent widespread endocardial scarring.

The rapidity with which this process may evolve in patients with hypereosinophilic syndrome is illustrated by patient 13, who had a cerebral embolus and severe mitral regurgitation at a time when he had 2-D echo evidence of left ventricular apical and inflow tract thrombus, with fixation of the posterior mitral leaflet on 2-D echo (fig. 6). Just 3 months previously, echocardiographic studies had failed to demonstrate thrombus in the left ventricle and the posterior mitral leaflet was normal.

Thus, marked limitation of posterior mitral leaflet motion by adherence to and eventual incorporation within thrombus and scar on the posterobasal endocardial surface of the left ventricle inflow tract is the mechanism by which mitral regurgitation occurs in patients with the hypereosinophilic syndrome. Posterobasal wall thickening and apical left ventricular echo densities suggest the presence of intraventricular thrombi, which are the source of systemic emboli and the cause of the subsequent development of a restrictive ventricle. These findings (fig. 8) may be reliably

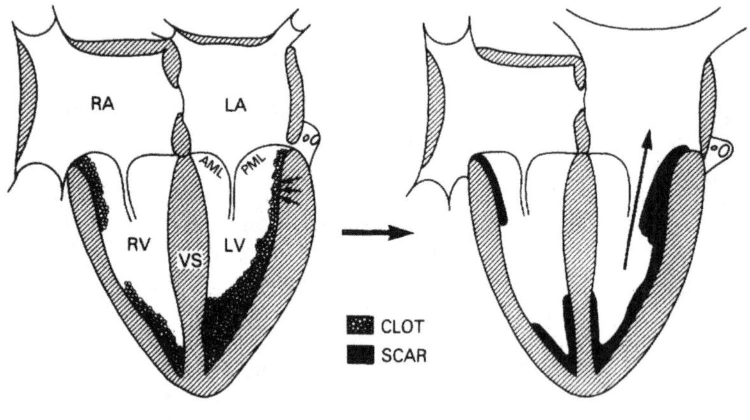

FIGURE 8. *The sequence of endocardial thrombus deposition and scar, resulting in mitral regurgitation, a restrictive ventricle and peripheral embolization. Postulated eosinophil-associated endocardial injury results in thrombus formation on endocardial surfaces of the right and left ventricles (RV and LV). Organization of thrombus in the left ventricular inflow tract behind the posterior mitral leaflet (PML, small arrows) results in adherence to and eventual incorporation of the leaflet within the material, with consequent mitral regurgitation (large arrow, right panel). Restrictive ventricle occurs as the right and left ventricular filling becomes impaired by endocardial scar (right panel). New and, hence, friable thrombus would be capable of dislodgment (embolization). AML = anterior mitral leaflet; LA = left atrium; RA = right atrium; VS = ventricular septum.*

detected by 2-D echo, which is, therefore, a useful adjunct in the cardiac evaluation of patients with the hypereosinophilic syndrome.

Acknowledgment

The authors thank Judy Easterly for her secretarial assistance in the preparation of this manuscript.

References

1. Hardy WR, Anderson RD: The hypereosinophilic syndrome. Ann Intern Med **68:** 1220, 1968
2. Chusid MJ, Dale DC, West BC, Wolff SM: The hypereosinophilic syndrome: analysis of fourteen cases with review of the literature. Medicine **54:** 1, 1975
3. Parrillo JE, Borer JS, Henry WL, Wolff SM, Fauci AS: The cardiovascular manifestations of the hypereosinophilic syndrome: prospective study of 26 patients, with review of the literature. Am J Med **67:** 572, 1979
4. Roberts WC, Leigler DG, Carbone PP: Endomyocardial diseases and eosinophilia. A clinical and pathologic spectrum. Am J Med **46:** 28, 1969
5. Fauci AS, Harley JB, Roberts WC, Ferrans VJ, Gralnick HR, Bjornson BH: The idiopathic hypereosinophilic syndrome: clinical, pathophysiologic and therapeutic considerations. Ann Intern Med. In press
6. Stack R, Kisslo J: Evaluation of the left ventricle with two-dimensional echocardiography. Am J Cardiol **46:** 1117, 1980
7. Tajik AJ, Seward JB, Hagler DJ, Mair DD, Lie JT: Two-dimensional real-time ultrasonic imaging of the heart and great vessels. Mayo Clin Proc **58:** 271, 1978
8. Silverman NH, Schiller NB: Apex echocardiography. A two-dimensional technique for evaluating congenital heart disease. Circulation **57:** 503, 1978
9. Davies JNP: Some considerations regarding obscure disease affecting the mural endocardium. Am Heart J **59:** 600, 1973
10. Brockington IF, Olsen EGJ: Löffler's endocarditis and Davies' endomyocardial fibrosis. Am Heart J **85:** 308, 1973
11. DeMaria AN, Bommer W, Neumann A, Grehl C, Wienert L, DeNardo S, Amsterdam EA, Mason DT: Left ventricular thrombi identified by cross-sectional echocardiography. Ann Intern Med **90:** 14, 1979
12. Asinger RW, Mikel FL, Sharma B, Hodges M: Observations on detecting left ventricular thrombus with two-dimensional echocardiography: emphasis on avoidance of false positive diagnoses. Am J Cardiol **47:** 145, 1981
13. Reeder GS, Tajik AJ, Seward JB: Left ventricular mural thrombus. Two-dimensional echocardiographic diagnosis. Mayo Clin Proc **56:** 182, 1981
14. Harley JB, McIntosh CL, Kirklin JW, Maron BJ, Gottdiener JS, Roberts WC, Fauci AS: Atrioventricular valve replacement in the idiopathic hypereosinophilic syndrome. Am J Med **73:** 77, 1982

Clinical and Morphologic Cardiac Findings After Anthracycline Chemotherapy

Analysis of 64 Patients Studied at Necropsy

JEFFREY M. ISNER, MD, VICTOR J. FERRANS, MD, PhD, STEVEN R. COHEN, MD, BRUCE G. WITKIND, MD, RENU VIRMANI, MD, JOHN S. GOTTDIENER, MD, J. ROBERT BECK, MD, and WILLIAM C. ROBERTS, MD

The relation between clinical evidence of and histologic signs of anthracycline cardiotoxicity was evaluated by reviewing the clinical and morphologic findings in 64 patients studied at necropsy, all of whom had received doxorubicin or daunorubicin chemotherapy during life. Of the 64 patients, 20 (31%) had documented clinical toxicity consisting of impaired left ventricular systolic performance; in 7 (35%) of these 20 patients, histologic signs of toxicity were absent. In the remaining 13 patients with clinical toxicity, histologic signs of toxicity ranged from mild to severe. Of the 44 (69%) patients without clinical signs of drug toxicity, 21 (48%) had no histologic sign of cardiotoxicity; in 23 (52%) of the patients without clinical toxicity, however, morphologic signs of cardiotoxicity were nevertheless present—mild in most patients, but extensive in 4. Signs of extensive histologic toxicity (19 [30%] of 64 patients) were associated with large doses (>450 mg/m^2) of the drug, mediastinal irradiation, and age >70 years. This study suggests that attempts to monitor cardiotoxicity by serial evaluation of cardiac histology in patients undergoing anthracycline chemotherapy may be seriously limited by the fact that clinical evidence of toxicity may be present without histologic signs of toxicity; likewise, histologic signs of anthracycline toxicity may be present without clinical evidence of toxicity.

The anthracycline drugs doxorubicin (Adriamycin™) and daunorubicin (Daunomycin™) are 2 of the most effective chemotherapeutic agents presently available for treatment of patients with solid tumors and leukemias.[1] Cardiac toxicity is a well-recognized complication of these agents and is frequently the dose-limiting factor in their administration.[2,3] Although endomyocardial biopsy has been used in several centers to monitor patients receiving anthracycline chemotherapy,[4] limited information is available regarding the results of necropsy examination of patients who have received these drugs.[5–7] The present study was designed to determine (1) the extent of morphologic cardiotoxicity at necropsy in patients treated with anthracycline compounds, and (2) the degree to which the results of morphologic examination of necropsy hearts correlated with clinical evidence of cardiac dysfunction.

From the Pathology and Cardiology Branches, National Heart, Lung, and Blood Institute, National Institutes of Health, Bethesda, Maryland. Manuscript received January 5, 1983, accepted January 6, 1983.

Address for reprints: Jeffrey M. Isner, MD, Tufts-New England Medical Center, 171 Harrison Avenue, Box 70, Boston, Massachusetts 02111.

Methods

Review of the clinical records of all patients with malignant neoplasms who died and underwent necropsy examination at the National Cancer Institute, Bethesda, Maryland, between January 1, 1970, and June 30, 1979, revealed 93 patients who had been treated with anthracyclines. In 11 patients, the gross and/or histologic material available for review was inadequate; in 18 additional patients, interpretation of both clinical and morphologic cardiac findings was complicated by medical problems such as severe anemia, renal failure, hemosiderosis, and myxedema. These 29 patients, therefore, were eliminated from further study. The remaining 64 patients form the basis of the present study. Review of gross and histologic findings and reexamination of the hearts from these 64 patients were performed without knowledge of the clinical cardiac findings.

The hearts of all 64 patients were evaluated grossly for pericardial disease, chamber dilatation, mural thrombus, and foci of fibrosis or necrosis. Histologic sections from the left ventricular free wall, ventricular septum, and right ventricular free wall were stained with hematoxylin-eosin and phosphotungstic acid hematoxylin. Each section was examined by 3 observers, who, by consensus, assigned to it a histologic score. Two characteristics were used to score the extent of histologic cardiotoxicity: vacuolization of cardiac muscle cells (Fig. 1a)

TABLE I Clinical and Morphologic Findings in 20 Patients With Clinical Evidence of Anthracycline Toxicity

Age (yr) & Sex	Interval Onset Sx to Death	Physical Examination			CXR		Echo		Hemodynamic Data		Cardiac Therapy		
		JVD	Rales	S_3	CE	PVH	LVd	FS	CVP	PAOP	Dig	Diur	Improved
Patients Without Histologic Signs of Anthracycline Toxicity													
5F	18 d	0	+	+	0	+	–	–	–	–	+	+	+
15M	1 d	+	+	+	+	+	50	0.16	20	–	+	+	0
18M	7 d	+	+	+	+	+	–	–	20	–	+	+	0
26F	1 d	0	+	+	0	+	–	–	18	–	+	+	0
37F	2 mo	+	+	+	+	+	–	–*	–	–	+	+	+
61M	7 mo	0	0	+	+	+	–	–	–	–	+	+	+
61M	14 mo	+	+	0	+	+	65	0.28	15	–	+	+	+
Patients with Histologic Signs of Anthracycline Toxicity													
13M	6 d	+	0	+	+	+	47	0.16	–	–	+	+	0
39M	4 mo	0	+	+	+	+	51	0.18	9	18	+	+	+
21M	15 d	+	+	+	+	0	58	0.19	20	20	+	0	0
22F	5 wk	0	+	0	+	0	52	0.19	18	–	+	+	+
35F	11 mo	+	+	+	+	+	54	0.19	–	22	+	+	+
78M	2 d	+	+	+	+	+	–	–	–	–	+	+	0
12M	9 d	+	+	0	+	+	46	0.30	17	–	+	+	+
15F	3 mo	0	0	+	+	0	61	0.10	–	18	+	+	+
29F	7 d	+	+	+	+	+	55	0.27	16	20	+	+	0
49F	1 mo	0	0	0	+	0	52	0.08	–	26	+	+	0
5M	17 d	+	0	+	0	0	–	–	–	–	+	+	+
33F	2 mo	+	0	+	0	0	44	0.23	–	–	+	+	+
11F	4 wk	+	+	+	+	+	46	0.13	–	–	+	+	+

* Preejection period/left ventricular ejection time = 0.61.

CE = cardiac enlargement; CVP = central venous pressure; DA = daunorubicin; DO = doxorubicin; DIG = digitalis; Diur = diuretic; FS = fractional shortening; Histo Tox = histologic toxicity; JVD = jugular venous distention; LVd = left ventricular end-diastolic dimension; Med Irrad = mediastinal

and myofibrillar dropout (Fig. 1b). The severity of each of these 2 histologic features was assessed for each section of the myocardium according to the following scale: 0 = none, 1 = mild, 2 = moderate, and 3 = extensive. The final score of histologic cardiotoxicity for a particular patient was arrived at by adding the highest grade for vacuolization and the highest grade for myofibrillar dropout observed on any of the various sections of myocardium from the patient. For example, a patient who received a score of 2+ for vacuolization and 1+ for myofibrillar dropout would receive a final score of 3+ for histologic cardiotoxicity.

The hospital records of all 64 patients were reviewed without knowledge of the necropsy findings. Echocardiograms performed in 26 patients also were reevaluated without knowledge of necropsy findings or of the original interpretation of the study.

Statistical significance regarding characteristics of groups with and without clinical or histologic toxicity was assessed by the chi-square test.

Results

Patients with clinical evidence of drug toxicity: Of the 64 patients, 20 (31%) had clinical evidence of cardiotoxicity (Table I). These 20 patients included 10 males and 10 females, aged 5–78 years (average 29). Their total dose of anthracycline drug ranged from 85 to 900 mg/m^2 (average 450), administered over a period of 4 to 156 weeks (average 41). Four patients also received mediastinal irradiation to a total dose of 4,000, 9,450, 12,450, and 12,600 rads, respectively. In 16 of these 20 patients, evidence of cardiotoxicity included hemodynamic documentation (12 patients) (elevated central venous pressure or elevated pulmonary capillary wedge pressure, or both) and/or echocardiographic documentation of decreased fractional shortening (11 patients); in the remaining 4 patients, the diagnosis of a drug-induced cardiomyopathy was based on a combination of physical signs of cardiac decompensation (jugular venous distention, inspiratory rales, S_3 gallop sound) and radiographic signs of pulmonary venous hypertension and cardiomegaly. All 20 patients with clinical signs of drug toxicity received digoxin and 10 also received diuretics.

In 7 of the 20 patients with clinical signs of drug toxicity, the pericardial sac contained >50 ml of fluid (average 186, range 80 to 300). Two of these 7 patients had received mediastinal irradiation, and in 1 the pericardial fluid was grossly hemorrhagic; in the remaining 6 the fluid was serosanguinous. None of the 7 patients had cardiac metastases. The average heart weight in the 17 adult patients with clinical signs of drug toxicity was 358 g (range 240 to 500) (Table I). In 18 of the 20 patients, the heart weight observed exceeded that predicted according to body weight[8] by an average of 106 g. In 11 of the 20 patients, both ventricular cavities were dilated, while in 4 other patients the left ventricle alone was dilated; in the remaining 5 patients, neither ventricular cavity was dilated. The presence or absence of cavity dilatation at necropsy was *not* a function of the interval between the onset of clinical signs of toxicity and death. In 2 patients, the dilated ventricular cavities contained mural thrombus (Fig. 2); neither patient had a history of peripheral embolic events.

Histologic signs of cardiotoxicity were observed in 13 of the 20 patients with clinical signs of drug toxicity (Tables I and II): these 13 patients included 10 of the 15 patients with and 3 of the 5 without cavity dilatation. The combined histologic scores for toxicity among these 13 patients ranged from 1 to 5 (average 2.3).

TABLE I (Continued)

Age (yr) & Sex	Oncologic Therapy: Total Anthracycline (mg/m²)	Duration Rx (wks)	Total Rads Med Irrad	Gross Findings: Heart Wt (g) Obs (Pred)	Dilated Ventricles	Histologic Findings: Myocyte Vacuoles	Myofibrillar Dropout	Histo Tox score
Patients Without Histologic Signs of Anthracycline Toxicity								
5F	345(DA)	26	0	150(99)	+	0	0	0
15M	530(DA)	32	0	450(253)	+	0	0	0
18M	630(DA)	32	0	295(297)	0	0	0	0
26F	330(DA)	12	0	320(258)	+	0	0	0
37F	550(DO)	88	0	270(260)	+	0	0	0
61M	210(DO)	4	0	396(350)	0	0	0	0
61M	250(DO)	8	0	500(352)	+	0	0	0
Patients With Histologic Signs of Anthracycline Toxicity								
13M	490(DA)	60	0	450(129)	+	0	1+	1
39M	180(DO)	4	4,000	350(300)	+	1+	0	1
21M	600(DO)	156	12,600	450(390)	+	1+	1+	2
22F	570(DO)	12	0	380(283)	0	0	2+	2
35F	900(DO)	60	12,450	240(249)	+	2+	0	2
78M	280(DO)	10	0	300(245)	0	2+	0	2
12M	195(DO)	3	0	300(253)	+	1+	2+	3
15F	510(DO)	20	0	380(155)	+	2+	1+	3
29F	550(DO)	28	0	280(189)	+	1+	2+	3
49F	550(DO)	42	0	310(249)	+	2+	1+	3
5M	500(DO)	12	0	90(54)	+	2+	2+	4
33F	85(DO)	16	9,450	270(258)	0	2+	2+	4
11F	750(DO)	132	0	200(120)	+	3+	2+	5

irradiation; Obs = observed; PAOP = pulmonary artery occlusion pressure; Pred = predicted; PVH = pulmonary vascular hypertension; Rx = treatment; Sx = symptoms; + = present; 0 = absent.

In contrast to the previous 13 patients, histologic signs of cardiotoxicity were absent from multiple sections of myocardium in 7 of the 20 patients with clinical signs of drug toxicity (Table I). These 7 patients included 5 patients with and 2 without cavity dilatation. The 7 patients in whom clinical evidence of anthracycline cardiotoxicity was *not* associated with histologic abnormalities ranged in age from 5 to 61 years. Four received up to 630 mg/m² of daunorubicin, while 3 received 210 to 500 mg/m² of doxorubicin. All had evidence on physical examination of congestive heart failure. On chest radiograms, signs of pulmonary venous hypertension were present in all, and 5 of 7 had an enlarged cardiac silhouette. Two patients had abnormal echocardiograms, 1 had abnormal systolic time intervals, and 4 had elevated venous pressures.

Patients without clinical evidence of drug toxicity: Of the 64 patients, 44 (69%) had no clinical signs of cardiotoxicity. These patients (23 males, 21 females) ranged in age from 2 to 70 years (average 44).

Three of these 44 patients had >50 ml of fluid in the pericardial sac (500, 400, and 100), while in 3 others the pericardial space was obilterated by dense, fibrous adhesions. One of the former 3 patients and all of the latter 3 had received >4,900 rads of mediastinal irradiation. The average heart weight, excluding 2 children, was 278 g (range 105 to 450). In 29 patients, the observed heart weight exceeded the predicted heart weight by an average of 65 g. Biventricular dilatation was observed in 4 patients, and mild left ventricular enlargement in 2. Left ventricular mural thrombus was found in 1 patient with no history of peripheral embolic events.

Histologic signs of cardiotoxicity were observed in 23 (52%) of the 44 patients, despite the fact that none of these 44 patients had clinical evidence of anthracycline cardiotoxicity (Table II). In 15 of the 23 patients, the histologic findings were limited to a mild degree (combined score 1/6) of vacuolization (14 patients) or myofibrillar dropout (1 patient). In the remaining 8 patients, however, more extensive morphologic changes were noted: 4 patients received combined scores of 2/6 for histologic cardiotoxicity.

TABLE II Relation of Clinical Toxicity to Type and Extent of Morphologic Toxicity

Clinical Toxicity	Patients (n)	Myocardial Vacuoles 0	1	2	3	Myofibrillar Loss 0	1	2	3
+	20	9	4	6	1	10	4	6	0
0	44	22	17	3	2	37	7	0	0
Totals									
n	64	31	21	9	3	47	11	6	0
%	...	48	33	14	5	74	17	9	0

(Columns 3–10: Type and Extent of Morphologic Toxicity.)

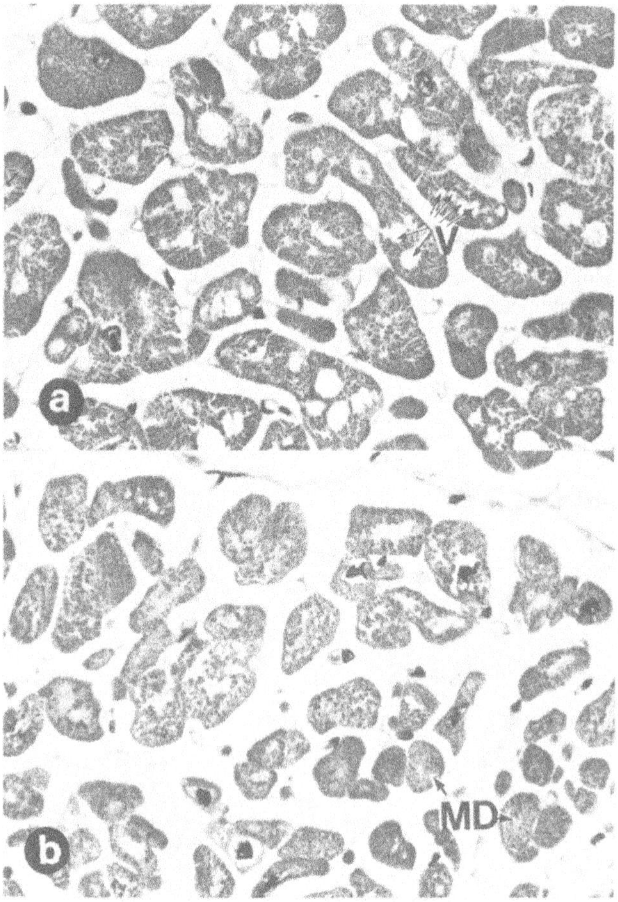

FIGURE 1. Findings used to score the extent of histologic cardiotoxicity: (a) vacuolization (V) of cardiac muscle cells, and (b) myofibrillar dropout (MD). This patient (15-year-old girl, Table I) received a histologic toxicity score of 3 (2+ vacuolization, 1+ myofibrillar dropout). (Hematoxylin and eosin stain; magnification ×500, reduced 33%.)

Patients grouped according to final (combined) scores for histologic cardiotoxicity (Fig. 3): The entire study group of 64 patients was analyzed from the standpoint of the combined score for histologic toxicity. Twenty-eight patients had a combined score of 0; 7 had clinical signs of toxicity while 21 did not. Seventeen patients received a histologic score of 1; clinical toxicity was present in 2 patients and absent in 15. Eight patients received a histologic score of 2; clinical toxicity was present in 4 and absent in 4. Seven patients received a histologic score of 3; 4 had clinical toxicity and 3 did not. Three patients received a histologic score of 4; 2 had clinical toxicity and 1 did not. Only 1 patient had a histologic score of 5 and this patient had overt clinical cardiotoxicity.

Relation between clinical cardiotoxicity and gross and histologic signs of toxicity (Fig. 4): Of the total 64 patients, 18 had neither clinical or structural evidence of cardiotoxicity. In 36 patients, histologic signs of toxicity were observed. Of these, 23 had no clinical evidence of toxicity, including 4 with dilated ventricles. Three patients had both clinical and histologic signs of toxicity unassociated with ventricular cavity dilatation. A complete "triad" of clinical, gross

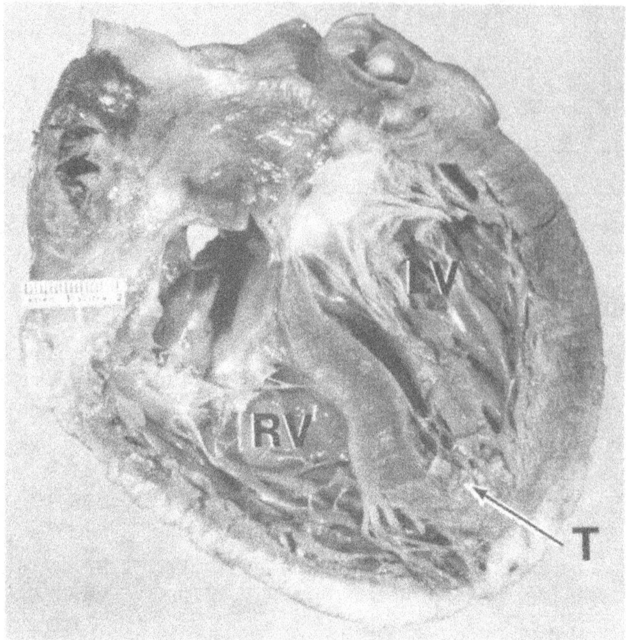

FIGURE 2. Biventricular cavity dilatation in 15-year-old girl (Table I) with clinical and histologic evidence of anthracycline cardiotoxicity. The apical portion of the dilated left ventricle (LV) contains antemortem thrombus (T). RV = right ventricle.

anatomic, and histologic signs of cardiotoxicity was observed in only 10 patients.

Of the remaining 10 patients of the study group of 64, 3 had ventricular cavity dilatation without histologic or clinical evidence of cardiotoxicity, 5 had clinical toxicity and cavity dilatation without histologic evidence of toxicity, and 2 had clinical signs of toxicity unassociated with either gross or histologic signs of toxicity. Thus, in 8 patients, cavity dilatation was not associated with histologic abnormalities.

Finally, in the entire study group of 64 patients, 20 had clinical signs of toxicity, and 2 of these patients showed no evidence of either cavity dilatation or histologic abnormalities. In 1, clinical evidence of toxicity consisted of jugular venous distention, inspiratory rales, and an S_3 gallop sound on physical examination; cardiomegaly and pulmonary venous hypertension on chest radiogram; and a central venous pressure of 20 mm Hg. The second patient also had an S_3 gallop sound, and cardiomegaly and pulmonary venous hypertension on chest radiogram. Both patients received treatment with digoxin and diuretics and 1 improved. Neither patient had pericardial fluid at necropsy.

The sensitivity of the histologic necropsy examination was calculated as follows: Patients with clinical and histologic toxicity/(patients with cardiotoxicity and histologic toxicity) + (patients with clinical toxicity without histologic toxicity) = 13/(13 + 7) = 0.65. The specificity of histologic necropsy examination was calculated as follows: Patients without clinical toxicity and without histologic toxicity/(patients without clinical toxicity and without histologic toxicity) + (patients with histologic toxicity without clinical toxicity) = 21/(21 + 23) = 0.48. The predictive value of the finding of his-

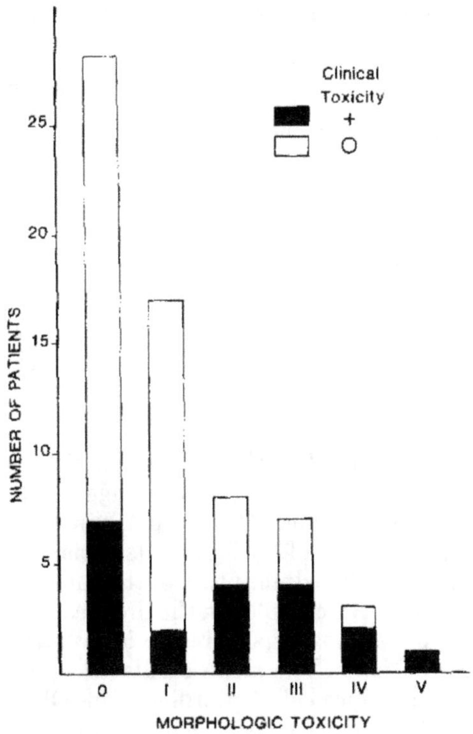

FIGURE 3. Number of patients with and without clinical evidence of cardiac toxicity in each category of histologic toxicity (see text for histologic toxicity grading system).

tologic toxicity was calculated as follows: Patients with clinical and histologic toxicity/(patients with clinical and histologic toxicity) + (patients with histologic toxicity without clinical toxicity) = 13/(13 + 23) = 0.36. This predictive value when tested proved not significantly different from random variation in toxicity (chi-square = 0.91, p >0.30).

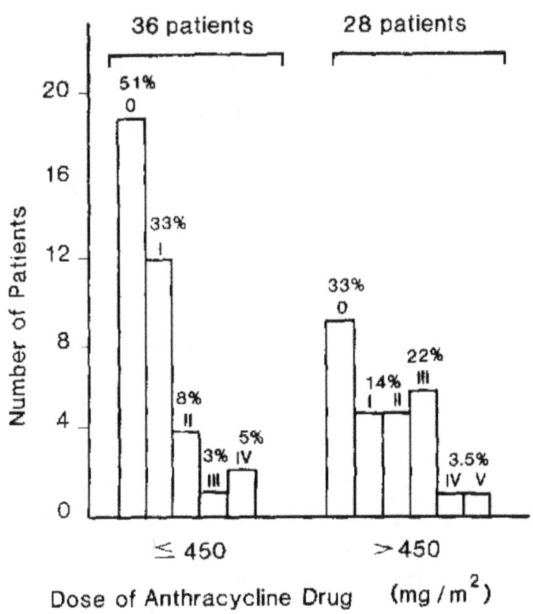

FIGURE 5. Scores for histologic toxicity grouped according to cumulative dose of anthracycline drug administered (≤450 or >450 mg/m²).

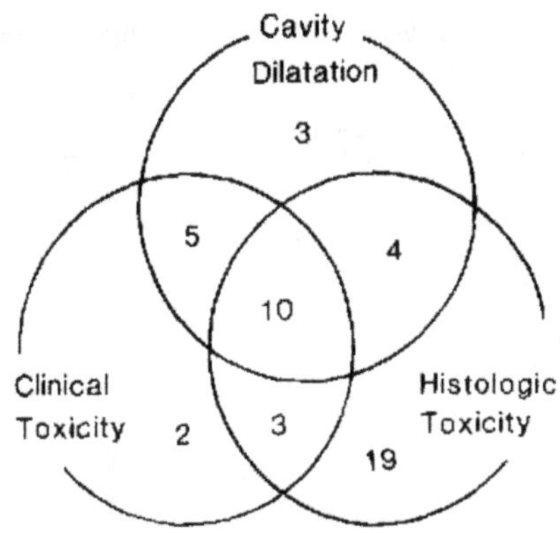

FIGURE 4. Relation of clinical cardiotoxicity to gross and histologic signs of cardiotoxicity. (Of the total 64 patients, 18 had neither clinical toxicity, cavity dilatation, nor morphologic toxicity and are not represented in this figure.)

Histologic toxicity as a function of cumulative dose of anthracycline drug: The relation between the extent of histologic signs of cardiotoxicity and the cumulative dose in mg/m^2 of anthracycline is illustrated in Figure 5. Of the 28 patients who received anthracycline therapy >450 mg/m^2, 13 (46%) had histologic scores of 2 to 5; in contrast, of 36 patients who received anthracycline therapy <450 mg/m^2, only 6 (17%) had histologic scores of ≥2 (p = 0.0097). Nevertheless, extensive histologic abnormalities were not limited to patients treated with >450 mg/m^2 of drugs: One patient treated with 100 mg/m^2 received a histologic toxicity score of 4 and had clinical signs of toxicity; 3 patients

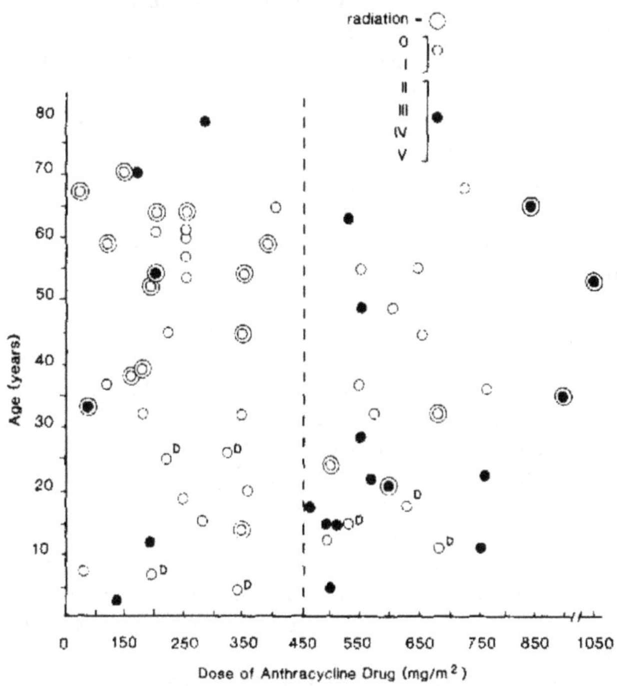

FIGURE 6. Morphologic toxicity as a function of cumulative dose of anthracycline drug, mediastinal irradiation, and age. All but 2 of the patients with scores of II to V received >450 mg/m^2, mediastinal irradiation, or were ≥70 years of age.

TABLE III Distribution of Histologic Changes (Morphologic Toxicity) in the Ventricular Walls of the Heart in 64 Necropsy Patients

Portion of Heart	Sections Examined (n)	Final Grade of Morphologic Toxicity						Nonrepresentative Sections
		0	I	II	III	IV	V	
Left ventricular free wall	62	26	14	8	7	3	1	3
Ventricular septum	36	12	7	6	5	0	1	5
Right ventricular free wall	50	22	7	3	5	3	1	9
Totals								
n	148	60	28	17	17	6	3	17
%	...	41	19	11	11	4	1	12

treated with 100 to 200 mg/m^2 received histologic toxicity scores of 2, 3, and 4, respectively, and 1 had clinical signs of toxicity; 2 patients treated with 200 to 300 mg/m^2 received a histologic toxicity score of 2.

Histologic toxicity as a function of cumulative drug, dose, age, and mediastinal irradiation: The effects of increasing age and mediastinal irradiation, in combination with cumulative drug dose, are illustrated in Figure 6. Of the 19 patients with combined histologic scores of 2 through 5, 13 received anthracycline therapy >450 mg/m^2. Of the 6 patients with extensive histologic changes who received <450 mg/m^2 of drug, 2 were treated with mediastinal irradiation (5,800 and 9,450 rads, respectively), and 2 were ≥70 years of age. Thus, all but 2 patients, in whom extensive histologic signs of anthracycline cardiotoxicity were recognized at necropsy, received >450 mg/m^2 of anthracycline therapy, or received combined mediastinal irradiation, or were ≥70 years of age.

Distribution of histologic abnormalities: The distribution of the histologic changes representing anthracycline cardiotoxicity is shown in Table III. Of 62 sections of left ventricular free wall from 64 patients, only 3 sections (5%) demonstrated histologic toxicity of lesser severity than was recognized in sections from either the ventricular septum or right ventricular free wall. Of 36 sections of ventricular septum taken from the 64 patients, only 5 (14%) were not representative of histologic lesions observed in sections taken from other sites of the myocardium. Of 50 sections taken from the right ventricular free wall, 9 (18%) were nonrepresentative. In those cases in which histologic toxicity was most extensive (histologic toxicity scores of 3, 4, and 5), these lesions were seen on sections taken from all 3 sites, that is, the right and left ventricular free walls and ventricular septum. The lesions corresponding to a histotoxicity score of 1 or 2 were more variable in distribution: In patients receiving a score of 1 or 2, the histologic abnormality was present in the left ventricle in 82 and 100%, respectively; in the ventricular septum in 64 and 64%; and in the right ventricular free wall in 54 and 50%.

Electrocardiographic findings in patients with and without clinical signs of drug toxicity: Electrocardiograms recorded between the time of onset of symptoms and the time of death were available in 9 of the 20 patients with clinical evidence of anthracycline toxicity. Two of the 9 patients had diminished amplitude of the QRS complex ("low voltage": ΣQRS amplitude [leads I, II, and III] ≤15 mm); in 1 of these 2 patients plus 1 other of the 9 patients, serial recordings demonstrated >30% diminution of the summated amplitude of the QRS complex in the limb leads. Pericardial heart disease was responsible for low voltage in only 1 of these patients. The mean cardiac weight of the 3 patients with reduced electrocardiographic QRS voltage was 248 g; the mean cardiac weight of the remaining 6 patients was 345 g.

Of the total group of 40 patients without clinical evidence of drug toxicity, 35 had electrocardiograms that were available for review: 11 (13%) had low voltage, including 1 with >30% diminution of the summated limb lead QRS amplitude on serial recordings. Their mean heart weight was 286 g, and none had pericardial heart disease, myxedema, cardiac amyloidosis, or hemochromatosis.

As a group, the 14 patients with low voltage and/or serial diminution in summated QRS amplitude did not differ significantly from the 30 patients with normal amplitude QRS complexes in terms of histologic findings: Vacuolar lesions were seen in 30% of the patients with and in 58% of the patients without low voltage; myofibrillar dropout in 20% of those with and in 28% of those without low voltage; interstitial fibrosis in 15% of those with and in 17% of those without low voltage; and attenuated myocytes ("fiber thinning") in 45% of the patients with versus 47% of those without low voltage.

Discussion

Anthracycline-induced cardiomyopathy was first reported by Tan et al[9] in 1967 in a 16-year-old girl treated with daunorubicin. Subsequent reports[10–14] confirmed the potential cardiotoxicity of daunorubicin and its derivative compound, doxorubicin. In the first detailed account of the morphologic findings of anthracycline-induced cardiomyopathy, Lefrak et al[5] described 2 patients in whom necropsy examination disclosed gross anatomic findings of biventricular dilatation with cavitary thrombus and histologic findings consisting of cytoplasmic hyaline transformation and cytoplasmic vacuolization. In both patients, clinical signs of a dilated cardiomyopathy had developed after they had received 720 and 825 mg/m^2 of doxorubicin.

Cortes et al[7] subsequently studied at necropsy 51 patients with doxorubicin, 17 (33%) of whom had signs of "toxic cardiopathy," defined as a combination of "intracellular edema, intracellular vacuolization, and myocardial fibrosis"; 5 had had congestive heart failure before death, and the remaining 12 never had overt cardiac failure.

Subsequent to these early necropsy observations, most published information regarding morphologic findings in patients receiving anthracycline drugs has been derived from analysis of myocardial biopsy specimens obtained from patients undergoing anthracycline chemotherapy.[4] Interest in this technique developed principally from 2 observations: (1) Although the development of anthracycline cardiotoxicity in general correlated with cumulative drug dose, in certain patients serious cardiotoxicity developed at relatively low doses,[15–19] while others, clearly in need of continuing chemotherapy, tolerated higher doses of the drug without adverse effects.[20] (2) Noninvasive methods contemporary to the early 1970s (electrocardiography, systolic-time intervals, echocardiography) proved unreliable for detecting latent, subclinical cardiac toxicity.[21–26] Thus, it was hoped that evaluation of serial biopsies might detect signs of potential cardiotoxicity before the time when cardiotoxicity became inevitable, and furthermore that biopsy analysis might predict how much longer a given patient could safely tolerate continued administration of anthracycline therapy.

The present study was designed to evaluate the correlation between clinical and morphologic signs of anthracycline cardiac toxicity in patients studied at necropsy. Examination of necropsy specimens eliminates the potential pitfalls posed by biopsy specimens, particularly the small size of tissue specimen,[27,28] limitation of sampling to subendomyocardial myocardium, and access to only 1 cardiac ventricle.[29] In addition, we hoped to extend the experience of Cortes et al[7] by (1) evaluating the pathologic material without knowledge of the clinical history, and (2) by establishing more rigid criteria for the definition of clinical and histologic signs of cardiotoxicity.

The present investigation suggests that prediction of clinical anthracycline cardiotoxicity on the basis of histologic changes is uncertain, because correlation between morphologic and functional changes is imperfect. Histologic signs of anthracycline cardiotoxicity may be absent, despite unequivocal clinical signs of a dilated cardiomyopathy: this situation was observed in 7 (35%) of our 20 patients. This finding has 3 important implications. The first, regarding therapy, is that in these 7 patients, an endomyocardial biopsy performed before the development of overt congestive heart failure would have suggested that treatment with anthracycline drugs could be continued safely. The second is that at least some of the "false-negative" results described in patients studied by the biopsy technique[22] are unlikely to have resulted simply from sampling errors. The third is that myofibrillar dropout and dilatation of the sarcoplasmic reticulum are not the only factors involved in the pathogenesis of anthracycline-induced cardiac failure. The concept that such failure is simply the result of structural damage to tissue represents an oversimplification of a very complex series of morphologic and biochemical changes.

The counterpart of the foregoing findings is that histologic signs of cardiotoxicity may be present without clinical signs of cardiac dysfunction: this situation was observed in 23 (52%) of 44 patients in the present report. Histologic signs of toxicity unassociated with clinical toxicity have been observed frequently in patients studied by endomyocardial biopsy, and, if extensive, have been interpreted as a contraindication to continued administration of anthracycline chemotherapy in these patients. The finding of morphologic toxicity in an asymptomatic patient—in the biopsy and, now, necropsy experience—suggests that such subclinical morphologic alteration may be the basis for the development of latent cardiac dysfunction described in long-term survivors of anthracycline therapy.[30,31] In nonhuman animal models of anthracycline toxicity, delayed development of cardiomyopathy has been observed as long as 6 months after discontinuation of therapy, and has been interpreted as evidence that the myocardial effects of anthracycline compounds are cumulative and irreversible.[32]

The serious discrepancies between morphologic and clinical evidence of toxicity found in the present investigation suggests that morphologic monitoring of patients receiving anthracycline drugs is of limited value for predicting the development of anthracycline cardiomyopathy. In contrast, physiologic evaluation of the cardiac response to exercise[26,31,33] or increased afterload[34] may improve the sensitivity of monitoring such patients for clinical evidence of latent cardiotoxicity. Long-term follow-up of such patients will determine whether such latent toxicity ultimately progresses to overt congestive heart failure.

Because this was a retrospective study and necropsy material from these patients had not been routinely preserved in glutaraldehyde fixative, examination of material was by necessity limited to gross anatomic and light microscopic studies. Nevertheless, as has been pointed out before, the morphologic lesions of anthracycline toxicity are evident by light microscopy.[27]

Electrocardiographic changes (low voltage or serial reduction ≥30% in limb lead voltage) previously proposed as evidence of anthracycline cardiotoxicity[35] correlated poorly with signs of morphologic toxicity in our patients, a finding noted previously by others.[23,36] The finding of low voltage was related to cardiac atrophy in patients with systemic cachexia, rather than to drug toxicity. The finding that cardiac atrophy frequently forms the morphologic basis for diminished QRS amplitude in such patients[37] makes this electrocardiographic feature particularly unsuitable for monitoring patients likely to be cachectic by virtue of their systemic illness.

Finally, our findings confirm observations made previously by Von Hoff,[2] Bristow,[33] and Billingham[38] regarding "risk factors" for anthracycline cardiotoxicity. Extensive morphologic toxicity was observed, with 2 exceptions, only in patients treated with >450 mg/m^2 of drug, or in patients in whom a smaller dose was administered in association with mediastinal irradiation or to a patient ≥70 years of age. These findings support the concept of empiric limitation of total dose of drug, if possible, to <450 mg/m^2, and to an even smaller total in patients likely to receive mediastinal irradiation and in patients ≥70 years of age. Nevertheless, the finding of clinical or morphologic toxicity in patients treated with lower total doses of drug unassociated with mediastinal irradiation or advanced age suggests that empiric limitation of total dose of anthracycline is not by itself adequate to protect against the cardiotoxic effects of these drugs and mandates some form of associated monitoring.

References

1. **Young RC, Ozols RF, Myers CE.** The anthracycline antineoplastic drugs. N Engl J Med 1981;305:139–153.
2. **Von Hoff DD, Layard MW, Basa P, Davis HL Jr, Von Hoff AL, Rozencweig M, Muggia FM.** Risk factors for doxorubicin-induced congestive heart failure. Ann Intern Med 1979;91:710–717.
3. **Von Hoff DD, Rozencweig M, Layard M, Slavik M, Muggia FM.** Daunomycin-induced cardiotoxicity in children and adults. A review of 110 cases. Am J Med 1977;62:200–206.
4. **Bristow MR, Mason JW, Billingham ME, Daniels JR.** Doxorubicin cardiomyopathy: evaluation of phonocardiography, endomyocardial biopsy, and cardiac catheterization. Ann Intern Med 1978;88:168–175.
5. **Lefrak EA, Pitha J, Rosenheim S, Gottlieb JA.** A clinicopathologic analysis of Adriamycin cardiotoxicity. Cancer 1973;32:302–314.
6. **Buja LM, Ferrans VJ, Mayer RJ, Roberts WC, Henderson ES.** Cardiac ultrastructural changes induced by daunorubicin therapy. Cancer 1973;32:771–788.
7. **Cortes EP, Lutman G, Wanka J, Wang JJ, Pickren J, Wallace J, Holland JF.** Adriamycin (NSC-123127) cardiotoxicity: a clinicopathologic correlation. Cancer Chermother Rep 1975;6:215–225.
8. **Smith HL.** Relation of the weight of the heart to the weight of the body and of the weight of the heart to age. Am Heart J 1928;4:79–93.
9. **Tan CL, Tasaka H, Yu KP, Murphy ML, Karnofsky D.** Daunomycin, an anti-tumor antibiotic, in the treatment of neoplastic disease. Clinical evaluation with specific reference to childhood leukemia. Cancer 1967;20:333–353.
10. **Malpas JS, Bodley Scott R.** Rubidomycin in acute leukemia in adults. Br Med J 1968;3:227–229.
11. **Bonadonna G, Monfardini S.** Cardiac toxicity of daunorubicin. Lancet 1969;1:837.
12. **Smith B.** Damage to the intrinsic cardiac neurones by rubidomycin (daunorubicin). Br Heart J 1969;31:607–609.
13. **Alnger LE, Bushore J, Johnson WW, Ito J.** Daunomycin: a cardiotoxic agent. J Natl Med Assoc 1971;63:261–267.
14. **Middleman E, Luce J, Frei E III.** Clinical trials with Adriamycin. Cancer 1971;28:844–850.
15. **Rinehart JJ, Lewis RP, Balcerzak SP.** Adriamycin cardiotoxicity in man. Ann Intern Med 1974;81:475–478.
16. **Starkebaum GA, Durack DT.** Early onset of daunorubicin (Daunomycin) cardiotoxicity. Lancet 1975;2:711–712.
17. **Ippoliti G, Casirola G, Marini, Invernizzi R.** Daunorubicin cardiotoxicity (letter). Lancet 1976;1:430.
18. **Harrison DT, Sanders LA.** Pericarditis in a case of early daunorubicin cardiomyopathy. Ann Intern Med 1976;85:339–341.
19. **Bristow MR, Thompson PD, Martin RP, Mason JW, Billingham ME, Harrison DC.** Early anthracycline cardiotoxicity. Am J Med 1978;65:823–832.
20. **Blum RH, Carter SK.** Adriamycin. A new anticancer drug with significant clinical activity. Ann Intern Med 1974;80:249–250.
21. **Minow RA, Benjamin RS, Gottlieb JA.** Adriamycin (NSC-123127) cardiomyopathy: an overview with determination of risk factors. Cancer Chemother Rep 1975;6:195–201.
22. **Mason JW, Bristow MR, Billingham ME, Daniels JR.** Invasive and noninvasive methods of assessing adriamycin cardiotoxic effects in man: superiority of histopathologic assessment using endomyocardial biopsy. Cancer Treat Rep 1978;62:857–864.
23. **Fulkerson PK, Talley R, Kleinman D, Weaver SK, Leier CV, Balcerzak SP, Lewis RP.** Noninvasive profile in the prospective monitoring of Adriamycin cardiomyopathy. Cancer Treat Rep 1978;62:881–886.
24. **Hutchinson RJ, Bailey C, Wood D, Donaldson MH.** Systolic time intervals in monitoring for anthracycline cardiomyopathy in pediatric patients. Cancer Treat Rep 1978;62:907–910.
25. **Henderson IC, Sloss LJ, Jaffe N, Blum RH, Frei E III.** Serial studies of cardiac function in patients receiving Adriamycin. Cancer Treat Rep 1978;62:923–929.
26. **Alexander J, Dainiak K, Berger HL, Goldman L, Johnstone D, Reduto L, Duffy T, Schwartz P, Gottschalk A, Zaret BL.** Serial assessment of doxorubicin cardiotoxicity with quantitative radionuclide angiocardiography. N Engl J Med 1978;300:278–283.
27. **Billingham ME, Mason JW, Bristow MR, Daniels JR.** Anthracycline cardiomyopathy monitored by morphologic changes. Cancer Treat Rep 1978;62:865–872.
28. **Isner JM, Maron BJ, Roberts WC.** Comparison of amount of myocardial cell disorganization in operatively excised septectomy specimens with amount observed at necropsy in 18 patients with hypertrophic cardiomyopathy. Am J Cardiol 1980;46:42–47.
29. **Ferrans VJ, Roberts WC.** Myocardial biopsy: a useful diagnostic procedure or only a research tool? Am J Cardiol 1978;41:965–967.
30. **Gottlieb SL, Edmiston WA Jr, Haywood LJ.** Late, late doxorubicin cardiotoxicity. Chest 1980;78:880–882.
31. **Gottdiener JS, Mathisen DJ, Borer JS, Bonow RO, Myers CE, Barr LH, Schwartz DE, Bacharach SL, Green MV, Rosenberg SA.** Doxorubicin cardiotoxicity: assessment of late left ventricular dysfunction by radionuclide cineangiography. Ann Intern Med 1981;94:430–435.
32. **Jaenke RS.** Delayed and progressive myocardial lesions after Adriamycin administration in the rabbit. Cancer Res 1976;36:2958–2966.
33. **Bristow MR, Mason JW, Billingham ME, Daniels JR.** Dose-effect and structure-function relationships in doxorubicin cardiomyopathy. Am Heart J 1981;102:709–718.
34. **Borow KM, Keane JF, Castaneda AR, Freed MD.** Systemic ventricular function in patients with tetralogy of Fallot, ventricular septal defect and transposition of the great arteries repaired during infancy. Circulation 1981;64:878–885.
35. **Minow RA, Benjamin RS, Lee ET, Gottlieb JA.** QRS voltage change with Adriamycin administration. Cancer Treat Rep 1978;62:931–934.
36. **Weaver SK, Fulkerson PK, Lewis RP, Leier C.** A paucity of chronic electrocardiographic changes with Adriamycin therapy. J Electrocardiog 1978;11:233–238.
37. **Isner JM, Fortin RV, Oliphant LH, Crisciticllo MG.** Cardiac atrophy is a frequent etiology for the electrocardiographic finding of low voltage (abstr). Circulation 1982;66:Suppl II:II-127.
38. **Billingham ME, Bristow MR, Glatstein E, Mason JW, Masek M, Daniels JR.** Adriamycin cardiotoxicity: endomyocardial biopsy evidence of enhancement by irradiation. Am J Surg Pathol 1977;1:17–23.

Amyloidosis Limited to Small Arteries Causing Angina Pectoris and Sudden Death

Jeffrey E. Saffitz, MD, PhD*
Kathleen Sazama, MD
William C. Roberts, MD

Amyloid deposits occur in 2 locations in body organs: *interstitium* and *blood vessels*. Of 54 patients with cardiac amyloid causing cardiac dysfunction studied in our laboratory, 53 (98%) had amyloid deposits involving both interstitium and blood vessels and 1 (2%) had amyloid deposits limited to blood vessels. Because only 2 other patients with amyloid limited to blood vessels have been reported, to our knowledge,[1,2] a brief summary of our case appears justified.

The patient was a 61-year-old woman who presented at age 56 years with inflamed eyelids, and work-up at that time disclosed the presence of immunoglobulin A (IgA)-myeloma. She received chemotherapy. At age 58 years (about 36 months before death), she developed chest pain diagnosed as angina pectoris and she was treated with isosorbide dinitrate and propranolol. She died suddenly at home.

Necropsy (SH#A81-47) disclosed amyloid deposits in blood vessels in virtually every body organ other than the brain without amyloid deposits in the interstitium of any body organ. The deposits involved the blood vessels in some organs—the heart, lungs, bowel, and skin—to a much greater extent than those in other organs. The deposits severely narrowed the lumens of many vessels but no organ infarcts occurred. The deposits were limited to the small intraorgan blood vessels (Fig. 1).

In the heart, amyloid was present not only in the intramural coronary arteries but also in the mural endocardium of all 4 chambers, particularly the atria, and in all 4 cardiac valves. (These structures may be considered modified

From the Pathology Branch, National Heart, Lung, and Blood Institute, National Institutes of Health, and the Department of Pathology, Suburban Hospital, Bethesda, Maryland. Manuscript received and accepted November 11, 1982.

* On leave of absence from the Department of Pathology, Washington University, St. Louis, Missouri.

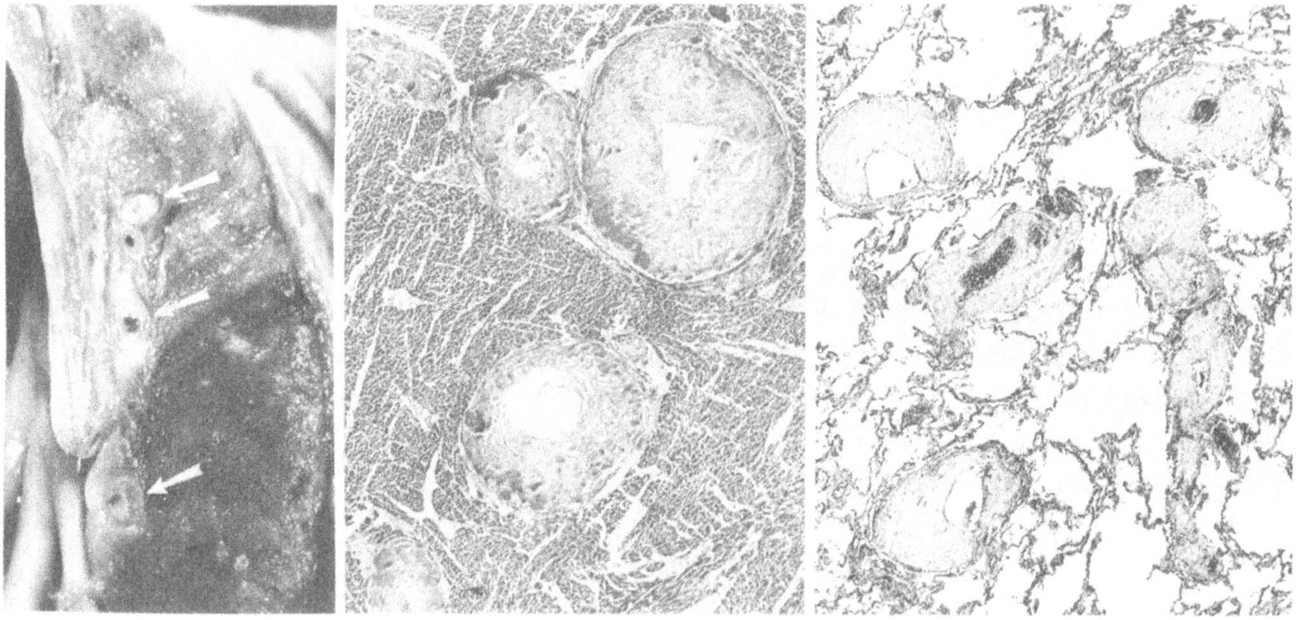

FIGURE 1. Longitudinal cut of ventricular septum (**left**) shows severe thickening of several intramural coronary arteries (**arrows**). Photomicrographs of left ventricular myocardium (**center**) and lung (**right**) reveal amyloid deposits in multiple arteries leading to luminal narrowing. No amyloid deposits are present in the interstitium. (Photographs by M.M.M. Moore.)

blood vessels because they are lined by endothelium.) In contrast, no deposits were located in the myocardial interstitium. The epicardial coronary arteries were free of significant narrowing and amyloid deposits.

Each of the 2 previously reported patients with amyloid confined to the vascular system also had angina pectoris without significant narrowing of the epicardial coronary arteries. Thus, amyloid confined to small (intramural) coronary arteries can cause angina pectoris and fatal cardiac arrest.

References

1. Case 23-1968. Case records of the Massachusetts General Hospital: weekly clinicopathological exercises. N Engl J Med 1968;278:1276–1286.
2. **Jennette JC, Sheps DS, McNeill DD.** Exclusively vascular systemic amyloidosis with visceral ischemia. Arch Pathol Lab Med 1982;106:323–327.

Cardiac Amyloidosis Causing Cardiac Dysfunction: Analysis of 54 Necropsy Patients

WILLIAM C. ROBERTS, MD and BRUCE F. WALLER, MD

Clinical and morphologic findings are described in 54 necropsy patients (32 men [59%]) aged 21 to 97 years (mean 64) with cardiac amyloid deposits extensive enough to cause fatal cardiac dysfunction. Chronic congestive heart failure (CHF) was present in 46 (85%). The duration of CHF, known in 39 patients, ranged from 1 to 108 months (mean 18) and lasted ≤12 months in 25 patients (64%). All 8 patients without CHF died suddenly and unexpectedly. Systemic arterial pressures were recorded in the last 3 months of life in 43 patients: the peak indirect systolic pressure was ≤130 mm Hg and the diastolic pressure <90 mm Hg in all. Electrocardiograms, recorded in the last 6 months of life in 40 patients, were abnormal in each: low voltage in 35 (63%); "myocardial infarction pattern" in 33 (83%); abnormal QRS axis in 29 (73%); arrhythmias in 29 (73%); first, second, or third degree heart block in 28 (45%); and complete bundle branch block in 7 (18%). In 30 patients, the QRS amplitude in all 12 leads was measured: in the 15 men it ranged from 60 to 197 mm (mean 99) (10 mm = 1 mV) and in the 15 women from 58 to 199 mm (mean 109). Diagnosis of amyloidosis was established by biopsy of noncardiac organs or tissues during life in only 18 (33%) patients. During life the condition simulated hypertrophic cardiomyopathy in 5 patients, constrictive pericardial disease in 3, and coronary heart disease (because of angina pectoris) in 4.

At necropsy, the hearts ranged in weight from 300 to 900 g (mean 554), and all but 1 had a "rubbery," noncompliant consistency. In addition to their presence in myocardial interstitium (53 patients) and in intramural coronary arteries (54 patients), amyloid deposits were present grossly in mural endocardium in all 54 patients and in valvular endocardium in 46 (85%). The cardiac ventricles were not dilated in 43 patients (80%), but both atria were dilated in all 54 patients. Intracardiac thrombi were present in 14 patients (26%). Cardiac amyloidosis must be considered in any elderly patient with chronic CHF unassociated with chest pain when blood pressure is normal and the electrocardiogram discloses low voltage and a pattern of "healed myocardial infarction."

In 1970, clinical and necropsy findings in 15 patients with cardiac dysfunction secondary to cardiac amyloidosis were reported from this laboratory.[1] During the past 13 years we have studied at necropsy an additional 39 patients with fatal cardiac amyloidosis. This report summarizes clinical and morphologic findings in these 54 patients with cardiac amyloid deposits extensive enough to cause cardiac dysfunction, with particular emphasis on electrocardiographic observations.

Patients Studied and Findings

Clinical findings: The 54 patients ranged in age at death from 21 to 97 years (mean 64). The 32 men (59%) ranged in age from 32 to 97 years (mean 65) and the 22 women (41%) from 21 to 93 years (mean 62) (Fig. 1). Thirty-eight (70%) were white and 16 (30%) were black. Of the 54 patients, 46 (85%) had clinical evidence of congestive heart failure (CHF) at some time. The duration of CHF was discernible in 39 of the 46 patients and ranged from 1 to 108 months (mean 18): for ≤12 months in 25 patients (64%), from >12 to 24 months in 6 patients (15%), from >24 to 36 months in 3 patients (8%), and from 60 to 108 months (mean 82) in 5 patients (13%). The duration of CHF in 18 women ranged from 1 to 72 months (mean 18) and in 25 men from 2 to 108 months (mean 22). Each of the 8 patients (15%) without clinical evidence of CHF died suddenly and unexpectedly: in 3 sudden death was the first evidence of amyloidosis, 2 had familial amyloidosis, 2 had multiple myeloma, and 1 clinically had presumed alcoholic cirrhosis (which at necropsy actually was massive hepatic amyloid infiltration). The 8 patients dying suddenly without ever having clinical evidence of CHF ranged in age from 21 to 88 years (mean 56) and the 46 patients with CHF from 32 to 97 years (mean 65). Chest pain was present at some time during amyloid illness in 8 patients (15%), 4 of whom were considered to have angina pectoris.[2,3] Of the 4 patients (aged

From the Pathology Branch, National Heart, Lung, and Blood Institute, National Institutes of Health, Bethesda, Maryland. Manuscript received and accepted April 12, 1983.

Address for reprints: William C. Roberts, MD, Building 10A, Room 3E30, National Institutes of Health, Bethesda, Maryland 20205.

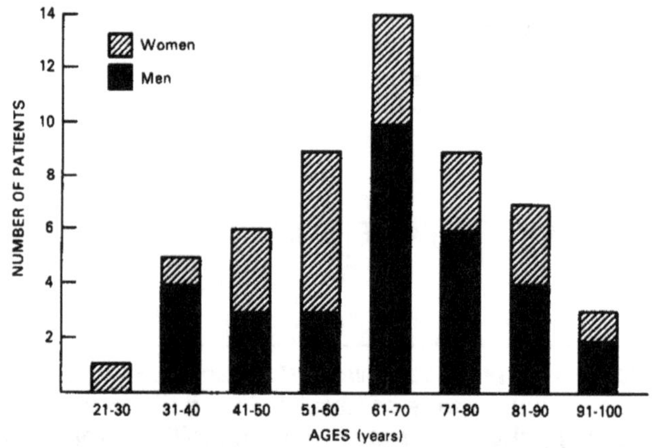

FIGURE 1. Age and sex distribution in the 54 necropsy patients with cardiac amyloidosis extensive enough to cause cardiac dysfunction.

67 to 89 years [mean 80]) with angina, 2 at necropsy had 1 or more of the 4 major (right, left main, left anterior descending, and left circumflex) epicardial coronary arteries narrowed 76 to 100% in cross-sectional area by atherosclerotic plaques.

Seven patients (13%) had histories of illnesses considered compatible with acute myocardial infarction that healed, but electrocardiographic and enzymatic documentation of myocardial necrosis at the time was unavailable. Grossly visible left ventricular scars, however, were absent at necropsy in all 7 patients, indicating that the histories of acute myocardial infarction in them were fallacious.

Four patients (7%) had 1 or more episodes of syncope. One patient was among the 4 with familial amyloidosis with peripheral neuropathy and postural hypotension. The mechanism of the syncope in the other 3 patients was not determined.

Systemic arterial pressure recordings during the last 3 months of life were available in 43 (80%) of the 54 patients. Although 24 (44%) of the 54 patients had a history of "hypertension," in none of the 43 patients (including the 24) with indirect blood pressure recordings available during the last 3 months of life was the systolic pressure >130 mm Hg or the diastolic pressure >90 mm Hg. The range of systolic arterial pressures during the last 3 months of life was 80 to 130 mm Hg (average 102) and of diastolic pressures 40 to 90 mm Hg (average 66).

TABLE I Cardiac Amyloid Causing Cardiac Dysfunction: Electrocardiographic Observations in 40 Patients*

Abnormality [No. (%)]	No. of Patients (%)
1. Low voltage (QRS ≤15 mm in I + II + III)	25 (63)
2. Myocardial infarct pattern	33 (83)
Anterior = 26 (79)	
Posterior = 2 (6)	
Both = 5 (15)	
3. Abnormal QRS axis	29 (73)
Right (+111 to +210°) = 6 (21)	
Left (−30 to −90°) = 23 (79)	
4. Arrhythmias	29 (73)
Atrial fibrillation = 9 (31)	
Atrial or junctional tachycardia = 10 (34)	
Ventricular premature complexes = 21 (72)	
5. Heart block	18 (45)
P-R interval >0.20 = 9 (50)	
2° AV block = 4 (22)	
3° AV block = 5 (28)	
6. Complete bundle branch block (QRS ≥0.12)	7 (18)
Right = 5	
Left = 2	

AV = atrioventricular.
* Numbers in parentheses represent percentages.

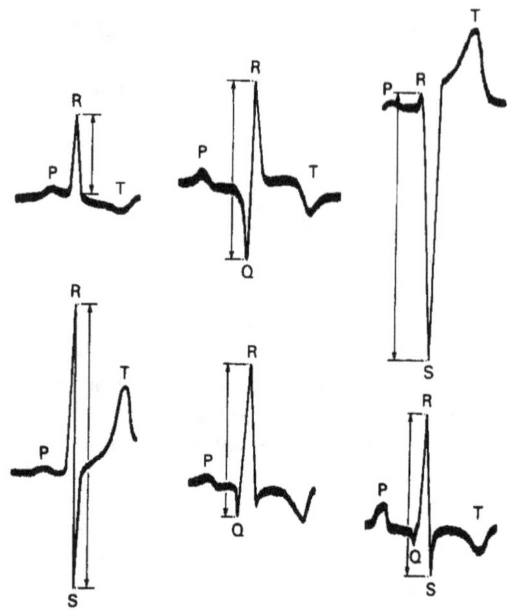

FIGURE 2. Various QRS complexes showing how each was measured.

The cardiac silhouette was enlarged on chest roentgenogram during the last few months of life in 39 (72%) of 54 patients. In several patients, however, earlier radiographs had shown the cardiac silhouette to be of normal size.

Adequate information on precordial examinations during the last few months of life was available in 44 of the 54 patients, 36 (82%) of whom had precordial murmurs. They were of a blowing type and consistent with mitral or tricuspid regurgitation, or both, in 35 (97%): grade 1 to 2/6 in 26, grade 3/6 in 7, and grade 4/6 in 2 patients. In addition, 1 patient had a murmur typical of valvular aortic stenosis (grade 3/6), which was confirmed to be present and was the type typically observed in the elderly.[4] At least 22 patients had third heart sounds (S_3) and at least 8 patients had fourth heart sounds (S_4).

Reports of 1 or more electrocardiograms recorded in the last 6 months of life were available in 40 patients, and all were abnormal (Table I). Of the 40 patients, electrocardiograms, recorded 0 to 160 days (mean 41) before death, were available for reexamination in 30 (Table II). In each of these 30 patients (15 women and 15 men), the QRS amplitude in all 12 leads was measured (Fig. 2). The total 12-lead QRS amplitude in the 15 men (mean age 52 years) ranged from 60 to 197 mm (mean 99) (10 mm = 1 mV) and in the 15 women (mean age 65 years) from 58 to 199 mm (mean 109). The heart weights in the 15 men ranged from 410 to 750 g (mean 570), and in the 15 women from 370 to 900 g (mean (494) (p <0.01). Some electrocardiograms are illustrated in Figures 3 to 6.

Information regarding digitalis therapy was available in 40 patients, and 31 of them received this drug. At least 12 (39%) of the 31 patients developed physical or electrical signs, or both, considered typical of digitalis toxicity.

M-mode echocardiograms were performed in the last few months of life in 11 patients. The findings are summarized in Table III and illustrated in Figures 6 and 7.

Cardiac catheterization was performed in the last few months of life in 10 patients (19%), and the findings are summarized in Table IV.

Of the 54 patients, the amyloidosis was primary in 42 (78%), associated with multiple myeloma in 7 (13%), and familial in 5 (9%). None of the 54 patients had "secondary" amyloidosis.

Diagnosis of amyloidosis was established by biopsy of noncardiac organs or tissues during life in 18 patients (33%), including 5 of the 8 patients without and in 13 (28%) of the 46 patients with chronic CHF. Of the 21 patients having undergone biopsy of noncardiac organs or tissues, findings in 18 were positive for amyloid: rectum, 6 of 6; gingiva, 3 of 4; liver, 3 of 3; tongue, 2 of 3; kidney, 1 of 2; and each of prostate gland, thyroid gland, and lymph node, 1 of 1. In addition, endomyocardial biopsy of the right ventricular aspect of the ventricular septum was performed in 1 patient, but amyloid was not observed on histologic examination.

Of the 46 patients with chronic CHF, biopsy of a noncardiac organ or tissue was performed in 10 and all findings were positive for amyloid. In addition to these 10 patients, amyloidosis was considered the most likely cause of chronic CHF in 9 other patients. The cause of chronic CHF was never established during life in the remaining 27 patients (59%). Of the 11 patients having undergone M-mode echocardiography, the maximal thickness of the ventricular septum was greater than that of the left ventricular free wall in 5, and as a consequence hypertrophic cardiomyopathy was the suspected diagnosis clinically in each of them (Fig. 8 and 9). One of these 5 patients also had undergone cardiac catheterization, and hypertrophic cardiomyopathy continued to be the most likely clinical cardiac diagnosis after that procedure. Inability to differentiate clinically between constrictive pericardial disease and restrictive cardiomyopathy led to thoracotomy in 3 patients. At operation, all 3 had normal visceral and parietal pericardia and normal amounts of pericardial fluid. Each of these 3 patients died within 5 days of thoracotomy.

Eight patients had transient episodes of chest pain. In 4 the pain was consistent with angina pectoris, and a diagnosis of coronary heart disease was made in each. At necropsy, however, only 2 of the 4 patients had significant narrowing of an epicardial coronary artery by atherosclerotic plaque. Of the 4 patients with chest pain not consistent with myocardial ischemia, 1 had significant narrowing of 1 or more epicardial coronary arteries by atherosclerotic plaques. One of the latter 4 patients was 1 of the 3 with clinical pericardial constriction syndrome. The cause of chest pain in the other 2 was unclear. All 8 patients with chest pain had chronic CHF, and 2 had a history of acute myocardial infarction in the remote past. All 8 patients had luminal narrowing of many intramural coronary arteries by amyloid deposits.

Morphologic findings: The hearts in all 54 patients were examined initially by 1 of us (WCR), and 40 were reexamined together by both of us. Heart weights, available in 50 of the 54 patients, ranged from 300 to 900 g (mean 554). Of the 22 women, heart weights, available in 19, ranged from 300 to 900 g (mean 484) and 17 (89%) of the 19 weighed >350 g (a weight considered the upper limit of normal in adult women). Of the 32 men, heart weights (available in 31) ranged from 410 to 900 g (mean 596) and all 31 weighed >400 g (a weight considered the upper limit of normal in men).

TABLE II Electrocardiographic QRS Voltage (mm) in Each of 12 Leads in 15 Men and 15 Women With Cardiac Amyloidosis Causing Fatal Cardiac Dysfunction

Case	Necropsy Number	Age (yr) at Death	Interval (Days) ECG to Death	Leads: I	II	III	R	L	F	V_1	V_2	V_3	V_4	V_5	V_6	Total QRS 12-Lead	Heart Weight (g)
Men																	
1	A63-125	32	88	6	10	6	8	4	7	11	23	16	14	11	9	125	700
2	Vt. MCV A75-174	35	56	4	4	3	4	3	4	5	9	9	11	13	8	77	750
3	A65-159	38	10	2	4	6	2	5	6	5	19	11	6	9	7	82	410
4	A70-254	38	2	2	2	5	1	3	3	4	18	16	16	9	5	84	600
5	A79-25	45	2	5	4	8	2	6	6	12	27	21	22	30	15	158	780
6	A81-6	46	13	5	5	5	4	4	3	2	10	17	19	19	13	106	545
7	NNMC 80A-15	49	107	6	3	4	3	6	3	14	20	15	12	9	4	99	850
8	A60-19	54	0	4	4	1	4	3	3	10	10	3	10	8	5	65	550
9	A56-81	55	23	2	3	2	2	1	3	5	9	11	11	7	4	60	480
10	A61-190	55	2	2	4	5	3	4	5	3	15	14	12	12	6	85	535
11	GT 74A-259	62	9	2	3	3	2	2	3	1	6	23	21	11	2	79	470
12	A65-232	65	103	7	20	12	11	3	15	8	15	24	32	27	23	197	560
13	A69-187	68	5	5	5	7	3	6	6	13	16	11	9	8	6	95	550
14	A67-241	68	35	9	5	6	7	7	3	11	7	13	15	12	6	101	420
15	A66-151	69	59	4	3	5	3	5	4	7	10	11	8	5	4	69	450
Mean		52	34	4.3	5.3	5.2	3.9	4.1	4.9	7.4	14.3	14.3	14.5	12.7	7.8	99	570
Women																	
1	A65-25	21	58	5	5	5	5	5	3	11	28	30	16	10	12	135	530
2	A68-23	48	50	4	3	3	3	3	3	5	7	9	8	9	8	65	450
3	GT 80A-262	50	91	4	3	3	2	3	3	11	24	20	18	11	14	116	460
4	A68-277	53	15	3	2	3	1	3	3	6	10	10	10	4	3	58	370
5	HU A77-19	54	51	5	2	8	2	7	6	7	15	15	4	7	6	84	420
6	Wil., D. WMC A79-24	55	8	1	8	9	4	5	9	14	21	17	9	9	5	110	430
7	SH A81-47	61	0	2	6	6	5	3	6	6	19	21	16	9	8	107	385
8	GT 71A-67	67	76	8	8	8	7	6	7	7	19	18	17	14	8	127	650
9	GT 81A-90	70	42	3	4	2	3	1	3	3	11	14	9	8	7	68	485
10	GT 71A-435	72	70	5	14	12	9	6	12	3	4	12	24	12	8	121	480
11	SH A79-76	75	30	7	10	7	6	12	5	16	18	17	17	15	15	145	510
12	GT 79A-127	78	49	3	5	4	4	2	3	4	9	16	17	21	9	97	520
13	WHC A82-120	82	6	5	8	12	4	7	10	8	18	34	41	25	27	199	900
14	GT 79A-195	89	160	3	5	1	4	2	3	3	9	14	18	20	9	91	440
15	Sibley A80-99	93	3	10	6	12	5	10	10	9	10	11	14	14	6	117	380
Mean		65	47	4.5	5.9	6.3	4.3	5.0	5.7	7.5	14.8	17.2	15.8	12.5	9.7	109	494
Total (mean)		58	41	4.4	5.6	5.8	4.1	4.6	5.3	7.5	14.5	15.8	15.2	12.6	8.7	104	532

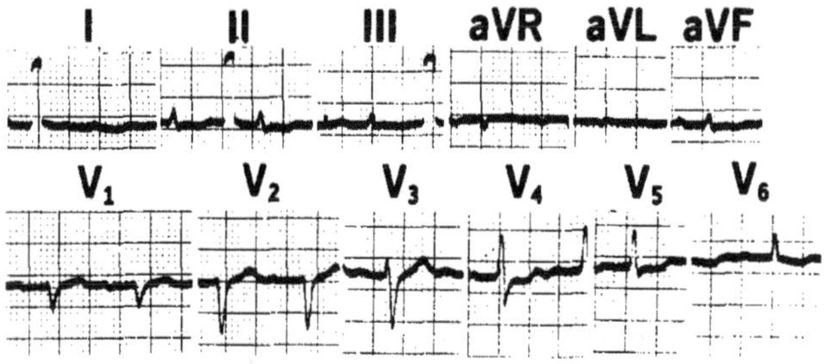

FIGURE 3. Electrocardiogram in a 55-year-old man (A56-81) recorded 23 days before death. The patient never had congestive heart failure. The heart weighed 480 g. The total 12-lead QRS voltage is only 60 mm. R waves are absent in leads V_1 and V_2 and small in V_3.

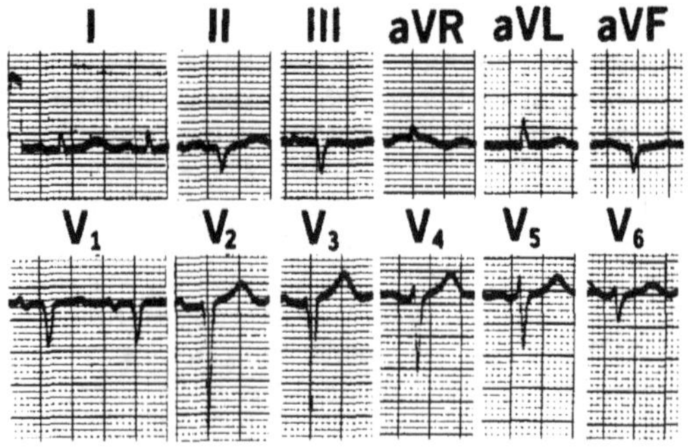

FIGURE 4. Electrocardiogram in a 55-year-old man (A61-190) recorded 2 days before death. The heart weighed 535 g and the total 12-lead QRS voltage is 85 mm. The voltage is decreased. The axis is leftward, Q waves are present in leads II, III, and aVF, and R waves are absent or small in the precordial leads.

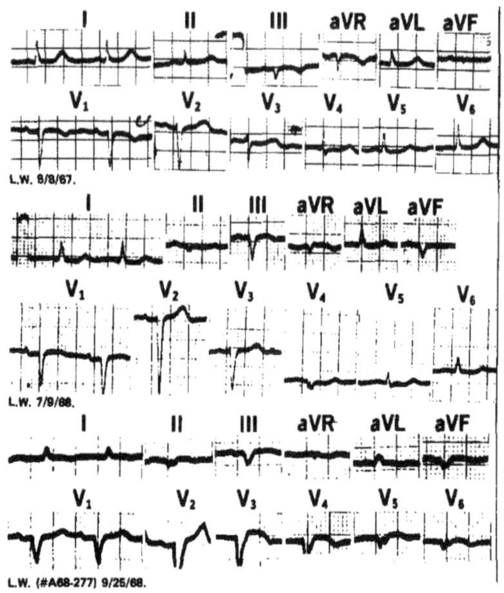

FIGURE 5. Electrocardiograms recorded over a 13-month period in a 53-year-old woman (A68-277) who had congestive heart failure for 5 months. The heart weighed 370 g. She died October 9, 1968. She had low voltage, left axis deviation, and absent R waves in the precordium. On the final electrocardiogram, the total 12-lead QRS voltage is 58 mm.

The hearts in 53 of the 54 patients were firm and rubbery, and this noncompliant consistency of the walls of all 4 cardiac chambers usually allowed the diagnosis of cardiac amyloidosis to be made immediately at necropsy without knowledge of clinical findings (Fig. 7 to 10). Both atria in all 54 patients on gross inspection were dilated, usually to a moderate degree. In contrast, the cardiac ventricles on gross inspection were of normal size in 43 patients (80%) and dilated in 11 (20%). The patients with dilated ventricles usually had other conditions that probably caused the dilatation: coronary heart disease

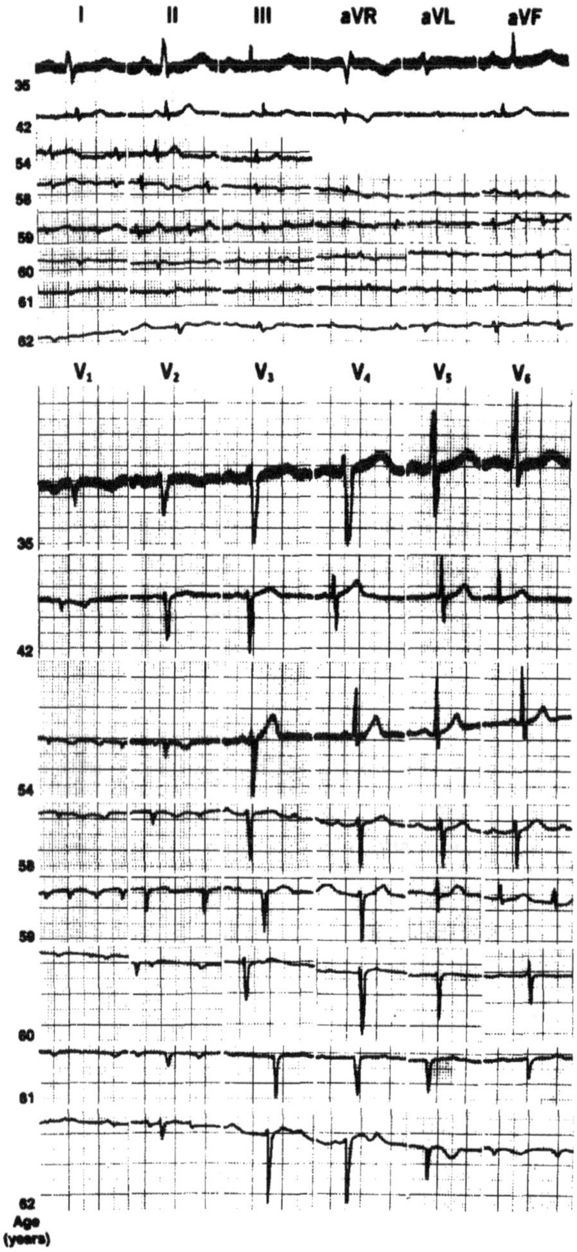

FIGURE 6. Electrocardiograms over a 27-year period in a 62-year-old man (GT 74A-259) who had congestive heart failure for 96 months and, at necropsy, a heart weighing 470 g. The QRS voltage progressively diminished, the axis changed, and R waves disappeared from the precordial leads. While taking digitalis, he developed atrial tachycardia with 2:1 block. The total 12-lead QRS voltage on the final electrocardiogram recorded 9 days before death was 79 mm.

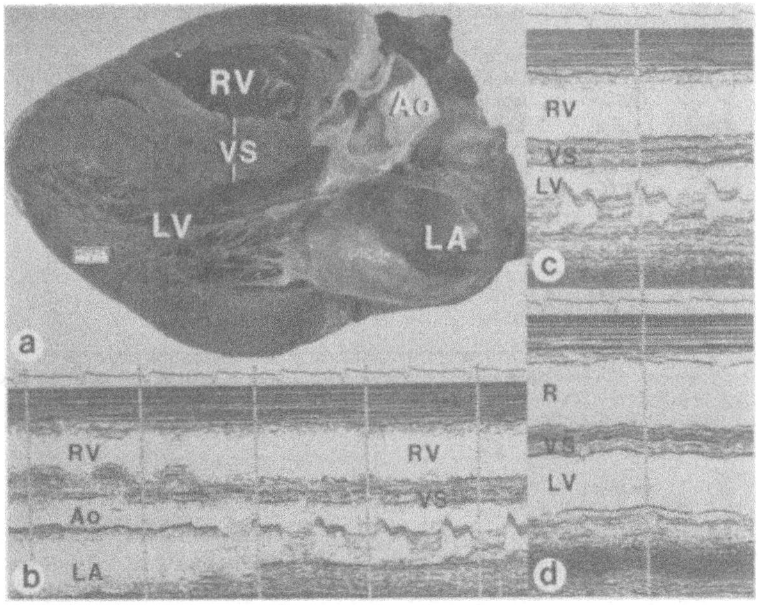

FIGURE 7. Cardiac amyloid with anasarca and pulmonary emboli. Longitudinal view of heart, weighing 545 g, in a 46-year-old man (A81-6) who had been well until 25 months before death, when parathesias and shoulder pain were noted. During his last 3 months he had severe congestive heart failure. When hospitalized 8 days before death, he had anasarca and third and fourth cardiac sounds. Electrocardiography showed a left atrial abnormality, right axis deviation, and poor R-wave progression over the precordium. Echocardiograms (**b, c, and d**) disclosed the ventricular septum (VS) and left ventricular (LV) free walls to be of similar thickness and each moved hardly at all. Both the left atrium (LA) and right ventricle (RV) were dilated. The pressures in mm Hg were: mean pulmonary artery wedge pressure, 27; pulmonary artery, 60/30; RV, 60/16; left ventricle, 90/26; and brachial artery, 90/60. He died from ventricular tachyarrhythmias. The heart in a longitudinal axis view is shown in **a.** The myocardium had the typical firm, rubbery appearance of extensive amyloidosis. Several pulmonary emboli may be the explanation of the right ventricular dilatation. Ao = aorta.

with left ventricular transmural scarring or chronic lung disease. The maximal thickness of the ventricular septum was identical or nearly so to the maximal thickness of the left ventricular free wall in 50 patients (93%); in the other 4 (7%) the septum was >1.3 times thicker than the free wall.

By gross examination, amyloid deposits (focal, tan, and waxy-appearing) were observed (and confirmed histologically) in the mural endocardium of 1 or both atria in all 54 patients and in valvular endocardium of 1 or more cardiac valves in 46 patients (85%) (Fig. 11): in the leaflets of the tricuspid valve in 45 patients (83%), the mitral valve in 43 patients (80%), the pulmonic valve in 29 patients (54%), and the aortic valve in 29 patients (54%). In 27 patients (50%), amyloid deposits were observed grossly in the leaflets of all 4 cardiac valves.

Focal transmural left ventricular lesions were observed grossly in 9 patients (17%) (Fig. 8); on histologic examination the lesions consisted entirely of fibrous tissue in 7 patients (13%) and of amyloid deposits in 2 (4%).

At least 3 histologic sections of heart were examined in each patient. In every patient, at least 1 section of left ventricular wall and at least 1 section of atrial wall were examined. Amyloid deposits, readily identified on hematoxylin-eosin stains, were confirmed by either congo red or crystal violet stains or both. In the chamber walls, the amyloid deposits were located in (1) interstitium, that is, between myocardial fibers, not within them in all but 1 patient,[4] (2) endocardium, often of all 4 chambers but always of 1 or both atria in all patients, and (3) within the walls of several intramural coronary arteries in all patients (Fig. 12). Additionally, amyloid deposits often were found in the lumina of some intramural coronary arteries, causing severe (>75% in cross-sectional area) narrowing of some lumina. Despite numerous sections of the major epicardial coronary arteries, no amyloid deposits were observed. At least 1 and usually multiple cardiac valves contained amyloid deposits, but none were judged to have deposits of sufficient quantity to cause valvular dysfunction. In several patients in whom histologic sections included coronary sinus, amyloid deposits were visible histologically in the wall of this structure.

In all 54 patients, amyloid deposits were observed in 1 or more other body organs. No patient had amyloid limited to the heart.

TABLE III M-Mode Echocardiographic Observations in 11 Necropsy Patients With Fatal Cardiac Amyloidosis*

Case	Age (yr) & Sex	Interval (Days) Cath to Death	VS		LV Wall		VS/LV Ratio		LV Cavity		LA Cavity		Ascending Aorta	
			ES	ED	ES	ED	ES	ED	ES	ED	ES	ED	ES	ED
1	21F	90	14	12	21	14	0.7	0.9	20	36	28	22	24	20
2	40M	...	...	20	...	20	...	1.0	...	...	...	36	...	41
3	45M	15	28	24	18	15	1.6	1.6	24	32	...	58	...	...
4	46M	62	14	14	18	14	0.7	1.0	36	40	36	40	34	30
5	54F	...	...	20	...	20	...	1.0	...	...	...	36	...	41
6	55F	334	30	26	18	15	1.7	1.7	26	36	...	30	...	27
7	55F	150	25	24	26	20	0.9	1.2	29	33	35	30	40	38
8	62M	300	19	19	22	18	0.9	1.1	38	42	20	18	38	30
9	63M	15	35	25	25	16	1.4	1.6	...	...	...	...	...	...
10	78F	169	12	9	13	8	0.9	1.1	36	48	45	40	35	31
11	89F	13	20	19	18	10	1.1	1.9	55	65	45	42	35	32

* All measurements in millimeters.
Cath = catheterization; ED = end-diastole; ES = end-systole; LV = left ventricular; VS = ventricular septum.

TABLE IV Hemodynamic Data in 9 Necropsy Patients With Fatal Cardiac Amyloidosis

Case	Age (yr) & Sex	Interval (Days) Cath to Death	Right Atrium* a	Right Atrium* v	Right Atrium* m	PAW* a	PAW* v	PAW* m	RV* (s/d)	PA* (s/d)	LV* (s/d)	SA* (s/d)	CI (liters/min/m²)
1	35M	90	...	...	11	...	...	25	52/16	48/28	100/24	100/70	...
2	38M	4	24	22	21	...	...	34	56/18	61/34	110/12	110/65	1.3
3	45M	14	12	13	11	28	38	30	60/11	65/33	100/28	100/64	1.7
4	46F	180	10	8	7	...	42	28	50/9	65/33	98/28	98/70	1.6
5	46M	360	...	...	20	...	...	27	60/16	60/30	90/26	90/65	...
6	47F	90	15	14	12	21	28	20	36/12	36/17	110/20	110/80	2.2
7	70M	7	...	...	...	...	...	30	50/	50/30	...	110/60	...
8	78F	150	14	11	10	...	30	26	70/2	70/30	100/20	100/60	2.3
9	96M	7	...	...	17	...	...	34	60/18	60/30	...	90/70	...

a = peak of a wave averaged for several beats; Cath = cardiac catheterization procedure; CI = cardiac index; LV = left ventricle; m = mean; PA = pulmonary artery; PAW = pulmonary arterial wedge; RV = right ventricle; SA = systemic artery; s/d = systolic/diastolic; v = peak of v wave averaged for several beats.
* Measurements in mm Hg.

Thrombi were observed grossly in 1 or more of the 4 cardiac chambers in 14 (26%) of the 54 patients: in 1 chamber only in 8 patients, in 2 chambers in 3 patients, in 3 chambers in 1 patient, and in all 4 chambers in 1 patient. Of the 22 cardiac chambers that contained thrombi (mainly fibrin in all) in the 14 patients, the right atrial appendage contained thrombi in 10 patients (isolated in 5); the left atrial appendage contained thrombi in 7 patients (isolated in 2); the right ventricle con-

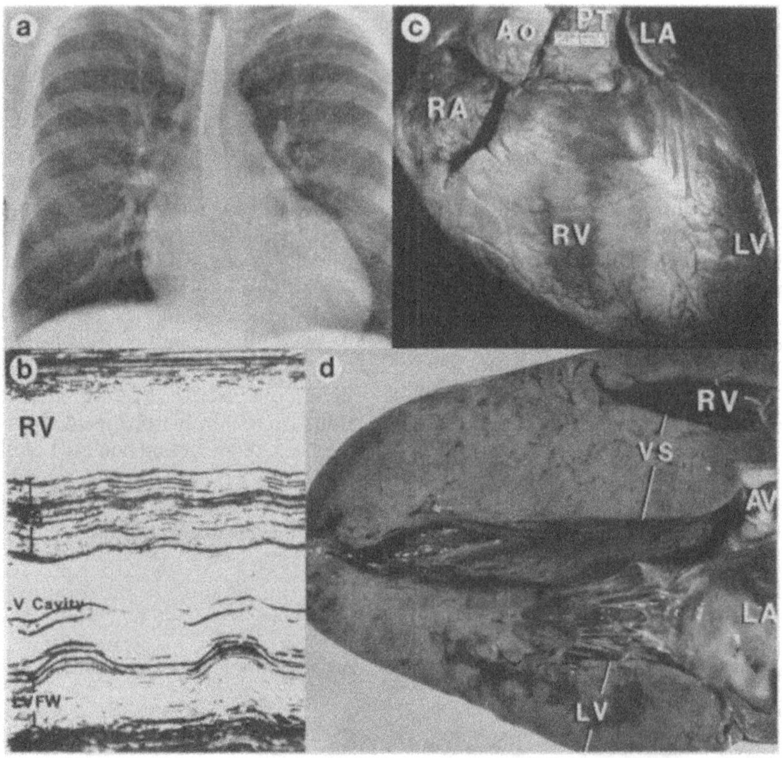

FIGURE 8. Cardiac amyloidosis simulating hypertrophic cardiomyopathy. Chest radiograph (**a**), M-mode echocardiogram just caudal to the tips of the mitral leaflets (**b**), exterior view of heart (**c**), and longitudinal axis view of heart (**d**) in a 46-year-old man (A79-25) who noted dyspnea while walking 24 months before death. M-mode echocardiography 1 month later disclosed the ventricular septum (VS) to be 1.7 times thicker than the left ventricular free wall (LVFW). The anterior mitral leaflet moved anteriorly during ventricular systole. The left atrial cavity was 30 mm in diameter. The pressures in mm Hg were: mean pulmonary arterial wedge, 5; pulmonary artery, 17/6; right ventricle (RV), 17/3; left ventricle (LV), 130/11; and aorta (Ao), 115/70. Clinically, the patient at that time was considered to have hypertrophic cardiomyopathy. Nine months before death, he had transient sudden left-sided weakness with slurred speech, worsened dyspnea, transient chest pain, and the carpal-tunnel syndrome was noted. Now the mean pulmonary arterial wedge pressure was 23; right ventricular pressure, 47/7; LV, 95/25; and Ao, 95/65 mm Hg. Echocardiogram now showed the ventricular septum to be 2.0 cm and the LVFW 1.5 cm; SAM now was absent. The left atrium (LA) now was 55 mm in diameter. A third catheterization performed 10 days before death showed the mean pulmonary wedge pressure to be 32 and that in the RV 65/11 mm Hg. The cardiac index was 1.4 liters/min/m². The heart was enlarged (**a**). M-mode echocardiogram (**b**) now showed the VS to be 2.6 cm and the LVFW 1.5 cm thick. Cardiac amyloidosis was never diagnosed clinically. At necropsy, the heart weighed 780 g. In addition to the usual interstitial myocardial amyloid, large deposits of amyloid were visible grossly on the LVFW (**d**). The VS is thicker than the free wall. The epicardial coronary arteries were virtually free of atherosclerotic plaques. AV = aortic valve; PT = pulmonary trunk; RA = right atrium; SAM = systolic anterior motion of the anterior mitral leaflet.

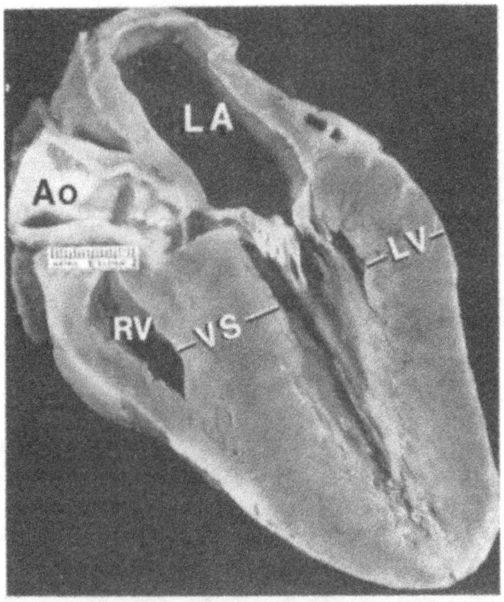

FIGURE 9. Cardiac amyloidosis simulating hypertrophic cardiomyopathy. Long-axis view of heart in a 55-year-old woman (WMC#A79-24) who had been well until 6 months before death when she developed periorbital purpura, pedal edema, and right-arm pain. When syncope occurred a month later, she was hospitalized and found to have multiple myeloma. Electrocardiography disclosed both atrial and ventricular arrhythmias and electrophysiologic studies disclosed distal H-V block. She never had congestive heart failure. On the day of death at home she fainted and soon thereafter had fatal cardiac arrest. The heart weighed 430 g and it had the typical amyloid consistency. A long-axis view is shown. The ventricular septum (VS) is thicker than the left ventricular (LV) free wall. The left atrium (LA) is dilated. Ao = aorta; RV = right ventricular cavity.

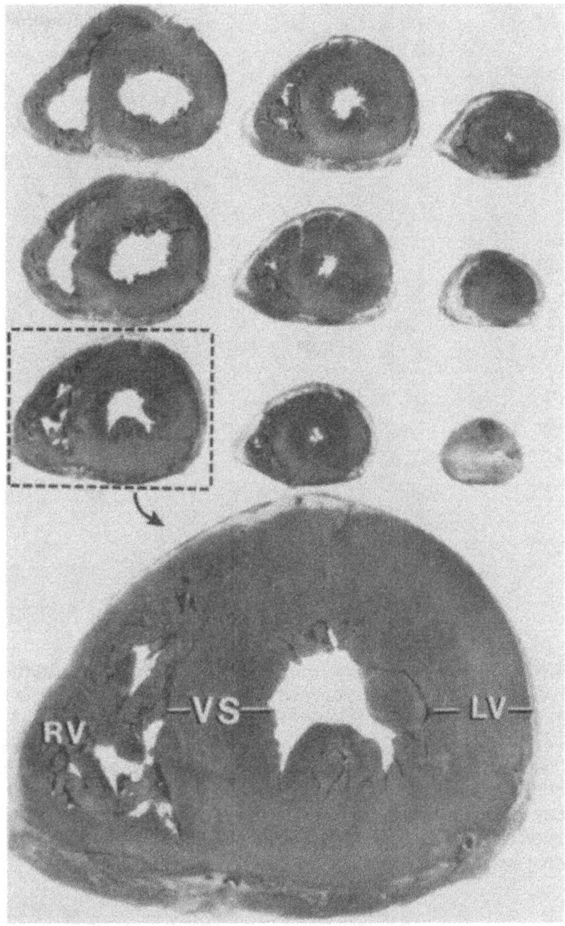

FIGURE 10. Massive ventricular amyloid deposits. Transverse cuts of the ventricles in the 49-year-old man (NNMC#A80-15), described in detail in Figure 3. This uniform appearance of the ventricular walls is the most common finding in extensive cardiac amyloidosis. LV = left ventricle; RV = right ventricle; VS = ventricular septum.

tained thrombi in 2 patients (none isolated), and the left ventricle contained thrombi in 3 patients (isolated in 2). Thus, of the 22 chambers with thrombi, 17 were atrial appendages and 5 were ventricles. None of the 5 ventricles containing thrombi appeared dilated by gross inspection. Of the 14 patients with intracardiac thrombi, 13 had clinical evidence of CHF and 1 died suddenly without evidence at any time of CHF: 2 (of 13) had chronic atrial fibrillation; 2 had clinical evidence of either pulmonary or systemic emboli, and 5 had severe narrowing of 1 or more epicardial cardiac arteries by either atherosclerotic plaque (4 patients) or fibrin-platelet embolus (1 patient). The latter patient was reported on previously.[2]

In addition to the extensive cardiac amyloid deposits, 8 patients (15%) had narrowing >75% in cross-sectional area by atherosclerotic plaques of 1 or more of the 4 major (right, left main, left anterior descending, and left circumflex) epicardial coronary arteries: in 5 patients, 3 of the 4 major arteries were so narrowed; in 1 patient 2 arteries, and in 2 patients 1 artery. The ages of these 8 patients ranged from 65 to 96 years (mean 78); 6 were men and 2 were women. Four had had periodic chest pain, considered angina pectoris in 2. One patient died suddenly and unexpectedly. At necropsy none had foci of myocardial necrosis, but 4 had healed transmural left ventricular infarcts, all of which had been clinically silent.

Calcific deposits were present in the mitral anulus in 7 patients (13%) and in 1 or more aortic valve cusps in 9 patients (17%). In 6 patients, the calcific deposits were present in both mitral anulus and in aortic valve cusps, in 3 patients they were limited to aortic valve cusps, and in 1 patient they were limited to mitral anulus. In 2 of the 9 patients with aortic valve calcium, the deposits appeared extensive enough to cause narrowing of the aortic valve orifice. In none of the 7 patients with mitral anulus calcium did the calcific deposits appear to cause clinically significant mitral dysfunction. All 10 patients (19%) with either mitral anular or aortic valve cuspal calcific deposits, or both, had calcific deposits in 1 or more of the 4 major epicardial coronary arteries, and in each patient they were within atherosclerotic plaques.

Discussion

Patients with cardiac amyloid deposits may readily be separated into 2 major groups: (1) those with amyloid deposits too small to produce cardiac dysfunction, and (2) those with amyloid deposits large enough to produce cardiac dysfunction which eventually is fatal. The finding of minute cardiac amyloid deposits in the heart in elderly persons at necropsy is common,[5–13] but patients with minute cardiac deposits, whether they be young or old, are not included in the present analysis. Each of our 54 patients had heavy cardiac amyloid deposits that caused fatal cardiac dysfunction. All but 1 had firm, rubbery ventricular and usually atrial walls with amyloid deposits in the interstitium (between myocardial cells) of the walls of all 4 chambers, in mural and usually in valvular endocardium, and in the in-

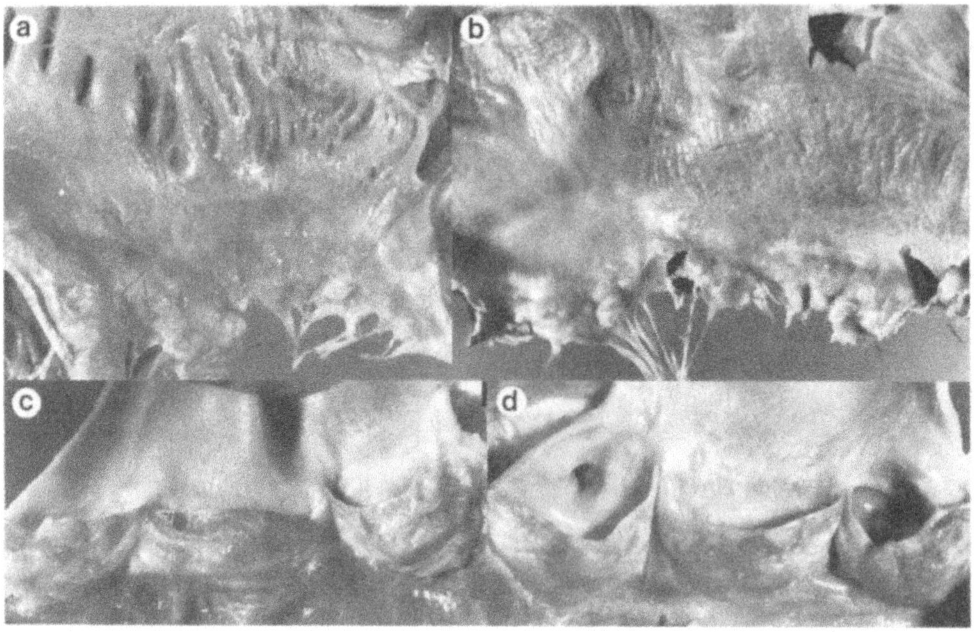

FIGURE 11. Endocardial amyloidosis. Opened right atrium and tricuspid valve (**a**), opened left atrium and mitral valve (**b**), opened pulmonic valve and pulmonary trunk (**c**), and opened aortic valve and aorta (**d**). The mural endocardium of each chamber and the cusps of all 4 cardiac valves contain amyloid deposits. The ventricular myocardium (shown in Figure 4) also contained massive quantities of amyloid, as did the pulmonary trunk. This 49-year-old man (NNMC#A80-15) had been well, but an automobile accident prompted an examination 10 months before death. Both pedal edema and hepatomegaly were found, the blood pressure was elevated (160/100 mm Hg), the heart was enlarged (cardiothoracic ratio 0.55), and electrocardiogram disclosed no R waves in leads V_1–V_3, nonspecific ST-T wave abnormalities, and low voltage. Echocardiogram was normal. Hepatic biopsy yielded amyloid. He remained asymptomatic until 4 months before death, when extensive subcutaneous edema appeared and pericardial effusion (700 ml) was found. The systemic blood pressure was then 120/80 mm Hg. His condition progressively worsened thereafter. He became acutely dyspneic at home and died.

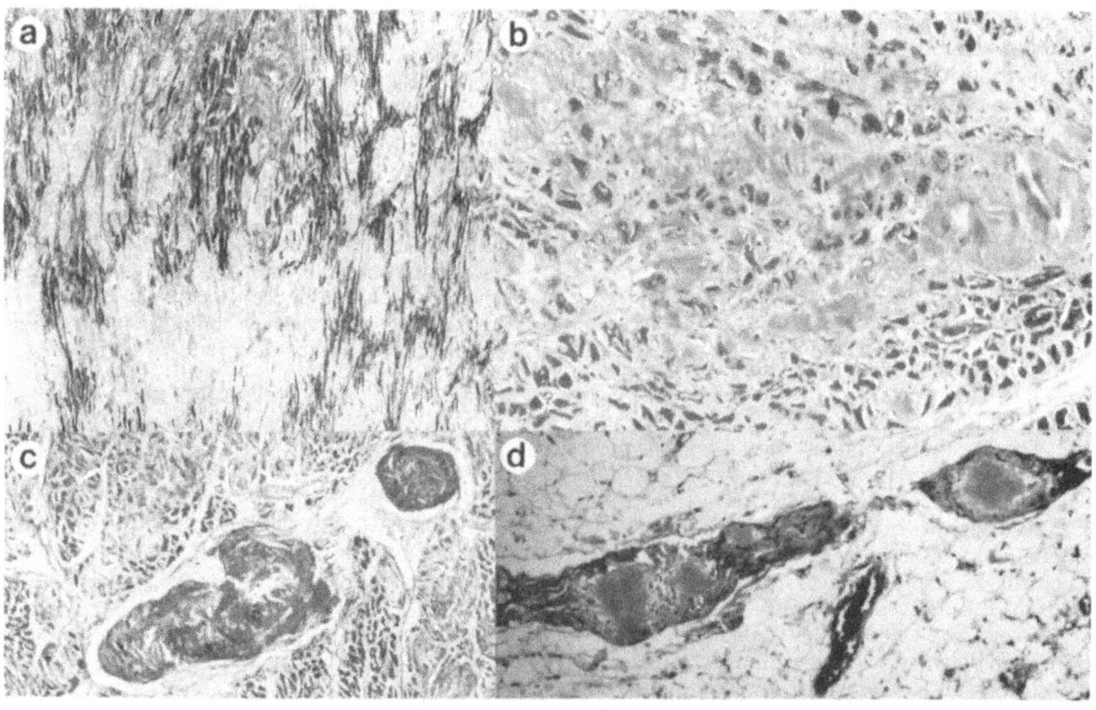

FIGURE 12. Location of amyloid in myocardium (**a** and **b**), intramural coronary artery (**c**) and epicardial nerve (**d**). **a,** massive interstitial myocardial amyloid observed in a longitudinal section in an 89-year-old man (A69-259) with chronic congestive heart failure (CHF) and a heart weighing 520 g. In this section, more amyloid than myocardial fibers are present. **b,** massive interstitial myocardial amyloid observed in cross section in a 68-year-old man (H-A76-143) who had CHF for 36 months. **c,** amyloid occluding the lumens of intramural coronary arteries in a 67-year-old man (A69-187) with chronic CHF and a heart weighing 550 g. **d,** amyloid in epicardial nerves in a 74-year-old man (A58-190) who died suddenly from familial amyloidosis and had a heart weighing 700 g. (Hematoxylin-eosin stain [**a**] ×25 and [**d**] ×100; Movat stain [**b**] ×100; Masson stain [**c**] ×39, all reduced 25%.)

tramural coronary arteries. The 1 patient without interstitial myocardial amyloid had amyloid filling the lumina of most intramural coronary arteries.[3] Additionally, several patients had amyloid in the epicardium but never in the walls or lumina of the major epicardial coronary arteries. All our 54 patients with cardiac amyloid had amyloid deposits in 1 or more noncardiac body organs. We suspect that cardiac amyloid severe enough to cause clinical evidence of cardiac dysfunction is never limited exclusively to the heart.

Although a diagnosis of cardiac amyloidosis was established clinically in less than half of our 54 patients, most were studied clinically before echocardiography and radionuclide angiography became commonly performed procedures. Echocardiography is now often one of the first clues to the diagnosis of cardiac amyloidosis,[14–19] and myocardial technetium-99m pyrophosphate scintigraphy may be diagnostic of this condition.[20–23] Thus, cardiac amyloidosis severe enough to cause cardiac dysfunction almost surely will be suspected hereafter in a majority rather than in a minority of patients. Clinically, diagnosis of cardiac amyloidosis should be suspected in an older patient with evidence of CHF, poorly responsive and/or particularly sensitive to digitalis, unassociated with chest pain or systemic hypertension, and in the presence of cardiomegaly by chest radiograph but low voltage by electrocardiogram. The echocardiogram, rather than showing dilatation of the left ventricle, shows this chamber to be of normal or near-normal size and the ventricular walls to move poorly, and these findings can be confirmed by hemodynamic and angiographic studies.[24–27] Biopsy of either noncardiac or cardiac[28] tissue is required for absolute diagnosis.

Severe cardiac amyloidosis is 1 of the causes of spontaneous cure of systemic hypertension. Although nearly half of our 54 patients had had either a history of systemic hypertension or recordings of elevated systemic arterial pressures, or both, all had systolic systemic pressures ≤130 mm Hg and diastolic systemic pressures ≤90 mm Hg in the last 3 months of life. The average recorded peak systolic arterial pressure in the last 3 months of life in our patients was 102 mm Hg and the diastolic pressure was 70 mm Hg. Thus, if the systemic arterial pressure is elevated in a patient with CHF, the chance that the CHF is the result of cardiac amyloidosis is minimal. Additionally, none of our patients had evidence of left ventricular hypertrophy by electrocardiogram in their final 3 months, although several had had left ventricular hypertrophy by electrocardiogram >1 year earlier.

The length of time necessary to develop cardiac amyloid deposits extensive enough to cause cardiac dysfunction is uncertain. One clue to the amount of time required can be gained by study of the systemic arterial pressures over several years. We have now observed several patients with systolic systemic pressures in the vicinity of 180 mm Hg; during a period of 4 to 5 years this pressure gradually decreased to about 100 mm Hg without use of antihypertensive agents. Thus, a gradual but spontaneous decrease in systemic arterial pressure also might be a clue to the development of cardiac amyloidosis.

Cardiac amyloidosis needs to be added to the list of great cardiac masqueraders. Initially, it was cardiovascular syphilis that was stated to frequently simulate other cardiac conditions. In recent years, hypertrophic cardiomyopathy has become the most prominent masquerader. The QRS and T-wave changes on the electrocardiogram in cardiac amyloidosis are similar to those produced by healed myocardial infarction secondary to coronary atherosclerosis. The presence of a nondilated left ventricle and the presence of a ventricular septum thicker than the left ventricular free wall by echocardiogram has suggested the presence of hypertrophic cardiomyopathy. Five of our 11 patients with echocardiograms were suspected of having hypertrophic cardiomyopathy because of the combination of these findings. Simulation of cardiac amyloidosis clinically to pericardial constriction has long been recognized.[1,24–27] Three of our 54 patients underwent thoracotomy because of suspected pericardial constriction. Cardiac amyloidosis may present as pericardial tamponade.[29] Its delayed left ventricular filling may simulate mitral stenosis on rare occasions.[30]

Although amyloid deposits are always more extensive in "working" than in "conducting" myocardium,[1,31,32] arrhythmias and conduction disturbances are common (Table I). Some of these disturbances, however, may be the result of aging rather than the result of extensive cardiac amyloidosis.[13,33] In our patients, left-axis deviation (58%), atrial fibrillation (23%), and bundle branch block (18%) were common, but these also are relatively common in elderly patients without cardiac amyloidosis.[13,33] The frequency of low voltage (63%) and a healed myocardial infarction pattern (83%), however, was striking in our patients, and each of these should raise the possibility of cardiac amyloidosis in a patient with CHF of unclear cause.

This report provides for the first time measurements of QRS voltages in each of the 12 leads of an electrocardiogram in patients with cardiac amyloidosis. Simonson[34] provided data on the upper and lower limits of amplitude of the QRS complexes in each of the 12 leads in normal men and women aged 20 to 59 years. (The mean for normal subjects is not available.) The upper and lower limits of normal for men aged 50 to 59 years were 277 and 36 mm and for women 248 and 27 mm, respectively. The upper and lower limits of amplitude in all leads in 30 of our 54 patients (Table II) were 199 and 58 mm, respectively, and averaged 104 mm. For our 15 women from whom the data were available, the total 12-lead QRS voltage ranged from 58 to 199 mm (mean 109) and for our 15 men from 60 to 197 mm (mean 99).

In comparison, Siegel and Roberts[35] determined the total 12-lead QRS voltage in 50 patients (aged 16 to 65 years) with severe and fatal isolated aortic valve stenosis. The upper and lower limits of amplitude in all 12 leads in their 50 patients were 417 and 144 mm, respectively, and averaged 260 mm. In their 14 women with aortic stenosis, the total 12-lead QRS voltage averaged 277 mm and in their 36 men, 249 mm. The average heart weight of their 14 women with aortic stenosis was 521 g, and the heart weight in our 15 women with severe cardiac amyloidosis and available total 12-lead

QRS voltage was 494 g. The difference, however, in average total 12-lead QRS voltage (277 mm versus 109 mm) was a factor of 2.5 times. The mean heart weight of the 36 men with aortic stenosis studied by Siegel and Roberts[35] was 639 g and that of our 15 men with fatal cardiac amyloidosis and available total 12-lead QRS voltage was 570 g. The average total 12-lead QRS voltage in the 36 men with aortic stenosis, however, was 249 mm compared with only 99 mm in our 15 men with fatal cardiac amyloid, again a 2.5-fold difference. Thus, although the sum of the QRS voltage in leads I, II, and III may not fulfill criteria of "low voltage," that is, ≤15 mm, the total QRS voltage in all 12 leads in severe cardiac amyloidosis is usually considerably lower than normal, and particularly small in proportion to the weight of the heart.

References

1. **Buja LM, Khoi NB, Roberts WC.** Clinically significant cardiac amyloidosis. Clinicopathologic findings in 15 patients. Am J Cardiol 1970;26:394–405.
2. **Barth RF, Willerson JT, Buja LM, Decker JL, Roberts WC.** Amyloid coronary artery disease, primary systemic amyloidosis and paraproteinemia. Arch Intern Med 1970;127:627–630.
3. **Saffitz JE, Sazama K, Roberts WC.** Amyloidosis limited to small arteries causing angina pectoris and sudden death. Am J Cardiol 1983;51:1234–1235.
4. **Roberts WC, Perloff JK, Costantino T.** Severe valvular aortic stenosis in patients over 65 years of age. A clinicopathologic study. Am J Cardiol 1971;27:497–506.
5. **Brandt K, Cathcart ES, Cohen AS.** A clinical analysis of the course and prognosis of forty-two patients with amyloidosis. Am J Med 1968;44: 955–959.
6. **Schwartz P.** Amyloidosis. Cause and manifestation of senile deterioration. Springfield, IL: Charles C Thomas, 1970:395.
7. **Kyle RA, Bayrd ED.** Amyloidosis: review of 236 cases. Medicine 1975; 54:271–300.
8. **Hodkinson HM, Pomerance A.** The clinical significance of senile cardiac amyloidosis: a prospective clinico-pathological study. Quart J Med 1977; 46:381–387.
9. **Smith RRL, Hutchins GM, Moore GW, Humphrey RL.** Type and distribution of pulmonary parenchymal and vascular amyloid. Correlation with cardiac amyloid. Am J Med 1979;66:96–104.
10. **Westermark P, Johansson B, Natvig JB.** Senile cardiac amyloidosis: evidence of two different amyloid substances in the aging heart. Scand J Immunol 1979;10:303–308.
11. **Cornwell GG III, Westermark P.** Senile amyloidosis: a protean manifestation of the aging process. J Clin Pathol 1980;33:1146–1152.
12. **Wright JR, Calkins E.** Clinical-pathological differentiation of common amyloid syndromes. Medicine 1981;60:429–448.
13. **Waller BF, Roberts WC.** Cardiovascular disease in the very elderly. Analysis of 40 necropsy patients aged 90 years or older. Am J Cardiol 1983;51: 403–421.
14. **Child JS, Levisman JA, Abbasi AS, MacAlpin RN.** Echocardiographic manifestations of infiltrative cardiomyopathy. A report of seven cases due to amyloid. Chest 1976;70:726–731.
15. **Borer JS, Henry WL, Epstein SE.** Echocardiographic observations in patients with systemic infiltrative disease involving the heart. Am J Cardiol 1977;39:184–188.
16. **Child JS, Krivokapich J, Abbasi AS.** Increased right ventricular wall thickness on echocardiography in amyloid infiltrative cardiomyopathy. Am J Cardiol 1979;44:1391–1395.
17. **Siqueira-Filho AG, Cunha CLP, Tajik AJ, Seward JB, Schattenberg TT, Giuliani ER.** M-mode and two-dimensional echocardiographic features in cardiac amyloidosis. Circulation 1981;63:188–196.
18. **St John Sutton MG, Reichek N, Kastor JA, Giuliani ER.** Computerized M-mode echocardiographic analysis of left ventricular dysfunction in cardiac amyloid. Circulation 1982;66:790–799.
19. **Bhandari AK, Nanda NC.** Myocardial texture characterization by two-dimensional echocardiography. Am J Cardiol 1983;51:817–825.
20. **Wizenberg TA, Muz J, Sohn YH, Samlowski W, Weissler AM.** Value of positive myocardial technetium-99m-pyrophosphate scintigraphy in the noninvasive diagnosis of cardiac amyloidosis. Am Heart J 1982;103: 468–473.
21. **Schiff S, Bateman T, Moffatt R, Davidson R, Berman D.** Diagnostic considerations in cardiomyopathy: unique scintigraphic pattern of diffuse biventricular technetium-99m-pyrophosphate uptake in amyloid heart disease. Am Heart J 1982;130:562–563.
22. **Sobol SM, Brown JM, Bunker SR, Patel J, Lull RJ.** Noninvasive diagnosis of cardiac amyloidosis by technetium-99m-pyrophosphate myocardial scintigraphy. Am Heart J 1982;103:563–566.
23. **Falk RH, Lee VW, Rubinow A, Hood WB Jr, Cohen AS.** Sensitivity of Technetium-99m-pyrophosphate scintigraphy in diagnosing cardiac amyloidosis. Am J Cardiol 1983;51:826–830.
24. **Chew C, Ziady GM, Raphael MJ, Oakley CM.** The functional defect in amyloid heart disese. The "stiff heart" syndrome. Am J Cardiol 1975;36: 438–444.
25. **Meaney E, Shabetai R, Bhargava V, Shearer M, Weidner C, Mangiardi, LM, Smalling R, Peterson K.** Cardiac amyloidosis, constrictive pericarditis and restrictive cardiomyopathy. Am J Cardiol 1976;38:547–556.
26. **Swanton RH, Brooksby IAB, Davies MJ, Coltart DJ, Jenkins BS, Webb-Peploe MM.** Systolic and diastolic ventricular function in cardiac amyloidosis. Studies in six cases diagnosed with endomyocardial biopsy. Am J Cardiol 1977;39:658–664.
27. **Tyberg TI, Goodyer AVN, Hurst VW III, Alexander J, Langou RA.** Left ventricular filling in differentiating restrictive amyloid cardiomyopathy and constrictive pericarditis. Am J Cardiol 1981;47:791–796.
28. **Schroeder JS, Billingham ME, Rider AK.** Cardiac amyloidosis. Diagnosis by transvenous endomyocardial biopsy. Am J Med 1975;59:269–273.
29. **Brodarick S, Paine R, Higa E, Carmichael KA.** Pericardial tamponade, a new complication of amyloid heart disease. Am J Med 1982;73:133–135.
30. **Shenoy UA, Peric-Golia L.** Primary cardiovascular amyloidosis manifesting as mitral stenosis. Hum Pathol 1982;13:768–770.
31. **Ridolfi RL, Bulkley BH, Hutchins GM.** The conduction system in cardiac amyloidosis. Clinical and pathologic features of 23 patients. Am J Med 1977;62:677–686.
32. **Bharati S, Lev M, Denes P, Modlinger J, Wyndham C, Bauernfeind R, Greenblatt M, Rosen KM.** Infiltrative cardiomyopathy with conduction disease and ventricular arrhythmia: electrophysiologic and pathologic correlations. Am J Cardiol 1980;45:163–173.
33. **Fisch C.** Electrocardiogram in the aged: an independent marker of heart disease? Am J Med 1981;70:4–6.
34. **Simonson F.** Differentiation between normal and abnormal in electrocardiography. St. Louis: CV Mosby, 1961:328.
35. **Siegel RJ, Roberts WC.** Electrocardiographic observations in severe aortic valve stenosis: correlative necropsy study to clinical, hemodynamic, and ECG variables demonstrating relation of 12-lead QRS amplitude to peak systolic transaortic pressure gradient. Am Heart J 1982;103:210–221.

Cardiac Involvement by Kaposi's Sarcoma in Acquired Immune Deficiency Syndrome (AIDS)

MARC A. SILVER, MD
ABE M. MACHER, MD
CHERYL M. REICHERT, MD, PhD
DAVID L. LEVENS, MD, PhD
JOSEPH E. PARRILLO, MD
DAN L. LONGO, MD
WILLIAM C. ROBERTS, MD

From the Pathology Branch, National Heart, Lung, and Blood Institute; Laboratory of Pathology, and Medicine Branch, National Cancer Institute, and Critical Care Medicine Department, The Clinical Center, National Institutes of Health, Bethesda, Maryland 20205. Manuscript received November 30, 1983, accepted December 16, 1983.

Acquired immune deficiency syndrome (AIDS), a recently described disease that affects primarily homosexuals and intravenous drug abusers, has generated considerable interest. At the National Institutes of Health we have performed autopsies on 18 patients with AIDS. General necropsy findings in the first 10 patients was recently reported.[1] This report focuses specifically on cardiac findings in the 18 patients.

Of the 18 patients, 5 (28%) had abnormalities in the heart, and in each they consisted of focal deposits of Kaposi's sarcoma (KS). All 5 patients were white men, aged 26 to 52 years (mean 41). The initial manifestation of AIDS in each was a dermal lesion which, on biopsy, was KS. The interval from the appearance of the dermal KS to death ranged from 6 to 22 months (mean 11). During life, no patient had symptoms attributable to cardiac dysfunction. ECGs recorded during the last 3.5 months of life were normal in all 5 patients. All 5 had normal-sized hearts by chest roentgenogram and all had normal-sized hearts at necropsy.

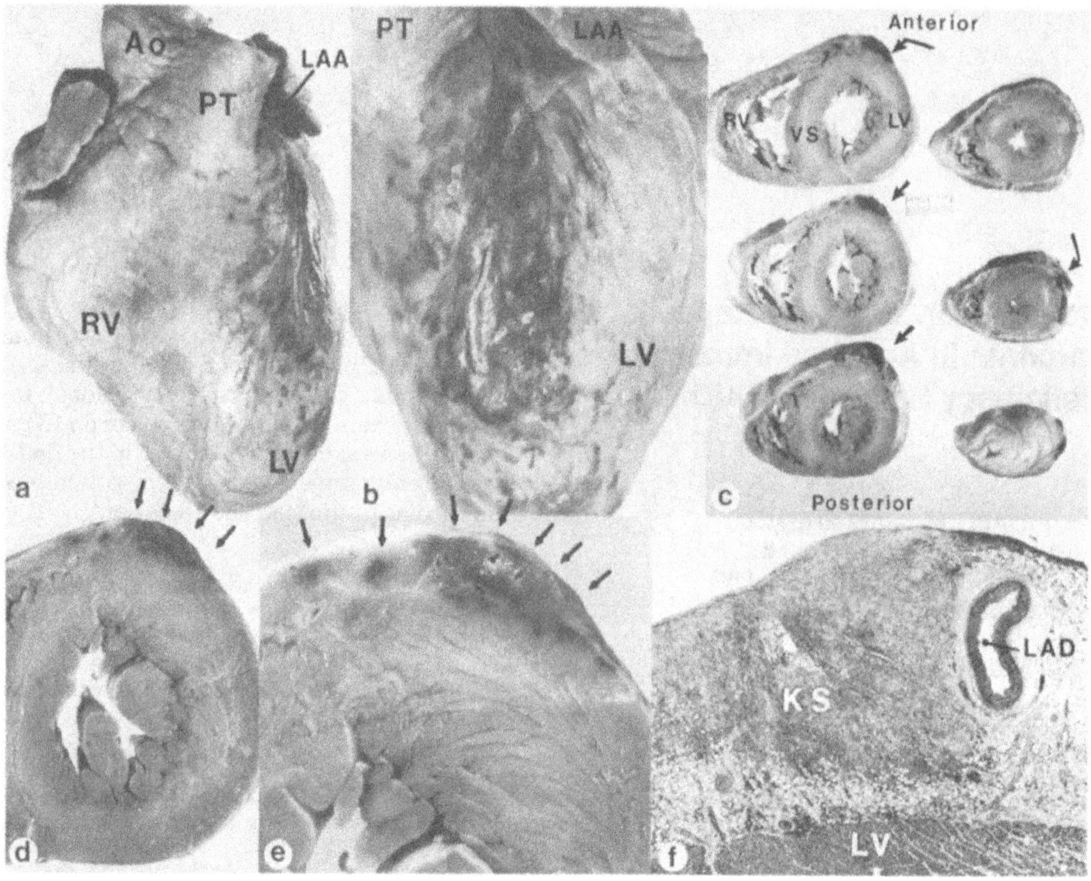

FIGURE 1. Gross and microscopic appearance of Kaposi's sarcoma (KS) in a 44-year-old man (A83-99) with symptomatic AIDS for 6 months before death. **a,** view of anterior surface of heart showing hemorrhagic area of KS involving subepicardial adipose tissue. Ao = ascending aorta; LAA = left atrial appendage; LV = left ventricle; PT = pulmonary trunk; RV = right ventricle. **b,** close-up view of **a**, showing KS surrounding the left anterior descending coronary artery. **c,** transverse slices of the cardiac ventricles showing tumor in subepicardial adipose tissue (**arrows**). VS = ventricular septum. **d** and **e,** close-up views showing tumor (**arrows**). **f,** photomicrograph demonstrating KS in adipose tissue adjacent to left anterior descending coronary artery (LAD) with uninvolved left ventricle below. Movat stain; magnification ×16, reduced 39%.

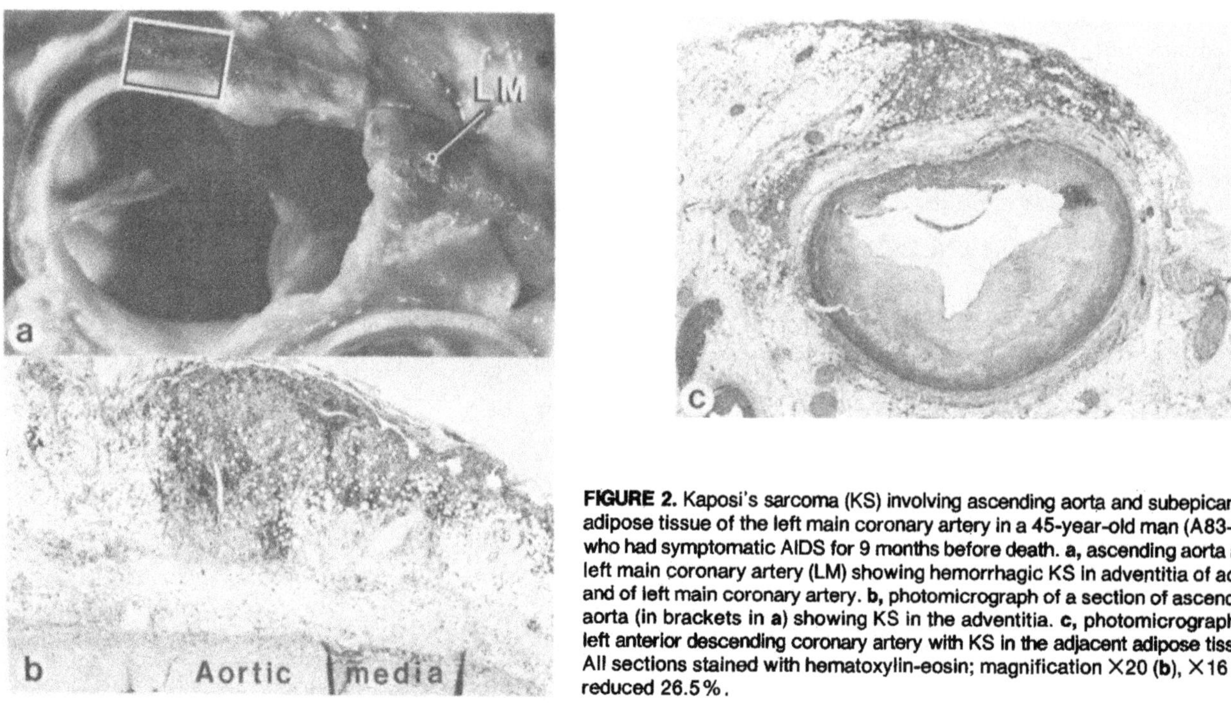

FIGURE 2. Kaposi's sarcoma (KS) involving ascending aorta and subepicardial adipose tissue of the left main coronary artery in a 45-year-old man (A83-94) who had symptomatic AIDS for 9 months before death. **a,** ascending aorta and left main coronary artery (LM) showing hemorrhagic KS in adventitia of aorta and of left main coronary artery. **b,** photomicrograph of a section of ascending aorta (in brackets in **a**) showing KS in the adventitia. **c,** photomicrograph of left anterior descending coronary artery with KS in the adjacent adipose tissue. All sections stained with hematoxylin-eosin; magnification ×20 (**b**), ×16 (**c**), reduced 26.5%.

At necropsy, small, focal, hemorrhagic areas involved subepicardial adipose tissue adjacent to 1 or more major coronary arteries in all 5 patients (Fig. 1). The KS was similar histologically to that seen in other anatomic sites, and was typical of what has been previously described.[1] *Three patients also had deposits of KS in the adventitia of ascending aorta, and 1 of them also had KS in the adventitia of the pulmonary trunk (Fig. 2). The myocardium and endocardium were free of KS. The lumens of the coronary arteries were normal in 4 patients, and 1 major coronary artery not involved by KS was narrowed 51 to 75% in cross-sectional area by atherosclerotic plaque in 1 patient. No infectious complications of AIDS were identified histologically.* Toxoplasma gondii, *however, was isolated in 1 patient from mice injected intraperitoneally with a homogenate of myocardium.*

Five of the 18 patients with AIDS studied at necropsy had cardiac abnormalities attributable to AIDS. In each, the abnormality consisted of KS in the subepicardial adipose tissue adjacent to a major coronary artery with or without involvement of the adventitia of ascending aorta or pulmonary trunk. In no patient did the KS compress or narrow the lumen of a coronary artery. No patient had clinical evidence of cardiac dysfunction. All 5 patients also had widely disseminated visceral, mucocutaneous and lymphatic KS. Disseminated KS, however, did occur in patients without cardiac involvement. Of the 18 necropsy patients with AIDS, 9 had KS: 5 had KS in the heart and 4 did not.

KS in the heart can occur in patients without AIDS, but its frequency and distribution is unclear, probably in part because at least 28 different terms have been used as synonyms for KS, including angiosarcoma.[2,3] We distinguish KS from angiosarcoma by the presence of cutaneous involvement with KS. Using this definition, patients with cardiac angiosarcoma, that is, without cutaneous involvement, usually have intracavitary tumor in the right atrium producing cardiac dysfunction. The pericardium and right ventricle also may be involved.[3,4]

Patients with cutaneous KS and cardiac involvement rarely have been reported. Lothe and Murray[5] described at necropsy 12 patients with cutaneous KS and 2 of them had cardiac involvement (Cases 8 and 9), which was epicardial in both, with extension to underlying myocardium in 1. Rarely, a patient with cutaneous KS may have extensive myocardial or intracavitary KS that produces dysfunction. In the case reported by Ayer et al,[6] cutaneous KS developed only 7 days before death, although cardiac dysfunction had been present for 11 years.

In patients with AIDS, however, as determined by examination of our 18 necropsy patients, asymptomatic cardiac involvement may occur, and that involvement in our patients was KS in subepicardial adipose tissue adjacent to 1 or more major coronary arteries with or without involvement of adventitia of ascending aorta or pulmonary trunk.

Addendum: Between submission of this manuscript and receipt of the galleys, we studied at necropsy 2 additional patients with AIDS. Both were white men, aged 28 and 33 years; both had cutaneous KS but neither had cardiac KS. One had focal acute myocarditis of undetermined etiology.

Acknowledgment: We appreciate the help of Drs. Carl C. Baker and Shyh-Ching Lo. Gross photography was done by M. M. M. Moore.

References

1. **Reichert CM, O'Leary TJ, Levens DL, Simrell CR, Macher AM.** Autopsy pathology in the acquired immune deficiency syndrome. Am J Pathol 1983;112:357–382.
2. **Choisser RM, Ramsey EM.** Angioreticuloendothelioma (Kaposi's disease) of the heart. Am J Pathol 1939;15:155–178.
3. **Glancy DL, Morales JB Jr, Roberts WC.** Angiosarcoma of the heart. Am J Cardiol 1968;21:413–419.
4. **Levison DA, Semple Pd'A.** Primary cardiac Kaposi's sarcoma. Thorax 1976;31:595–600.
5. **Lothe F, Murray JF.** Kaposi's sarcoma: autopsy findings in the African. Acta Unio Internationalis Contra Cancrum 1962;18:429–452.
6. **Ayer JP, Paul O, Capps RB.** Clinical pathologic conference. Am Heart J 1962;63:566–572.

Idiopathic Dilated Cardiomyopathy: Analysis of 152 Necropsy Patients

WILLIAM C. ROBERTS, MD, ROBERT J. SIEGEL, MD, and BRUCE M. McMANUS, MD, PhD

Certain clinical and cardiac necropsy findings are described in 152 patients aged 16 to 78 years (mean 45) with idiopathic dilated cardiomyopathy: 109 (72%) were men and 43 (28%) were women. Compared with the women, the men had a significantly (p <0.05) shorter mean duration of chronic congestive heart failure (CHF) (43 vs 69 months), a higher percentage of habitual alcoholism (40 vs 24%) and a higher mean heart weight (632 vs 551 g). The male to female ratio among the 58 known alcoholics was 7.3:1 and among the 70 known nonalcoholics, 1.5:1 (p <0.05). The mean duration of clinical evidence of CHF was similar among the known alcoholics and the known nonalcoholics (each 50 months). Of the 152 patients, 148 (97%) had clinical evidence of chronic CHF; in 114 patients it was the initial manifestation of idiopathic dilated cardiomyopathy, and in most it became intractable and caused death. The interval from onset of chronic CHF to death (known in 120 patients) ranged from 1 to 264 months (mean 54). Comparison of the 27 patients surviving >72 months after onset of chronic CHF to the 64 patients surviving ≤36 months disclosed a significantly higher frequency in the longer survival group of older patients, of women, of habitual alcoholics, of patients with chest pain syndromes, diabetes mellitus, pulmonary emboli, of patients treated with warfarin and of patients with larger hearts at necropsy. Each of the 4 patients without chronic CHF died suddenly and sudden death was the initial manifestation of idiopathic dilated cardiomyopathy in them. An additional 33 patients also died suddenly, but each of them previously had had chronic CHF. Of the 79 patients (of the 131 for whom information was available) with either pulmonary or systemic emboli or both, 67 (85%) had either right- or left-sided thrombi or mural endocardial plaques or both, whereas of the 52 patients without emboli, 36 (69%) had intracardiac thrombi or plaques (p <0.05). Electrocardiograms in the last 6 months of life in 101 patients disclosed atrial fibrillation in 25; complete left (41 patients) or right (6 patients) bundle branch block or indeterminate intraventricular conduction delay (4 patients) in 51 patients; QRS voltage indicative of ventricular hypertrophy in 44 patients (left ventricular in 39 patients). The patients with left bundle branch block compared with those without had a significantly longer duration of CHF, (83 vs 43 months), larger mean heart weights (628 vs 590 g) and a higher frequency of grossly visible scars (44 vs 13%). The total 12-lead QRS amplitude in 35 men ranged from 74 to 250 mm (mean 147) (10 mm = 1 mV) and in the 14 women from 75 to 243 mm (mean 167). The hearts at necropsy in the women ranged from 360 to 860 g (mean 551) and in the men from 400 to 940 g (mean 632) (p <0.05). Grossly visible left ventricular scars were observed in 22 (14%) patients. Histologic examination (96 patients) of sections of the ventricular myocardium disclosed interstitial or replacement fibrosis in 55 patients (57%), and inflammatory cell infiltrates in 5 patients.

(Am J Cardiol 1987;60:1340–1355)

Idiopathic dilated cardiomyopathy (IDC) is a well-recognized condition both clinically and morphologically. It is characterized by dilatation of both ventricular cavities and manifested clinically by chronic congestive heart failure (CHF), which usually becomes intractable and eventually fatal. Despite the relative frequency of this condition, few studies focusing on a large number of necropsy patients have been reported. Herein, we describe certain clinical and morphologic features in 152 necropsy patients fulfilling a rigorous definition of IDC.

Patients Studied

Criteria for inclusion: All 152 patients were older than 15 years of age, all had dilated right and left ventricular cavities and all had hearts of increased weight (>350 g in women and >400 g in men). None had narrowing of any of the epicardial coronary arteries of >75% in cross-sectional area, none had a significant congenital cardiac anomaly, none had an anatomically abnormal cardiac valve (except for minimal focal thickening of the margins of the anterior mitral leaflet), none had a defect in the atrial or ventricular septum other than possibly a valvular competent patent foramen ovale, none had an infiltrative myocardial disease (such as amyloid, sarcoid, iron, calcium or glycogen), none had a systemic disease other than possibly adult-onset diabetes mellitus, none had a neurologic disease, none had extensive cystic or interstitial pulmonary parenchymal disease and none had a major grossly visible abnormality of the pericardium. During the last 3 months of life, the systemic arterial systolic pressure was <140 mm Hg and the systemic arterial diastolic pressure was <90 mm Hg. Additionally, none had clinical evidence in the past of hypertrophic cardiomyopathy and none had other family members who had hypertrophic cardiomyopathy. Patients with complete heart block from birth were excluded, and patients who had received a drug known to be capable of causing a dilated cardiomyopathy, such as doxorubicin, were excluded. Patients with a history of habitual alcoholism were included and considered to have idiopathic dilated cardiomyopathy.

From the Pathology Branch, National Heart, Lung, and Blood Institute, National Institutes of Health, Bethesda, Maryland. Manuscript received July 22, 1987, revised manuscript received and accepted August 18, 1987.

Address for reprints: William C. Roberts, MD, Building 10, Room 2N-258, National Institutes of Health, Bethesda, Maryland 20892.

Dr. Siegel's present address is Division of Cardiology, Department of Medicine, Cedars-Sinai Medical Center, Los Angeles, California.

Dr. McManus's present address is Cardiovascular Registry, Department of Pathology and Microbiology, University of Nebraska Medical Center, Omaha, Nebraska.

Selection of cases: All hearts and clinical and morphologic records of cases classified as IDC in the files of the Pathology Branch, National Heart, Lung, and Blood Institute, were reviewed. Of nearly 200 cases so classified, nearly 50 were eliminated from this study because they did not fulfill the aforementioned clinical and morphologic criteria. A total of 152 patients fulfilled the criteria and form the basis of this report. The clinical and necropsy records were reviewed in all 152 patients. Detailed data on the electrocardiograms recorded in the last 6 months of life were available in 101 of the 152 patients, and in 55 the electrocardiograms themselves were reexamined. All 152 hearts were examined initially by 1 of us (WCR) and most were examined later by RJS and BMM. All patients were studied at necropsy from 1959 through April 1981. The patients were studied clinically at 14 different hospitals, mainly those located in the Washington, DC, area, and the hearts were subsequently brought to one of us (WCR) for examination. In addition to the gross examination of each heart, at least 2 histologic sections of left ventricular wall extending from endocardium to epicardium and measuring ≥2 cm in circumferential length were examined in 96 of the 152 cases. A least 1 full-thickness histologic section of ventricular septum and right ventricular free wall also was examined in 80 and 88 of these 96 patients, respectively.

Statistics: Comparisons of all parametric data were made using the 2-tailed *t* test for independent samples when comparisons between 2 groups were made, and using a 1-way analysis of variance when comparisons among ≥3 groups were made. The level of significance was 0.05. Comparisons of nonparametric data were made using the chi-square method with a level of significance of 0.05. Correlations were tested using Spearman's rho and linear regression coefficients and calculated when deemed useful.

Clinical Findings

Age, race, sex and duration of congestive heart failure: The 152 patients ranged in age from 16 to 78

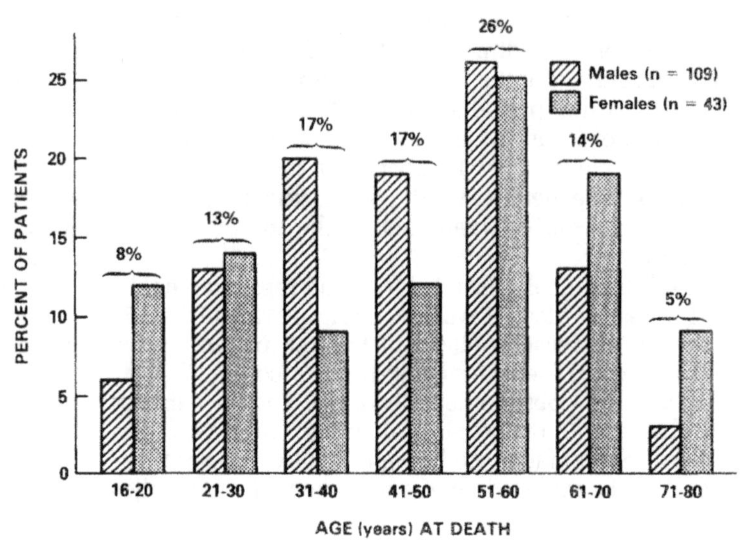

FIGURE 1. Bar graph showing the percent of patients with idiopathic dilated cardiomyopathy dying during various decades.

TABLE I Certain Clinical and Necropsy Characteristics of 152 Patients with Idiopathic Dilated Cardiomyopathy and Comparisons Between 109 Men and 43 Women

	Total (n = 152)	Men (n = 109)	Women (n = 43)	p Value
Age (yr) (mean)	16–78 (45)	16–73 (45)	16–78 (49)	NS
Black:white	90:47 (1.9:1)	63:36 (1.8:1)	27:11 (2.5:1)	NS
Duration (mo) CHF	0–240 (54)	6–204 (43)	1–240 (69)	<0.05
Pulmonary edema	34/86 (40%)	21/61 (34%)	13/25 (52%)	NS
Angina pectoris	15/105 (14%)	11/75 (15%)	4/30 (13%)	NS
Nonanginal chest pain	40/114 (35%)	29/82 (35%)	11/32 (34%)	NS
"AMI" (history)	25/113 (22%)	17/80 (21%)	8/33 (24%)	NS
Alcoholism	49/136 (36%)	40/99 (40%)	9/37 (24%)	NS
Emboli				
Pulmonary, clinical	49/126 (39%)	31/89 (35%)	18/37 (49%)	NS
Pulmonary, necropsy	39/101 (39%)	29/72 (40%)	10/29 (34%)	NS
Systemic, clinical	24/122 (20%)	20/88 (23%)	4/34 (12%)	NS
Pulmonary, necropsy	23/90 (26%)	19/65 (29%)	4/25 (16%)	NS
Mode of death				
Chronic CHF	81/139 (58%)	55/98 (56%)	26/41 (63%)	NS
Sudden	38/139 (27%)	28/98 (29%)	10/41 (24%)	NS
Pulmonary embolus	12/139 (9%)	8/98 (8%)	4/41 (10%)	NS
Other	8/139 (6%)	7/98 (7%)	1/41 (2%)	NS
Heart weight (g)	400–940 (605)	400–940 (632)	360–860 (551)	<0.05
Intracavitary thrombi (T) only	42/148 (28%)	30/105 (29%)	12/43 (28%)	NS
Endocardial plaques (P) only	32/148 (22%)	22/105 (21%)	10/43 (23%)	NS
Both T and P	37/148 (25%)	28/105 (27%)	9/43 (21%)	NS
Transmural LV scars (gross)	9/148 (6%)	9/105 (9%)	5/43 (12%)	NS
LV replacement fibrosis (microscopic only)	71/96 (73%)	50/74 (68%)	21/22 (95%)	<0.05

AMI = acute myocardial infarction; CHF = chronic congestive heart failure; LV = left ventricular; NS = not significant (p >0.05); SD = sudden death.

years (mean 45) (Figure 1). Of the 137 in whom race was known, 90 (66%) were black and 47 (34%) were white. Of the 152 patients, 109 (72%) were men and 43 (28%) were women. Comparison of various clinical and morphologic findings between the men and women is summarized in Table I. Of the 16 factors analyzed, 3 were significantly (p <0.05) different between the 2 groups. Compared with women, men had a shorter mean duration of chronic CHF (43 vs 69 months), a higher percentage of habitual alcoholism (40 vs 24%) and a higher mean heart weight (632 vs 551 g).

Relation to pregnancy: Of the 43 women, the relation of onset of symptoms of chronic CHF to pregnancy was known in 39. In 13 (33%) of them, symptoms of CHF appeared either during pregnancy (2 patients) or within 12 months after delivery (11 patients). In 7 of the latter 11 patients, the onset of symptoms of cardiac dysfunction was within 3 months of delivery. Comparison of findings in the 13 women with onset of CHF in the peripartum period to those in 26 women in whom the onset of CHF was known not to be related to pregnancy disclosed only 1 statistically significant factor (Table II): the mean age of the peripartum patients was younger (p <0.001) than that of the nonperipartum patients.

Habitual alcoholism: Information regarding habitual intake of alcohol was available in 128 of the 152 patients. At least 58 (45%) of the 128 patients were considered by their physicians to be "alcoholic." Comparison of 15 observations in the 58 known habitual alcoholics with those in the 70 nonalcoholic cases disclosed several factors to be significantly different (Table III). The male to female ratio among the alcoholics was 7.3:1 and in the nonalcoholics, 1.5:1 (p <0.05). The mean duration of symptoms of CHF was the same (50 months); the mean heart weight (631 vs 593 g) was significantly (p <0.05) greater in the alcoholics compared with the nonalcoholics, a reflection of the greater proportion of men in the alcoholic group.

Diabetes mellitus: Information regarding the presence or absence of diabetes mellitus was available in 110 of the 152 patients. Of that number, 8 patients (7%) (4 men, 4 women) had known diabetes mellitus beginning after age 35. Their ages at death ranged from 37 to 71 years (mean 55) and their ages at onset of diabetes from 36 to 64 years (mean 51). Two patients were treated with insulin and 4 with hypoglycemic agents; the type of diabetic treatment received in the other 2 patients is uncertain. Two of the 8 patients were habitual alcoholics. The duration of chronic CHF in the 8 patients ranged from 24 to 204 months (mean 105). At necropsy, 2 of the 8 patients had grossly visible left ventricular scars, and on histologic examination, none had abnormalities of the intramural coronary arteries.

Familial cardiomyopathy: At least 1 other family member had a similar fatal cardiac condition in 9 (6%) of the 152 patients. Of these 9 patients, at least 20 family members were affected by a similar cardiac condition, and all of the 20 affected relatives died before age 50 years, most before age 40 years. The 9 patients with familial dilated cardiomyopathy ranged in age from 17 to 58 years (mean 37); 7 were men and 2 were women. Only 2 were habitual alcoholics. The duration of the chronic CHF in 8 of the 9 patients ranged from 3 to 72 months (mean 46); the ninth patient had evidence of CHF for only 10 days. Six of the 9 patients died from chronic CHF and 3 died suddenly.

TABLE II *Idiopathic Dilated Cardiomyopathy in Women: Comparison of Findings in 13 Necropsy Patients with Onset in Peripartum Period to Those in 26 Necropsy Patients with Onset in Nonperipartum Period*

	Peripartum Onset (n = 13)	Nonperipartum Onset (n = 26)	p Value
Age (yr) (mean)	18–61 (32)	21–78 (57)	<0.001
Black:white	10:3	18:8	NS
Systemic hypertension	1 (8%)	8 (31%)	NS
Habitual alcoholism	2 (15%)	7 (27%)	NS
Duration CHF (mo) (mean)	2–264 (65)	1–240 (65)	NS
Embolic events	7 (54%)	18 (69%)	NS
Pulmonary	6 (46%)	13 (50%)	NS
Systemic	1 (8%)	5 (19%)	NS
Sudden death	3 (23%)	7 (26%)	NS
Heart weight (g) (mean)	370–770 (512)	360–810 (567)	NS
Transmural LV scars	1 (8%)	8 (31%)	NS
Intracardiac thrombi (only)	3 (23%)	8 (31%)	NS
Endocardial plaques (only)	3 (23%)	6 (22%)	NS
Both plaques and thrombi	2 (15%)	7 (27%)	NS
Either plaques or thrombi	8 (61%)	21 (81%)	NS

CHF = congestive heart failure; LV = left ventricular; NS = not significant.

TABLE III **Clinical and Necropsy Characteristics of 58 Alcoholic and 70 Nonalcoholic Patients with Idiopathic Dilated Cardiomyopathy**

	Alcoholic (n = 58)	Nonalcoholic (n = 70)	p Value
Age (yr) (mean)	21–78 (46)	16–75 (45)	NS
Male:female	51:7 (7.3:1)	42:28 (1.5:1)	<0.05
Black:white	37:14 (2.6:1)	34:29 (1.2:1)	NS
Duration (mo) CHF	0–144 (50)	1–168 (50)	NS
Pulmonary edema	9/33 (27%)	18/46 (39%)	<0.05
Angina pectoris	8/43 (19%)	7/59 (12%)	NS
"AMI" (history)	14/43 (32%)	8/61 (13%)	<0.05
Emboli			
Pulmonary, clinical	18/39 (46%)	24/59 (41%)	NS
Pulmonary, necropsy	16/36 (44%)	26/41 (63%)	<0.05
Systemic, clinical	12/41 (29%)	6/71 (8%)	<0.05
Systemic, necropsy	13/35 (37%)	8/38 (21%)	<0.05
Mode of death			
Chronic CHF	26/46 (57%)	39/67 (58%)	NS
Sudden death	14/46 (30%)	19/67 (28%)	NS
Pulmonary embolus	5/46 (11%)	5/67 (7%)	NS
Other	1/46 (2%)	4/67 (6%)	NS
Heart weight (g) (mean)	360–940 (631)	370–940 (593)	<0.05
Intracavitary thrombi (T) only	16/58 (28%)	18/70 (26%)	NS
Endocardial plaques (P) only	12/58 (21%)	14/70 (20%)	NS
Both T and P	16/58 (28%)	15/70 (21%)	NS
Transmural LV scars (gross)	8/58 (14%)	3/69 (4%)	NS
Replacement fibrosis (microscopic)	20/34 (59%)	19/31 (61%)	NS

AMI = acute myocardial function; CHF = congestive heart failure; LV = left ventricular; NS = not significant.

None of the 9 and none of the affected family members had evidence either clinically or morphologically of hypertrophic cardiomyopathy.

Congestive heart failure: Of the 152 patients, 148 (97%) had clinical evidence of chronic CHF; in 114 patients, it was the initial manifestation of their illness, and in most it became intractable and caused death. Good information on the interval from onset of chronic CHF to death was available in 120 of the 148 patients and it ranged from 1 to 264 months (mean 54) (Table I and Figure 2). From onset of CHF to death in these patients, 29 (24%) lived ≤12 months; 54 (45%), 13 to 60 months; 20 (17%) 61 to 120 months and 16 (14%), >120 months. These 120 patients were divided into 3 survival periods and 13 factors were compared (Table IV). Comparison of the 27 patients surviving >72 months after onset of chronic CHF to the 64 patients surviving ≤36 months disclosed a significantly ($p < 0.05$) higher frequency in the longer survival group of older patients, of women, of habitual alcoholics, of patients with chest pain syndromes, diabetes mellitus and pulmonary emboli, of patients treated with warfarin and of patients with bigger hearts at necropsy.

Sudden death: Each of the 4 patients without clinical evidence of chronic CHF died suddenly and unexpectedly and sudden death in them was the initial manifestation of IDC. All 4 were men aged 23 to 43 years (mean 31) with hearts weighing 480 to 780 g

TABLE IV Duration of Survival in Idiopathic Dilated Cardiomyopathy: Clinical and Necropsy Findings

	Duration (mo) of Survival			
	≤36	>36–72	>72	p value
Number of patients	64 (53%)	29 (24%)	27 (23%)	—
Age (yr) (mean)	16–75 (40)	20–71 (49)	16 –75 (51)	<0.05
Black:white	35/60(58%):25/60(42%)	16/27(59%):11/27(41%)	13/22(59%):9/22(41%)	NS
Male:female	49(77%):15(23%)	21(72%):8(28%)	13(48%):14(52%)	<0.05
Duration (mo) CHF (mean)	0–36 (15)	38–72 (58)	84–264 (131)	<0.05
Mode of death				
CHF	33 (52%)	17 (59%)	18 (67%)	<0.05
Sudden	12 (18%)	5 (17%)	3 (11%)	NS
Pulmonary emboli	6 (9%)	2 (7%)	4 (15%)	NS
Other	5 (7%)	4 (14%)	2 (7%)	NS
History				
Pulmonary edema	15 (21%)	9 (31%)	5 (36%)	<0.05
Angina pectoris	5 (7%)	4 (14%)	4 (20%)	<0.05
AMI	9 (14%)	5 (17%)	8 (33%)	<0.05
Hypertension	9 (14%)	2 (7%)	4 (17%)	NS
Diabetes mellitus	6 (8%)	3 (10%)	6 (26%)	<0.05
Emboli				
Pulmonary, clinical	21 (33%)	8 (28%)	13 (54%)	<0.05
Pulmonary, necropsy	23 (36%)	7 (24%)	9 (47%)	<0.05
Systemic, clinical	10 (16%)	6 (21%)	4 (17%)	NS
Systemic, necropsy	11 (17%)	4 (14%)	6 (32%)	NS
Warfarin therapy				
≥3 mo <12 mo	9 (14%)	5 (17%)	9 (33%)	<0.05
≥12 mo	3 (4%)	2 (7%)	6 (22%)	NS
Heart weight (g) (mean)	400–940 (586)	360–940 (615)	400–860 (625)	<0.05
LV scar				
Transmural	7 (11%)	3 (10%)	2 (7%)	NS
Subendocardial	9 (14%)	3 (10%)	5 (18%)	NS
Intracardiac				
Thrombi only	24 (36%)	7 (24%)	6 (22%)	NS
Plaques only	12 (18%)	3 (10%)	12 (44%)	<0.05
Both thrombi and plaques	14 (22%)	6 (21%)	7 (26%)	NS
Replacement fibrosis (microscopic)	7/25 (28%)	5/14 (36%)	3/18 (17%)	NS

Abbreviations as in Table III.

(mean 640). Three were habitual alcoholics. None had histories of systemic hypertension or evidence of diabetes mellitus. Thirty other patients died suddenly, but each of them previously had had CHF; of them, 19 had fatal cardiac arrest outside the hospital and the other 14 patients, while in the hospital.

Emboli: Information regarding the presence or absence of pulmonary or systemic emboli or both was available in 131 of the 152 patients, and of them 79 patients (60%) had either clinical or necropsy evidence or both of embolic events. Of the 79 patients, 40 (51%) had pulmonary emboli only, 13 (16%) had systemic emboli only and 26 (33%) had both. Thus, of the 79 patients, there were 66 (84%) with pulmonary emboli or infarcts and 39 (49%) with systemic emboli or infarcts. The manner in which the emboli were diagnosed, either clinically or morphologically or both, and their relation to intracardiac thrombi and to mural en-

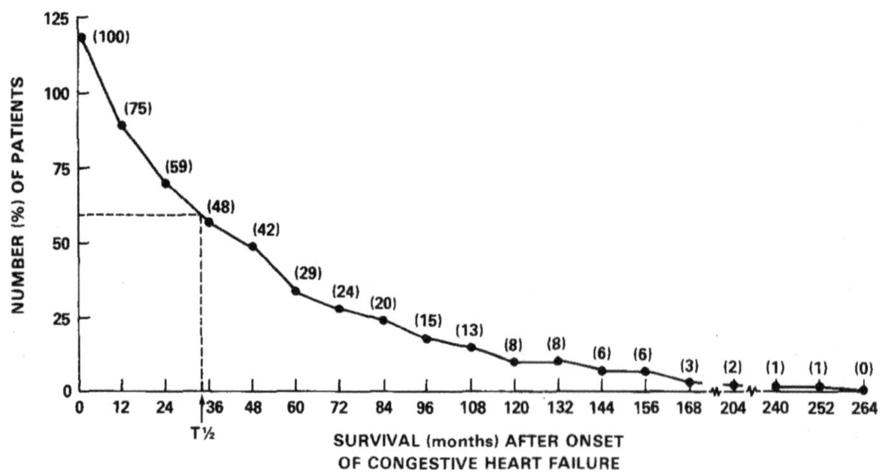

FIGURE 2. Cumulative survival of 118 patients with idiopathic dilated cardiomyopathy after onset of congestive heart failure. One-half of the patients were dead in <36 months ($T_{1/2}$).

TABLE V Frequency of Pulmonary and Systemic Emboli and Infarcts and Relation to Intracardiac Thrombi and Mural Endocardial Plaques in Idiopathic Dilated Cardiomyopathy

Present	Pt	Diagnosis: Clinically Only	Diagnosis: Necropsy Only	Diagnosis: Both	RV T Only	RV Plaques Only	Both	RAA T	RV or RAA T	Right-Sided T or Plaque	LV T Only	LV Plaques Only	Both	LAA T	LV or LAA T	Left-Sided T or Plaque	Either Right- or Left-Sided T or Plaque or Both	WS Rx
Pulmonary Emboli or Infarcts																		
+	66	19 (29%)	17 (20%)	30 (45%)	26 (39%)	8 (12%)	5 (8%)	20 (30%)	37 (56%)	45 (68%)	19 (29%)	11 (17%)	19 (29%)	10 (15%)	39 (59%)	50 (76%)	54 (82%)	12 (18%)
0	65	0	0	0	11 (17%)	4 (6%)	4 (6%)	15 (23%)	21 (32%)	26 (40%)	11 (17%)	14 (22%)	11 (17%)	11 (17%)	28 (43%)	45 (69%)	48 (74%)	11 (17%)
Systemic Emboli or Infarcts																		
+	39	15 (39%)	11 (28%)	13 (33%)	15 (22%)	7 (18%)	4 (10%)	13 (33%)	20 (51%)	29 (74%)	11 (28%)	8 (21%)	14 (36%)	6 (3%)	26 (66%)	34 (87%)	39 (100%)	10 (26%)
0	92	0	0	0	21 (23%)	5 (5%)	5 (5%)	20 (22%)	36 (39%)	40 (43%)	14 (15%)	22 (24%)	13 (14%)	13 (14%)	37 (40%)	59 (64%)	63 (68%)	13 (14%)
Total: Pulmonary or Systemic Emboli or Both																		
+	79	24 (30%)	20 (25%)	28* (35%)	29 (37%)	12 (15%)	6 (8%)	24 (30%)	41 (52%)	47 (59%)	33 (42%)	14 (18%)	28 (35%)	11 (14%)	64 (81%)	59 (75%)	67 (85%)	17 (22%)
0	52	0	0	0	8 (15%)	1 (27%)	3 (6%)	9 (17%)	15 (29%)	17 (33%)	9 (17%)	15 (29%)	8 (15%)	9 (17%)	20 (38%)	34 (65%)	36 (69%)	6 (12%)

* In an additional 2 patients with both pulmonary and systemic emboli, one was diagnosed clinically only and the other was diagnosed only at necropsy.
LAA = left atrial appendage; LV = left ventricular; RAA = right atrial appendage; RV = right ventricular; Rx = treatment; T = thrombus; WS = warfarin sodium.

docardial plaques (almost surely the result of organization of thrombi) are summarized in Table V. Comparison of the 66 patients with pulmonary emboli or infarcts to the 64 without disclosed a significantly higher frequency of right-sided intracardiac thrombi or endocardial plaques or both in the former (68 vs 40%, p <0.05). Comparison of the 39 patients with systemic emboli or infarcts to the 92 without also disclosed a significantly higher frequency of left-sided intracardiac thrombi or endocardial plaques or both in the former (87 vs 64%, p <0.05). Of the 79 patients with either pulmonary or systemic emboli or both, 67 (85%) had either right- or left-sided thrombi or mural endocardial plaques or both, whereas of the 52 without emboli, 36 (69%) had intracardiac thrombi or plaques (p <0.05). The numbers of patients treated with warfarin sodium were not large enough to make meaningful conclusions.

Electrocardiographic findings: Electrocardiographic observations during the last 6 months of life were available in 101 of the 152 patients and the findings are summarized in Table VI. Of the 101 patients, 25 had atrial fibrillation, and findings in them are summarized in Table VII and compared with observations in 25 age- and sex-matched patients with sinus rhythm: no significant differences were noted with regard to race, history of habitual alcoholism, duration of chronic CHF or mode of death. The patients with atrial fibrillation had a lower frequency of embolic events (64 vs 80%) and a lower frequency of intracardiac thrombi (13 vs 18 patients). The frequency of atrial thrombi among the 2 groups of patients was identical. P-wave abnormalities (in addition to their absence in 25% of the patients) were present in 49 of the 101 patients; left only in 35, right only in 6 and both in 8.

Either left ventricular (38 patients) or right (5 patients) ventricular hypertrophy or both (1 patient) were observed electrocardiographically in 44 patients. Complete bundle branch block occurred in 51 patients: left in 41, right in 6 and indeterminate intraventricular conduction delay in 4. Comparison of 32 patients with complete left bundle branch block to 33 with left ventricular hypertrophy and 15 with neither bundle branch block nor left ventricular hypertrophy disclosed that the patients with left bundle branch block had an older mean age (55 vs 45 years vs 42 years [p <0.05]), a longer mean duration of chronic CHF (83 vs 32 months vs 43 months [p <0.05]), larger mean heart weights (628 vs 605 vs 590 g [p <0.05]) and higher frequencies of grossly visible left ventricular scars (44 vs 21 vs 13% [p <0.05]). These observations are summarized in Table VIII and in Figure 3.

In 49 patients in whom electrocardiograms were recorded in the last year of life and available for reexamination, the QRS amplitude in all 12 leads was measured (Table IX, Figure 4). The total 12-lead QRS amplitude in the 35 men (mean age 46 years) ranged from 74 to 250 mm (10 mm = 1 mV) (mean 147) and in the 14 women (mean age 54 years), from 75 to 243 mm (mean 167). The heart weights in the 35 men ranged from 400 to 940 g (mean 620), and in the 14 women, from 400 to 860 g (mean 602). The maximal width of the QRS complex in the 35 men averaged 0.104 second and in 19 patients (54%) was ≥0.12 second; the width in the 14 women averaged 0.122 second and in 11 (79%) patients it was ≥0.12 second. The mean PR interval and QT interval were identical in both men and women (0.19 and 0.39 second, respectively).

The mean 12-lead QRS amplitude among 18 patients with complete left bundle branch block, in 22 patients with electrocardiographic evidence of left ventricular hypertrophy and in 10 patients with neither left bundle branch block nor electrocardiographic left ventricular hypertrophy did not correlate with heart weight (Figure 3). Comparison of total 12-lead QRS amplitude in all 12 leads to heart weight within each group, however, disclosed a striking positive correlation between total 12-lead QRS amplitude and heart weight in the group with complete left bundle branch block (r = +0.81). Because the coefficient of determination was 0.66, approximately two-thirds of the total QRS amplitude in all 12 leads are presumed to be determined by heart weight in our patients with IDC and left bundle block branch. The correlation coefficients between total 12-lead QRS voltage and either voltage criteria of left ventricular hypertrophy or left bundle branch block or neither electrocardiographic criteria for left ventricular hypertrophy nor left bundle branch block were +0.09 and +0.15, re-

TABLE VI Electrocardiographic Findings in 101 Necropsy Patients with Idiopathic Dilated Cardiomyopathy*

	Number (= %)
Rhythm	
Sinus	76
Atrial fibrillation	25
QRS axis abnormality	50
Left (−30 to −90°)	43
Right (110 to 270°)	7
Atrial abnormality	49
Left†	35
Right‡	6
Both	8
Ventricular hypertrophy	44
Left§ only	38
Without strain pattern	21
With‖ strain pattern	17
Right§ only	5
Both	1
Conduction abnormality¶	
Prolonged (>0.20 s) P-R interval	23
Second degree atrioventricular block	1
Complete atrioventricular block	1
Complete bundle branch block	51
Left	41
Right	6
Indeterminant intraventricular conduction delay	4
Arrhythmias, episodic	
Atrial premature complexes	12
Ventricular premature complexes	41
Supraventricular tachycardia	7
Ventricular tachycardia	5
Low voltage (sum QRS in I, II + III ≤ 15 mm)	22
Myocardial damage pattern	38
A. Poor R-wave progression precordial leads**	22
B. Q wave II, III, aVF	7
C. Q wave I, AVL, V_{4-6}	2
D. Combinations A. + B. =	5
B. + C. =	2
Nonspecific ST-T wave changes	12

* Based on analysis of electrocardiograms in 55 patients and detailed reports in 46 patients.

† P terminal force in V_1 is equal to or more negative than −0.04 mm-s.

‡ P wave has height 2.5 mm in leads II, III or AVG.

§ Criteria of Chou.

‖ ST-segment depressed with upward convexity and final downward slope ends in an inverted T wave.

¶ Eleven patients had neither complete bundle branch block nor left ventricular hypertrophy.

** R wave in lead V_3 ≤4 mm.

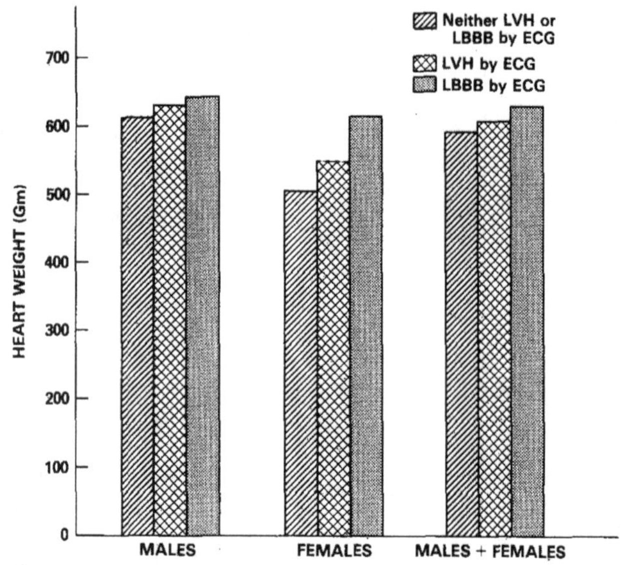

FIGURE 3. Bar graph showing relation of heart weight to electrocardiographic evidence of left ventricular hypertrophy (LVH) or left bundle branch block (LBBB) or neither in both sexes.

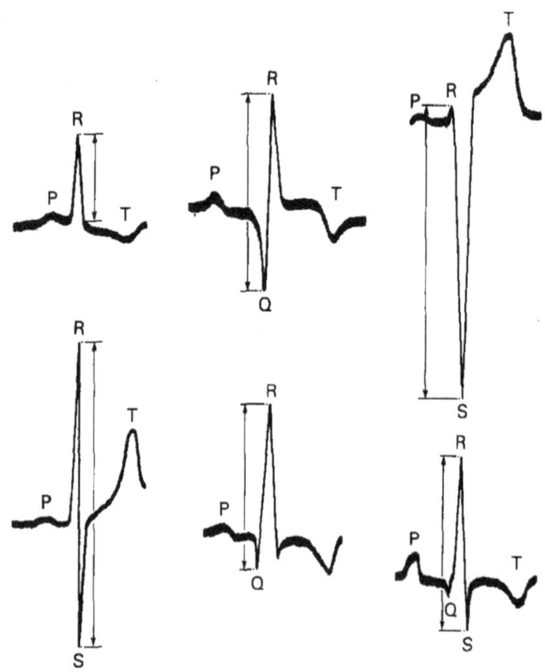

FIGURE 4. Various electrocardiographic QRS complexes showing how the voltage (in mm) was measured. Reproduced with permission from C.V. Mosby.[52]

TABLE VII Clinical and Necropsy Characteristics of 50 Patients with Idiopathic Dilated Cardiomyopathy: 25 with Atrial Fibrillation and 25 with Sinus Rhythm

	Sinus Rhythm (n = 25)	Atrial Fibrillation (n = 25)	p Value
Age (yr) (mean)	20–75 (49)	22–73 (53)	NS
Black:white	14:11 (56%:44%)	16:9 (64%:36%)	NS
Male:female	17:8 (68%:32%)	20:5 (80%:20%)	NS
Habitual alcoholism	12 (48%)	10 (40%)	NS
Duration (mo) CHF (mean)	8–168 (53)	1–264 (52)	NS
Mode of death			
CHF	17 (68%)	14 (60%)	NS
Emboli	3 (12%)	1 (4%)	NS
Sudden	4 (16%)	6 (26%)	NS
Other	1 (4%)	2 (8%)	NS
Emboli	20 (80%)	14 (64%)	NS
Pulmonary	15 (62%)	11 (44%)	NS
Systemic	10 (40%)	8 (32%)	NS
Electrocardiogram			
LV hypertrophy	3 (12%)	4 (16%)	NS
With strain	12 (48%)	2 (8%)	<0.01
Left BBB	9 (36%)	11 (44%)	NS
Right BBB	0	3 (12%)	NS
Heart weight (g)			
Total (mean)	400–940 (627)	370–770 (593)	NS
Male (mean)	440–940 (654)	390–760 (604)	NS
Female (mean)	400–860 (560)	370–770 (552)	NS
Cardiac thrombi			
RA-LA-RV-LV	10-6-12-15	10-6-6-7	<0.05
Thrombi only	7 (28%)	12 (48%)	NS
Mural plaque			
RA-LA-RV-LV	2-1-8-13	1-1-3-5	0.05
Plaque only	4 (16%)	4 (16%)	NS
Thrombi + plaque	11 (44%)	1 (4%)	0.001
Either:neither	22:3 (88%:12%)	17:8 (68%:32%)	NS
LV scars			
S:T	4:6	2:8	NS

BBB = bundle branch block; CHF = congestive heart failure; LA = left atrium; LV = left ventricular or left ventricle; NS = not significant; RA = right atrium; RV = right ventricle; S = subendocardial; T = transmural.

TABLE VIII Clinical and Necropsy Characteristics of Patients with Idiopathic Dilated Cardiomyopathy and Left Bundle Branch Block (BBB), Left Ventricular (LV) Hypertrophy or Neither by Electrocardiogram

	Left BBB (n = 32)	LV Hypertrophy (n = 33)	Neither (n = 15)
Ages (yr) (mean)	27–71 (55)	20–75 (45)	22–66 (42)
Male:female	21:11	27:6	8:7
Duration (mo) CHF (mean)	1–168 (83)	2–96 (32)	2–84 (43)
Heart weight (g) (mean)			
Male + female	400–860 (628)	400–870 (605)	370–940 (590)
Male only	400–860 (642)	400–870 (629)	410–940 (613)
Female only	460–800 (613)	440–650 (548)	370–680 (503)
Left ventricular scar			
Transmural (T):non-T	4:10 (12%:30%)	3:4 (9%:12%)	2:0 (13%:0)

spectively, indicating an insignificant relation between total 12-lead QRS amplitude and heart weight in these latter 2 groups.

Myocardial damage patterns unassociated with complete bundle branch block were observed by electrocardiogram in 38 (38%) of the 101 patients (Table VI). Thus, of the 50 patients without complete bundle branch block, 37 (76%) had myocardial damage patterns, including 22 with poor R-wave progression in the precordial leads, 7 with Q waves in leads II, III and aVF, 2 with Q waves in leads I, AVL and V_4 through V_6 and 7 with combinations of these 3. Comparison of the 38 patients to the 12 patients without a myocardial damage pattern on electrocardiogram (all 50 without complete bundle branch block) disclosed no significant differences in mean age, sex, mode of death, duration of CHF, frequency of chest pain syndromes, habitual alcoholism, diabetes mellitus, left ventricu-

TABLE IX Electrocardiographic Measurements in 35 Necropsy Men and in 14 Necropsy Women with Idiopathic Dilated Cardiomyopathy

Pt	Age (yr) at ECG	Days ECG to Death	Heart Weight (g)	QRS Voltage (mm) All 12	Leads I,II,III	A,L,F.	V_1–V_6	QRS Width (s)	P-R Interval (s)	Q-T Interval (s)	QRS Axis (degrees)	Ventricular Rate (beats/min)
						Men						
1	19	30	550	97	16	14	67	0.08	0.16	0.40	+120	80
2	20	3	610	250	35	29	186	0.08	0.16	0.40	+30	75
3	21	30	460	113	13	6	94	0.14	0.16	0.36	−45	110
4	22	9	700	109	13	12	84	0.08	0.22	0.36	+45	105
5	27	10	700	219	46	46	127	0.08	0.16	0.36	+30	115
6	28	240	540	197	24	20	153	0.08	0.16	0.36	−20	80
7	28	120	460	196	43	36	117	0.08	0.20	0.50	−15	65
8	32	990	—	133	15	16	102	0.08	0.19	0.40	−30	80
	35	5	940	114	10	9	95	0.06	0.20	0.48	−15	120
9	35	3	870	152	18	17	117	0.08	0.24	—	−20	105
10	36	60	750	135	10	8	107	0.08	0.18	0.32	+40	90
11	36	350	730	149	26	22	101	0.12	0.16	0.40	120	80
12	38	60	400	90	18	14	58	0.12	—	0.36	−30	80
13	41	426	—	145	16	13	116	0.10	0.23	0.40	0	76
	42	3	500	131	13	14	104	0.11	0.24	0.40	−90	90
14	42	9	630	103	13	12	78	0.12	0.14	0.44	—	90
15	42	117	550	188	21	19	148	0.08	0.22	0.36	−45	100
16	45	840	—	148	20	21	107	0.13	0.22	0.36	−90	120
	47	60	620	159	19	15	125	0.13	0.21	0.40	−90	105
17	46	60	500	144	22	17	105	0.08	0.24	0.40	−60	75
18	47	180	550	148	14	12	122	0.09	0.24	0.36	+30	90
19	47	30	760	281	28	19	234	0.08	0.22	0.40	−40	80
20	48	240	650	172	25	20	127	0.09	0.18	0.40	−15	75
21	50	15	650	112	12	11	89	0.08	0.20	0.36	−60	100
22	51	45	—	179	20	17	142	0.08	0.16	0.56	−20	50
	51	20	500	115	20	18	77	0.10	0.16	0.52	−40	45
23	51	71	650	74	9	10	55	0.09	0.22	0.40	−110	80
24	53	450	—	103	13	10	80	0.12	0.23	0.41	—	58
	54	3	—	106	14	14	78	0.13	0.10	0.32	—	110
25	54	1,500	—	164	24	19	121	0.09	0.16	0.40	+40	75
	58	6	610	107	12	13	82	0.14	0.24	0.40	−60	105
26	56	20	830	202	50	44	108	0.12	0.20	0.42	—	—
27	53	1,100	—	179	33	27	119	0.14	0.12	0.36	−80	75
	56	80	460	136	18	17	101	0.14	0.16	0.36	−75	110
28	58	90	440	114	15	11	88	0.08	0.16	0.36	−40	115
29	59	10	690	146	12	13	123	0.16	0.24	—	−60	95
30	62	450	—	178	22	16	140	0.12	0.16	0.40	−15	120
	63	37	700	185	19	15	151	0.16	0.18	0.38	−30	100
31	62	60	600	141	21	15	105	0.12	0.20	0.40	−40	100
32	63	9	500	123	27	28	68	0.12	0.21	0.40	−70	72
33	67	1	—	137	6	3	128	0.16	—	0.44	0	70
34	70	210	—	128	25	27	76	0.13	—	0.40	−40	77
35	73	4	725	182	31	26	125	0.08	—	0.40	−30	70
Mean	46	64*	620	147	21	18	109	0.104	0.192	0.39		90
						Women						
1	22	165	440	221	22	22	177	0.09	0.18	0.32	+60	90
2	32	12	650	195	18	17	160	0.08	0.16	0.36	+60	130
3	50	24	700	187	26	17	144	0.16	—	0.38	−45	75
4	51	270	570	75	16	13	46	0.06	—	0.36	−30	75
5	52	18	500	151	25	31	95	0.14	0.28	0.40	−80	110
6	53	20	400	155	18	17	120	0.08	0.18	0.42	0	70
7	54	900	—	154	15	13	126	0.13	0.20	0.36	+45	130
	57	9	550	108	12	8	88	0.14	0.22	0.40	+45	115
8	58	22	640	180	32	33	115	0.12	0.14	0.40	−40	110
9	58	180	—	196	55	54	87	0.18	0.22	0.40	−40	80
	58	30	860	241	48	48	145	0.20	0.24	0.44	−45	70
10	58	7	620	160	21	21	118	0.12	—	0.36	−70	120
11	59	15	750	243	25	18	200	0.14	0.20	0.42	−40	80
12	60	1	490	91	9	9	73	0.16	0.16	0.40	1	95
13	64	30	—	154	13	11	130	0.14	0.18	0.36	−60	90
14	75	7	650	182	28	26	128	0.08	0.21	0.40	−60	75
Mean	54	45*	602	167	22	21	124	0.122	0.195	0.39		93

* In the 9 patients with 2 ECGs analyzed, the mean utilizes the interval from the second ECG to death.
ECG = electrocardiogram.

TABLE X Hemodynamic Data in 26 Necropsy Patients with Idiopathic Dilated Cardiomyopathy

			Duration (mo)			Pressures (mm Hg)													Thrombus		
						RA					PAW										
Pt	Age (yr)	Sex	CHF	CHF → CC	CC → Death	a	v	m	RV (s/d)	PA (s/d)	a	v	m	LV (s/d)	SA (s/d)	CI	HW (g)	RV	LV	PE
1	17	M	36	9	27	9	8	5	26/10	26/14	20	22	16	100/14	100/60	4.1	585	0	+	0
2	18	F	5	2	3	—	—	—	—	36/22	—	—	—	80/25	80/40	—	—	0	0	+
3	20	M	46	4	2	10	8	5	26/7	26/12	10	12	9	102/13	115/60	3.0	610	0	0	+
4	22	M	12	1	11	—	—	—	—	—	—	—	—	100/26	100/50	—	600	+	+	+
5	26	M	16	4	12	9	4	2	17/13	17/10	8	12	5	110/10	110/75	1.4	700	0	+	0
6	26	M	4	1	3	—	—	—	—	27/14	—	—	14	100/12	100/60	1.4	460	0	0	0
7	26	M	5	4	1	—	—	13	—	45/20	—	—	32	—	—	1.5	—	0	+	−
8	29	F	108	103	5	—	—	—	90/-	90/-	—	—	32	90/25	90/60	—	460	0	+	+
9	30	M	5	3	2	18	17	13	70/22	70/26	26	22	18	150/28	140/70	1.5	410	0	0	+
10	32	M	96	84	12	2	3	2	26/2	24/17	—	—	22	120/27	120/70	—	550	+	+	+
11	37	F	23	22	5 days	16	18	17	51/23	51/37	—	—	28	—	—	—	—	0	0	+
12	37	M	36	22	14	AF	8	6	58/6	58/30	—	45	30	126/28	102/80	2.5	400	+	+	0
13	39	M	18	5	13	—	—	0	20/2	20/12	—	—	6	100/18	105/70	2.1	720	0	+	+
14	42	M	72	71	7 days	—	—	16	77/15	77/37	—	—	16	—	100/80	—	650	0	+*	+
15	42	M	30	25	5	30	27	23	40/20	43/32	—	—	35	—	100/60	1.6	550	+	+	0
16	42	M	24	11	13	—	—	7	55/10	55/30	—	—	35	95/35	95/60	1.6	510	0	0	+
17	47	M	12	6	6	9	6	5	45/7	45/20	26	38	25	85/25	85/60	1.5	550	0	+	+
18	48	M	60	48	12	—	—	—	45/8	45/30	—	—	30	85/30	85/55	—	—	0	+	0
19	49	M	48	41	7	AF	—	27	78/28	78/-	—	54	40	—	80/60	—	700	+	+	0
20	50	F	60	60	14 days	AF	30	25	74/24	70/40	—	45	36	100/30	110/75	1.1	700	+	+*	+
21	51	M	72	20	52	AF	10	9	50/9	52/24	—	—	15	120/20	120/75	1.85	570	0	0	0
22	55	M	60	59	1	AF	—	7	40/7	—	—	40	26	110/26	110/80	—	500	0	0	0
23	56	M	36	34	2	—	—	23	—	55/30	—	—	25	—	85/55	—	460	+	+	+
24	58	F	168	165	3	8	7	6	60/10	60/30	32	30	23	140/32	140/80	2.3	860	0	0	+
25	58	F	12	11	21 days	—	12	4	40/6	40/20	—	—	20	95/20	95/70	1.6	620	+	+*	+
26	62	F	62	24	1 day	—	—	4	55/24	55/35	—	—	25	108/23	110/90	2.4	760	0	0	+
27	63	M	—	—	5 days	AF	—	—	70/10	70/27	—	—	28	—	130/75	1.9	—	+	+	0
28	70	M	60	50	10	AF	—	4	60/10	60/20	—	9	7	150/8	150/60	—	580	+	+	+
Mean	41		44	33	8	12	12	11	51/12	50/25	20	30	28	108/23	106/67	2.0	587			

* Thrombus was not visualized on left ventricular angiogram performed 1 month or less before death.

a = a wave; AF = atrial fibrillation; CC = cardiac catheterization; CI = cardiac index (in liters/min/m²); CHF = congestive heart failure; HW = heart weight; LV = left ventricle; m = mean; PA = pulmonary artery; PE = pulmonary emboli (at necropsy); Pt = patient; RA = right atrium; RV = right ventricle; SA = systemic artery; s/d = peak systole/end diastole; V = V wave.

lar hypertrophy on electrocardiogram or intracardiac thrombi. The frequencies of atrial fibrillation and grossly visible left ventricular scars, however, were different. Of the 38 patients with myocardial damage patterns on electrocardiogram, 1.0 (26%) had atrial fibrillation and 10 (26%) had left ventricular scars; in contrast, all 12 patients without myocardial damage patterns were in sinus rhythm and none had left ventricular scars.

Hemodynamic data: Cardiac catheterization data were available in 28 of the 152 patients (Table X). The mean atrial or ventricular end-diastolic pressures or both were elevated in all 28 patients. The right ventricular end-diastolic pressure was >6 mm Hg in 18 (82%) of 22 patients, the left ventricular end-diastolic pressure was >12 mm Hg in 18 (86%) of 21 patients and the mean pulmonary arterial wedge pressure was >12 mm Hg in 22 (85%) of 26 patients. The pulmonary arterial systolic pressure was >30 mm Hg in 20 (77%) of 26 patients, including 8 in whom this pressure was ≥60 mm Hg. Of the 28 patients who had cardiac catheterization, 17 had necropsy evidence of pulmonary emboli or infarcts, and 12 (71%) had pulmonary arterial systolic pressures >30 mm Hg, including 10 (59%) in whom this pressure was >50 mm Hg. A left ventricular to aortic peak systolic pressure gradient of 23 mm Hg was observed in 1 patient, and this patient at necropsy had a thrombus in the left ventricular outflow tract. The cardiac indexes were <2.5 liters/min/m² in 14 (82%) of 17 patients. Left ventricular angiograms in 18 patients disclosed global hypokinesia in all 18 and mitral regurgitation in 6 of 13 in whom it was mentioned. No significant correlation was observed between total duration of chronic CHF or duration of CHF from the time of catheterization to death and the pulmonary arterial systolic pressure ($r = +0.39$ and $r = -0.20$), but a significant correlation was observed between the total duration of CHF and the mean pulmonary arterial wedge pressure ($r = +0.65$) ($p < 0.002$). The left ventricular end-diastolic pressure did not correlate with heart weight ($r = -0.08$), total duration of CHF ($r = -0.14$) or duration of CHF from catheterization to death ($r = -0.17$).

Necropsy Findings

Heart weights and chamber sizes: The hearts at necropsy ranged in weight from 360 to 940 g (mean 615): in the women the range was from 360 to 860 g (mean 551) and in the men, from 400 to 940 g (mean 632) ($p < 0.05$). By definition, both right and left ventricular cavities were dilated in all patients (Figures 5 through 7). So were both atria. The frequency of intracavity thrombi and mural endocardial plaques have been described previously.

Ventricular scars: Grossly visible left ventricular or right ventricular scars or both (excluding isolated papillary muscle scars) were found in 22 (14%) patients: 21 scars involved, at some point, greater than the inner one-half of the myocardial wall, that is, transmural, and 1 was limited to the inner one-half, that is, subendocardial. The scars were small in 14 patients, moderate in 4 and large in 4. The scars involved left ventricular free wall in all 22 patients, the ventricular septum also in 20 and the right ventricular free wall in 5. The frequency of intraventricular thrombi and endocardial plaques was similar in the patients with and without grossly visible ventricular wall scars. The 22 patients with ventricular scars ranged in age from 17 to 67 years (mean 56), which is an average of 13 years older than the mean (43 years) of the 130 patients without grossly visible left ventricular scars ($p < 0.05$). Of these 22 patients, 21 had chronic CHF an average of 44 months, which is significantly ($p < 0.05$) less than the mean duration (65 months) of chronic CHF in the 99 patients in whom no grossly visible ventricular scars were present and information on the duration of chronic CHF was available. Of the 22 patients, 4 had clinical events during life considered to be compatible with "acute myocardial infarction." None, of course, had significantly (>75% in cross-sectional area) narrowed coronary arteries at necropsy. Of the 22 patients, 11 had histories of habitual alcoholism and 2 had adult-onset diabetes mellitus. Electrocardiograms, available in 21 of the 22 patients, disclosed voltage criteria for left ventricular hypertrophy in 6 (29%), complete bundle branch block in 9 (43%) and myocardial infarct or damage patterns in 6 (29%). The mean heart weight (available in 19 patients) in the patients

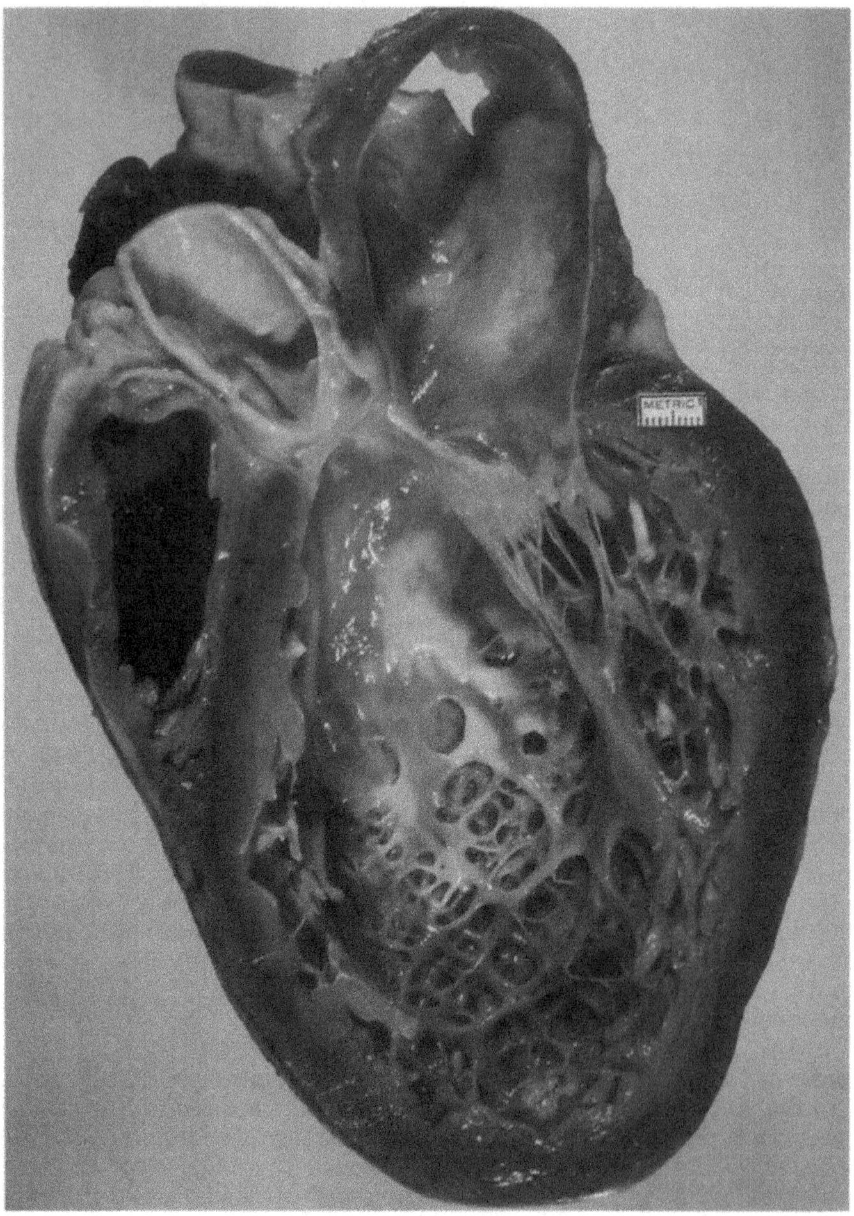

FIGURE 5. Longitudinal view of left side of the heart from a 54-year-old man (SH A81-57) with idiopathic dilated cardiomyopathy. Shown is the outflow portion of right ventricle and much of the left ventricle. The white plaques on the left ventricular aspect of the ventricular septum probably are residua of organization of thrombi. The mitral valve occupies a small portion of the very dilated left ventricular cavity. The heart weighed 920 g. Congestive heart failure had been present for 3.5 years.

with grossly visible scars was similar to that in the patients without (607 vs 615 g).

Histology of ventricular myocardium: A total of 1,422 histologic sections of myocardial wall from 96 patients were examined: 508 sections of left ventricle, 215 of ventricular septum, 355 of right ventricle and 344 of atrium. Additionally, 967 sections of cross-sections of major (right, left main, left anterior descending and left circumflex) epicardial coronary arteries were examined. The ventricular myocardium contained multiple patchy areas of replacement fibrosis in 29 (35%) of 83 sections of right ventricle and in 55 (57%) of 96 sections of left ventricle from the 96 patients. The replacement fibrosis often was accompanied by in-

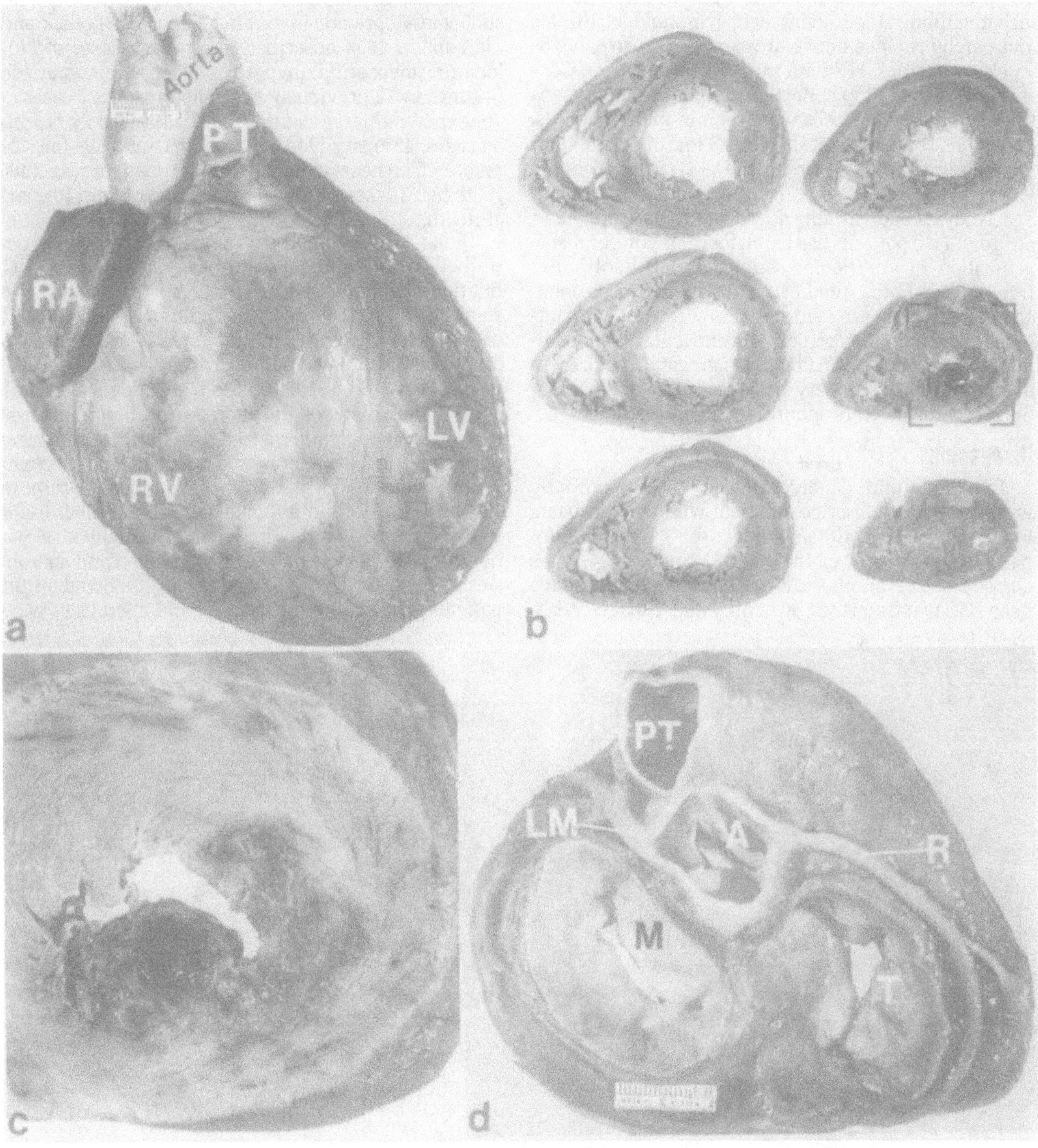

FIGURE 6. Heart from a 58-year-old woman (SH A78-7) with congestive heart failure for 10 years due to idiopathic dilated cardiomyopathy. *A*, exterior view of the heart. LV = left ventricle; PT = pulmonary trunk; RA = right atrium; RV = right ventricle. *B*, sections of the dilated cardiac ventricles after transverse sectioning. *C*, close-up view of the section shown in brackets in *B*. A thrombus is present. *D*, view of the mitral (M), tricuspid (T) and aortic (A) valves and of pulmonary trunk after removal of the atrial walls. R = right; LM = left main coronary arteries.

creased perivascular fibrous tissue and perimyocytic fibrosis in the left ventricle: it was present in 22 (23%) of 96 and 27 (28%) of 96 patients, respectively (Figure 8). In addition, in 13 (16%) of 83 sections of right ventricle and in 32 (33%) of 96 sections of left ventricle extensive subendocardial scarring was present. Interstitial inflammatory cell infiltrates were present in ventricular myocardium in 5 patients: 4 had prominent mononuclear infiltrates without associated myocardial necrosis and 1 had multiple small foci of necrotizing inflammation. One patient with lymphoid infiltrates and patchy replacement fibrosis had a progressive 5-week course of CHF with positive serology for Coxsackie B_3 virus. Tiny collections of perivascular "sentinal" mononuclear cells were seen in many patients. Seven (8%) of 83 patients had small foci of coagulation necrosis in the right ventricle and 11 (11%) of 96 in the left ventricle.

Myocytes had variable degrees of hypertrophy and atrophy. Two patients had small foci of myofiber disorganization in ventricular septum or left ventricular free wall or both. Another 2 patients had occasional calcified myocytes in ventricular myocardium and another 2 had subendocardial left ventricular foci of colliquative myocytolysis. Platelet aggregate was present in an intramural coronary artery in 1 patient. No infectious organisms were identified in any section.

Discussion

Josserand and Gallavardin[1] in 1901 apparently were the first to describe a patient with what appears to have been IDC, although they used the term "idiopathic hypertrophy of the heart." Another 24 years elapsed before another case of what appears to have been IDC was described by Laubry and Walser.[2] Whittle[3] in 1929 added another case. By 1944, Levy and Von Glahn[4] reported 10 necropsy cases of "cardiac hypertrophy of unknown cause" and they described the usual clinical features: "marked cardiac hypertrophy; occurrence of various types of arrhythmia; frequent emboli to the pulmonary and systemic circulations; rapidly progressive course after the onset of symptoms; and death from gradual cardiac failure or in sudden fashion." In 1955 Serbin and Chojnacki[5] reported 3 more cases of "idiopathic cardiac hypertrophy" and collected 46 previously published cases. Spodick and Littman[6] in 1958 described 8 necropsy cases of "idiopathic myocardial hypertrophy" and summarized findings in 72 previously published necropsy cases of "unexplained large hearts." Of the previously reported cases, 42% survived <12 months and 65% for <24 months. The heart weight in all but 1 patient was ≥400 g. Of the 72 cases, 62 (86%) were younger than 50 years at death.

Since 1958, numerous publications[7-47] have described various clinical features in patients with IDC, but none have focused on findings at necropsy. Massumi et al[11] in 1965 described clinical features of 50 cases of "primary myocardial disease" seen in a 41-month period; 13 died and necropsies were performed in 10. Goodwin[13] in 1970 studied 70 patients with IDC; 41 (55%) had died and the average duration from onset of symptoms to death was 3.5 years; necropsies were performed in 26 patients and all had heart weights ≥400 g. Hamby[14] in 1970 described clinical features in 100 cases; 44 died in a 5-year period, and necropsies were performed in 23. Shugoll et al[17] followed 50 patients for 3 to 72 months (mean 30); 10 died and necropsies were performed in 5. Hatle et al[22] followed up 106 patients for 2 to 12 years; 50 died and necropsies were

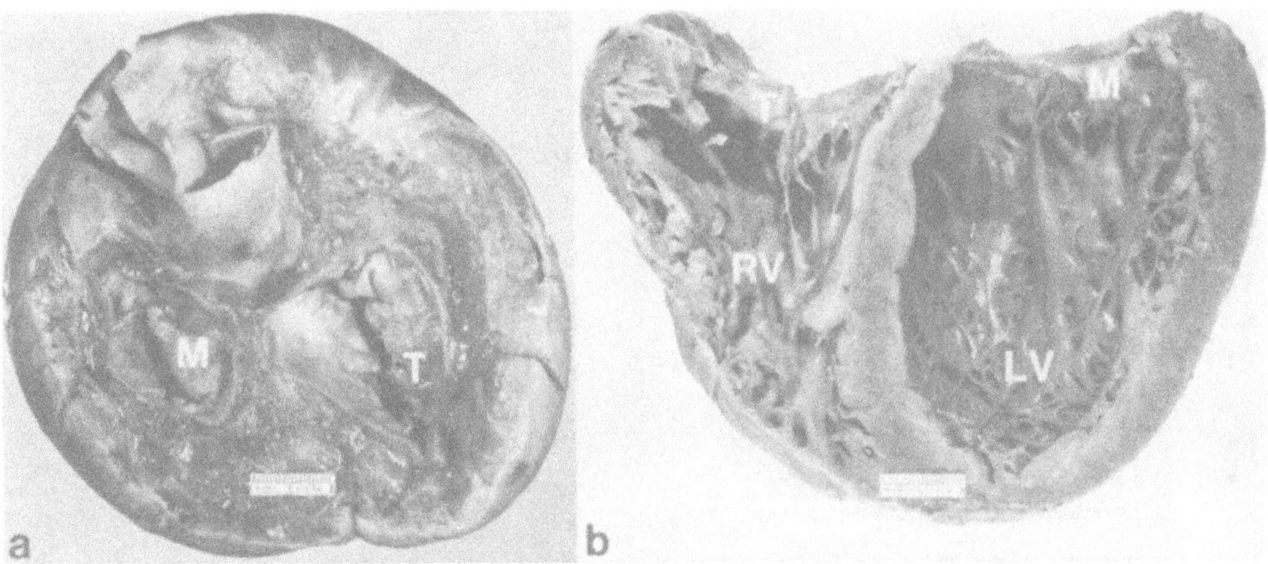

FIGURE 7. Heart (*A* and *B*) from a 34-year-old woman (DCGH 74A-65) with congestive heart failure for 5 years from idiopathic dilated cardiomyopathy. The mitral (M) anulus is only mildly dilated, whereas the tricuspid (T) valve anulus is considerably dilated, as are both ventricular cavities. The usual mechanism of tricuspid regurgitation in patients with idiopathic dilated cardiomyopathy is dilatation of the tricuspid valve anulus. In contrast, the usual mechanism of mitral regurgitation in idiopathic dilated cardiomyopathy is altered papillary muscle anchoring due to dilatation of the left ventricular cavity, mainly in its more central portion. The heart in this patient weighed 870 g.

TABLE XI Certain Reported Studies Since 1960 in Idiopathic Dilated Cardiomyopathy

	First Author	Year	No. Cases (males)	Period Patients Seen	Age Range (yr) (mean) When First Seen or When Studied	Age (yr) at Death (mean)	Race B	Race W	Range of Follow-up (mo) (mean)	Duration (mo) S → Death (mean)	History of Alcoholism	Peripartum (no. women)	Familial	Diabetes Mellitus	No. Having Coronary Angiography	No. Died in Follow-Up	No. Having Necropsy
1	Fowler et al[7,8]	1962	29 (25)	—1964	8–62 (36)	18–68 (45)	10	19	1–312 (—)	6–312 (120)	8/23	1 (4)	1	0	0	26	26
2	Dye et al[9,10]	1963	32 (32)	—	20–68 (43)	—	14	18	—48 (—)	— (44)	21	0 (0)	—	—	0	12	9
3	Massumi et al[11]	1965	50 (40)	1960–1963	20–79 (—)	28–79 (54)	45	5	—41 (—)	— (10)	30	— (10)	0	—	0	13	10
4	Alexander[12]	1966	83 (83)	1949–1960	19–67 (44)	— (47)	—	—	—	— (2)	24	0 (0)	—	—	0	27	—
5	Goodwin[13]	1970	70 (—)	—	—	—	—	—	—	— (42)	16	7 (—)	—	—	9	41	26
6	Hamby[14]	1970	100 (71)	1954–1968	20–61 (45)	— (45)	71	29	2–60 (15)	— (55)	40	— (29)	—	3	24	35	23
7	McDonald and Rahimtoola[15]	1971	48 (47)	1959–1969	21–57 (38)	—	42	6	0.2–108 (52)	— (45)	48	0 (1)	—	—	0	19	14
8	Demakis[16]	1971	27 (0)	—	—	—	—	—	12–252 (97)	—	0	27 (27)	0	—	0	13	—
9	Shugoll et al[17]	1972	50 (50)	—1961	22–50 (—)	—	46	4	3–72 (30)	12–108 (38)	31	0 (0)	0	—	23	10	5
10	Kreulen et al[18]	1973	33 (24)	—	20–69 (43)	—	—	—	—	—	7	— (9)	—	—	33	9	—
11	Feild et al[19]	1973	36 (23)	—	18–66 (46)	—	—	—	—56 (—)	3–144 (38)	5	— (13)	0	5	15	19	5
12	Damakis et al[20]	1974	57 (49)	1962–1970	23–50 (41)	—	47	10	4–96 (41)	— (36)	57	0 (8)	—	—	4	24	7
13	Bashour et al[21]	1975	65 (56)	1969–1974	21–66 (42)	—	—	—	— (21)	—	65	— (9)	—	—	—	—	—
14	Hatle et al[22,23]	1976	91 (—)	1962–1972	<10–>60 (—)	—	—	—	2–12 (—)	—	2	— (—)	5	0	81	50	36
15	Hess et al[24]	1976	30 (24)	—	— (43)	—	—	—	10–34 (24)	—	—	— (6)	—	—	30	8	—
16	Segal et al[25]	1978	115 (71)	1961–1976	1–65 (—)	1–65 (46)	37	78	60–192 (96)	— (74)	0	0 (44)	0	0	—	77	48
17	Shirey et al[26]	1980	113 (—)	—	—	—	—	—	—96 (60)	0.5–90 (25)	8	— (—)	—	12	113	44	—
18	Koide et al[27]	1980	36 (29)	1965–1978	(44 ± 13)	— (53)	—	—	1–216 (—)	— (53)	10	3 (7)	3	—	—	17	11
19	Convert et al[28]	1980	132 (110)	1969–1977	15–71 (46)	—	—	—	(40 ± 24)	<6–>36 (—)	77	— (22)	—	—	79	48	—
20	Fuster et al[29]	1981	104 (64)	1960–1973	— (49)	—	—	—	72–240 (132)	—	22	3 (40)	—	0	46	80	39
21	Lengyel and Kokeny[30]	1981	98 (88)	1973–1979	17–66 (41)	17–66 (40)	—	—	6–70 (18)	6–60 (13)	34	2 (10)	5	—	15	39	15
22	Engler et al[31]	1982	18 (—)	—	32–71 (54)	—	—	—	6–49 (25)	—	—	— (—)	—	—	18	—	—
23	Kuhn et al[32]	1982	258 (187)	1971–1980	8–68 (44)	(44 ± 10)	—	—	(36 ± 24)	(60 ± 36)	40	— (71)	—	—	258	69	18
24	Franciosa et al[33]	1983	87 (—)	1974–1981	—	—	—	—	1–41 (12)	(45 ± 43)	—	— (—)	—	—	22	30	—
25	Huang et al[34]	1983	35 (24)	1976–1980	22–72 (51)	—	—	—	4–74 (34)	—	—	— (11)	—	—	35	4	—
26	von Olshausen et al[35]	1984	60 (54)	1981–1982	18–60 (45)	—	—	—	1–18 (12)	—	—	— (6)	—	—	60	7	—
27	Meinertz et al[36,37]	1984	74 (—)	—	—	— (50)	—	—	2–21 (11)	(60 ± 37)	0	— (—)	—	—	74	19	—
28	Poll et al[38]	1984	11 (6)	1975–1983	27–74 (49)	—	—	—	— (21)—	—	—	— (5)	—	—	—	4	—
29	Unverferth et al[39,40]	1984	69 (49)	1979–1982	19–79 (45)	19–79 (45)			—12 (—)	(31 ± 46)	15	2 (20)	4	5	69	24	—
30	Wallis et al[41]	1984	50 (32)	1981–1983	11–68 (47)	—	—	—	1–26 (11)	—	—	— (18)	—	—	47	10	—
31	Holmes et al[42]	1985	15 (12)	1981–1983	34–66 (50)	—	—	—	6–21 (11)	—	3	1 (3)	0	0	5	5	—
32	Anderson et al[43,44]	1985	50 (33)	1981–1984	25–75 (50)	—	—	—	1–38 (19)	—	0	—	—	—	All > 30	11	—
33	Sanderson et al[45]	1985	20 (9)	—	— (34)	—	—	—	—	—	—	—	—	—	<9	—	—
34	Michels et al[46]	1985	169 (119)	1976–1982	<50	—	—	—	—	—	—	—	11	—	~80	—	—
35	O'Connell et al[47]	1986	69 (—)	—	— (44)	—	—	—	—	—	—	14 (—)	—	—	—	—	—

B = black; M = men; S = symptoms of cardiac dysfunction; W = white; — = no information available.

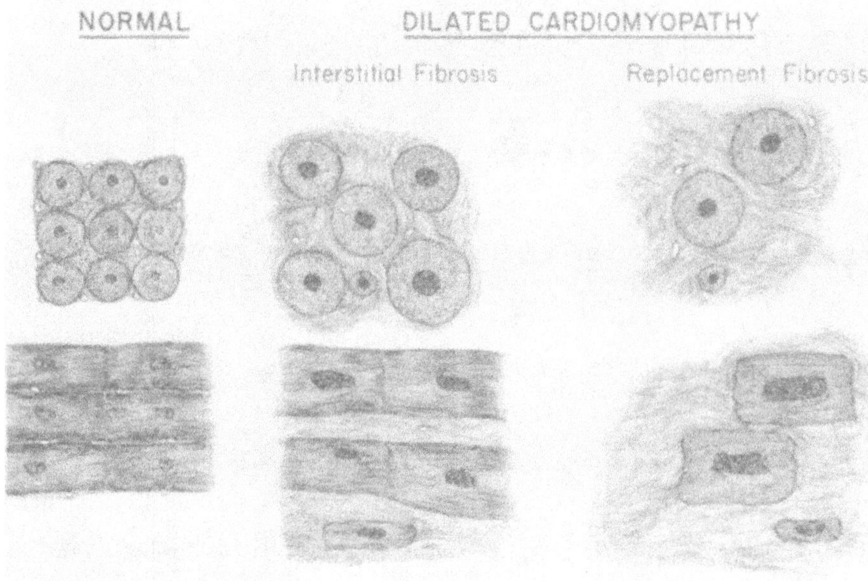

FIGURE 8. Diagram showing the various findings commonly observed in sections of left ventricular wall in the patients with idiopathic dilated cardiomyopathy. Some myocardial cells are larger than normal, others are smaller than normal and others have been replaced by fibrous tissue, which also is increased in the interstitum between the myocardial cells.

performed in 36. Segal et al[25] followed 115 patients with presumed IDC for a minimum of 5 years (median 8); 77 died and necropsies were performed in 48. Only 35 of the 48 had cardiomegaly at necropsy, an observation suggesting that some of the cases may not have been IDC. Shirey et al[26] studied 113 patients with IDC (only 48 of whom had CHF), following them up to 8 years (mean 5); 44 died but the number who had necropsy is unclear. Fuster et al[29] followed 104 patients from 6 to 20 years (median 11); 80 died and necropsy was performed in 39. Franciosa et al[33] followed 87 patients from 1 to 41 months (mean 12); 30 died but the number who had necropsy is unclear. These studies and many others are summarized in Table XI.

In contrast to the studies just mentioned, the starting point in the present study was the finding at necropsy of cardiac abnormalities fulfilling a rigorous definition of IDC. All 152 patients had hearts that were enlarged (>350 g in women and >400 g in men), all had dilated cardiac ventricular cavities, all had anatomically normal cardiac valves and pericardia, all had insignificant narrowing of the epicardial coronary arteries and none had an abnormality of a noncardiac body organ sufficient to cause the cardiac abnormalities. None during life had a systemic arterial indirect pressure >140/90 mm Hg during their last 3 months of life. Of the 148 patients with chronic CHF, the diagnosis of IDC was either made or suspected clinically. In the 4 patients whose initial manifestation of IDC was sudden death, diagnosis of IDC, of course, was not made until necropsy.

The findings in the present study are shown in detail in Tables I through X. This study provides the most extensive data for the natural history of IDC thus far presented. Clues to the cause of the IDC were not provided by this morphologically based study. Despite current interest in myocardial biopsy for identification of inflammatory myocardial injury in patients with IDC, this technique if applied shortly before death in the 152 patients included in this study probably would not have produced a diagnosis of "myocarditis" in a single patient. Our findings are in keeping with other observations regarding the infrequency of significant inflammatory cells in ventricular myocardium in patients with IDC.[48,49]

Although numerous reports have described electrocardiographic changes in patients with IDC (see references compiled by Perloff[50]), the present study is the first to describe total 12-lead QRS voltage in patients with IDC. A recent study by Odom et al[51] provided total 12-lead QRS voltage in a group of necropsy patients with no evidence of cardiac or pulmonary dysfunction or myocardial ischemia during life and all had normal-sized hearts at necropsy. Only 1 of the 30 subjects with normal-sized hearts had total 12-lead QRS voltage >175 mm (10 mm = 1 mV). The total 12-lead QRS voltage in 49 patients with IDC included in this study ranged from 75 to 250 mm (mean 153), a mean number within normal limits despite a mean heart weight for the group of >550 g. For comparison, Siegel and Roberts[52] determined total 12-lead QRS voltage in 50 patients aged 16 to 65 years with severe and fatal isolated aortic valve stenosis. The total 12-lead QRS voltage in these 50 patients ranged from 144 to 417 mm (mean 260), and the heart weights were similar to those in the present study of patients with IDC. In a study of total 12-lead QRS voltage in 30 patients with severe and fatal cardiac amyloidosis, Roberts and Waller[53] found total 12-lead QRS voltage to range from 60 to 199 mm (mean 104) despite a mean heart weight of the 30 patients of 532 g. Thus, by total 12-lead QRS voltage criteria, few IDC patients in the present study or patients with severe cardiac amyloidosis have "left ventricular hypertrophy" despite the occurrence of considerable cardiomegaly at necropsy.

References

1. Josserand E, Gallavardin L. *De l' a systolie progressive des jeunes sujets par myocardite subaigue primitive. Arch Gen Med 1901;6:513–548.*
2. Laubry C, Walser J. *Sur un cas d'insuffisance cardiaque primitive. Les*

myocardies. Bull Mem Soc Med Hop Paris 1925;49:409–418.
3. Whittle CH. "Idiopathic" hypertrophy of heart in young man. Lancet 1929;1:1354–1355.
4. Levy RL, Von Glahn WC. Cardiac hypertrophy of unknown cause. A study of the clinical and pathologic features in ten adults. Am Heart J 1944;28:714–741.
5. Serbin RA, Chojnacki B. Idiopathic cardiac hypertrophy. Report of 3 cases. N Engl J Med 1955;252:10–13.
6. Spodick DH, Littman D. Idiopathic myocardial hypertrophy. Am J Cardiol 1958;1:610–623.
7. Fowler NO, Gueron M, Rowlands DT Jr. Primary myocardial disease. Dis Chest 1962;41:593–602.
8. Fowler NO, Gueron M. Primary myocardial disease. Circulation 1965;32: 830–836.
9. Dye CL, Rosenbaum D, Lowe JC, Behnke RH, Genovese PD. Primary myocardial disease: part I. Clinical features. Ann Intern Med 1963;58:426–441.
10. Dye CL, Genovese PD, Daly WJ, Behnke RH. Primary myocardial disease. Part II. Hemodynamic alterations. Ann Intern Med 1963;58:442–453.
11. Massumi RA, Rios JC, Gooch AS, Nutter D, De Vita VT, Datlow DW. Primary myocardial disease. Report of fifty cases and review of the subject. Circulation 1965;31:19–41.
12. Alexander CS. Idiopathic heart disease: I. Analysis of 100 cases, with special reference to chronic alcoholism. Am J Med 1966;41:213–228.
13. Goodwin JF. Congestive and hypertrophic cardiomyopathies. A decade of study. Lancet 1970;1:732–739.
14. Hamby RI. Primary myocardial disease. A prospective clinical and hemodynamic evaluation in 100 patients. Medicine 1970;49:55–78.
15. McDonald CD, Burch GE, Walsh JJ. Alcoholic cardiomyopathy managed with prolonged bed rest. Ann Intern Med 1971;74:681–691.
16. Demakis JG, Rahimtoola SH. Peripartum cardiomyopathy. Circulation 1971;44:964–968.
17. Shugoll GI, Bowen PJ, Moore JP, Lenkin ML. Follow-up observations and prognosis in primary myocardial disease. Arch Intern Med 1972;129:67–72.
18. Kreulen TH, Gorlin R, Herman MV. Ventriculographic patterns and hemodynamics in primary myocardial disease. Circulation 1973;47:299–308.
19. Feild BJ, Baxley WA, Russell RO Jr, Hood WP Jr, Holt JH, Dowling JT, Rackley CE. Left ventricular function and hypertrophy in cardiomyopathy with depressed ejection fraction. Circulation 47:1022–1031.
20. Demakis JG, Proskey A, Rahimtoola SH, Jamil M, Sutton GC, Rosen KM, Gunnar RM, Tobin JR Jr. The natural course of alcoholic cardiomyopathy. Ann Intern Med 1974;80:293–297.
21. Bashour TT, Fahdul H, Cheng TO. Electrocardiographic abnormalities in alcoholic cardiomyopathy. A study of 65 patients. Chest 1975;68:24–27.
22. Hatle L, Orjavik O, Storstein O. Chronic myocardial disease. I. Clinical picture related to long-term prognosis. Acta Med Scand 1976;199:399–405.
23. Hatle L, Stahe G, Storstein O. Chronic myocardial disease. II. Hemodynamic findings related to long-term prognosis. Acta Med Scand 1976;199: 407–411.
24. Hess OM, Turina J, Goebel NH, Krayenbuhl HP. Clinical course of congestive cardiomyopathy. Schweiz Med Wochenschr 1976;106:1577–1579.
25. Segal JP, Stapleton JF, McClellan JR, Waller BF, Harvey WP. Idiopathic cardiomyopathy: clinical features, prognosis and therapy. Curr Probl Cardiol 1978;3:1–49.
26. Shirey EK, Proudfit WL, Hawk WA. Primary myocardial disease. Correlation with clinical findings, angiographic and biopsy diagnosis. Follow-up of 139 patients. Am Heart J 1980;99:198–207.
27. Koide T, Kato A, Takabatake Y, Iizuka M, Uchida Y, Ozeki K, Morooka S, Kakihana M, Serizawa T, Tanaka S, Ohya T, Momomura S, Murao S. Variable prognosis in congestive cardiomyopathy. Role of left ventricular function, alcoholism, and pulmonary thrombosis. Jpn Heart J 1980;21:451–463.
28. Convert G, Delaye J, Beaune J, Biron A, Gonin A. Prognosis of primary nonobstructive cardiomyopathies. Arch Mal Coeur 1980;73:227–237.
29. Fuster V, Gersh BJ, Giuliani ER, Tajik AJ, Brandenburg RO, Frye RL. The natural history of idiopathic dilated cardiomyopathy. Am J Cardiol 1981; 47:525–531.
30. Lengyel M, Kokeny M. Follow-up study in congestive (dilated) cardiomyopathy. Acta Cardiol 1981;36:35–48.
31. Engler R, Ray R, Higgins CB, McNally C, Buxton WH, Bhargava V, Shabetai R. Clinical assessment and follow-up of functional capacity in patients with chronic congestive cardiomyopathy. Am J Cardiol 1982;49:1832–1837.
32. Kuhn H, Becker R, Fischer J, Curtius JM, Losse B, Hort W, Loogen F. Studies on the etiology, the clinical course and the prognosis of patients with dilated cardiomyopathy (DCM). Z Kardiol 1982;71:497–508.
33. Franciosa JA, Wilen M, Ziesche S, Cohn JN. Survival in men with severe chronic left ventricular failure due to either coronary heart disease or idiopathic dilated cardiomyopathy. Am J Cardiol 1983;51:831–836.
34. Huang SK, Musser JV, Denes P. Significance of ventricular tachycardia in idiopathic dilated cardiomyopathy: observations in 35 patients. Am J Cardiol 1983;51:507–518.
35. Von Olshausen K, Schäfer A, Mehmel HC, Schwarz F, Senges J, Kübler W. Ventricular arrhythmias in idiopathic dilated cardiomyopathy. Br Heart J 1984;51:195–201.
36. Meinertz T, Hofmann T, Kasper W, Treese N, Bechtold H, Stienen U, Pop T, Leitner E-RV, Andresen D, Meyer J. Significance of ventricular arrhythmias in idiopathic dilated cardiomyopathy. Am J Cardiol 1984;53:902–907.
37. Meinertz T, Treese N, Kasper W, Geibel A, Hofmann T, Zehender M, Bohn D, Pop T, Just H. Determinants of prognosis in idiopathic dilated cardiomyopathy as determined by programmed electrical stimulation. Am J Cardiol 1985;56:337–341.
38. Poll DS, Marchlinski FE, Buxton AE, Doherty JU, Waxman HL, Josephson ME. Sustained ventricular tachycardia in patients with idiopathic dilated cardiomyopathy; electrophysiologic testing and lack of response to antiarrhythmic drug therapy. Circulation 1984;70:451–456.
39. Unverferth DV, Mehegan JP, Magorien RD, Unverferth BJ, Leier CV. Regression of myocardial cellular hypertrophy with vasodilator therapy in chronic congestive heart failure associated with idiopathic dilated cardiomyopathy. Am J Cardiol 1983;51:1392–1398.
40. Unverferth DV, Magorien RD, Moeschberg ML, Baker PB, Fetters JK, Leier CV. Factors influencing the one-year mortality of dilated cardiomyopathy. Am J Cardiol 1984;54:147–152.
41. Wallis DE, O'Connell JB, Henkin RE, Costanzo-Nordin MR, Scanlon PJ. Segmental wall motion abnormalities in dilated cardiomyopathy: a common finding and good prognostic sign. JACC 1984;4:674–679.
42. Holmes J, Kubo SH, Cody RJ, Kligfield P. Arrhythmias in ischemic and nonischemic dilated cardiomyopathy: prediction of mortality by ambulatory electrocardiography. Am J Cardiol 1985;55:146–151.
43. Anderson JL, Lutz JR, Gilbert EM, Sorensen SG, Yanowitz FG, Menlove RL, Bartholomew M. A randomized trial of low-dose beta-blockade therapy for idiopathic dilated cardiomyopathy. Am J Cardiol 1985;55:471–475.
44. Anderson JL, Carlquist JF, Lutz JR, DeWitt CW, Hammond EH. HLA A, B and DR typing in idiopathic dilated cardiomyopathy: a search for immune response factors. Am J Cardiol 1984;53:1326–1330.
45. Sanderson JE, Koech D, David I, Ojiambo HP. T-lymphocyte subsets in idiopathic dilated cardiomyopathy. Am J Cardiol 1985;55:755–758.
46. Michels VV, Driscoll DJ, Miller FA Jr. Familial aggregation of idiopathic dilated cardiomyopathy. Am J Cardiol 1985;55:1232–1233.
47. O'Connell JB, Costanzo-Nordin MR, Subramanian R, Robinson JA, Wallis DE, Scanlon PJ, Gunnar RM. Peripartum cardiomyopathy: clinical, hemodynamic, histologic and prognostic characteristics. JACC 1986;8:52–56.
48. Cassling RS, Linder J, Sears TD, Waller BF, Rogler WC, Wilson JE, Kugler JD, Kay HD, Dillon JC, Slack JD, McManus BM. Quantitative evaluation of inflammation in biopsy specimens from idiopathically failing or irritable hearts: experience in 80 pediatric and adult patients. Am Heart J 1985; 110:713–720.
49. Tazelaar HD, Billingham ME. Leukocytic infiltrates in idiopathic dilated cardiomyopathy. Am J Surg Pathol 1986;10:405–412.
50. Perloff JK. The cardiomyopathies: dilated and restrictive. Circulation 1981;63:1189–1198.
51. Odom H II, Davis JL, Dinh H, Baker BJ, Roberts WC, Murphy ML. QRS voltage measurements in autopsied men free of cardiopulmonary disease: a basis for evaluating total QRS voltage as an index of left ventricular hypertrophy. Am J Cardiol 1986;58:801–804.
52. Siegel RJ, Roberts WC. Electrocardiographic observations in severe aortic valve stenosis: correlative necropsy study to clinical, hemodynamic, and ECG variables demonstrating relation of 12-lead QRS amplitude to peak systolic transaortic pressure gradient. Am Heart J 1982;103:298–301.
53. Roberts WC, Waller BF. Cardiac amyloidosis causing cardiac dysfunction: analysis of 54 necropsy patients. Am J Cardiol 1983;52:137–146.

Sudden Death in Hemochromatosis After Closed-Chest Catheter Ablation of the Atrioventricular Junction

ROBERT LEMERY, MD
PEDRO BRUGADA, MD
MICHAEL HAVENITH, MD
DEBORAH BARBOUR, MD
WILLIAM C. ROBERTS, MD
HEIN J.J. WELLENS, MD

In patients with supraventricular tachycardia refractory to antiarrhythmic drugs or antitachycardia pacemakers, closed-chest catheter ablation of the atrioventricular (AV) junction is an alternative to surgery.[1,2] We report clinical and necropsy findings in a patient who died suddenly 1 week after catheter ablation of the AV junction.

A 47-year-old man with hemochromatosis since age 25 had evidence of congestive heart failure since age 44 and paroxysmal atrial fibrillation with recorded heart rates of up to 160 beats/min since age 45. He had been unsuccessfully treated with digitalis, disopyramide, propafenone and amiodarone. The ejection fraction by echocardiography was 24%. No family members had hemochromatosis and he had never received blood transfusions. Serum ferritin was 5,430 μg/liter (normal 34 to 310 μg/liter); hemoglobin, 7.4 mmol/liter and potassium 5.1 mmol/liter.

Catheter ablation of the AV junction was performed 1 day after admission. Atrial fibrillation was present. The electrogram of the His bundle measured 0.4 mV (Figure 1). Four shocks were given, but atrial fibrillation returned immediately after ablation. A second session 4 days later, using 6 shocks (300 J each), failed to produce complete heart block. The serum creatine kinase rose to 332 U/liter (3% MB) after the first session and to 365 U/liter after the second. Following the second ablation session, paroxysmal atrial fibrillation was present with episodes of escape beats at 40 beats/min when the pacemaker was turned off. A permanent rate-responsive pacemaker was implanted 3 days after the second ablation session. That same day, however, recurrent episodes of paroxysmal atrial fibrillation with rates of up to 140 beats/min prompted therapy with sotalol (160 mg/day) and digitalis (0.375 mg/day). Electrocardiographic monitoring showed a 3-beat run of ventricular tachycardia (Figure 2A) at 180 beats/min (Holter monitoring before the present admission had revealed ventricular couplets). Continuous monitoring revealed no further ventricular ectopic activity (Figure 2B). No abnormal pacemaker

From the Departments of Cardiology and Pathology, University of Limburg, University Hospital, Maastricht, the Netherlands, and the Pathology Branch, National Heart, Lung, and Blood Institute, National Institutes of Health, Bethesda, Maryland.
Manuscript received June 8, 1987; revised manuscript received and accepted November 25, 1987.

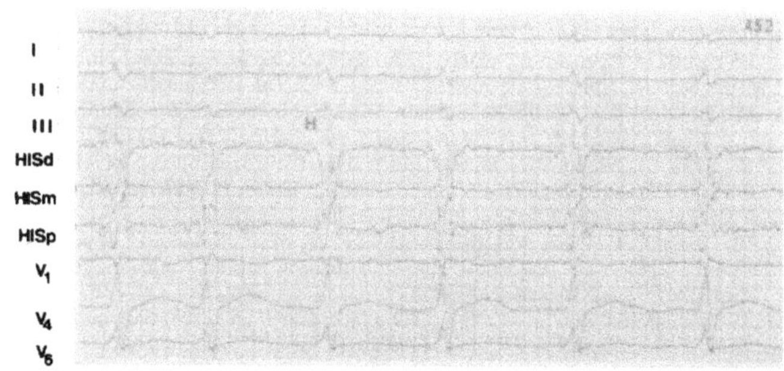

FIGURE 1. His bundle recording before catheter ablation. From top to bottom: standard electrocardiographic leads I, II, III, unipolar recordings from each electrode of a tripolar catheter positioned in the region of the His bundle and precordial leads V_1, V_4, and V_6. The amplitude of the His electrogram measured 0.4 mV and the rhythm is atrial fibrillation.

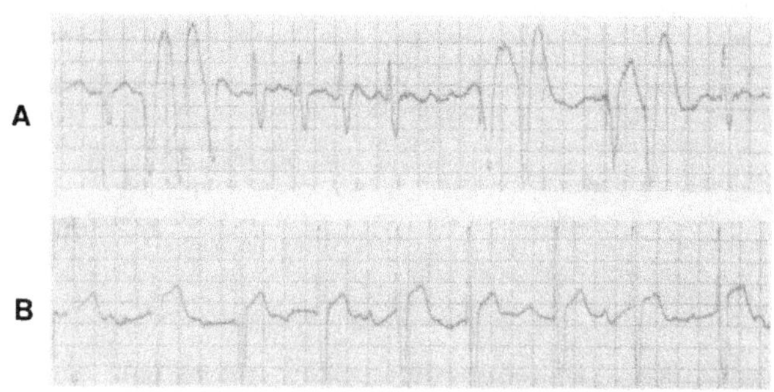

FIGURE 2. *A* shows a 3-beat run of nonsustained ventricular tachycardia, 3 days after catheter ablation. *B* shows sinus rhythm with first-degree atrioventricular block, taken 10 hours before death.

behavior was observed and electrocardiographic monitoring was discontinued during the evening of his tenth day in the hospital. The patient was found dead in bed 7 hours later.

Necropsy disclosed heavy iron deposits in the liver (weight 2,650 g), spleen (350 g), thyroid gland and pancreas. The heart weighed 530 g. The coronary arteries were normal. Foci of subendocardial hemorrhage were present in the area of the AV bundle. Iron deposits were present in numerous myocardial cells in the walls of all 4 chambers, but heaviest in the left ventricular wall. No grossly visible foci of myocardial necrosis or fibrosis were seen.

A total of 3,140 sections were cut from the AV node and bundle area. Every twentieth section was stained with hematoxylin and eosin, and every two hundredth was stained with Prussian blue. The iron deposits were far less extensive in the conducting tissue than in the "working" myocardium. The myocardial cells in the area of the AV bundle and in the subendocardial portion of the ventricular septum, right ventricular aspect, were lysed and some inflammatory cells were present. The AV node and bundle were intact. The junction between the AV bundle and the right bundle branch was interrupted (Figure 3).

Sudden death has been reported in approximately 2% of patients after catheter ablation.[3] Detailed histopathologic studies have been reported in single patients dying at 6 weeks,[4] 5 months[5] and 5.5 months,[6] respectively, after catheter ablation. Histopathologic changes in patients dying after catheter ablation have shown replacement of AV nodal tissue by fibrous tissue.[4-6] The caudal part of the AV bundle and the bun-

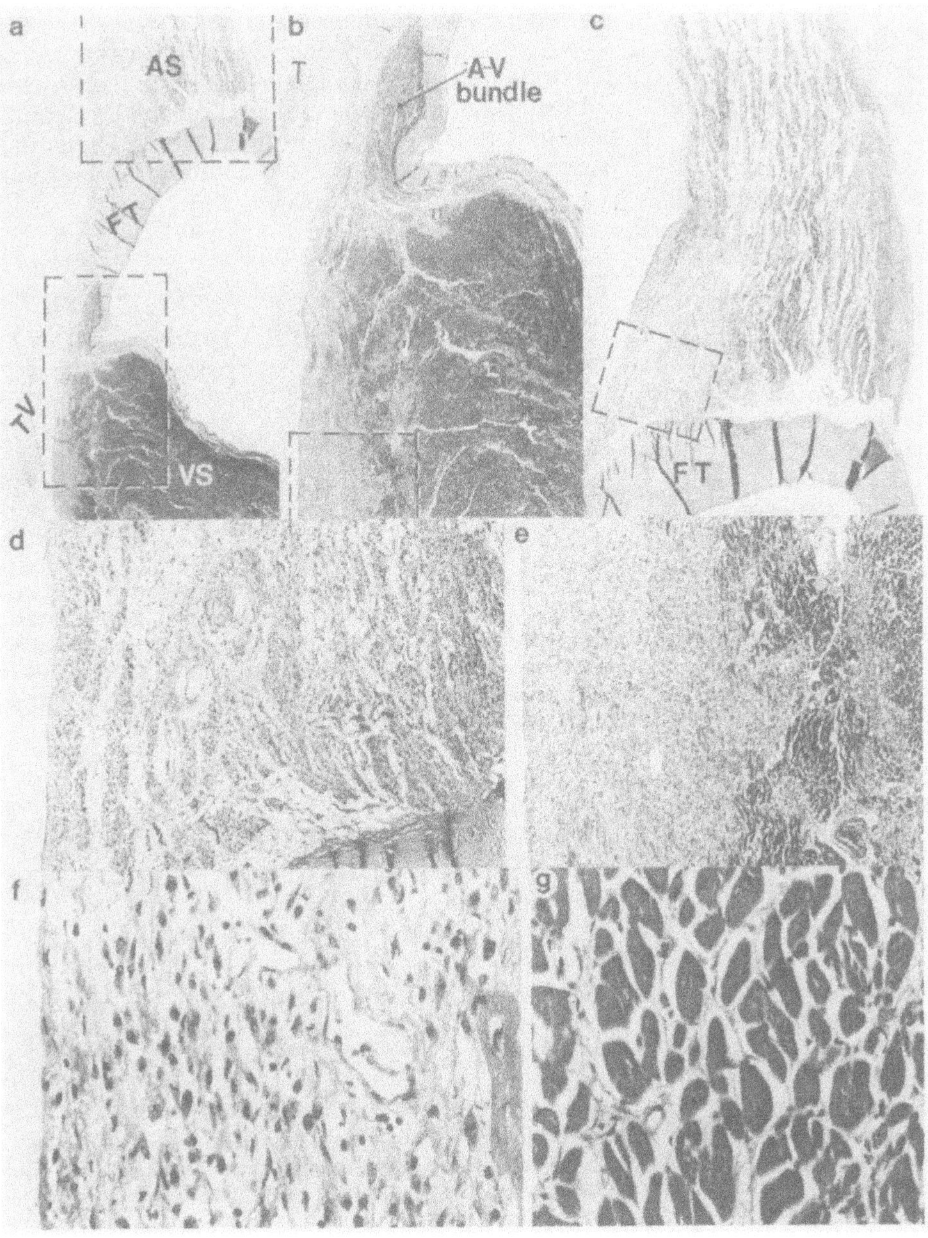

FIGURE 3. Photomicrographs from the area of the atrioventricular (AV) bundle in the patient. All sections were stained by hematoxylin and eosin. *A*, low-power (× 6.5) view of the atrial septum (AS) and the fibrous trigone (FT), within which is the AV bundle and to which is attached the septal leaflet of the tricuspid valve (TV) and the ventricular septum (VS) below. *B*, a closer view (× 16) of one of the areas in brackets shown in *A*. The myocardium beneath the mural endocardium on the right ventricular aspect of the ventricular septum is extensively damaged and a close-up (× 54) of a portion of this damaged myocardium in brackets in *B* is shown in *E*. The connection between the AV bundle and the left bundle branch is intact, but the connection between the AV bundle and the right bundle branch is interrupted. *C*, closer view (× 11.5) of the atrial septum above the fibrous trigone. A portion of this area also is visible in the brackets in *A*. An even closer view (× 54) of the area in brackets in *C* is shown in *D*. The myocardial fibers are extensively damaged. *F*, a high-power view (× 430) of a portion of the damaged myocardial fibers shown in *E*. The myocardial fibers have disappeared. *G*, a high-power view (× 430) of preserved or undamaged myocardium of the ventricular septum for comparison to *F*.

dle branch showed no abnormalities in 2 of the previously reported patients.[5,6] Both had received a single shock (280 J in 1 patient[5] and 275 J in the other[6]). In the report by Bharati et al,[4] the patient received 2 shocks of 500 J each and damage was present in the left and right bundle branch, with scarring seen in the summit of the muscular ventricular septum. In our patient, the AV node was spared and the AV bundle was interrupted at the take-off of the right bundle branch. The continuity of the AV bundle and left bundle branch is in agreement with the symptomatic recurrence of AV conduction in our patient.

The cause of our patient's sudden death is uncertain. Nonsustained ventricular tachycardia occurs occasionally after catheter ablation of the AV junction. Our patient received a new antiarrhythmic agent 3 days before death and its proarrhythmic effect could have contributed to his death.

1. Scheinman MN, Morady F, Hess DS, Gonzalez R. *Catheter induced ablation of the atrioventricular junction to control refractory supraventricular arrhythmias. JAMA 1982;248:851–855.*

2. Gallagher JJ, Svenson RH, Kasell JH, German LD, Bardy GH, Broughton A, Critelli G. *Catheter technique for closed chest ablation of the atrioventricular conduction system. N Engl J Med 1982;306:194–200.*

3. Scheinman MM, Davis JC. *Catheter ablation for treatment of tachyarrhythmias: present role and potential promise. Circulation 1986;73:10–13.*

4. Bharati S, Scheinman MM, Morady F, Hess DS, Lev M. *Sudden death after catheter-induced atrioventricular junctional ablation. Chest 1985;88:883–889.*

5. Critelli G, Gallagher JJ, Thieve G, Perticane F, Marda V, Rossi L. *Histologic observations after closed chest ablation of the atrioventricular conduction system. JAMA 1984;252:2604–2606.*

6. Ward DE, Davies M. *Transvenous high energy shock for ablating atrioventricular conduction in man: observations in the histological effects. Br Heart J 1984;51:175–178.*

Serial Electrocardiographic Changes in Idiopathic Dilated Cardiomyopathy Confirmed at Necropsy

Robert L. Wilensky, MD, Paul Yudelman, MD, Andrew I. Cohen, MD, Ross D. Fletcher, MD, James Atkinson, MD, PhD, Renu Virmani, MD, and William C. Roberts, MD

Serial electrocardiographic changes in necropsy-proven idiopathic dilated cardiomyopathy are evaluated and a method of predicting heart weight using QRS amplitudes is described. In 34 patients with multiple electrocardiograms (mean 3/patient) progressive prolongation of PR interval (0.18 ± 0.03 to 0.21 ± 0.03, $p < 0.001$) and QRS duration (0.10 ± 0.02 to 0.13 ± 0.03, $p < 0.0001$) was noted. Progressive conduction abnormalities were common (82%). QTc interval and QRS- and T-wave axes did not change. In 50 patients with electrocardiograms within 60 days of death, total 12-lead QRS and V_1 through V_6 QRS amplitude correlated better with heart weight ($r = 0.51$, $p < 0.0001$ and $r = 0.55$, $p < 0.0001$) than the Estes-Romhilt score did. The mean total 12-lead QRS amplitude was 138 mm with a mean of 106 for V_1 through V_6. In 31 patients cardiac mass index was calculated and showed significant correlation with 12-lead and V_1 through V_6 QRS amplitudes ($r = 0.68$, $p < 0.0001$ and $r = 0.75$, $p < 0.0001$, respectively). The QRS amplitudes remained constant during the illness. By using total 12-lead QRS or frontal plane QRS amplitude, heart weight can be predicted as early as 2 years before death. Use of body surface area and QRS amplitude criteria increases the accuracy of heart weight prediction. Thus, progressive electrocardiographic changes are common in patients with idiopathic dilated cardiomyopathy and QRS amplitude criteria are more accurate in the prediction of left ventricular hypertrophy than standard criteria.

(Am J Cardiol 1988;62:276–283)

From the Department of Medicine and Division of Cardiology, Veterans Administration Medical Center and the Armed Forces Institute of Pathology, Washington, DC, Department of Pathology, Vanderbilt University, Nashville, Tennessee, and the Pathology Branch, National Heart, Lung, and Blood Institute, National Institues of Health, Bethesda, Maryland. Manuscript received March 3, 1988; revised manuscript received and accepted April 4, 1988.

Address for reprints: Robert L. Wilensky, MD, Krannert Institute of Cardiology, 1001 West 10th Street, Indianapolis, Indiana 46202.

Although electrocardiographic abnormalities are common in patients with idiopathic dilated cardiomyopathy (IDC),[1-4] no studies have looked at serial changes. In the present study we describe electrocardiographic findings in 56 patients with necropsy-proven IDC; 34 had multiple electrocardiograms. The progressive electrocardiographic changes are evaluated and a method of predicting heart weight in IDC using QRS amplitudes is described.

METHODS

The following criteria for diagnosis of IDC had to be met[4,5]: (1) increased heart weight (>350 g in women and >400 g in men), (2) increased size of both right and left ventricular cavities, (3) absence of significant (>75% cross-sectional area) narrowing of an epicardial coronary artery, (4) absence of significant valvular and pericardial abnormalities, (5) absence of a major congenital cardiac malformation, (6) absence of obstructive pulmonary disease, (7) absence of infiltrative and inflammatory diseases affecting the heart and (8) absence of renal lesions consistent with systemic hypertension.

Pathology reports of 197 patients with IDC were reviewed. Electrocardiograms or clinical records could not be retrieved in 89 cases. Of the remaining 108 cases, 23 did not die of their cardiomyopathy, 11 had acute dilated cardiomyopathy and 18 did not have an electrocardiogram in the last 60 days of life or multiple electrocardiograms spanning >50% of their illness or the last year of their life. The 56 patients remaining (138 electrocardiograms) make up the study population. Death resulted from complications of IDC (i.e., low cardiac output failure, arrhythmias or thromboembolism). No patient had another concomitant life-threatening disease or systemic hypertension at least in the last 3 months of life. The Pathology Branch of the National Heart, Lung, and Blood Institute, National Institutes of Health, provided 40 cases; Vanderbilt University Hospital, 7 cases; and the Nashville Veterans Administration Hospital, 9 cases. Each heart was examined by 1 of 3 investigators (WCR, RV or JA).

Records were retrieved from the hospitals in which the patients had died. Duration of symptoms of cardiac dysfunction was the time from onset of symptoms of congestive heart failure or significant arrhythmias to death. The body surface area was calculated from height and weight.

Serial electrocardiograms—spanning either >50% of the duration of the clinical illness with the last electrocardiogram within 180 days of death or the year before death—were available in 34 patients; 50 patients had electrocardiograms within 60 days of death. Electrocardiograms were reviewed by 2 investigators (RLW and AIC) independently and discrepencies in interpretation were resolved by consensus opinion. Results from 18 cases (21 electrocardiograms) have been published previously.[4]

Conduction abnormalities were defined according to previously defined standards.[6] Any Q-wave >40 ms was considered abnormal. Poor R-wave progression was defined as an absence of progressively increasing R-wave amplitudes in leads V_1 through V_4. Left atrial abnormality was defined as a wide, biphasic or downward directed P wave in leads V_1 and V_2 with an increased P-wave duration to PR-interval ratio.[7] Right atrial abnormality was the presence of peaked P waves in leads II, III and aVF with a voltage >2.5 mV.[7]

Left ventricular hypertrophy was determined by Estes and Romhilt criteria and by a method using QRS voltage criteria.[8] Patients with bundle branch block were included in both determinations. The amplitude of QRS waves, defined as the number of millimeters between the point of maximum inflection (top of the R wave) and deflection (bottom of the Q or S wave, whichever was greater), was measured for each lead (Figure 1). Total V_1 through V_6 and total 12-lead QRS amplitudes were obtained by adding the amplitudes of the individual leads. Amplitudes were standardized to 10 mm equaling 1 mV.

Statistical analysis in the correlation of heart weight and cardiac mass index with electrocardiographic determinations of left ventricular hypertrophy used linear regression. The paired *t* test was used in determining change in PR intervals, QRS duration, QTc interval, QRS and T-wave axis between the initial and final electrocardiogram. In addition, paired *t* test evaluated change in voltages and Estes-Romhilt score between the initial and final electrocardiogram.

RESULTS

The 56 patients ranged in age from 17 to 73 years (mean 49); 33 were white (27 men and 6 women) and 23 were black (19 men and 4 women). Duration of symptoms of cardiac dysfunction ranged from 180 to 7,660 days (mean 1,755). In 3 cases the exact disease duration could not be discerned but was >1 year.

Heart weight ranged from 400 to 1,050 g (mean 675) in men and from 400 to 860 g (mean 650) in women. Heart weight did not correlate with disease duration. Ventricular wall thickness was obtained in 31 cases. The left ventricular free wall thickness was 0.9 to 2.5 cm (mean 1.6). The right ventricular free wall thickness was 0.2 to 1.0 cm (mean 0.8). In 13 patients grossly visible left ventricular scars were present.

In the 34 patients (28 men and 6 women) with multiple electrocardiograms (Table I) the last electrocardiogram was recorded within 60 days of death in 28 patients and within 180 days in the remaining 6 (average 32). Duration of symptoms of cardiac dysfunction averaged 1,601 days (1,507 days in men and 2,391 days in women) and ranged from 365 to 4,015 days in men and from 1,065 to 7,665 days in women. Available electrocardiograms spanned 865 days in men (57% of disease duration) and 1,924 days in women (80%). For men and women combined electrocardiograms spanned an average of 1,057 days, representing the latter 65% of the disease. Digoxin was prescribed in 27 patients, procainamide in 5 (1 patient had both procainamide and mexiletine), quinidine in 3 and phenytoin in 1. Heart weight averaged 681 g in men (range 400 to 940) and 623 g in women (range 400 to 800).

Of 34 patients, 24 (71%) remained in sinus rhythm throughout their illness; 4 patients had atrial fibrillation on all electrocardiograms, 4 other patients developed atrial fibrillation and 2 additional patients developed other atrial tachyarrhythmias. Heart rate averaged 94 beats/min on the initial electrocardiogram and remained constant.

Of the 24 patients in sinus rhythm, the PR interval lengthened in 16 patients (67%), decreased in 4 (17%) and did not change in 4 (17%). Mean PR interval (Table II) increased from 0.18 second on the initial electrocardiogram to 0.21 second on the final electrocardiogram ($p < 0.001$). QRS duration increased in 26 patients (76%), decreased in 4 (12%) and did not change in 4 (12%). The average QRS duration increased from 0.10 to 0.13 second ($p < 0.0001$). Progression of PR and QRS intervals did not correlate with disease duration or changes in medications. QTc increased in 18 patients (53%), decreased in 8 (24%) and remained constant in 8 (24%). Average QTc increased insignificantly ($p = 0.06$). QRS axis remained constant as did T-wave axis.

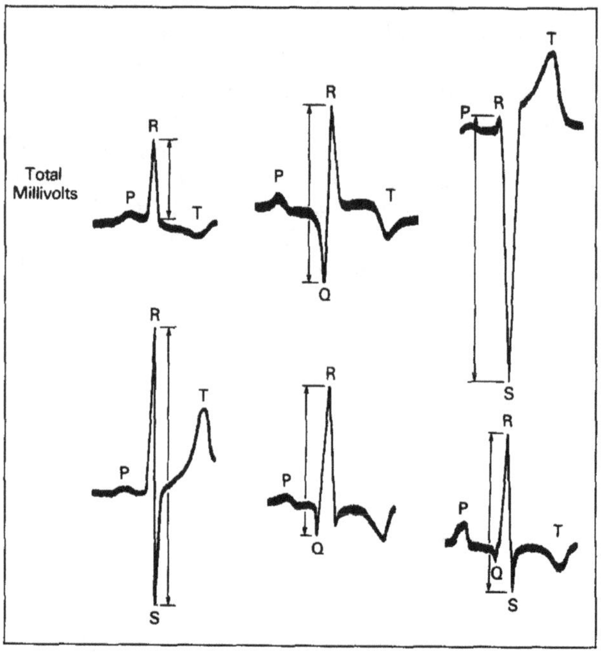

FIGURE 1. The method of QRS amplitude measurement (in mm). From Siegel and Roberts[8] reproduced with permission from C.V. Mosby.

TABLE IA Serial Electrocardiographic Changes in 28 Men with Autopsy-Proven Idiopathic Dilated Cardiomyopathy

Age at Death (yrs), Race	Duration (days) Symptoms of CD	Interval (days) ECG to Death	HR (bpm)	Rhythm	Interval(s)			Axis(°)		Conduction Abnormality	QRS Voltage (mm)			Estes-Romhilt Score	VPC	Atrial Abnormality		HW (g)	LV Scar
					PR	QRS	QTc	QRS	T		Total	V_{1-6}	I, II, III R, L, F			Right	Left		
22, W	365	190	100	S	0.21	0.08	0.41	I	I	0	73	56	17	3	0	0	0	700	0
		9	115	S	0.21	0.08	0.48	15	I	0	99	77	22	3	0	0	0		
28, W	540	280	82	S	0.16	0.08	0.42	−45	−120	LAFB	191	143	48	3	+	0	0	540	0
		88	88	S	0.19	0.12	0.45	−30	I	LAFB	190	145	45	3	0	0	0		
		1	100	S	0.19	0.12	0.45	−75	75	LAFB	147	110	37	6	0	0	0		
35, W	1,095	990	125	S	0.20	0.09	0.47	60	I	0	92	82	10	0	+	0	0	940	+
		5	77	S	0.19	0.08	0.48	−30	I	0	138	115	23	5	0	0	+		
39, W	?	425	110	AF	—	0.10	0.48	−45	135	IVCD, LAFB	84	58	26	5	+	—	—	400	—
		60	80	AF	—	0.16	0.48	−30	120	IVCD, LAFB	75	52	23	5	+	—	—		
43, W	?	400	76	S	0.22	0.12	0.45	−15	90	0	164	136	28	6	0	0	0	500	0
		3	88	S	0.25	0.14	0.45	−45	90	IVCD, LAFB	194	154	40	7	0	0	+		
44, B	600	2,000	84	S	0.16	0.05	0.50	10	80	0	124	80	44	1	0	0	0	700	+
		580	115	S	0.16	0.08	0.48	−30	I	LAFB	140	96	44	6	0	0	+		
		265	95	S	0.16	0.08	0.42	−45	130	LAFB	146	107	39	6	+	0	+		
		55	96	S	0.16	0.09	0.41	−70	50	LAFB	125	100	25	6	0	0	+		
44, W	4,015	591	102	AF	—	0.10	0.44	45	90	0	135	108	27	2	+	—	—	750	+
		440	74	AF	—	0.11	0.44	−15	I	Left BBB	116	95	21	2	+	—	—		
		120	85	AF	—	0.12	0.44	−15	I	Left BBB	113	95	18	2	0	—	—		
47, W	2,190	917	120	S	0.21	0.14	0.45	−130	90	Right BBB	116	86	30	3	+	0	0	620	0
		54	110	S	0.20	0.16	0.50	−120	I	Right BBB, LAFB	145	115	30	3	+	0	0		
48, B	699	1,095	98	S	0.16	0.08	0.41	0	−120	0	241	192	49	4	0	0	+	900	0
		530	96	S	0.24	0.10	0.46	−30	−130	LAFB	206	152	54	7	0	0	+		
		350	102	S	0.24	0.12	0.43	−40	−90	IVCD, LAFB	225	158	67	10	0	0	+		
		28	75	S	0.28	0.12	0.43	−45	90	Left BBB	313	242	71	11	0	0	+		
48, B	1,035	1,023	102	S	0.16	0.06	0.44	−10	I	0	144	110	34	6	0	0	+	660	0
		684	98	S	0.17	0.08	0.41	−5	I	0	174	145	29	5	0	0	+		
		399	112	S	0.19	0.10	0.44	0	I	Inc Left BBB	151	135	16	6	+	0	+		
		180	89	S	0.20	0.11	0.49	5	I	Inc Left BBB	140	125	15	6	0	0	+		
48, W	2,980	2,130	74	S	0.21	0.09	0.48	45	90	0	160	120	40	0	+	0	0	650	+
		1,400	60	S	0.20	0.10	0.42	10	90	Left BBB	196	158	39	5	+	0	0		
		1,030	62	S	0.21	0.12	0.43	−15	90	Left BBB	159	124	35	3	+	0	0		
		330	66	S	0.20	0.16	0.47	−45	90	Left BBB	111	70	41	4	+	0	0		
		95	70	S	0.21	0.14	0.49	−90	90	Left BBB	117	80	37	5	+	0	0		
49, W	2,355	1,625	105	S	0.16	0.11	0.43	−30	90	Right IVCD	190	158	32	4	0	0	+	705	+
		913	90	S	0.17	0.11	0.44	−15	90	Right IVCD	163	148	15	6	0	0	+		
		180	90	S	0.20	0.12	0.44	−15	90	Right IVCD	166	148	18	7	0	0	+		
50, B	2,190	430	100	S	0.18	0.10	0.49	−60	I	LAFB	78	61	17	4	+	0	+	650	0
		1	105	AT	—	0.10	0.47	−60	I	LAFB	86	65	21	1	+	0	+		
50, B	1,825	395	124	AF	—	0.12	0.46	100	I	0	114	100	14	0	0	0	0	710	+
		9	100	AF	—	0.12	0.45	90	I	IVCD	92	76	16	0	0	0	0		
50, W	2,190	380	59	S	0.24	0.10	0.44	−5	170	0	191	141	50	1	0	0	0	790	+
		74	74	S	0.28	0.12	0.55	−5	170	0	192	150	42	1	0	0	0		
		19	80	S	0.29	0.13	0.42	5	175	IVCD	219	165	54	4	0	0	0		
51, B	1,825	1,660	80	S	0.18	0.11	0.45	−120	I	LAFB	61	51	10	4	+	0	0	650	0
		400	73	S	0.22	0.12	0.40	−120	90	LAFB	93	76	17	2	+	0	+		
		1	65	S	0.21	0.14	0.45	−120	I	IVCD, LAFB	70	56	14	4	+	0	+		
56, B	1,460	556	70	S	0.14	0.12	0.48	−90	I	Right BBB	75	55	20	3	0	0	0	475	0
		56	95	S	0.19	0.16	0.44	−120	I	Right BBB	45	37	8	6	0	0	+		
		1	67	S	0.28	0.16	0.45	−130	I	Right BBB	43	35	8	6	0	0	+		
56, B	600	500	90	S	0.16	0.11	0.46	0	65	IVCD	218	178	40	8	+	0	+	670	0
		230	74	S	0.17	0.10	0.52	−10	−30	IVCD	218	175	43	8	+	0	+		
		1	105	S	0.21	0.12	0.46	90	35	IVCD	151	137	14	4	+	+	+		

TABLE IA (continued)
Serial Electrocardiographic Changes in 28 Men with Autopsy-Proven Idiopathic Dilated Cardiomyopathy

Age at Death (yrs), Race	Duration (days) Symptoms of CD	Interval (days) ECG to Death	HR (bpm)	Rhythm	Interval(s) PR	Interval(s) QRS	Interval(s) QTc	Axis(°) QRS	Axis(°) T	Conduction Abnormality	QRS Voltage (mm) Total	QRS Voltage (mm) V_{1-6}	QRS Voltage (mm) I, II, III R, L, F	Estes-Romhilt Score	VPC	Atrial Abnormality Right	Atrial Abnormality Left	HW (g)	LV Scar
57, B	450	440	98	S	0.24	0.13	0.43	−45	90	Left BBB	130	102	28	8	0	0	+	710	0
		5	130	S	0.22	0.12	I	−90	I	Left BBB	141	123	17	8	0	0	+		
57, B	1,460	1,200	98	S	0.17	0.12	0.44	−90	I	Left BBB	197	148	49	7	0	0	0	760	0
		835	92	S	0.16	0.14	0.44	−90	90	Left BBB	141	110	31	7	0	0	+		
		77	115	S	0.18	0.15	0.45	−85	90	Left BBB	185	94	91	8	0	0	+		
58, W	2,500	1,500	84	S	0.16	0.10	0.41	30	90	0	152	116	36	1	+	0	0	610	0
		1	102	S	0.22	0.12	0.43	−60	110	Left BBB	101	78	23	6	+	0	0		
58, B	540	430	125	S	0.20	0.09	0.49	30	I	0	188	163	25	7	0	0	+	720	0
		120	115	AF	—	0.12	0.55	70	I	IVCD	171	131	40	5	+	0	0		
		1	90	AF	—	0.12	0.49	90	I	IVCD	130	103	27	2	+	0	0		
61, B	1,970	990	82	S	0.20	0.06	0.44	−15	−30	0	104	90	14	3	0	0	+	570	+
		600	75	S	0.21	0.08	0.45	−15	I	0	82	69	13	3	+	0	+		
		57	82	AF	—	0.12	0.49	−75	−30	IVCD, LAFB	118	101	17	2	0	—	—		
		1	100	AF	—	0.12	0.49	−60	−30	IVCD, LAFB	91	78	13	1	+	—	—		
61, W	730	335	105	S	0.17	0.09	0.40	80	I	0	157	111	46	4	0	0	+	655	0
		1	90	S	0.16	0.10	0.74	90	I	0	112	91	21	4	+	0	+		
61, B	1,900	720	100	S	0.18	0.10	0.48	−30	115	IVCD	275	181	94	7	0	0	0	780	+
		335	97	S	0.20	0.12	0.50	−30	130	IVCD, LAFB	251	176	75	7	0	0	0		
		1	65	AT	—	0.19	0.55	−45	195	Right BBB, LAFB	176	134	42	8	+	—	—		
63, W	1,460	470	82	S	0.18	0.16	0.48	−15	I	Left BBB	168	100	68	6	+	0	0	770	0
		40	94	S	0.20	0.16	0.50	−30	I	Left BBB	152	124	28	6	0	0	+		
65, W	2,300	2,190	68	S	0.16	0.08	0.43	−15	90	0	153	112	41	4	0	0	+	645	0
		3	76	S	0.19	0.10	0.47	30	I	0	159	120	39	1	+	0	+		
70, W	540	360	75	S	0.30	0.08	0.45	80	I	0	133	95	38	1	0	0	0	840	0
		19	125	AF	—	0.09	0.43	90	I	0	125	95	30	0	0	0	0		

TABLE IB Serial Electrocardiographic Changes in Six Women with Autopsy-Proven Idiopathic Dilated Cardiomyopathy

Age at Death (yrs), Race	Duration (days) Symptoms of CD	Interval (days) ECG to Death	HR (bpm)	Rhythm	Interval(s) PR	Interval(s) QRS	Interval(s) QTc	Axis(°) QRS	Axis(°) T	Conduction Abnormality	QRS Amplitude (mm) Total	QRS Amplitude (mm) V_{1-6}	QRS Amplitude (mm) I, II, III R, L, F	Estes-Romhilt Score	VPC	Atrial Abnormality Right	Atrial Abnormality Left	HW (g)	LV Scar
33, B	1,065	910	90	AF	—	0.09	0.44	75	90	0	63	58	5	1	+	—	—	400	0
		590	68	AF	—	0.11	0.49	120	−90	IVCD	98	76	22	3	+	—	—		
		4	120	AF	—	0.14	0.53	I	90	IVCD	47	26	21	3	0	—	—		
53, W	1,065	520	105	S	0.18	0.06	0.45	−30	90	LAFB	117	68	49	2	0	0	+	750	0
		399	120	S	0.18	0.08	0.51	−60	90	LAFB	108	60	48	3	0	0	+		
		30	112	S	0.20	0.10	0.54	−60	90	IVCD, LAFB	114	67	47	8	0	0	+		
		6	127	S	0.20	0.13	0.43	−60	90	Left BBB	143	76	65	4	+	0	+		
55, W	1,095	635	90	S	0.18	0.11	0.44	−130		0	80	63	17	5	0	0	+	615	0
		180	80	S	0.20	0.12	0.49	−120		0	93	81	12	6	0	0	+		
		1	90	S	0.24	0.16	0.58	−45		IVCD, LAFB	84	59	25	5	0	0	0		
56, W	?	900	136	S	0.20	0.12	0.48	30	90	IVCD	164	142	22	6	+	0	+	550	0
		5	105	S	0.20	0.12	0.43	−30	90	Left BBB	144	114	30	6	+	0	+		
63, W	7,665	7,600	96	S	0.16	0.13	0.50	−30	90	Left BBB	98	66	32	8	0	0	+	800	+
		3,650	72	S	0.19	0.20	0.45	−15	90	Left BBB	210	163	47	8	0	0	+		
		700	94	S	0.12	0.16	0.52	−30	90	Left BBB	264	203	39	6	0	0	+		
		2	92	S	0.20	0.20	0.54	−40	90	Left BBB	225	177	48	6	0	0	+		
67, B	1,065	980	118	S	0.16	0.12	0.47	30	30	0	195	136	59	3	+	0	0	620	0
		85	86	AF	—	0.12	0.47	30	I	0	120	89	31	1	+	0	0		

AF = atrial fibrillation, AT = atrial tachyarrhythmia, B = black, BBB = bundle branch block, bpm = beats/min, CD = cardiac dysfunction, HR = heart rate, HW = heart weight, I = indeterminate, inc = incomplete, IVCD = intraventricular conduction delay, LAFB = left anterior fascicular block, LV = left ventricular, S = sinus, VPC = ventricular premature complex; W = white, + = present, 0 = absent, — = unknown.

TABLE II Electrocardiographic Changes in Chronic Dilated Cardiomyopathy

	No.	Initial Determination	Determination at Death	p Value
PR interval (s)	24	0.18 ± 0.03	0.21 ± 0.03	0.0007
QRS interval (s)	34	0.10 ± 0.02	0.13 ± 0.03	<0.0001
QTc interval (s)	33	0.45 ± 0.03	0.49 ± 0.06	NS
QRS axis (degrees)	33	−15 ± 60	−27 ± 64	NS
Total QRS amplitude (mm)	34	142 ± 53	133 ± 54	NS
V_1 to V_6 amplitude (mm)	34	108 ± 41	104 ± 43	NS

NS = not significant.

Of the 34 patients, 28 (82%) developed conduction abnormalities (Table I). Bundle branch block was seen in 13 patients (38%) with 10 having left and 3 having right bundle branch block. Six patients developed left bundle branch block within the period studied and 1 developed a right bundle branch block in his final year. Two of 3 patients with right bundle branch block also had left anterior fascicular block.

Anterior Q waves were present on the last electrocardiogram in 19 of 56 patients. Poor R-wave progression was seen in 49 patients. Of the 13 patients with left ventricular scars, 4 had anterior Q waves (31%); of the 43 patients without left ventricular scars, 15 (35%) had Q waves. All 13 patients with left ventricular scars had poor R-wave progression (100%) and 36 of 43 (84%) patients without scars had poor R-wave progression.

In the period examined, the latter 65% of the patient's clinical disease, the V_1 to V_6 and total QRS amplitude remained constant (Table II, Figure 2). The Estes-Romhilt score increased insignificantly from 3.7 to 4.5.

Table III lists results of 50 electrocardiograms obtained within 60 days of death. V_1 to V_6 ($r = 0.55$, $p < 0.0001$) and total 12-lead QRS ($r = 0.51$, $p < 0.0001$) amplitudes correlated significantly with heart weight at death (Figure 3). Estes-Romhilt score did not correlate.

In 31 of 56 patients the heights and weights at the time of the last electrocardiogram were available and cardiac mass index (g/m^2) was calculated. Mean V_1 through V_6 and 12-lead total QRS amplitude correlated significantly with the cardiac mass index at necropsy ($r = 0.75$, $p < 0.0001$ and $r = 0.68$, $p < 0.0001$, respectively) as shown in Figure 4.

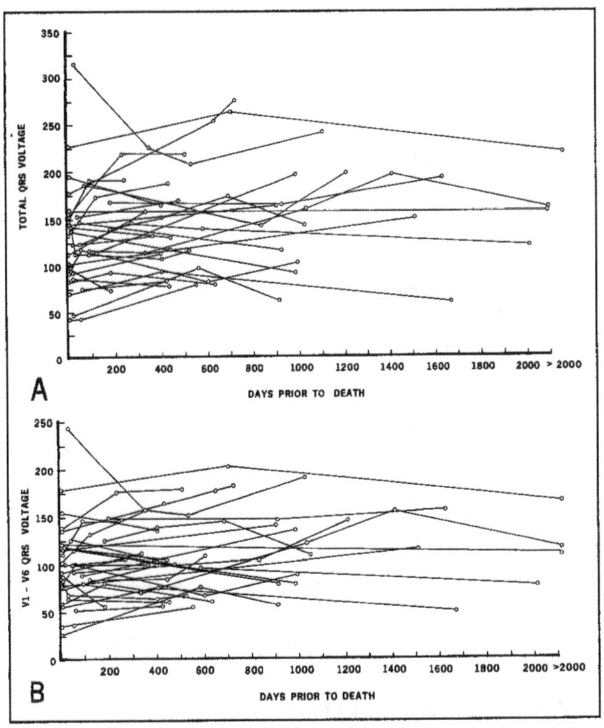

FIGURE 2. The stability of QRS amplitude over time in 34 patients. *A*, total 12-lead QRS amplitude progression; *B*, V_1 through V_6 QRS amplitude progression.

TABLE III Abnormalities on the Last 12-Lead Electrocardiogram Recorded Within 60 Days of Death in 50 Adults with Idiopathic Dilated Cardiomyopathy

Age (yrs): range (mean)	17–73 (50)
Men/women	41/9
White/black	30/20
Duration of symptoms of cardiac dysfunction (mos): range (mean)	8–256 (57)
Interval ECG to death (days): Range (mean)	1–60 (18)
Heart weight (g): range (mean)	400–1,050 (684)
Left ventricular scar (%)	9 (18)
Heart rate (beats/min): range (mean)	58–150 (96)
Rhythm	
Atrial fibrillation (%)	7 (14)
Atrial flutter (%)	2 (4)
Atrial tachyarrhythmia (%)	2 (4)
PR interval (s): range (mean)	0.14–0.29 (0.20)
QRS interval (s): range (mean)	0.08–0.20 (0.12)
QTc interval (s): range (mean)	0.36–0.74 (0.48)
QRS axis (degrees): range (mean)	−130 to +130 (−21)
T-wave axis (degrees): range (mean)	−90 to +195 (76)
Conduction abnormalities	41
Left BBB only (%)	18 (36)
Right BBB only (%)	2 (4)
RBBB + left anterior fascicular block (%)	1(2)
LAFB only (%)	7 (14)
IVCD only (%)	8 (16)
LAFB + IVCD (%)	5 (10)
Ventricular premature complexes (%)	22 (44)
Atrial abnormality	
Right alone (%)	1/39 (3)
Left alone (%)	20/39 (51)
Both (%)	3/39 (8)
Abnormal Q waves (%)	18 (36)
Poor R-wave progression (%)	43 (86)
QRS voltage (mm)	
Total: range (mean)	43–313 (138)
I + II + III + R + L + F: range (mean)	8–71 (32)
V_2 to V_6: range (mean)	26–242 (106)
Estes-Romhilt score: range (mean)	0–11 (4.7)

BBB = bundle branch block; IVCD = intraventricular conduction delay; LAFB = left anterior fascicular block.

DISCUSSION

This is the first study analyzing more than one 12-lead electrocardiogram in patients with autopsy-proven IDC. Our results show a progressive increase in PR interval and QRS duration (Figure 5). Many electrocardiograms had ventricular premature complexes, anterior Q waves and poor R-wave progression (Table I and III). Anterior Q waves and poor R-wave progression appear unrelated to left ventricular scarring. Progressive conduction disturbances were common. Both 12-lead and V_1 to V_6 QRS amplitude correlated better with heart weight than did the Estes-Romhilt criteria for left ventricular hypertrophy. Significant increases in PR interval and QRS duration were seen during the disease process. While prolonged PR interval and QRS duration have been noted previously,[1,4] our study is the first to show the progressive nature of the increase. While the administration of digitalis invariably increased PR interval the progressive nature of the increase argues for an underlying organic cause of PR prolongation. The increase in QRS duration was not due to medications as only 9 of 34 patients were prescribed medications that prolong QRS intervals. Fibrotic infiltration of the conduction pathways could prolong the PR interval and fibrous tissue infiltration of the ventricular myocardium[9,10] could prolong the QRS complex. Myocardial cell hypertrophy also may play a role in increasing the con-

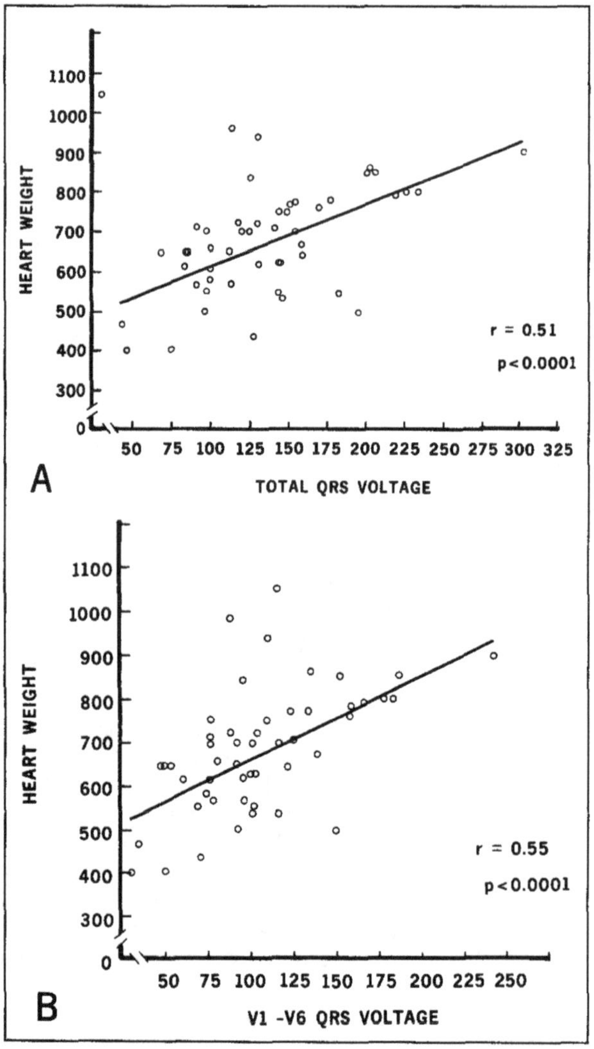

FIGURE 3. The relation between QRS amplitude criteria and heart weight at necropsy in 50 patients with chronic idiopathic dilated cardiomyopathy with electrocardiograms recorded within 60 days of death. *A*, correlation of total 12-lead QRS amplitudes and heart weight; *B*, correlation of V_1 through V_6 QRS amplitude and heart weight.

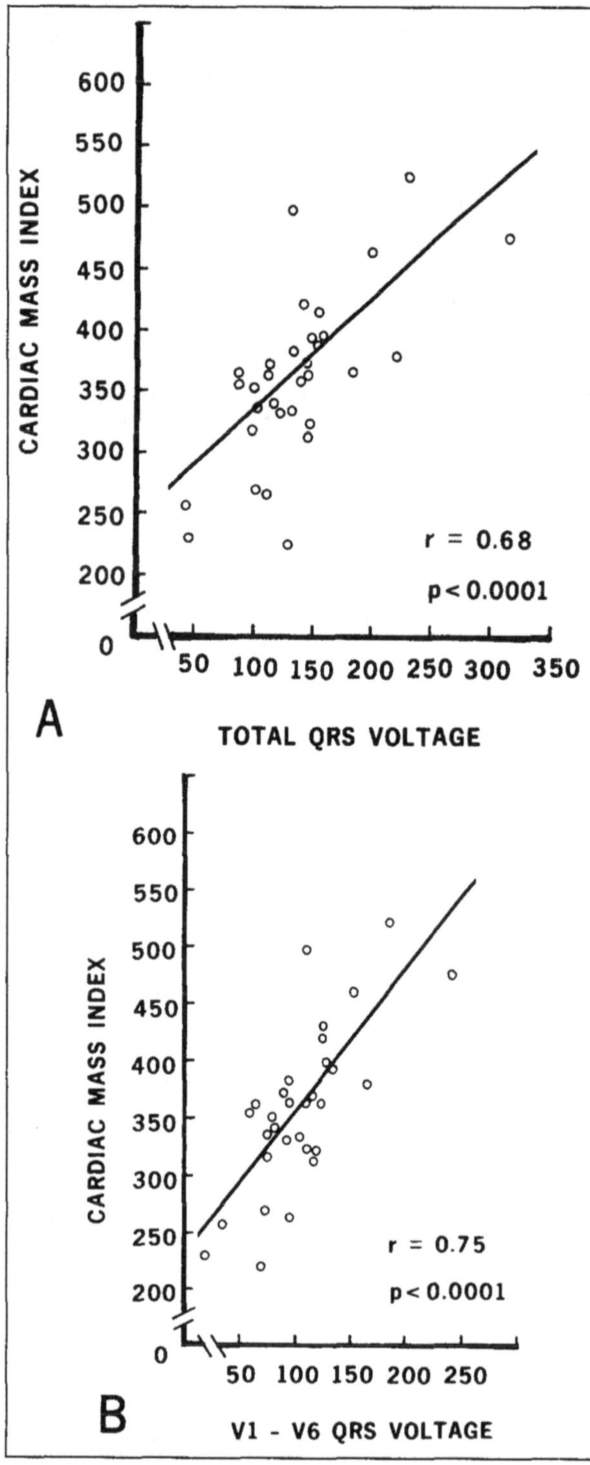

FIGURE 4. The correlation between QRS amplitude criteria, on the last recorded electrocardiogram before death, and cardiac mass index at necropsy in 31 patients. *A*, total 12-lead QRS amplitude and cardiac mass index; *B*, V_1 through V_6 QRS amplitude and cardiac mass index.

duction time. Progressive prolongation of the PR interval and QRS duration may indicate continued fibrous tissue infiltration.

Conduction abnormalities were common (82%). Left bundle branch block, left anterior fascicular block and intraventricular conduction delay occurred often while few hearts had right intraventricular conduction disturbances. This finding is similar to results published earlier.[3,4] Of our patients with conduction abnormalities, 68% had progressive disturbances in the time period studied. This observation supports evidence that conduction abnormalities in IDC are more common in patients with clinical courses >1 year.[11] The conduction abnormalities may be an electrocardiographic marker of increasing interstitial myocardial fibrosis[12–14] or due to increasing left ventricular hypertrophy.

Frontal plane and total 12-lead QRS amplitudes correlated with heart weight better than the Estes-Romhilt score did and they were unchanged during the period of study. Correlating V_1 to V_6 or total 12-lead QRS amplitudes with the cardiac mass index yields a more accurate indication of heart weight at necropsy. Recent studies have shown that Estes-Romhilt criteria are inadequate in evaluating left ventricular hypertrophy in chronic aortic regurgitation[15] and in amyloidosis.[16] A new method of using total 12-lead QRS amplitude has been applied[7] and correlated with heart weight in aortic regurgitation,[15] amyloidosis[16] and IDC.[4] Odom et al[17] established standards in normal hearts. Total QRS amplitude averaged 127 mm, ranging from 80 to 185 mm with values remaining constant the last 5 years of life. Roberts and Day[15] suggested that 175 mm might be considered the upper limit of normal with values >175 mm representing left ventricular hypertrophy (93% specificity). Roberts et al[4] have shown that total electrocardiogram amplitude in IDC ranges from 75 to 250 mm (mean 153), similar to the results of the present study. No studies have looked at V_1 through V_6 amplitude as a marker of left ventricular hypertrophy but in 1 study[17] the mean was 90 mm (range 54 to 134). In the present study total QRS amplitude in IDC was 138 mm and the V_1 to V_6 voltage was 106; these values are only slightly higher than the amplitude in normal patients. No studies have correlated 12-lead QRS amplitude criteria with cardiac mass index. It would be difficult to diagnose IDC purely on amplitude criteria, but the criteria can be an indicator of heart weight.

Although virtually all patients with IDC have biatrial enlargement only 11% had right atrial abnormality and 59% left atrial abnormality on electrocardiogram. Previous studies have shown that P-wave amplitude does not correlate with either left or right atrial weights at autopsy[18] and only 53% with left atrial abnormality on electrocardiogram had echocardiographic evidence of increased left atrial dimension.[19] Our results support the conclusion that the electrocardiogram is insensitive in diagnosing atrial abnormalities.

A limitation of this study is its retrospective nature. We were, therefore, unable to determine exactly when electrocardiographic changes occurred. In addition, criteria for entering this study included the presence of electrocardiograms recording >50% of the disease duration with the last electrocardiogram within 6 months of death or electrocardiograms spanning the last year of life. Thus, a number of patients dying suddenly may not have had an electrocardiogram in the time period necessary for inclusion.

Because some investigators believe that left conduction delay and ventricular arrhythmias represent significant risk factors for early death,[20] our results may underestimate the degree of conduction abnormalities or ventricular arrhythmias present in patients with IDC.

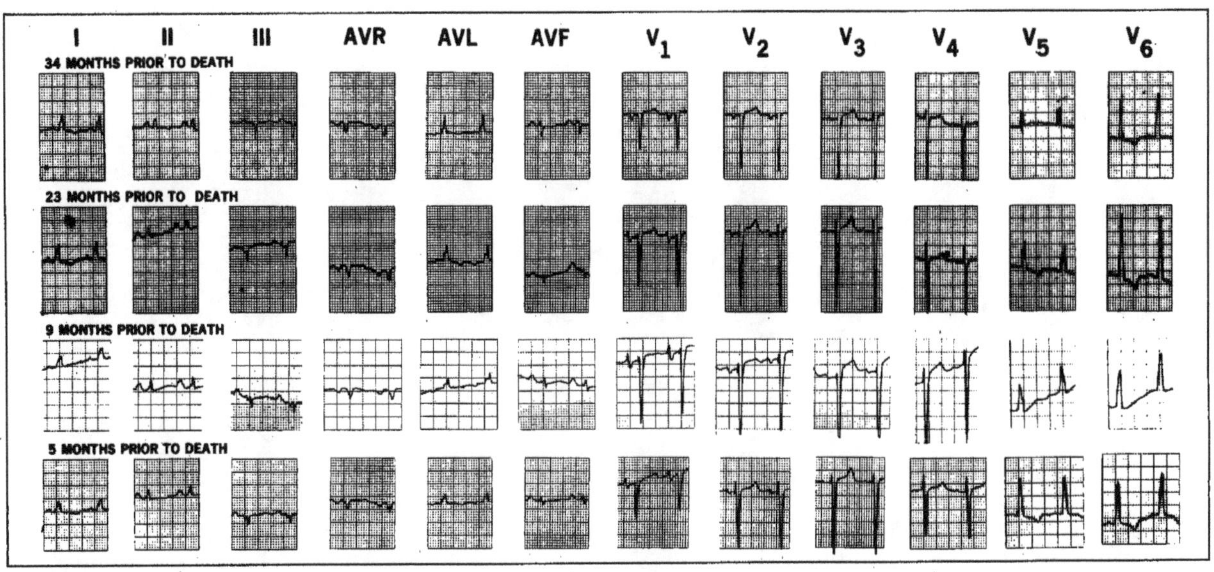

FIGURE 5. Serial electrocardiograms from a patient with idiopathic dilated cardiomyopathy. Onset of symptoms of cardiac dysfunction occurred 34 months before death.

Our study did not correlate the degree of interstitial myocardial fibrosis with the PR interval, QRS duration or conduction abnormalities. It has been well documented, however, that interstitial fibrosis is a common finding in IDC[4,9,10] and the presence of interstitial myocardial fibrosis has been correlated previously with conduction abnormalities.[12-14]

Acknowledgment: The authors gratefully acknowledge William Green, MD, for his assistance in obtaining patient records and Elisabeth Alcenius-W for her excellent graphic skills.

REFERENCES

1. Hamby RI, Raia F. *Electrocardiographic aspects of primary myocardial disease in 60 patients. Am Heart J 1968;76:316–328.*
2. Stapleton JF, Segal JP, Harvey WP. *The electrocardiogram of myocardiopathy. Prog Cardiovasc Dis 1970;13:217–239.*
3. Segal JP, Stapleton JF, McClellan JR, Waller BF, Harvey WP. *Idiopathic cardiomyopathy. Clinical features, prognosis and therapy. Curr Probl Cardiol 1978;3:1–49.*
4. Roberts WC, Siegel RJ, McManus BM. *Idiopathic dilated cardiomyopathy: analysis of 152 necropsy patients. Am J Cardiol 1987;60:1340–1355.*
5. Roberts WC, Ferrans VJ. *Pathologic anatomy of the cardiomyopathies. Idiopathic dilated and hypertrophic types, infiltrative types, and endomyocardial disease with and without eosinophilia. Hum Pathol 1975;6:287–342.*
6. Willems JL, Robles de Medina EO, Bernard R, Coumel P, Fisch C, Krikler D, Mazur NA, Meijer FL, Morgensen L, Moret P, Pisa Z, Rautaharju PM, Surawicz B, Watanabe Y, Wellens HJJ. *Criteria for intraventricular conduction disturbances and pre-excitation. JACC 1985;5:1261–1275.*
7. Surawicz B. *Electrocardiographic diagnosis of chamber enlargement. JACC 1986;8:711–724.*
8. Siegel RJ, Roberts WC. *Electrocardiographic observations in severe aortic valve stenosis: correlative necropsy study to clinical, hemodynamic, and ECG variables demonstrating relation of 12-lead QRS amplitude to peak systolic transaortic pressure gradient. Am Heart J 1982;103:298–301.*
9. Dick MR, Unverferth DV, Baba N. *The pattern of myocardial degeneration in nonischemic congestive cardiomyopathy. Hum Pathol 1982;13:740–744.*
10. Factor SM, Sonnenblick EH. *The pathogenesis of clinical and experimental congestive cardiomyopathies: recent concepts. Prog Cardiovasc Dis 1985;27:395–420.*
11. Benjamin IJ, Schuster EH, Buckley BH. *Cardiac hypertrophy in idiopathic dilated congestive cardiomyopathy: a clinicopathic study. Circulation 1981; 64:442–447.*
12. Unger PN, Greenblatt M, Lev M. *The anatomic basis of the electrocardiographic abnormality in incomplete left bundle branch block. Am Heart J 1968;76:486–497.*
13. Lev M, Unger PN, Rosen KM, Bharati S. *The anatomic substrate of complete left bundle branch block. Circulation 1974;50:479–486.*
14. Kulbertus HE, Demoulin JC. *Pathological basis of concept of left hemiblock. In: Wellens HJJ, Lie LI, Janse MJ, eds. The Conduction System of the Heart. Structure, Function and Clinical Implications. Philadelphia: Lea and Febiger, 1976:287–296.*
15. Roberts WC, Day PJ. *Electrocardiographic observations in clinically isolated, pure, chronic, severe aortic regurgitation: analysis of 30 necropsy patients aged 19 to 65 years. Am J Cardiol 1985;55:431–438.*
16. Roberts WC, Waller BF. *Cardiac amyloidosis causing cardiac dysfunction: analysis of 54 necropsy patients. Am J Cardiol 1983;52:137–146.*
17. Odom H II, Davis JL, Din H, Baker BJ, Roberts WC, Murphy ML. *QRS voltage measurements in autopsied men free of cardiopulmonary disease: a basis for evaluating total QRS voltage as an index of left ventricular hypertrophy. Am J Cardiol 1986;58:801–804.*
18. Mazzoleni A, Wolff R, Wolff L, Reiner L. *Correlation between component cardiac weights and electrocardiographic patterns in 185 cases. Circulation 1964;30:808–829.*
19. Josephson ME, Kastor JA, Morganroth J. *Electrocardiographic left atrial enlargement. Electrophysiologic, echocardiographic and hemodynamic correlates. Am J Cardiol 1977;39:967–971.*
20. Unverferth DV, Magorien RD, Moeschberger ML, Baker PB, Fetters JK, Leier CV. *Factors influencing the one-year mortality of dilated cardiomyopathy. Am J Cardiol 1984;54:147–152.*

Frequency of Myocarditis, Left Ventricular Dysfunction and Ventricular Tachycardia in the Acquired Immune Deficiency Syndrome

Joseph M. Reilly, MD, Robert E. Cunnion, MD, David W. Anderson, MD, PhD, Timothy J. O'Leary, MD, PhD, J. Thayer Simmons, MD, H. Clifford Lane, MD, Anthony S. Fauci, MD, William C. Roberts, MD, Renu Virmani, MD, and Joseph E. Parrillo, MD

To evaluate possible relations between clinical and histopathologic cardiac findings in patients with the acquired immune deficiency syndrome (AIDS), 58 consecutively autopsied AIDS patients were reviewed retrospectively. Twenty-six (45%) had histopathologic myocarditis. Fifteen of these 26 (58%) had ≥1 clinical cardiac abnormalities: 6 had congestive heart failure or left ventricular (LV) dysfunction, or both, 4 had ventricular tachycardia (VT), 10 had electrocardiographic abnormalities and 4 had pericardial abnormalities. Of the 32 patients without myocarditis, 6 (19%) had pericardial or electrocardiographic abnormalities, or both, but none had congestive heart failure, LV dysfunction or VT. Overall, clinical cardiac abnormalities were found in 21 patients (36%). Patients with myocarditis had a significantly higher incidence of clinical cardiac abnormalities than patients without myocarditis (58 vs 19%, $p < 0.01$). All patients with congestive heart failure, LV dysfunction or VT had myocarditis. Thus, serious clinical cardiac abnormalities were common in patients with AIDS and were associated with myocarditis.

(Am J Cardiol 1988;62:789–793)

From the Critical Care Medicine, Pathologic Anatomy and Radiology Departments, Clinical Center, National Institute of Allergy and Infectious Diseases, and National Heart, Lung, and Blood Institute, National Institutes of Health, Bethesda, Maryland, and the Armed Forces Institute of Pathology, Washington, DC. Manuscript received April 11, 1988; revised manuscript received and accepted May 31, 1988.

Address for reprints: Joseph M. Reilly, MD, Critical Care Medicine Department, Building 10, Room 10D48, National Institutes of Health, Bethesda, MD 20892.

Limited data are available describing clinical cardiac abnormalities in patients with acquired immune deficiency syndrome (AIDS). One study emphasized the ability of echocardiography to identify pericardial effusions and ventricular hypokinesis.[1] Recently, a brief report described 3 patients with dilated cardiomyopathy and AIDS.[2] In the 2 patients autopsied, dilated cardiomyopathy and focal myocarditis were found. The prevalence of such cardiac involvement in AIDS is unknown. We retrospectively reviewed 58 consecutively autopsied AIDS patients to evaluate possible relations among cardiac abnormalities, myocarditis and patients' clinical courses.

METHODS

Patients: Between October 1981 and July 1986, 403 patients with human immunodeficiency virus infection were evaluated and followed at the Clinical Center of the National Institutes of Health. Almost 200 of these patients have died, and 58 of them were autopsied at the National Institutes of Health. The hearts were studied in detail and reported elsewhere.[3]

Data collection: All patient charts were reviewed by a clinician blinded to the gross and histopathologic autopsy data. The information collected from the charts included: age, sex, race, risk factors for contracting AIDS, date of initial diagnosis, neoplasms and opportunistic infections, date of death, hematologic and biochemical parameters, conventional and experimental therapies and coexisting disease processes. Cardiac symptoms and signs, cardiac medications and exposure to known cardiotoxins were also noted.

Definitions: CONGESTIVE HEART FAILURE: The diagnosis of congestive heart failure required a compatible clinical syndrome (dyspnea with pulmonary rales, systemic venous hypertension or an S_3 gallop) or a pulmonary artery wedge pressure ≥20 mm Hg, or both.

LEFT VENTRICULAR DYSFUNCTION: The diagnosis of left ventricular (LV) dysfunction required an ejection fraction of ≤44% (normal 45 to 72). All ejection fractions were obtained at rest from electrocardiographically gated technetium-99m cardiac blood pool scans. Patients received an injection of stannous pyrophosphate and 30 minutes later each received 0.3 mCi/kg technetium-

TABLE I Clinical Cardiac Abnormalities in 58 AIDS Patients	
Abnormalities	No. Positive/Total
Major	7/58 (12%)
Congestive heart failure and ventricular tachycardia	3
Congestive heart failure alone	1
Left ventricular dysfunction alone	1
Ventricular tachycardia and sudden death	1
Left ventricular dysfunction and sudden death	1
Minor	
Electrocardiogram	14/43 (33%)
ST-T wave changes	12
Low voltage	1
Intraventricular conduction delay	1
Pericardial	9/58 (16%)
Clinical pericarditis	2
Effusion by echocardiography	7
Total with major or minor abnormalities	21/58 (36%)

TABLE II Cardiac Abnormalities in AIDS Patients With and Without Myocarditis

Clinical Characteristics	Myocarditis Present (n = 26)	Myocarditis Absent (n = 32)	p Value
Congestive heart failure or left ventricular dysfunction	6	0	<0.01
Ventricular tachycardia	4	0	<0.05
Abnormal electrocardiogram	10	4	<0.02
Pericardial abnormalities	4	5	NS
Major clinical cardiac abnormalities	7	0	<0.01
Any clinical cardiac abnormality	15	6	<0.01

NS = difference not significant.

99m to accomplish in vivo labeling of the patient's erythrocytes. All radionuclide scans were performed in the critical care unit using a portable Elscint gamma camera.

VENTRICULAR TACHYCARDIA: Ventricular tachycardia (VT) was verified by analysis of rhythm strips from patients' clinical charts. Diagnosis of VT required a QRS complex duration of ≥130 ms and >3 consecutive beats. Repetitive VT was defined as >3 episodes and sustained VT as >30 seconds. Ventricular arrhythmias occurring preterminally (within 24 hours of death) were excluded from analysis if the patient clearly was dying from shock, respiratory failure or another nonarrhythmic process.

MAJOR CLINICAL CARDIAC ABNORMALITIES: Major clinical cardiac abnormalities include congestive heart failure, LV dysfunction, VT and sudden death.

MINOR CLINICAL CARDIAC ABNORMALITIES: Minor clinical cardiac abnormalities include electrocardiographic and pericardial abnormalities.

After the clinical data were determined, each patient was then classified according to the presence or absence of histopathologic myocarditis at necropsy examination.

Pathologic evaluation: The pathologic data have been described elsewhere.[3] Hematoxylin and eosin-stained myocardial sections were reviewed by pathologists blinded to the clinical data. Myocarditis was diagnosed by the Dallas criteria[4] and required an inflammatory infiltrate with adjacent myocyte necrosis or degeneration. At least 2 foci per case and ≥5 inflammatory cells present per focus were required for the diagnosis of myocarditis. The presence of inflammation alone did not fulfill the criteria for myocarditis. Clinically important findings such as ventricular dilation, valvular disease, presence of and extent of coronary artery narrowing and pericardial disease also were noted.

Statistical analysis: For continuous variables, groups were compared using a 2-tailed, unpaired sample Student t test. For categorical variables, groups were compared by chi-square analysis. A p value of <0.05 was regarded as statistically significant.

RESULTS

Fifty-eight patients (mean age 37 years [range 23 to 58]) were analyzed in this study; 55 were men and 3 were women. Forty-nine were white, 8 were black and 1 was Oriental. Risk factors for AIDS included homosexuality (53 patients), hemophilia (1 patient), intravenous drug abuse (1 patient), heterosexual contact with intravenous drug abusers (2 patients) and heterosexual contact with a bisexual male (1 patient). The mean interval from diagnosis of AIDS to death was 340 days (range 17 to 1,044). Thirty-three patients had Kaposi's sarcoma and 41 had *Pneumocystis carinii* documented at some time. Forty-three patients had characteristic cytomegaloviral inclusion bodies demonstrated in ≥1 organ at necropsy. As part of immunomodulation therapy protocols, 21 patients received interferon alpha or gamma[5] and 7 received interleukin-2.[6] Doxorubicin (Adriamycin) was administered to 17 patients as part of a chemotherapeutic protocol for Kaposi's sarcoma.[7] No patient received interferon or doxorubicin within 1 week of clinical cardiac evaluation.

Clinical cardiac abnormalities: Table I lists the clinical cardiac abnormalities noted among the 58 patients. Of the 58 patients, 21 (36%) had ≥1 abnormality (33 abnormalities in 21 patients). Major clinical cardiac abnormalities occurred in 7 patients; 4 had congestive heart failure, 2 had LV dysfunction and 3 had VT. Review of the 43 available electrocardiograms revealed that 14 patients had abnormalities. Ten of these 14 cases had had normal electrocardiograms earlier in their clinical courses. Pericardial abnormalities included pericarditis diagnosed clinically (chest pain and pericardial friction rub) and pericardial effusions documented by echocardiography. No patient developed pericardial tamponade.

Table II summarizes the associations between the presence or absence of myocarditis at necropsy and the presence of clinical cardiac abnormalities. Major clinical cardiac abnormalities, i.e., congestive heart failure, LV dysfunction and VT, occurred only in the presence of myocarditis (p <0.01). Electrocardiographic, but not pericardial, abnormalities were associated with myocarditis. Of the 26 patients with myocarditis, 15 (58%) had

TABLE III Characteristics of Seven AIDS Patients with Histopathologic Myocarditis and Major Clinical Cardiac Abnormalities

Pt	Age (yrs)	AIDS OI	AIDS KS	Cardiac Diagnoses	Hemodynamics CI	Hemodynamics PAWP	Scan EF	Experimental Protocols	Survival (days)	Cause of Death
1	36	+	0	VT (Rep, Sus, Ref)	2.4	8	NA	None	3	VT
2	27	0	+	CHF, VT (Rep)	2.1	28	41	Interferon, doxorubicin (100 mg/m²)	15	LV failure
3	40	0	+	CHF, VT (Rep)	3.2	20	31	Doxorubicin (20 mg/m²)	44	Respiratory failure
4	40	+	0	CHF, VT	3.7	20	64	None	24	Septic shock
5	38	0	+	CHF	3.1	25	63	Interferon	25	Respiratory failure
6	31	0	+	LVD	4.9	14	40	Interferon, doxorubicin	11	Respiratory failure
7	24	0	+	LVD	4.0	10	31	Interleukin-2	0	Sudden death

CHF = congestive heart failure; CI = cardiac index; EF = ejection fraction (%); KS = Kaposi's sarcoma; LV = left ventricular; LVD = left ventricular dysfunction; NA = not available; OI = opportunistic infections; PAWP = pulmonary artery wedge pressure (mm Hg); Ref = refractory; Rep = repetitive; Survival = days from onset of cardiac dysfunction until death; Sus = sustained; VT = ventricular tachycardia.

clinical cardiac abnormalities; of the 32 patients without myocarditis, 6 (19%) had clinical cardiac abnormalities ($p < 0.01$).

Seven patients had major clinical cardiac abnormalities, and all 7 patients had myocarditis at necropsy. Their clinical characteristics, including experimental protocols received, are shown in Table III. The mean interval between onset of cardiac dysfunction and death was 17 days. Four patients had VT. In 1 patient, VT was repetitive, sustained and refractory to antiarrhythmic therapy, directly causing the patient's death. In 3 of these 4 patients, no obvious metabolic abnormality could be implicated in either initiating or sustaining the arrhythmia, i.e., arterial oxygen saturation was >90%, potassium, magnesium and calcium determinations were normal, arterial pH was between 7.35 and 7.45 and mean arterial pressure was >60 mm Hg. The fourth patient was receiving an intravenous infusion of dopamine hydrochloride (2 μg/kg/min) and various dosages of intravenous levarterenol (8 to 15 μg/min) during the episodes of VT. Three of these 4 patients had congestive heart failure at the time of the arrhythmia.

Four patients were treated for congestive heart failure with diuretic or inotropic agents, or both (patients 2, 3, 4 and 5, Table III). Patients 2 and 3 had episodes of pulmonary edema, with reduced LV ejection fraction and elevated pulmonary artery wedge pressure. Patients 4 and 5 had elevated pulmonary artery wedge pressure with normal LV ejection fraction. Patient 2 responded poorly to inotropic therapy; patients 3 and 4 improved clinically with digoxin and furosemide. The last 2 patients (6 and 7) had abnormal resting LV ejection fractions, but normal pulmonary artery wedge pressure; patient 7 died suddenly, without apparent cause. No patient with VT or LV dysfunction had a history of significant alcohol ingestion.

Table IV compares demographic and laboratory characteristics of AIDS patients with and without congestive heart failure or LV dysfunction. Also listed are concurrent disease processes and the number of patients in each group exposed to experimental therapeutic protocols, specifically interferon, interleukin-2 and doxorubicin. All 6 patients with congestive heart failure or LV dysfunction had right-sided heart catheterization studies and radionuclide gated blood pool scans. Of the 52 patients without congestive heart failure or LV dysfunction, 20 had right-sided heart catheterization and 11 had radionuclide blood pool scans. No significant differences were observed between the groups in age, duration of illness or any of the laboratory parameters. No significant differences could be detected between the groups in terms of exposure to experimental therapeutic protocols or concurrent disease processes. A significant difference was noted only in pulmonary artery wedge pressure (20 ± 3 vs 9 ± 1, $p < 0.01$); a near-significant difference was noted in LV ejection fraction (45 ± 6 vs 55 ± 2, $p = 0.06$).

TABLE IV Characteristics of AIDS Patients With and Without Congestive Heart Failure or Left Ventricular Dysfunction

Characteristics	CHF or LVD (n = 6)	No CHF or LVD (n = 52)	p Value
General			
Age (yrs)	33 ± 3*	37 ± 1	NS†
Disease interval (days)	291 ± 96	346 ± 30	NS†
Laboratory			
Calcium (mEq/liter)	4.0 ± 0.1	4.1 ± 0.4	NS†
Phosphorus (mg/dl)	3.3 ± 0.3	3.5 ± 0.1	NS†
Creatinine (mg/dl)	1.2 ± 0.2	1.2 ± 0.1	NS†
Albumin (g/dl)	2.2 ± 0.3	2.7 ± 0.1	NS†
Total protein (g/dl)	5.5 ± 0.5	5.7 ± 0.2	NS†
Lymphocytes (mm⁻³)	474 ± 359	548 ± 65	NS†
Experimental protocols‡			
Interleukin-2	1	6	NS§
Interferon	3	18	NS§
Doxorubicin (Adriamycin)	3	14	NS§
Concurrent diseases‡			
Kaposi's sarcoma	5	28	NS§
Pneumocystis carinii	3	38	NS§
Cytomegalovirus	4	39	NS§

* Mean ± standard error.
† By Student *t* test.
‡ Number of patients in each group.
§ By chi square.
CHF = congestive heart failure; LVD = left ventricular dysfunction.

Pathology: Using strict diagnostic criteria,[4] 26 of the 58 patients (45%) had myocarditis. In 2 cases, cytomegaloviral inclusion bodies were found in the myocardium at autopsy. One of these cases had histopathologic myocarditis and the other did not. Among the 58 patients, only 3 had ≥50% cross-sectional area narrowing of ≥1 major coronary artery, and only 1 of these 3 (patient 2, Table III) had significant clinical cardiac abnormalities. This patient had 50 to 75% cross-sectional area narrowing of all major coronary arteries. There was no evidence of acute or healed myocardial infarcts in any patient. No patient with major clinical cardiac abnormalities had valvular heart disease. Biventricular dilation was found in 3 patients, 2 of whom had major clinical cardiac abnormalities (patients 2 and 4, Table III). All 3 patients with biventricular dilation had myocarditis.

Histopathology slides were reviewed blindly for evidence of doxorubicin cardiotoxicity. The characteristic dose-dependent myocardial degeneration that occurs includes myofibrillar loss and vacuolar degeneration.[8] Three patients had myocardial degeneration indicative of doxorubicin toxicity, but none had major clinical cardiac abnormalities.

DISCUSSION

Clinical cardiac abnormalities: The principal findings of this study are that clinical cardiac abnormalities occur in critically ill patients who die of AIDS and that these abnormalities frequently are associated with the presence of myocarditis at postmortem examination. In this series, major cardiac dysfunction (VT, sudden, death, congestive heart failure and LV dysfunction) occurred only in cases with myocarditis.

VT was documented in 4 patients in this series. Three of these 4 patients had congestive heart failure. One patient manifested repetitive, sustained VT that was refractory to antiarrhythmic therapy and caused his death. Further, malignant arrhythmias probably caused the sudden death of patient 7 (Table III). This patient had LV dysfunction and died suddenly minutes after last being seen. The 2 cases of sudden death noted in this series could not be explained on the basis of gross postmortem findings. However, both patients had myocarditis.

Three cases of dilated cardiomyopathy in AIDS have been reported in a recent series.[2] Our data confirm the occurrence of congestive heart failure in AIDS. Six of 58 patients (10%) had congestive heart failure or LV dysfunction and all 6 had myocarditis at necropsy. Two patients had high pulmonary artery wedge pressures but normal LV ejection fractions; the mechanism of their congestive heart failure may have been related to an abnormality of LV compliance.[9] None of the abnormal radionuclide gated blood pool scans were obtained during an episode of septic shock, which has been demonstrated previously to cause transient decreases in LV ejection fraction.[10]

Experimental protocols: An alternative explanation for the congestive heart failure or LV dysfunction in our patients could be cardiotoxicity from an experimental protocol drug. Doxorubicin is a known cardiotoxin that causes a dose-related congestive cardiomyopathy. There is a fairly constant progression of myocardial damage as a function of dose, with drug-associated degenerative changes identified at doses greater than 240 mg/m^2.[8] Clinical dilated cardiomyopathy is directly related to the degree of myocyte damage and usually occurs with doses greater than 450 mg/m^2. Congestive heart failure also can occur acutely after 1 dose of this drug, usually affecting patients with borderline cardiac reserve.[11] Doxorubicin is unlikely to be the cause of our patients' congestive heart failure or LV dysfunction for the following reasons: (1) No patient received >210 mg/m^2 cumulative dose of this drug, (2) the doses received by the 3 patients with cardiac dysfunction were not >100 mg/m^2 (Table III), (3) no patient received the drug within 1 week of cardiac evaluation and (4) no patient in Table III had evidence of doxorubicin cardiotoxicity on histopathologic study.

Interferon is the only other experimental or conventional therapy suspected of being cardiotoxic that was administered to our patients. Acute administration of interferon has been reported to cause hypotension, supraventricular arrhythmias and myocardial infarctions in a few patients.[12–14] In general, most of these toxicities have occurred with high doses (>30 million U/m^2 daily) of interferon.[14] Also, most of these patients were older, with evidence of preexisting heart disease or with limited cardiac reserve.[12,14] The doses of interferon administered to our patients ranged from 6 to 15 million U/m^2 daily. No patient developed clinical cardiac abnormalities during the acute administration of interferon and necropsy failed to reveal any cases of acute or healed myocardial infarctions. Thus, it is unlikely that interferon caused the congestive heart failure or LV dysfunction in our patients.

Myocarditis: The cause of the major cardiac abnormalities in our patients was probably myocarditis. Most cases of myocarditis may be subclinical, but patients may have significant arrhythmias, conduction disturbances, heart failure and sudden death.[9] Correlation between histologic findings and clinical course suggests that many cases of unexplained dilated cardiomyopathy result from myocarditis.[15] The cause of myocarditis in AIDS remains unknown. No statistical association could be demonstrated between the presence of myocarditis and exposure to any therapy, conventional or experimental (data not shown). There is little evidence to support bacterial, fungal or protozoan causes for this myocarditis. Virus-induced myocarditis remains the single most likely possibility. Despite the high frequency of documented cytomegaloviral infection in our patients, the frequency of myocarditis was not significantly higher among patients with cytomegalovirus.

Clinical implications: We attempted to establish the mechanism of death in all patients in this study. Three of the 7 patients with major clinical cardiac abnormalities had clear evidence that cardiac disease was the principal cause of death. Cardiac abnormalities appeared to be contributing causes, although not principal causes, of death in 3 of the 4 remaining patients. It is not clear whether cardiac abnormalities caused, or contributed to, any of the deaths in the remaining patients.

The abnormalities of cardiac function all occurred late in the course of these patients' illnesses. In AIDS patients with dyspnea and diffuse pulmonary infiltrates, the differential diagnosis must include congestive heart failure. If a cardiac abnormality is suspected on clinical or roentgenographic grounds, an echocardiogram should be done to evaluate cardiac function and to look for pericardial fluid. Although most AIDS patients with diffuse lung infiltrates and dyspnea will be found to have a primary pulmonic process, a few will have clinically important cardiac dysfunction.

Acknowledgment: The authors thank Kathy Kiefer for her excellent secretarial help.

REFERENCES

1. Fink L, Reichek N, St. John Sutton M. Cardiac abnormalities in acquired immune deficiency syndrome. *Am J Cardiol 1984;54:1161–1163.*

2. Cohen I, Anderson D, Virmani R, Reen B, Macher A, Sennesh J, DiLorenzo P, Redfield R. Congestive cardiomyopathy in association with the acquired immunodeficiency syndrome. *N Engl J Med 1986;315:628–630.*

3. Anderson D, Virmani R, Reilly J, O'Leary T, Cunnion R, Rubinowitz M, Macher A, Punja U, Villaflor J, Parrillo J, Roberts W. Prevalent myocarditis at necropsy in the acquired immunodeficiency syndrome. *JACC 1988;11:792–799.*

4. Aretz H, Billingham M, Edwards W, Factor S, Fallon J, Fenoglio J, Olsen E, Schoen F. Myocarditis: histopathologic differentiation and classification. *Am J Cardiovasc Pathol 1986;1:3–14.*

5. Gelmann E, Preble O, Steis R, Lane H, Rook A, Wesley M, Jacob J, Fauci A, Masur H, Longo D: Human lymphoblastoid interferon treatment of Kaposi's sarcoma in the acquired immune deficiency syndrome. *Am J Med 1985;78:737–741.*

6. Lane H, Siegel J, Rook A, Masur H, Gelmann E, Quinnan G, Fauci A. Use of interleukin-2 in patients with acquired immunodeficiency syndrome. *J Biol Response Mod 1984;3:512–516.*

7. Gelmann E, Longo D, Lane H, Fauci A, Masur H, Wesley M, Preble O, Jacob J, Steis R. Combination chemotherapy of disseminated Kaposi's sarcoma in patients with the acquired immunodeficiency syndrome. *Am J Med 1987;82:456–462.*

8. Bristow M, Mason J, Billingham M, Daniels J. Doxorubicin cardiomyopathy: evaluation by phonocardiography, endomyocardial biopsy, and cardiac catheterization. *Ann Intern Med 1978;88:168–175.*

9. Johnson R, Palacios I. Dilated cardiomyopathies of the adult. *N Engl J Med 1982;307:1051–1058;1119–1126.*

10. Parker M, Shelhamer J, Bacharach S, Green M, Natanson C, Frederick T, Damske B, Parrillo J. Profound but reversible myocardial depression in patients with septic shock. *Ann Intern Med 1984;100:483–490.*

11. Bristow M, Billingham M, Mason J, Daniels J. Clinical spectrum of anthracycline antibiotic cardiotoxicity. *Cancer Treat Rep 1978;62:873–879.*

12. Oldham R. Toxic effects of interferon (letter). *Science 1983;219:902.*

13. Kirkwood J, Ernstoff M, Davis C, Reiss M, Ferraresi R, Rudnick S. Comparison of intramuscular and intravenous recombinant alpha-2 interferon in melanoma and other cancers. *Ann Intern Med 1985;103:32–36.*

14. Quesada J, Talpaz M, Rios A, Kurzrock R, Gutterman J. Clinical toxicity of interferon in cancer patients: a review. *J Clin Oncol 1986;4:234–243.*

15. Dec G, Palacios I, Fallon J, Aretz H, Mills J, Lee D, Johnson R. Active myocarditis in the spectrum of acute dilated cardiomyopathies: clinical features, histologic correlates, and clinical outcome. *N Engl J Med 1985;312:885–890.*

Frequency of Acute and Healed Myocardial Infarcts in Fatal Cardiac Amyloidosis

Deborah J. Barbour, MD, and William C. Roberts, MD

Transmural (involvement of more than the inner one-half of the myocardial wall) left ventricular necrosis or fibrosis is most often secondary to severe (>75% cross-sectional area) narrowing by atherosclerotic plaques of 1 or more of the major epicardial coronary arteries. Myocardial infarction also may occur without significant narrowing of an epicardial coronary artery in several conditions, including hypertrophic cardiomyopathy,[1,2] dilated cardiomyopathy,[3] left or right ventricular outflow obstruction[4–10] and anomalies of coronary arterial origin or course.[11] Another condition associated with myocardial infarction without significant narrowing of 1 or more of the epicardial coronary arteries is cardiac amyloidosis. Our necropsy experience with myocardial infarction associated with cardiac amyloidosis is summarized here.

Of 61 necropsy patients aged 21 to 97 years (mean 64) with cardiac amyloidosis severe enough to cause cardiac dysfunction studied in this laboratory during the past 28 years,[12] 3 (5%) had transmural necrosis, 5 (8%) had transmural fibrosis of the left ventricular wall and 53 (87%) had neither necrosis nor fibrosis (Figure 1). One patient with necrosis, 3 with fibrosis and 9 with neither necrosis nor fibrosis had 1 or more epicardial coronary arteries severely narrowed by atherosclerotic plaque. Two patients with necrosis and 2 with fibrosis, plus 44 with neither, had no epicardial coronary artery narrowed >75% in cross-sectional area by atherosclerotic plaque.

In all 61 patients whose cardiac amyloid deposits were severe enough to cause dysfunction, amyloid depos-

From the Pathology Branch, National Heart, Lung, and Blood Institute, National Institutes of Health, Bethesda, Maryland 20892. Manuscript received June 9, 1988, and accepted July 13.

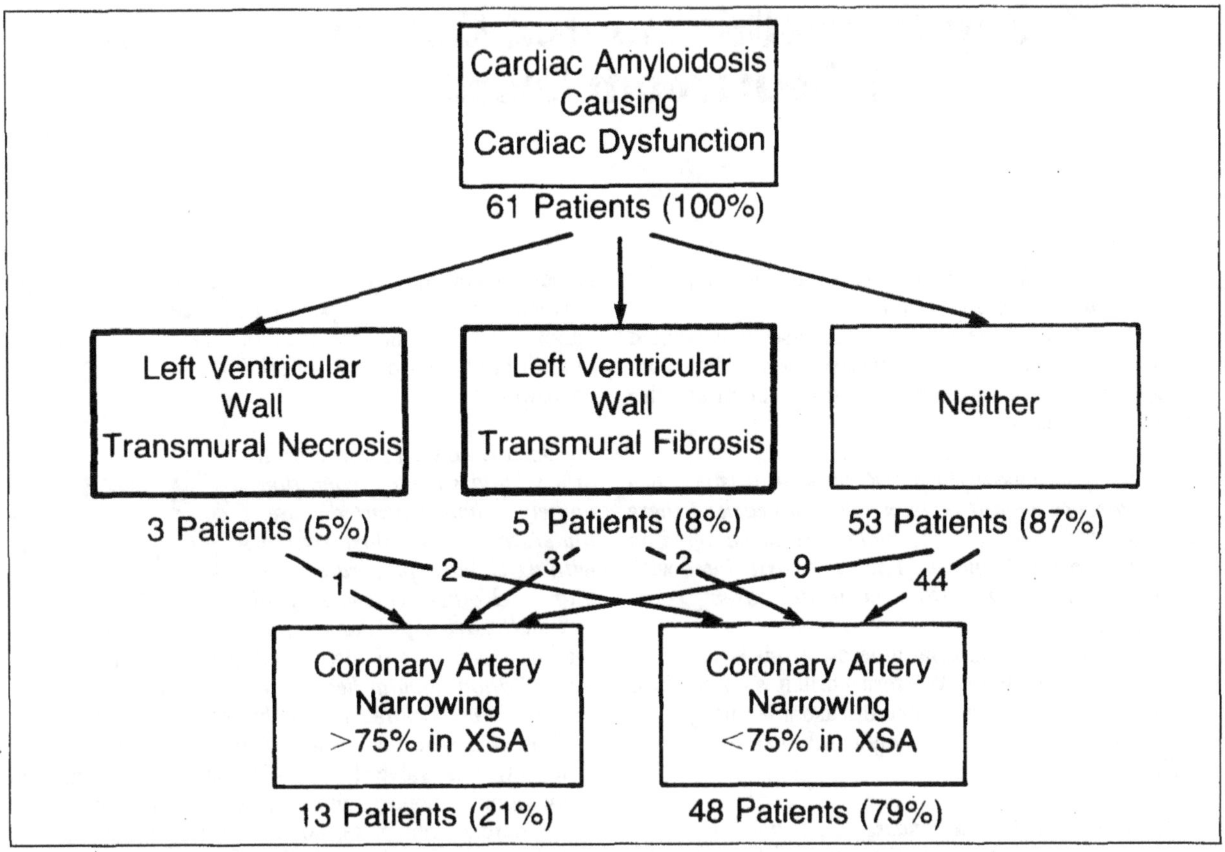

FIGURE 1. Diagram showing the frequency of left ventricular necrosis, the frequency of fibrosis and the frequency of coronary arterial narrowing in 61 necropsy patients with fatal cardiac amyloidosis. XSA = cross-sectional area.

its were present in the walls and lumens of the intramural coronary arteries, but the narrowing of the small coronary arteries by amyloid deposits did not appear to be greater in the patients with left ventricular necrosis and/or fibrosis than in those patients without myocardial lesions.

Of our 8 patients with transmural necrosis or fibrosis, none had clinical evidence of acute myocardial infarction. Of the 108 necropsy patients with cardiac amyloidosis reported by Smith and Hutchins[13], 5 (aged 54 to 89 years) had "severe . . . amyloid deposition" in the intramyocardial coronary arteries associated with myocardial necrosis or fibrosis. In all 5, the epicardial coronary arteries were free of atherosclerotic narrowing. No comment was made regarding the severity of intramural coronary artery amyloid deposits in those without myocardial necrosis or fibrosis or in those with concurrent atherosclerotic narrowing of the epicardial coronary arteries.

Jennette et al[14] reported a 70-year-old man with amyloidosis who had a clinically diagnosed fatal acute myocardial infarction. At necropsy, his epicardial coronary arteries were free of atherosclerotic narrowing; however, the lumens of the intramural coronary arteries were severely narrowed by amyloid deposits and the myocardium had multiple small areas of necrosis and fibrosis.

Thus, cardiac amyloidosis needs to be added to the list of conditions associated with transmural left ventricular necrosis or fibrosis unassociated with significant narrowing of 1 or more major epicardial coronary arteries.

1. McReynolds RA, Roberts WC. The intramural coronary arteries in hypertrophic cardiomyopathy (abstr). *Am J Cardiol 1975;35:120.*
2. Maron BJ, Wolfson JK, Epstein SE, Roberts WC. Intramural (small vessel) coronary artery disease in hypertrophic cardiomyopathy. *JACC 1986;8:545–557.*
3. Roberts WC, Siegel RJ, McManus BM. Idiopathic dilated cardiopathy: analysis of 152 necropsy patients. *Am J Cardiol 1987;60:1340–1355.*
4. Roberts WC. The structure of the aortic valve in clinically-isolated aortic stenosis. An autopsy study of 162 patients over 15 years of age. *Circulation 1970;42:91–97.*
5. Roberts WC. The congenitally bicuspid aortic valve. A study of 85 autopsy cases. *Am J Cardiol 1970;26:72–83.*
6. Roberts WC. Anatomically isolated aortic valvular disease. The case against its being of rheumatic etiology. *Am J Med 1970;49:151–159.*
7. Falcone MW, Roberts WC, Morrow AG, Perloff JK. Congenital aortic stenosis resulting from a unicommissural valve. Clinical and anatomic features in twenty-one adult patients. *Circulation 1971;44:272–280.*
8. Maron BJ, Redwood DR, Roberts WC, Henry WL, Morrow AG, Epstein SE. Tunnel subaortic stenosis. Left ventricular outflow tract obstruction produced by fibromuscular tubular narrowing. *Circulation 1976;54:406–416.*
9. Muna WFT, Ferrans VJ, Pierce JE, Roberts WC. Discrete subaortic stenosis in Newfoundland dogs: association of infective endocarditis. *Am J Cardiol 1978; 41:746–754.*
10. Roberts WC, Shemin RJ, Kent KM. Frequency and direction of interatrial shunting in valvular pulmonic stenosis with intact ventricular septum and without left ventricular inflow or outflow obstruction. An analysis of 127 patients treated by valvulotomy. *Am Heart J 1980;99:142–148.*
11. Roberts WC. Major anomalies of coronary arterial origin seen in adulthood. *Am Heart J 1986;111:941–963.*
12. Roberts WC, Waller BF. Cardiac amyloidosis causing cardiac dysfunction: analysis of 54 necropsy patients. *Am J Cardiol 1983;52:137–146.*
13. Smith RRL, Hutchins GM. Ischemic heart disease secondary to amyloidosis of intramyocardial arteries. *Am J Cardiol 1979;44:413–417.*
14. Jennette JC, Sheps DS, McNeill DD. Exclusively vascular systemic amyloidosis with visceral ischemia. *Arch Pathol Lab Med 1982;106:323–327.*

Defining Idiopathic Dilated Cardiomyopathy: A Courtroom Discussion

Doctor, how do you define the condition idiopathic dilated cardiomyopathy (IDC)?

I define IDC as heart muscle disease unassociated with coronary, valvular, hypertensive, pericardial, congenital or pulmonary heart disease or with an infiltrative myocardial disease.

Doctor, you have defined IDC by what it is not. Before we discuss what it is, let's delve into each of these "unassociated conditions" to make certain we agree on what "unassociated" means. You say unassociated with coronary artery disease? Does this mean "absent" coronary disease?

Because coronary arterial atherosclerosis is so prevalent in adults living in the Western world it is not realistic to believe that coronary artery disease is actually "absent". It is better to say "insignificantly narrowed" epicardial coronary arteries.

Then neither the word "unassociated" nor "absent" is appropriate in characterizing the status of the epicardial coronary arteries in patients with IDC. What degree of luminal narrowing do you consider "significant"?

Because flow through an artery is not compromised until >75% of the lumen's cross-sectional area is obliterated, it is reasonable to consider >75% cross-sectional area narrowing as "significant" and lesser degrees of narrowing as "insignificant".

At present the only means of determining coronary arterial narrowing during life is by angiography, and the unit of angiographic narrowing is diameter reduction, not cross-sectional area reduction. Thus, what is a 75% cross-sectional area narrowing equivalent to in terms of diameter narrowing?

In general, a 75% cross-sectional area narrowing is equivalent to a 50% diameter narrowing. This equivalency assumes that the coronary artery is relatively straight (and obviously the right and left circumflex coronary arteries are not straight) and that the lumen is central or nearly so (and the lumen is central in only about 30% of significantly narrowed epicardial coronary arteries). Nevertheless, some demarcation definition is needed and the 50% diameter reduction is reasonable.

Therefore, doctor, if 1 or more epicardial coronary arteries is narrowed at some point >50% in diameter at angiography, then the diagnosis of IDC cannot be made. Is that correct?

Yes. But, because coronary arterial disease is so common in our society a few patients with "IDC" will have associated coronary artery disease. Nevertheless, it is improper to diagnose IDC in the presence of "significant" coronary arterial narrowing.

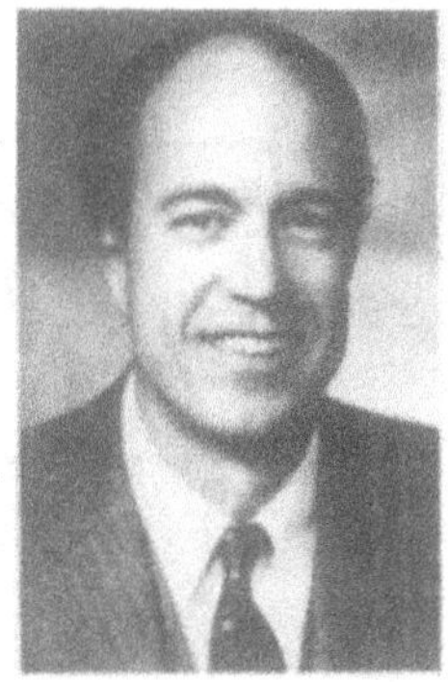

Doctor, now let's move to another "unassociated condition", namely valvular heart disease. I understand that most patients with IDC have precordial murmurs and other evidences of mitral and/or tricuspid valve regurgitation sometime during their courses? Thus, is not atrioventricular valve regurgitation valvular heart disease? What do you mean then by "unassociated with valvular heart disease"?

Yes, it is true that most patients with IDC develop atrioventricular valve regurgitation but this regurgitation is functional or nonorganic; i.e., it is caused by the dilation of the cardiac ventricles, not by primary disease of the valvular leaflets and/or chordae tendineae.

Then "unassociated valvular heart disease" means lack of intrinsic disease of the valvular leaflets and/or chordae, even though the degree of valvular regurgitation may be equal to or even greater than in patients with primary valvular disease. Is that correct?

Yes. But quantitating the degree of tricuspid or mitral valve regurgitation is difficult. Furthermore, valvular repair or replacement is contraindicated in patients with IDC although at times the degree of regurgitation might be considerable.

If atrioventricular valve regurgitation in patients with IDC is not due to primary valve disease, then what is the mechanism of the regurgitation?

The mechanism of the tricuspid valve regurgitation is different from that of the mitral regurgitation. The tricuspid valve regurgitation results from dilatation of the tricuspid valve anulus. Normally the tricuspid valve anulus is ≤11 cm in circumference; in patients with IDC the circumference may increase to as much as 16 cm, depending on the original size of the heart. Whenever the right ventricular cavity dilates the tricuspid valve anulus dilates, and the amount of anular circumference dilatation is roughly proportional to the amount of right ventricular cavity dilatation.

The mitral regurgitation in IDC, in contrast, is never the result of mitral anular dilatation.[1,2] Normally, the mitral anulus is about 9 cm in circumference, and in IDC, the anular circumference rarely increases to more than about 11 cm. The maximal transverse dilatation of the left ventricle takes place in the midportion of the cavity or about half way between the mitral valve anulus and the left ventricular apex. The midcavity dilatation causes the papillary muscles to move outwardly from the cavity's center and this outward movement pulls the chordae tendineae toward the ventricle's mural endocardium which in turn pulls the margins of the posterior and anterior mitral leaflets away from one another with resulting regurgitation. An additional factor is the elongation of the left ventricular cavity from the mitral anulus to apex, a distance equivalent to that distance from the base of the right aortic valve cusp to left ventricular apex. As this longitudinal distance increases the stumps of both left ventricular papillary muscles move away from the mitral anulus or toward the left ventricular apex. This movement, in turn, pulls the chordae tendineae and their attached leaflets closer to the left ventricular mural endocardium, further increasing the regurgitant area of the mitral orifice during ventricular systole.

Doctor, how is secondary atrioventricular valvular regurgitation as occurs in patients with IDC distinguished clinically from primary valvular regurgitation as occurs, for example, in patients with mitral valve prolapse?

Sometimes this distinction is not easy clinically, especially if the murmur of mitral regurgitation is present when the patient with IDC is first seen. In general, the intensity of the precordial murmur of primary mitral regurgitation is louder than that of secondary mitral regurgitation. The echocardiogram is helpful in this distinction. In IDC, the left ventricular wall contracts poorly whereas in primary mitral regurgitation, left ventricular contraction usually is good. In chronic primary mitral regurgitation, the left atrial cavity is usually larger than in secondary mitral regurgitation associated with IDC. If there is associated aortic valve regurgitation, diagnosis of IDC is inappropriate, and mitral regurgitation when present in this circumstance is more liable to be primary rather than secondary. Any dysfunction of a semilunar cardiac valve is incompatible with IDC. Neither the ascending aorta nor the pulmonary trunk dilate in IDC whereas one or both may dilate in patients with primary valve disease. In the Western world mitral valve prolapse is now the most common cause of primary, pure (no associated valve stenosis) mitral regurgitation and when the regurgitation is severe the mitral anulus is usually considerably dilated.[3–5] Thus, in contrast to earlier teachings, the only condition associated with severe mitral anular dilatation is mitral valve prolapse and IDC is rarely if ever associated with a functionally significant increase in mitral anular circumference.

Doctor, now let's move to another "unassociated condition", namely systemic hypertension. You stated earlier that systemic hypertension was absent in patients with IDC and yet some patients with IDC have histories of systemic hypertension or actually elevated systemic arterial pressures early in their courses or during periods of particularly severe congestive heart failure. How do you explain these apparent discrepancies?

Yes, all of your statements about systemic hypertension in IDC are true. Most patients with systemic hypertension who develop severe chronic congestive heart failure, however, have underlying atherosclerotic coronary artery disease and usually one or more healed myocardial infarcts, which may or may not have been clinically apparent. As the cardiac output in these patients with "ischemic cardiomyopathy" progressively falls the systemic arterial pressure also progressively falls because systemic hypertension requires both an increased peripheral vascular resistance and a normal or increased cardiac output. Although nearly 10% of patients with IDC may also have grossly visible left ventricular scars, the scars are small, in contrast to the patients with ischemic cardiomyopathy, and focal wall motion abnormalities are uncommon in IDC whereas they are common in ischemic cardiomyopathy. In contrast to ischemic cardiomyopathy, the epicardial coronary arteries are not significantly narrowed in IDC and clinical events characteristic of acute myocardial infarction are nearly nonexistent in IDC, whereas, of course, they are common in patients with ischemic cardiomyopathy.[7,8] As the congestive heart failure worsens in both IDC and in ischemic cardiomyopathy the systemic arterial pressure falls so that during the last 3 months of life the systemic arterial pressure in both conditions is typically about 90/60 mm Hg. The distinction between IDC and ischemic cardiomyopathy, therefore, is not on the basis of previous or present levels of systemic arterial pressure but on the basis of the presence or absence of coronary arterial narrowing and a history of an event characteristic of acute myocardial infarction that healed.

Doctor, are there any circumstances where the systemic arterial pressure progressively increases along with a progressive increase in congestive heart failure?

Yes. The most common is chronic renal disease. Typically, as the renal disease worsens the systemic arterial pressure progressively rises and, finally, features of congestive heart failure appear and progress. Some of these latter features may be consequences of retained body fluids as renal output diminishes. Hemodialysis is changing this picture a bit. Nevertheless, the heart in chronic renal failure is one of increased mass and increased ventricular cavity size, features characteristic of IDC. Diagnosis of IDC, however, is inappropriate in the presence of chronic renal disease either clinically or at necropsy.

Doctor, now let's move to another "unassociated cardiac condition", namely pericardial heart disease. Are pericardial effusions common in patients with IDC?

Yes. Pericardial effusions are common in patients with chronic congestive heart failure from any cause, just as effusions into pleural spaces and into abdominal cavity are common in patients with heart failure. The effusions are serous and those into the pericardial cavity rarely are more than 200 ml, and they are never associated with tamponade. Normally, the pericardial sac contains up to 50 ml of serous fluid ("the oil of the heart" to decrease friction between the visceral and parietal pericardia) and an increase of 3 or 4 times over several months is of no functional consequence.

Thus, doctor, it is not correct to say "absent" pericardial disease. Some abnormality is present, namely serous effusions, but the abnormality is of no functional consequence. Are there any other pericardial abnormalities in patients with IDC?

No. Fibrin deposits on the pericardial surfaces and pericardial friction rubs are absent in patients with IDC. Likewise, neither the parietal nor the visceral pericardia are thickened in IDC. Nevertheless, particularly before the advent of echocardiography, patients with IDC sometimes were misdiagnosed as having "constrictive pericarditis" (better termed "constrictive pericardial disease") and thoracotomy was performed. Hemodynamically, constrictive pericardial disease can mimic IDC. Thoracotomy and pericardiectomy are the treatments for the former, but thoracotomy obviously is contraindicated in IDC. Thus, clinically significant pericardial heart disease is absent in IDC, but pericardial heart disease often is a diagnostic consideration in these patients.

Doctor, now let's move to another "unassociated condition", namely congenital heart disease. Does the absence of congenital heart disease indicate that IDC cannot be present at birth? Is IDC ever of congenital origin?

Yes. In a rare patient IDC manifests itself early in life and when this occurs it is possible that IDC was present from birth and is therefore congenital in origin in this circumstance. Furthermore, IDC occurs occasionally in more than 1 family member and in this circumstance it is "familial" and therefore possibly congenital. In contrast to IDC, which is rarely congenital or familial, hypertrophic cardiomyopathy is usually familial and occasionally manifests itself from the time of birth. Therefore, although hypertrophic cardiomyopathy is usually classified under myocardial diseases of uncertain origin, it is also congenital heart disease and indeed one of the more common varieties of congenital heart disease. Although the cardiac abnormality usually is present from the time of birth, it usually does not manifest itself until adulthood.

Doctor, now let's move to another "unassociated condition", namely pulmonary parenchymal or vascular disease. How much lung disease do you allow to be present and still diagnose IDC?

Sometimes a lot and sometimes very little. Many men, and in some studies most men,[6] with IDC are habitual alcoholics and the frequency of heavy cigarette smoking is much higher in chronic alcoholics than in nonalcoholics. Accordingly, the frequency of parenchymal pulmonary disease is fairly frequent in older adults with IDC. In general, parenchymal pulmonary disease may increase pulmonary arterial pressure and lead to cor pulmonale. Although cor pulmonale typically causes dilation of only the right side of the heart, an occasional patient with cor pulmonale also has a dilated left ventricular cavity and this circumstance can lead to confusion with IDC. The patient with severe parenchymal lung disease should be excluded from consideration of having IDC.

Pulmonary emboli with and without pulmonary infarcts are common in patients with IDC and this complication of IDC obviously should not exclude diagnosis of the underlying condition. Thrombi in the right ventricular cavity and in the right atrial appendage are common in IDC and are the likely sources of the pulmonary emboli. Elevation of the pulmonary arterial pressure may also occur in IDC as a consequence of the elevated pulmonary venous pressures from elevated left ventricular filling pressures.

Doctor, now let's move to another "unassociated condition", namely infiltrative heart disease. Obviously, the presence of amyloid fibrils, sarcoid granulomas or iron in the heart excludes the diagnosis of IDC. Which of the infiltrative diseases is most commonly confused with IDC?

Cardiac *sarcoidosis*.[9] This infiltrative cardiomyopathy may cause severe dilatation of both ventricular cavities, ventricular arrhythmias and conduction disturbances in the absence of palpable lymph nodes or radiographically visible pulmonary lesions, and, therefore, it can readily mimic IDC. It is important not to misdiagnose cardiac sarcoidosis as IDC because the sarcoid granuloma usually are responsive to corticosteroid therapy, whereas, short of cardiac transplantation, there is no specific therapy for IDC. Biopsy of a lymph node more likely will lead to diagnosis of sarcoidosis than will endomyocardial biopsy. Cardiac *hemosiderosis*,[10] even though it too may produce severe ventricular cavity dilatation, is rarely confused with IDC because of a history of repeated blood transfusions unassociated with bleeding diastasis or evidence of hemochromatosis (hepatic cirrhosis, diabetes mellitus, etc.) Cardiac *amyloidosis* is rarely confused with IDC because the cardiac ventricular cavities are not dilated in this condition (unless another cardiac disease is also present like atherosclerotic coronary artery disease) and these patients are generally much older than the IDC patients. Amyloid heart disease is far more likely to be confused with hypertrophic cardiomyopathy than with IDC.

Doctor, does the presence of inflammatory infiltrates in the interstitium of the ventricular walls exclude the diagnosis of IDC?

No. For years many investigators believed that myocarditis (interstitial inflammatory cells associated with necrotic myocardial fibers) was a precursor of IDC. With some exceptions, endomyocardial biopsy in patients with IDC has failed to disclose the presence of interstitial inflammatory cells in patients with IDC. In 1 necropsy study of 152 patients with IDC, only 5 had interstitial myocardial inflammatory cell infiltrates and in them the infiltrates were small, mononuclear and located in areas where fibrous tissue was increased.

Doctor, does the presence of certain systemic diseases or diseases that affect primarily noncardiac organs or tissues prevent the diagnosis of IDC?

Yes and no. The presence of *diabetes mellitus* does not. It is generally believed that patients with diabetes have an increased frequency of clinically significant atherosclerosis compared to nondiabetics of similar age and sex. Of 152 recently reported necropsy patients with IDC,[6] 8 had associated diabetes mellitus, and none, of course, had significant narrowing of a major epicardial coronary artery and none had abnormalities of the intramural coronary arteries.

Three neurologic conditions—namely, Duchenne's type of muscular dystrophy, Friedreich's ataxia and myotonia congenita—occasionally are associated with dilatation of both cardiac ventricles, depressed ventricular function, arrhythmias and conduction disturbances, and abnormalities of some intramural coronary arteries. The dilated cardiomyopathy observed in these 3 neurologic conditions is probably related to the neurologic disease, and, therefore, the use of the word "idiopathic" to precede the phrase "dilated cardiomyopathy" in them is inappropriate.

Some patients with chronic anemia, for example, congenital hemolytic anemia or sickle-cell anemia, develop dilated ventricular cavities, precordial murmurs consistent with tricuspid and/or mitral regurgitation, and depressed ventricular function. Despite a similar morphologic appearance of the heart, diagnosis of IDC in the setting of chronic severe anemia is inappropriate.

Doctor, let's move the discussion from what IDC is not to what it is. What has to be present before IDC is present?

Both ventricular cavities must be dilated, the cardiac mass must be increased and the cardiac output must be decreased. Also, the dilatation of both ventricles is roughly to the same degree. The circumstance where 1 cardiac ventricle is enormously dilated and the other one is only slightly dilated is not IDC. A condition that causes dilatation of only 1 cardiac ventricle is not IDC. Both atrial cavities also are dilated. It is likely that the atrial dilatation simply follows the ventricular dilatation.

The weight of the heart at necropsy in IDC is always increased. Although total cardiac mass is increased, the thickness of the left and right ventricular walls may not be greater than normal. Indeed, in IDC usually the maximal thickness of the right ventricular free wall is ≤ 5 mm and that of the left ventricular free wall is ≤ 15 mm. The maximal thickness of the left ventricular free wall and ventricular septum in IDC is similar.

Some athletes have hearts with dilated ventricular cavities and increased mass but in them the cardiac output is normal or even supernormal. In IDC, cardiac output is depressed. The ventricles dilate in IDC as systolic function worsens, which in turn causes increased end-systolic volume, and this leads to further ventricular dilatation.

Doctor, could you summarize your definiton of IDC?

IDC is a heart muscle disease of uncertain origin characterized by dilatation of both ventricular cavities, by increased cardiac mass and by depressed cardiac output. IDC is unassociated with significant narrowing of 1 or more epicardial coronary arteries; with primary valvular heart disease; with systemic hypertension; with functionally significant pericardial heart disease; with congenital defects or anomalies of cardiac septa or great arteries or veins; or with myocardial infiltrative diseases, such as sarcoid, amyloid and iron. IDC should not be considered in the presence of severe parenchymal pulmonary disease or in the presence of conditions that affect primarily noncardiac organs or tissues such as chronic anemia and the neurogenic heart diseases.

Doctor, is the "definition of a disease" the same as "criteria for diagnosis of a disease"?

No. A definition of a disease is a description of what the disease is and is independent of the means by which the disease is diagnosed. A definition may change as more information is gained about the disease. Criteria for diagnosis of a disease, in contrast, are dependent on the symptoms and physical signs produced by a disease and on the findings produced by laboratory tests and various "instruments of precision" that are helpful in diagnosing the disease. The laboratory tests and "instruments of precision" change periodically and when they do the criteria for diagnosis of a disease also may change.

Thank you doctor.

William C. Roberts

William C. Roberts, MD
Editor in Chief

1. Roberts WC, Cohen LS. Left ventricular papillary muscles. Description of the normal and a survey of conditions causing them to be abnormal. *Circulation 1972;46:138–154.*

2. Roberts WC, Perloff JK. Mitral valvular disease. A clinicopathologic survey of the conditions causing the mitral valve to function abnormally. *Ann Intern Med 1972;77:939–975.*

3. Waller BJ, Morrow AG, Maron BJ, Del Negro AA, Kent KM, McGrath FJ, Wallace RB, McIntosh CL, Roberts WC. Etiology of clinically isolated, severe, chronic, pure mitral regurgitaton: analysis of 97 patients over 30 years of age having mitral valve replacement. *Am Heart J 1982;104:276–288.*

4. Roberts WC, McIntosh CL, Wallace RB. Mechanisms of severe mitral regurgitation in mitral valve prolapse determined from analysis of operatively excised valves. *Am Heart J 1987;113:1316–1323.*

5. Roberts WC, Honig HS. The spectrum of cardiovascular disease in the Marfan syndrome: a clinico-morphologic study of 18 necropsy patients and comparison to 151 previously reported necropsy patients. *Am Heart J 1982;104:115–135.*

6. Roberts WC, Siegel RJ, McManus BM. Idiopathic dilated cardiomyopathy: analysis of 152 necropsy patients. *Am J Cardiol 1987;60:1340–1355.*

7. Ross EM, Roberts WC. Severe atherosclerotic coronary artery disease, healed myocardial infarction and chronic congestive heart failure: analysis of 81 patients studied at necropsy. *Am J Cardiol 1986;57:44–50.*

8. Ross EM, Roberts WC. Severe atherosclerotic coronary arterial narrowing and chronic congestive heart failure without myocardial infarction: analysis of 18 patients studied at necropsy. *Am J Cardiol 1986;57:51–56.*

9. Roberts WC, McAllister HA Jr, Ferrans VJ. Sarcoidosis of the heart. A clinicopathologic study of 35 necropsy patients (group I) and review of 78 previously described necropsy patients (group II). *Am J Med 1977;63:86–108.*

10. Buja LM, Roberts WC. Iron in the heart. Etiology and clinical significance. *Am J Med 1971;51:209–221.*

11. Roberts WC, Waller BF. Cardiac amyloidosis causing cardiac dysfunction: analysis of 54 necropsy patients. *Am J Cardiol 1983;52:137–146.*

Pathologic Findings Associated With Interleukin-2–Based Immunotherapy for Cancer: A Postmortem Study of 19 Patients

AMY H. KRAGEL, MD, WILLIAM D. TRAVIS, MD, LAURIE FEINBERG, MD, STEFANIA PITTALUGA, MD, LILIANE M. STRIKER, MD, WILLIAM C. ROBERTS, MD, MICHAEL T. LOTZE, MD, JAMES J. YANG, MD, AND STEVEN A. ROSENBERG, MD

The use of interleukin-2 (IL-2), either alone or in combination with lymphokine-activated killer cells, tumor infiltrating lymphocytes, or other immunotherapeutic agents has added a new list of alternatives to conventional antineoplastic regimens. Little information is available about the pathologic changes occurring in patients treated with these agents. In this study, we reviewed the necropsy materials from 19 patients, 12 men and 7 women, with a variety of malignancies including melanoma, renal cell carcinoma, gastrointestinal and pulmonary adenocarcinoma, and metastatic gastrinoma, who died after receiving IL-2–based immunotherapy. Death occurred at intervals ranging from less than 1 hour to 143 days following the last dose of therapy. All patients dying at or less than 43 days following cessation of therapy had lymphoid infiltrates of varying intensity in residual tumor. At necropsy, the major cause of death unrelated to the presence of metastatic tumor was bacterial sepsis. In addition, we found evidence of significant cardiac and pulmonary toxicity: two patients with acute myocardial infarction, one with and one without significant coronary artery disease, two cases of unexplained lymphocytic myocarditis, and one case of fatal pulmonary capillary plugging following an infusion of lymphokine-activated killer cells. Thus, not unlike other forms of therapy for cancer, IL-2–based immunotherapy does not appear to be without significant toxicity. HUM PATHOL 21:493–502. This is a US government work. There are no restrictions on its use.

The use of interleukin-2 (IL-2) as an immunotherapeutic agent for the treatment of metastatic carcinoma has been under evaluation since the early 1980s when methods for producing recombinant IL-2 were developed.[1,2] Several clinical trials have shown that immunotherapy with IL-2, alone and in combination with other agents including lymphokine-activated killer (LAK) cells, is capable of inducing partial and complete remissions in patients with various types of cancer.[3-5] At the same time, clinical toxicity associated with IL-2 has been recognized, and several publications have described the frequency of various manifestations of IL-2 toxicity.[3-8] Reported side effects have included nausea, vomiting, malaise, altered mental status, somnolence, skin rash, weight gain, hypotension, angina pectoris, cardiac arrhythmias, acute myocardial infarction, myocarditis, increased serum creatinine, decreased urinary output, hyperbilirubinemia, anemia, eosinophilia, thrombocytopenia, serious bacterial infections, and alterations in thyroid gland function.[3-18]

The use of IL-2, either alone or in combination with LAK cells, tumor infiltrating lymphocytes (TILs), or other immunotherapeutic agents has added a new list of alternatives to existing conventional antineoplastic regimens. As the use of these agents increases, it becomes increasingly important to study the effects which IL-2–based immunotherapy has on various organ systems and to develop an understanding of the impact of therapy on the ultimate causes of death in these patients. Little published information is available regarding the pathologic changes in patients who have received IL-2. In this article, we describe morphologic findings at necropsy in 19 patients who had received IL-2 based immunotherapy.

METHODS

Patients Studied

Nineteen consecutive patients were identified in the files of the Laboratory of Pathology, National Cancer Institute, as having received IL-2–based immunotherapy treatment. These included IL-2 alone and IL-2 in combination with either LAK cells (mononuclear cells obtained by leukopheresis and subsequently incubated with IL-2 for 2 to 3 days), alpha interferon, cyclophosphamide, monoclonal antibodies, or TILs.

Materials Examined

The autopsy protocols and clinical records were reviewed. The following items from these records were noted: (1) specific immunotherapy regimen received; (2) interval from the last dose of therapy to death; (3) signs and symptoms of adverse reactions during therapy; and (4) cause of death.

The following organs were studied in detail: heart, lungs, thyroid, liver, kidney and skin. In 16 of the 19 cases, the heart specimen was available for review and was reexamined. In these cases, two to four additional 2 cm sections

From the Pathology Branch, National Heart, Lung, and Blood Institute, the Laboratory of Pathology and Surgery Branch, National Cancer Institute, and Metabolic Disease Branch, National Institute of Diabetes and Digestive and Kidney Diseases, National Institutes of Health, Bethesda, MD; and Mayo Medical School, Mayo Clinic, Rochester, MN. Accepted for publication September 5, 1989.

Key words: myocarditis, acute myocardial infarction, diffuse alveolar damage, thyroiditis, lymphoid infiltrate, lymphokine activated killer cells.

Address correspondence and reprint requests to William D. Travis, MD, Laboratory of Pathology, Building 10, Room 2N212, National Cancer Institute, National Institutes of Health, Bethesda, MD 20892.

0046-8177/90/2105-0005$0.00/0

of both right and left ventricle (including papillary muscle) were taken, fixed in formalin, processed, sectioned, and stained with hematoxylin and eosin. Hematoxylin and eosin-stained sections were available for review in 18 of 19 cases. Formalin-fixed sections of kidney, lung, and liver were reviewed in all cases. In addition, sections of kidney stained by the periodic acid-Schiff method were examined. In 18 of 19 cases, sections of thyroid were reviewed, In three cases, sections of skin were available for review. All other hematoxylin and eosin-stained sections taken at the time of autopsy were reviewed. The extent and location of tumor and the presence or absence of a lymphoid infiltrate within or around that tumor was noted in each case. The lymphoid infiltrate, if present, was graded on a scale of 1 to 3.

RESULTS

Clinical Features

The clinical features of the 19 patients studied are summarized in Table 1. Twelve men and seven women, aged 22 to 67 years (mean 50), with a variety of malignancies, including renal cell carcinoma (eight cases), malignant melanoma (six cases), adenocarcinoma of the lung (two cases), adenocarcinoma of the stomach (one case), colorectal carcinoma (one case), and gastrinoma (one case) were studied. All patients received IL-2. Lymphokine-activated killer cells were included in the treatment protocols of 11 patients, alpha interferon in those of two patients, TILs in those of two patients, cyclophosphamide in that of one patient, and monoclonal antibodies in that of one patient.

Tumor Pathology

Metastatic disease at necropsy was extensive in 18 (95%) patients. Tumor was identified in lungs (18 cases), lymph nodes (10 cases), liver (10 cases), heart (seven cases), adrenal glands (six cases), bone marrow (five cases), brain (five cases), gastrointestinal tract (four cases), spleen (three cases), pancreas (two cases), thyroid gland (two cases), skin (two cases), gall bladder (two cases), urinary bladder (two cases), bone (two cases), testes (two cases), uterus and ovary (one case), breast (one case), and other soft tissue sites in five cases. One patient (patient no. 1, Table 1), who received IL-2 as adjuvent therapy following resection of lymph nodes containing metastatic melanoma, had no detectable tumor at either the initiation of therapy or at necropsy.

Lymphoid infiltrates were identified either at the periphery of or within the tumor in 14 patients (Table 1, Fig 1). All of these 14 patients died within 43 days of the last dose of therapy. The amount of infiltrate varied from 1+ to 3+. No correlation was found between the severity of the infiltrate and the interval between the last dose of therapy and death. No apparent correlation was noted between the type of malignancy and the presence or severity of the lymphoid infiltrate.

Cardiac Findings

The clinical signs and symptoms of cardiac dysfunction or ischemia and the gross and microscopic findings in the hearts of the patients studied are sum-

TABLE 1. Certain Clinical and Necropsy Findings in 19 Patients Receiving Immunotherapy

Case No.	Age/Race/Sex (yr)	Type of Malignancy	Immunotherapy Regimen	Interval From Last Rx to Death (d)	Tumor-associated Lymphocytes at Necropsy (1-3+)	Cause of Death
1	22/W/F	Melanoma	IL2/LAK	0	NA	Respiratory Failure*
2	67/W/M	Renal cell CA	IL2	1	1+	AMI
3	51/W/M	Renal cell CA	IL2	4	2-3+	Sepsis
4	24/W/M	Melanoma	IL2/LAK	4	1+	Sepsis
5	45/W/M	Adeno CA, colorectal	IL2/LAK	4	1+	Sepsis
6	65/W/M	melanoma	IL2/MoAb	6	3+	Metastatic disease
7	55/W/M	Renal cell CA	IL2/aIFN	8	1+	Metastatic disease
8	34/W/F	Melanoma	IL2/TILs	13	1+, focal	Metastatic disease
9	53/W/F	Renal cell CA	IL2/Cytoxan	16	1+, focal	Sepsis, GI bleed
10	59/W/M	Adeno CA, lung	IL2/LAK	17	1+, focal	Sepsis
11	57/W/M	Renal cell CA	IL2/aIFN	20	3+	Anoxic encephalopathy†
12	25/W/M	Melanoma	IL2/TILs	20	1+, focal	Sepsis, metastatic disease
13	58/B/M	Renal cell CA	IL2/LAK	42	1+	Sepsis/multi-system failure
14	59/W/M	Adeno CA, GE jct	IL2/LAK	43	1+	Sepsis, GI bleed
15	58/B/F	Renal cell CA	IL2/LAK	47	0	Metastatic disease
16	67/W/M	Gastrinoma	IL2/LAK	67	0	Metastatic disease
17	53/W/M	Renal cell CA	IL2/LAK	71	0	Cardiac failure secondary to AMI
18	40/W/F	Adeno CA, lung	IL2/LAK	74	0	Metastatic disease
19	43/W/F	Melanoma	IL2/LAK	143	0	Metastatic disease

Abbreviations: aIFN, alpha interferon; AMI, acute myocardial infarction; CA, carcinoma; GE jct, gastroesophageal junction; GI, gastrointestinal; IL-2, interleukin 2; LAK, lymphokine-activated killer cells; MoAb, antimelanoma antibodies; NA, not applicable, no tumor present at necropsy; Rx, immunotherapy; TILs, tumor infiltrating lymphocytes.

* Pulmonary capillary engorgement and interstititial infiltration by lymphocytes.

† Anoxic encephalopathy followed a cardiac arrest after aspiration of gastric contents during a period of altered mental status associated with therapy.

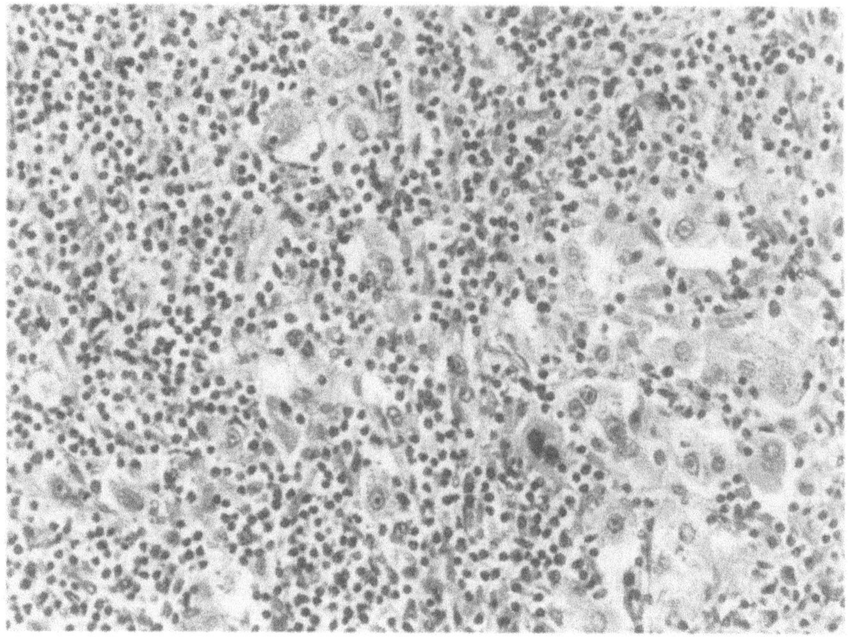

FIGURE 1. Section of liver (case no. 11) entirely replaced by metastatic renal cell carcinoma with dense lymphocytic infiltrate. (Hematoxylin and eosin stain; original magnification × 250.)

marized in Table 2. Significant weight gain during therapy occurred in all 19 patients and varied from 2% to 29% of the admission weight (mean 10%). Significant hypotension occurred in 17 patients (89%) and was severe enough to warrant vasopressor therapy in 13 patients. Arrhythmias (atrial in four and ventricular in eight) were noted in nine patients (47%), eight of whom had some form of right or left ventricular necrosis or fibrosis. The presence of or severity of weight gain, hypotension, or arrhythmias did not correlate with any specific pathologic finding at necropsy.

A lymphocytic myocarditis (Fig 2) was present in two of the four patients dying less than 5 days from the last dose of therapy in whom the heart was available for review. Both of these (patients no. 1 and 3, Table 2) had a patchy inflammatory infiltrate in the walls of both ventricles (predominately lymphocytic, with a few polymorphonuclear leukocytes and eosinophils). There was associated myocyte degeneration and necrosis. No infectious etiology was identified in either case.

Septic myocarditis was observed in three patients who had acute inflammatory infiltrates in the myocardium associated with bacterial sepsis. Patient no. 4 had an acute inflammatory infiltrate and minute abscesses in the myocardium. This patient had evidence of severe and generalized sepsis at necropsy. The other two patients had focal interstitial inflammatory infiltrates without associated necrosis or myocyte degeneration. In patient no. 11, the infiltrate was mixed (polymorphonuclear leukocytes, lymphocytes, and eosinophils) and in the second patient (patient no. 16), it was predominantly polymorphonuclear. Isolated lymphoid aggregates were found in the myocardium of two additional patients (patient nos. 18 and 19).

Acute myocardial infarction was present in one case (patient no. 2) and a healed myocardial infarct was present in a second (patient no. 17). In both cases, the clinically recognized events compatible with acute myocardial infarcts occurred while on therapy or immediately after it was halted. At necropsy, the heart in case no. 2 weighed 520 g and there was > 75% cross-sectional-area narrowing of at least one of the major epicardial coronary arteries. The age of the infarct as evaluated histologically was compatible with the clinical event which occurred less than 24 hours before death. Patient no. 17 had a massive transmural circumferential healed myocardial infarct which extended from the apex to the base of the left ventricle (Fig 3). The major epicardial coronary arteries were virtually devoid of atherosclerotic plaque. The age of the infarct was compatible histologically with a clinically recognized event 71 days before death.

Renal Findings

Selected clinical parameters of renal dysfunction including peak blood urea nitrogen, creatinine, and blood urea nitrogen-to-creatinine ratio while on therapy were tabulated. Virtually all patients had elevated blood urea nitrogen and creatinine during therapy. The peak urea nitrogen/creatinine ratio while on therapy ranged from 8 to 31 (mean 17).

Autolysis was quite pronounced in several cases, and the tubular lesions observed may be largely related to postmortem artifacts. The glomeruli and blood vessels were better preserved. The following tubular lesions were observed: tubular dilation (13 cases), tubular atrophy (eight cases), casts (15 cases), and loss of brush border of the tubular proximal segment (seven cases). Necrosis and regeneration could not be evaluated in the autopsy specimens. No correlation was found between the presence or severity of acute tubular lesions and either the peak blood urea nitrogen/creatinine ratio during therapy or the interval between death and the last dose of therapy. Of the

TABLE 2. Cardiac Findings, Clinical and Anatomic, in 19 Patients Who Received Immunotherapy

		Signs and Symptoms of Clinical Toxicity While on Therapy						Right or Left Ventricular			
					Arrhythmias						
Case No.	Interval Last Rx to Death (d)	Weight Gain (% of adm wt)	Hypotension*	Ischemia†	Atrial‡	Ventricular§	Maximum CA % CSA Narrowing	Myocytolysis (0-4+)	Contraction Band Necrosis (0-4+)	Nontransmural Fibrosis (0-4+)	Lymphocytic Myocarditis (0-4+)
1	0	9	4+	3+	4+	4+	0-25	0	0	0	2+
2[‖]	1	3	4+	4+	4+	4+	>75	0	1+	1+	0
3	4	3	2+	0	2+	1+	0-25	0	0	1+	1-2+
4	4	7	4+	0	0	4+	0-25	0	3-4+	2+	0
5	4	2	4+	0	0	0	—	—	—	—	—
6	6	10	3+	0	0	0	—	1+	0	0	0
7	8	9	3+	0	1+	0	26-50	1+	1+	1+	0
8	13	25	3+	0	0	0	26-50	0	0	0	0
9	16	7	0	0	0	0	—	1+	0	0	0
10	17	6	3+	0	0	0	—	0	0	0	0
11	20	10	2+	4+	4+	2+	51-75	0	0	1-2+	0
12	20	21	3+	0	0	0	0-25	0	0	0	0
13	42	3	3+	0	0	0	0-25	0	0	1+	0
14	43	3	0	0	0	1+	51-75	0	0	1+	0
15	47	9	3+	0	0	0	0-25	1-2+	0	0	0
16	67	8	3+	0	3+	0	0-25	0	0	1+	0
17[¶]	71	8	4+	4+	0	4+	0-25	1-2+	0	1+	0
18	74	13	3+	0	0	0	0-25	0	0	0	0
19	143	29	2+	0	0	1+	0-25	0	0	0	0

Note: 0 = negative.

Abbreviations: adm wt, admission weight; CA, coronary artery; CSA, cross-sectional area; d, days; RV, right ventricular; LV, left ventricular.

* Hypotension: 1+, hypotension not requiring therapy; 2+, hypotension responding to fluid therapy; 3+, hypotension requiring and responsive to pressors; 4+, hypotension unresponsive to pressors.

† Ischemia: 2+, nonspecific electrocardiographic (ECG) changes, elevated creatinine kinase; 3+, angina, ischemic changes in ECG, elevated MB band, 4+, myocardial infarction.

‡ Atrial arrhythmias: 1+, sinus tachycardia >110 beats per minute; 2+, premature atrial contractions, 3+, atrial fibrillation or sinus tachycardia >150 beats per minute; 4+, atrial arrhythmia with hypotension.

§ Ventricular arrhythmias: 1+, unifocal ventricular premature contractions; 2+, multifocal ventricular premature contractions, bigeminy, trigeminy; 3+, nonsustained ventricular tachycardia (VT); 4+, sustained VT.

‖ Acute transmural myocardial infarct, <24 hours.

¶ Circumferential transmural left ventricular infarct, >6 weeks.

19 patients, six had interstitial lymphoid infiltrates unassociated with glomerular or tubular lesions. No correlation was found between evidence of clinical toxicity while on therapy (peak blood urea nitrogen or creatinine or their ratio) or interval from last dose of therapy to death, and the presence of an interstitial lymphoid infiltrate. Three patients with renal cell carcinoma had other renal lesions including acute pyelonephritis (patient no. 3), increased cellularity within the mesangial areas (patient no. 2), and diffuse severe mesangial sclerosis (patient no. 11). One patient (patient no. 1) with malignant melanoma had focal glomerulosclerosis.

Pulmonary Findings

Clinical and morphologic findings are summarized in Table 3. Pulmonary toxicity was severe enough in 10 patients to necessitate intubation during the course of therapy. Despite this, no correlation was found between the severity of pulmonary toxicity while on therapy and the survival from the last dose of therapy.

Lung weight, reflecting pulmonary edema, congestion, pneumonia, tumor, and other infiltrates, was heavy in the five patients who died less than 5 days from the last dose of therapy, but it was equally heavy in other patients dying at prolonged intervals after therapy was halted and when clinical evidence of pulmonary toxicity was reversed (Table 3).

The lungs disclosed variable histologic changes. The most striking changes were seen in patient no. 1, a 22-year-old white woman who received IL-2 and LAK cells for treatment of melanoma (Fig 4). She died in severe respiratory distress less than 1 hour after an infusion of LAK cells and 1 week following a course of high dose IL-2 treatment. The lungs contained marked numbers of lymphoid cells in the pulmonary capillaries. The cells were mostly large lymphocytes, with a high nuclear-to-cytoplasmic ratio and hyperchromatic nuclei. In addition, a marked perivascular and interstitial lymphoid infiltrate, occasional small fibrin microthrombi, and focal hyaline membranes were found. While perivascular and interstitial lymphoid infiltrates were seen in two patients each, in none was it nearly as prominent as in this patient. Hyaline membranes were seen in two other patients, both with diffuse alveolar damage. No specific pulmonary findings at necropsy seemed to correlate with the degree of clinical toxicity during therapy or with the interval from the last dose of

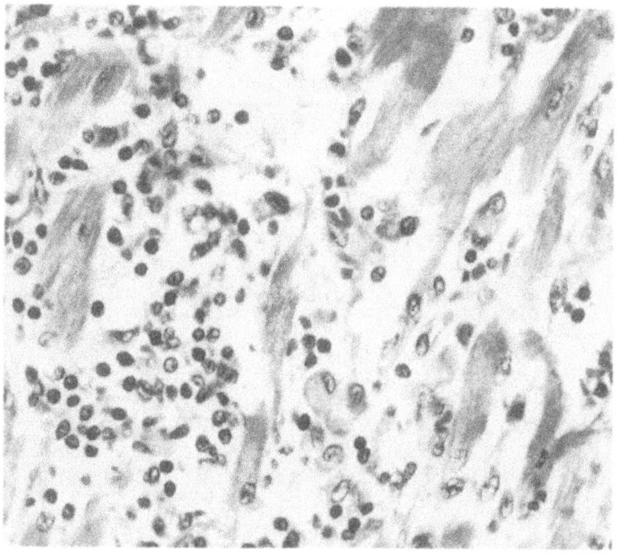

FIGURE 2. Section of left ventricular myocardium (case no. 3) showing a lymphocytic myocarditis. Individual myocytes show degenerative changes. (Hematoxylin and eosin stain; original magnification × 204.)

therapy to death. Bronchopneumonia was found in nine patients and in six it appeared to contribute significantly to the patient's terminal course.

Hepatic Findings

Evidence of hepatobiliary toxicity as reflected in the serum bilirubin and morphologic findings in the liver are outlined in Table 4. Peak serum bilirubin while on therapy ranged from 0.5 to 10.6 mg/dL. No correlation was found between peak bilirubin and the survival from the last dose of therapy. Almost all patients had some degree of centrilobular congestion at necropsy.

All seven patients dying within 8 days of the last dose of therapy had a lymphocytic portal infiltrate, which was more prominent in the two patients dying within 24 hours (Fig 5). Patient no. 2 had extension of this infiltrate beyond the limiting plate with rare foci of associated single-cell hepatocyte necrosis. Patient no. 4 had a mixed lymphocytic, eosinophilic, and polymorphonuclear portal infiltrate and acute cholangitis. Five of the six patients dying within 6 days of the last dose of therapy had lymphocytic sinusoidal infiltrates (Fig 5). Sinusoidal infiltrates were seen in no patients dying later than 6 days from the last dose of therapy.

Three patients dying 20 days or later after cessation of therapy had lymphocytic portal infiltrates. In patients no. 13 and 14 portal fibrosis and extensive metastases also were present. These changes were consistent with chronic biliary obstruction.

At least six patients had other foci of hepatic necrosis, considered to be secondary to either congestion or metastatic tumor.

Steatosis was seen in three patients dying within 5 days of therapy, and in three patients at longer intervals from therapy.

Acute or chronic cholangitis in four patients was either associated with generalized sepsis or extensive hepatic metastases. Severe cholestasis was associated with acute cholangitis in two patients, and with extrahepatic biliary obstruction secondary to tumor in one patient.

A bile duct adenoma and a hemangioma were incidental findings in two patients. Foci of extramedullary hematopoesis were identified in two other patients dying long after cessation of therapy.

Thyroid Gland Findings

Three of the four patients (nos. 1, 2, and 4) dying within 5 days had lymphoid infiltrates in the thyroid

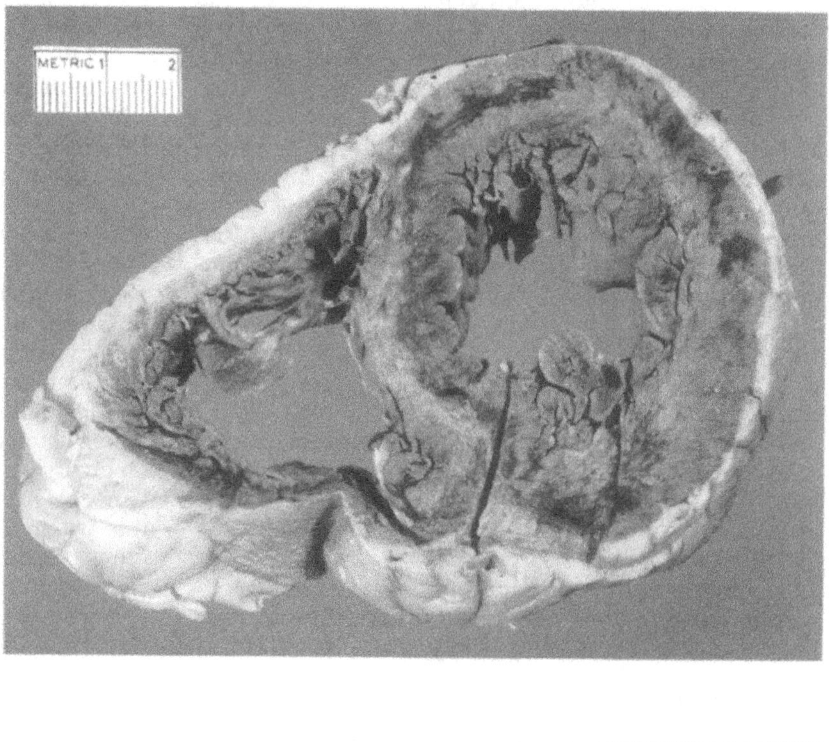

FIGURE 3. Transverse section of the ventricular chambers of the heart (case no. 17) with circumferential left ventricular scarring and biventricular dilatation. The infarct is both subendocardial and transmural. The dark staining of the myocardium corresponds to foci of intracellular calcific deposits. The coronary arteries were essentially devoid of atherosclerotic plaque in this case.

TABLE 3. Pulmonary Findings, Clinical and Anatomic, in Patients Receiving Immunotherapy

Case No.	Interval Last Rx to Death	Clinical Toxicity on Therapy*	Lung Weight (combined, g)	Interstitial Lymphocytes (0-4+)	Perivascular Lymphocytes (0-4+)	Hyaline Membranes (+/−)	Fibrin Microthrombi +/−	Pneumonia +/1
1	0	4+	1,350	3+	3+	focal	+	0
2	1	4+	1,350	0	0	0	+	0
3	4	2+	2,800	0	0	0	0	+
4	4	4+	>1,850	0	0	+	0	+
5	4	4+	2,900	1+ focal	0	0	0	+
6	6	3+	1,100	0	0	0	+	0
7	8	0	1,350	0	0	0	0	0
8	13	4+	700	0	1+	0	0	+
9	16	0	1,410	0	0	0	0	0
10	17	4+	2,000	0	0	0	0	+
11	20	4+	1,450	0	1+	0	+	+
12	20	2+	900	0	0	0	+	+
13	42	4+	2,650	0	0	+	0	0
14	43	0	2,160	0	0	0	0	+
15	47	3+	850	0	0	0	0	0
16	67	0	1,410	0	0	0	0	0
17	71	4+	1,130	0	0	0	0	0
18	74	4+	1,500	1+	0	0	0	0
19	143	0	660	0	0	0	0	+

Abbreviation: Rx, immunotherapy.

* Clinical pulmonary toxicity while on therapy: 1+, Exertional dyspnea; 2+, Dyspnea at rest; 3+, Severe respiratory distress; 4+, Intubation required.

gland, and in one (patient no. 1, Fig 6) they were severe and associated with parenchymal destruction. Two patients (nos. 14 and 17) dying late also had lymphoid infiltrates: several isolated lymphoid aggregates in one patient and moderate lymphoid infiltrates and associated mild parenchymal fibrosis in one patient.

Dermal Findings

Hematoxylin and eosin-stained sections of skin lesions were reviewed in three cases. Subepidermal bullae associated with minimal inflammation were present in one patient, a mild superficial lymphocytic perivascular infiltrate in one patient, and a pustular dermatitis in one patient.

Miscellaneous Findings

With the exception of case no. 1, who in addition to the previously described myocardial, renal, pulmonary, hepatic, and thyroid glandular lesions had lymphoid hyperplasia of ileum, spleen, and lymph nodes, no other significant lesions were noted in sections of the gastrointestinal, reproductive, or hematopoietic organs. (Changes within hematopoietic organs were not assessed systematically because of postmortem changes in these organs.)

Cause of Death

The cause of death (Table 1) was considered the direct result of the presence of metastatic disease in eight patients (one of whom was septic terminally): cerebral metastases (three cases), lung metastases (three cases), lung and liver metastases (one case), and liver and inferior vena cava metastases (one case). In seven other patients, sepsis was considered the cause of death: antemortem blood cultures and/or postmortem cultures of blood and/or lung were positive for *Escherichia coli* and *Klebsiella pneumoniae* in two; *E. coli* and *Enterobacter* sp in one; *Pseudomonas aeruginosa* in one; and *Bacteroides fragilis* in one. In one patient, micro-abscesses containing colonies of gram-positive cocci suggestive of *Staphylococcus* species were identified in multiple organs at necropsy. In one patient, no specific organism was identified as a source of sepsis. In none of these seven patients was a mycobacterium, fungus, or protozoal organism considered responsible for the sepsis. Candida species *fungemia* was seen in one terminal patient (no. 17) who died with severe congestive heart failure secondary to an acute myocardial infarction. The fungemia occurred approximately 6 weeks after cessation of therapy and was not felt to be a consequence of therapy. In eight cases, death was considered directly or indirectly related to the consequences of immunotherapy. Two of these patients died from complications of an acute myocardial infarct (nos. 2 and 17, Table 1); one died with severe respiratory distress and plugging of pulmonary vessels with large atypical lymphoid cells (no. 1, Table 1), three died of sepsis (nos. 3 to 5, Table 1), one died of multisystem failure which developed during therapy and was associated with terminal sepsis (no. 13, Table 1), and one death was secondary to anoxic encephalopathy 20 days after aspiration-induced cardiac arrest (no. 11, Table 1). The latter patient was believed to have aspirated because of an altered mental status associated with therapy.

DISCUSSION

Sepsis was the major cause of death not directly related to the presence of metastatic disease in this

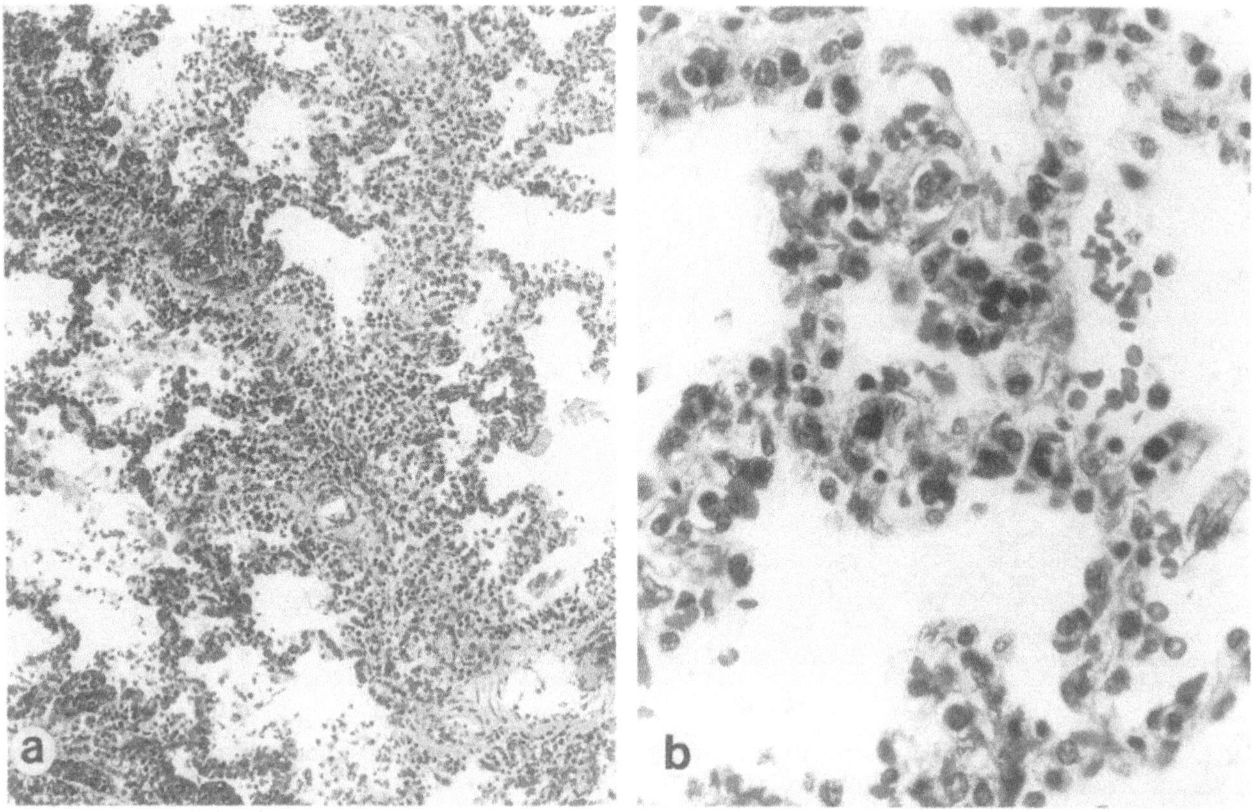

FIGURE 4. Sections of lung (case no. 1) from a 22-year-old female with malignant melanoma who died within 1 hour of infusion of LAK cells and 1 week following high-dose IL-2 therapy. (a) Low-power view showing an extensive interstitial lymphoid infiltrate and congestion of capillaries [original magnification × 125.] (b) High-power view showing engorgement of capillaries with both large and small lymphocytes [original magnification × 500.]

series of 19 patients who received IL-2–based therapy for cancer. It is remarkable that bacterial organisms were responsible for the seven cases of fatal sepsis rather than one of the opportunistic agents associated with conventional chemotherapy and T cell immunosuppression. The paucity of opportunistic infection and the high frequency of serious bacterial infections in patients treated with IL-2 have been previously noted.[11,15,17] Potential explanations for the high frequency of bacterial sepsis may be found in recent evidence that IL-2–based therapy may cause neutrophil dysfunction including depressed Fc receptor expression and decreased chemotactic response.[19] Other recognized alterations in immune function include the development of anergy and decreased proliferative response to soluble antigens.[20] While additional studies are currently underway to further evaluate the immunologic defenses of patients treated with these regimens, it seems clear that the immunologic alterations induced by these agents are not solely directed at the tumor and that they may have serious consequences.

Our study demonstrates the evidence of acute myocardial infarction and lymphocytic myocarditis in patients receiving IL-2–based treatments. Patients receiving IL-2 have been shown to develop a variety of clinical cardiac side effects including profound hypotension, a decrease in systemic vascular resistance, a decrease in ejection fraction, and an increase in heart rate, findings similar to those seen in patients with sepsis.[12,13,16] A small percentage of patients have either atrial or ventricular arrhythmias while on therapy.[3-5] Clinical evidence of acute myocardial infarction or angina pectoris while on therapy has been reported,[3-5,13] and the presence of myocarditis in patients receiving immunotherapy had been documented.[18] Acute myocardial infarction occurred in two of our patients in the face of profound hypotension secondary to immunotherapy. One patient had severe coronary artery disease and the second had widely patent coronary arteries. Two of the four patients dying less than 5 days from the last dose of immunotherapy had a lymphocytic myocarditis without an apparent infectious etiology. All of our patients who had either atrial or ventricular arrhythmias during therapy had either an acute myocardial infarct, a lymphocytic or bacterial myocarditis, or died late with patchy nontransmural fibrosis. Whether or not this nontransmural fibrosis represents a healed myocarditis remains speculative.

Pulmonary toxicity associated with IL-2–based therapy appears primarily to be a consequence of the development of pulmonary edema and to be a transient phenomenon. In a recent review[5] some degree of respiratory distress occurred in 10%, and respiratory distress severe enough to warrant intubation occurred in 4% of 1,039 courses of IL-2–based therapy. The one fatality in this series of 19 patients, which was due to respiratory failure associated with early diffuse alveolar damage and LAK-cell congestion of

TABLE 4. Clinical and Necropsy Findings Pertaining to Liver Pathology

Case No.	Interval Last Rx to Death	Peak Bilirubin on Therapy (mg/dl)	Lymphocytic Portal Inflammation 0-4+	Lymphocytic Sinusoidal Infiltrate 0-4+	Necrosis 0-4+	Cholestasis 0-4+	Steatosis 0-4+	Cholangitis +/−
1	0	2.3	2+	3+	0	0	2+	0
2	1	0.9	2+	1+	1+	0	0	0
3	4	1.1	1+*	2+	0	0	2+	0
4	4	10.6	1+	1+	0	0	2+	+, acute
5	4	0.8	1+	0	0	0	0	0
6	6	0.5	1+	1+	0	0	0	0
7	8	4	1+	0	0	0	0	0
8	13	4.8	0	0	2+	3+	2+	0
9	16	1	0	0	0	0	0	0
10	17	3.8	0	0	0	0	0	0
11	20	5.2	1+	0	0	0	2+	+
12	20	2.6	0	0	0	0	3+	0
13	42	3.8	1+†	0	4+	3+	0	+, acute and chronic
14	43	4.7	2+†	0	3+	0	0	+, chronic
15	47	4.4	0	0	2+	0	0	0
16	67	2.7	0	0	0	0	0	0
17	71	6.5	0	0	focal	3+	0	0
18	74	5.3	0	0	0	0	0	0
19	143	1	0	0	0	0	0	0

Abbreviation: Rx, immunotherapy.
* Eosinophils and polymorphonuclear leukocytes were also present.
† Consistent with chronic biliary obstruction.

pulmonary capillaries, demonstrates the potential for serious pulmonary toxicity associated with administration of LAK cells. The perivascular lymphoid infiltrate which was seen in this patient resembles that which has been observed in rat and mice IL-2 toxicity experiments.[21,22]

The high incidence of portal lymphocytic infiltrates and hepatic sinusoidal infiltrates in patients dying at short intervals after therapy suggests that these findings are directly related to immunotherapy. The accumulation of LAK cells in the liver shortly after infusion of these cells has also been documented by rectilinear scanning.[23] Lymphocytic portal infiltrates, seen in many patients dying shortly after therapy, and the associated necrosis which was seen in one patient have been described in studies of IL-2 toxicity in rats.[21] While reversible cholestasis is a recognized complication of IL-2–based therapy,[8] bile stasis was not appreciated except in patients with other evidence of obstructive jaundice.

Alterations in thyroid function have been reported.[10] We observed a high frequency of lymphoid infiltrates in the thyroid gland of patients dying shortly after cessation of therapy, suggesting that these may be immediate sequelae of therapy. The clinical significance of these findings is not clear, as

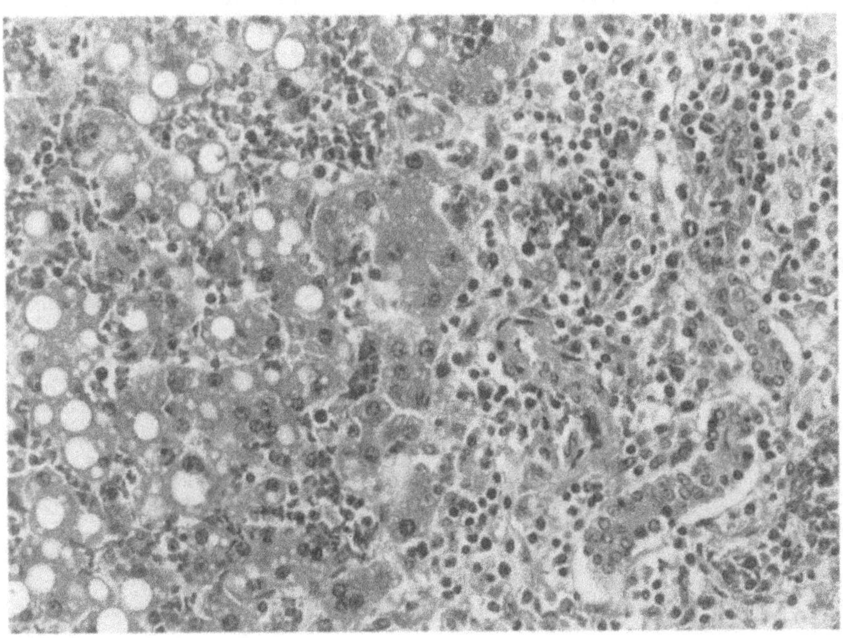

FIGURE 5. Section of liver (case no. 1) from a 22-year-old female who died shortly after an infusion of LAK cells and 1 week following a course of high-dose IL-2. There is a dense portal and sinusoidal lymphoid infiltrate. Hepatocytes show microvesicular steatosis. (Hematoxylin and eosin stain; original magnification × 250.)

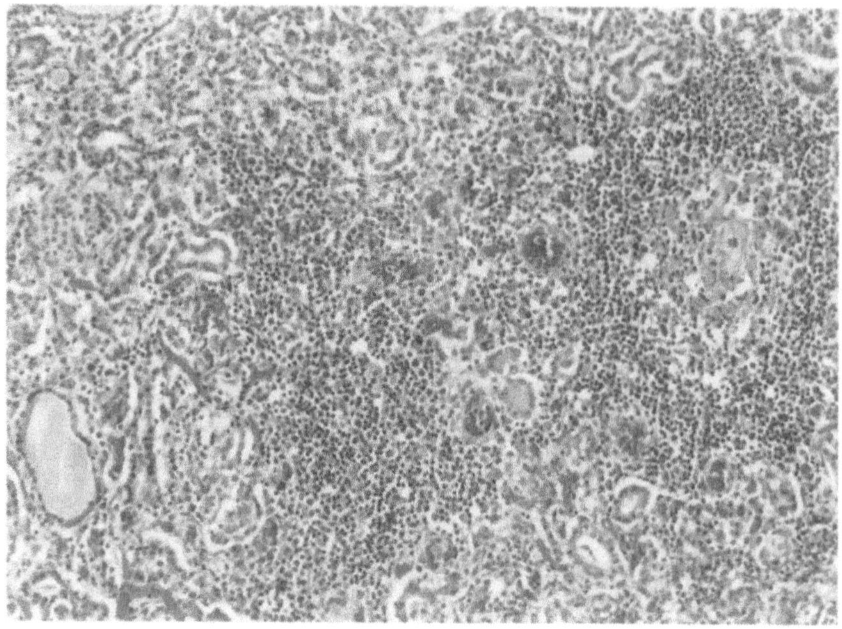

FIGURE 6. Section of thyroid gland (case no. 1) showing a lymphocytic thyroiditis. There is extensive lymphocytic infiltration of the thyroid gland with destruction of follicles. (Hematoxylin and eosin stain; original magnification × 125.)

tests of thyroid function were not available for review in all patients.

Renal dysfunction, attributed to prerenal azotemia.[6] is uniformly present in patients receiving IL-2. No consistent renal findings were present at necropsy which could be related to immunotherapy. Likewise, despite the high frequency of dermal changes[3-5,9] in patients receiving IL-2–based therapies, no pathologic correlates were identified at autopsy.

In summary, in addition to the uniform finding of lymphoid infiltrates in the tumors of patients dying less than 43 days after cessation of therapy which, presumably, is related to its beneficial effects, IL-2–based immunotherapy, not unlike other forms of therapy for the treatment of malignancy, is associated with serious side effects. Despite this, in only 10 of the more than 650 patients who have been treated with these agents at this institution (including eight of the patients described in this report) was death felt to be a direct consequence of therapy. In the 19 patients described in this report there may be an increased frequency of fatal bacterial infections as well as significant cardiac and pulmonary toxicity. As these 19 patients represent a small fraction of the more than 650 patients who have received IL-2–based immunotherapy at this institution,[5] continued follow-up is necessary to document the frequency and confirm the significance of our findings.

REFERENCES

1. Taniguchi T, Matsui H, Fujita T, et al: Structure and expression of a cloned cDNA for human interleukin-2. Nature 302:305-310, 1983
2. Rosenberg SA, Grimm EA, McGrogan M, et al: Biological activity in recombinant human interleukin-2 produced in E coli. Science 223:1412-1415, 1984
3. Rosenberg SA, Lotze MT, Muul LM, et al: A progress report on the treatment of 157 patients with advanced cancer using lymphokine-activated killer cells and interleukin-2 or high dose interleukin-2 alone. N Engl J Med 316:889-897, 1987
4. Fisher RI, Coltman CA, Doroshow JH, et al: Metastatic renal cancer treated with interleukin-2 and lymphokine-activated killer cells. A phase II clinical trial. Ann Intern Med 108:518-523, 1988
5. Rosenberg SA, Lotze MT, Yang JC, et al: Experience with the use of high dose interleukin-2 in the treatment of 652 patients with cancer. Ann Surg 210:474-485, 1989
6. Belldegrun A, Webb DE, Austin HA, et al: Effects of interleukin-2 on renal function in patients receiving immunotherapy for advanced cancer. Ann Intern Med 106:817-822, 1987
7. Marolda R, Belli F, Prada A, et al: A phase I study of recombinant interleukin-2 in melanoma patients. Toxicity and clinical effects. Tumori 73:575-584, 1987
8. Fisher B, Keenan AM, Garra BS, et al: Interleukin-2 induces profound reversible cholestasis: A detailed analysis in treated patients. J Clin Oncol 7:1852-1862, 1989
9. Gaspari AA, Lotze MT, Rosenberg SA, et al: Dermatologic changes associated with interleukin-2 adminsitration. JAMA 258:1624-1629, 1987
10. Atkins MB, Mier JW, Parkinson DR, et al: Hypothyroidism after treatment with interleukin-2 and lymphokine-activated killer cells. N Engl J Med 318:1557-1563, 1988
11. Begley MG, Shawker TH, Robertson CN, et al: Fournier gangrene: Diagnosis with scrotal US. Radiology 169:387-389, 1988
12. Gaynor ER, Vitek L, Sticklin L, et al: The hemodynamic effects of treatment with interleukin-2 and lymphokine-activated killer cells. Ann Intern Med 109:953-958, 1988
13. Nora R, Abrams JS, Tait NS, et al: Myocardial toxic effects during recombinant interleukin-2 therapy. JNCI 81:59-63, 1989
14. Osanto S, Cluitmans FH, Franks CR, et al: Myocardial injury after interleukin-2 therapy. Lancet 2:48-49, 1988
15. Schwartzentruber D, Lotze MT, Rosenberg SA: Colonic perforation. An unusual complication of therapy with high dose interleukin-2. Cancer 62:2350-2353, 1988
16. Lee RE, Lotze MT, Skibber JM, et al: Cardiorespiratory effects of immunotherapy with interleukin-2. J Clin Oncol 7:7-20, 1989
17. Bock SN, Lee RE, Fisher B, et al: A prospective randomized trial evaluating prophylactic antibiotics to prevent catheter-related sepsis in patients treated with immunotherapy. J Clin Oncol 8:161-169, 1990

18. Samlowski WE, Ward JH, Craven CM, et al: Severe myocarditis following high dose interleukin-2 administration. Arch Pathol Lab Med 113:838-841, 1989

19. Jablons D, Bolton E, Mertins S, et al: In vivo administration of interleukin-2 to humans alters circulating neutrophil Fc receptor expression and chemotaxis. J Immunol (in press)

20. Wiebke EA, Rosenberg SA, Lotze MT: Acute immunologic effects of interleukin-2 therapy in cancer patients: Decreased delayed type hypersensitivity response and decreased proliferative response to soluble antigens. J Clin Oncol 6:1440-1449, 1988

21. Matory YL, Chang AE, Lipford EH III, et al: Toxicity of recombinant human interleukin-2 in rats following intravenous infusion. J Biol Response Mod 4:377-390, 1985

22. Puri RK, Travis WD, Rosenberg SA: Decrease in Interleukin-2 induced vascular leakage in the lungs of mice by administration of recombinant Interleukin-1 in vivo. Cancer Res 49:969-976, 1989

23. Rosenberg SA: Adoptive immunotherapy: Accomplishments and prospects. Cancer Treat Rep 68:233-255, 1984

Myocarditis or Acute Myocardial Infarction Associated With Interleukin-2 Therapy for Cancer

Amy H. Kragel, MD,* William D. Travis, MD,† Ronald G. Steis, MD,‡
Steven A. Rosenberg, MD,§ and William C. Roberts, MD*

The hearts of eight patients aged 22 to 67 years (mean, 41 years) who died during or within 4 days of interleukin-2 (IL-2) based immunotherapy for treatment of renal cell carcinoma or melanoma were studied at necropsy. Death resulted from combined cardiorespiratory failure in two patients, sepsis in four patients, acute myocardial infarction in one patient, and myocarditis in one patient. Transmural left ventricular necrosis was present in one of the two patients with significant atherosclerotic coronary artery narrowing. Noninfectious myocarditis was present in five patients: the inflammatory infiltrate was lymphocytic in four and composed of a mixture of eosinophils and lymphocytes in one. Although treatment-related deaths associated with high-dose IL-2 therapy are uncommon (1.5% in 652 consecutive patients), the potential for significant myocardial ischemia or myocarditis exists, and careful monitoring for arrhythmias or myocardial failure is warranted. *Cancer* 66:1513–1516, 1990.

INTERLEUKIN-2 (IL-2) BASED immunotherapy for the treatment of cancer has been associated with a variety of hemodynamic and cardiac alterations, including hypotension, tachycardia, decreased systemic vascular resistance, decreased ejection fraction, variable changes in pulmonary arterial wedge pressure, and peripheral edema.[1–3] In addition, atrial and ventricular arrhythmias, angina pectoris, myocarditis (noninfectious), and acute myocardial infarction have been reported.[4–8] Some of these abnormalities can be explained by the development of a "capillary leak syndrome" with profound hypotension. We studied the hearts at necropsy of eight patients who died during or within 4 days of cessation of IL-2-based immunotherapy to identify anatomic cardiac abnormalities associated with IL-2 administration.

Patients and Methods

The autopsy records of the Pathology Laboratory, National Cancer Institute, were searched for patients in whom IL-2-based immunotherapy had been administered and in whom death had occurred within 5 days of the cessation of therapy. Nine such patients were identified; in one patient, however, neither the heart nor histologic sections were available for review. The remaining eight cases are the subject of this report. In each case, the clinical records, necropsy report, heart specimen, and multiple hematoxylin and eosin stained sections of right and left ventricular myocardium were examined.

Results

The clinical and morphologic features of the five men and three women are summarized in Table 1. Certain features of patients 1, 2, 6, and 8 were reported previously.[8] Therapy was administered for the treatment of melanoma in six patients and for renal cell carcinoma in two. In

From the *Pathology Branch, National Heart, Lung, and Blood Institute, and the †Laboratory of Pathology, ‡Clinical Research Branch, Biological Response Modifiers Program, and §Surgery Branch, National Cancer Institute, National Institutes of Health, Bethesda, Maryland.

The authors thank all of the many people involved in the care of the patients included in this study, including Dr. Mario Sznol, Clinical Research Branch, National Cancer Institute, Frederick Memorial Hospital, and the physicians and nurses of the Clinical Center, National Institutes of Health, Bethesda, Maryland.

Address for reprints: Amy H. Kragel, MD, Pathology Branch, National Heart, Lung, and Blood Institute, Building 10, Room 2N258, Bethesda, MD 20892.

Accepted for publication February 22, 1990.

TABLE 1. Clinical and Cardiac Necropsy Findings in 8 Patients Receiving Interleukin-2-Based Immunotherapy

Case no.	Age (yr)	Sex	Immunotherapy regimen	Interval treatment to death (days)	Mode of death	Evidence of toxicity while on therapy: Hypotension*	Ischemia†	Arrhythmias: Atrial‡	Arrhythmias: Ventricular§	HW (g)	Dilated cavity: RV	Dilated cavity: LV	CA narrowing (% CSA)	Myocarditis
1	22	F	IL2/LAK	0	CR Failure	4+	3+	4+	4+	295	+	0	0–25	+
2	24	M	IL2/LAK	4	Sepsis	4+	0	0	4+	355	+	0	0–25	+
3	30	M	IL2/TILs/C	4	Sepsis	–	–	–	–	440	+	0	0–25	+
4	34	M	IL2/TILs/C	4	Sepsis	–	–	–	–	430	0	0	0–25	0
5	50	F	IL2/LAK	1	CR Failure	0	0	0	0	330	+	0	0–25	+
6	51	M	IL2	4	Sepsis	2+	0	2+	1+	365	0	0	0–25	+
7	53	F	IL2	1	Sudden Death	1+	0	–	–	415	0	0	76–95	+
8	67	M	IL2	1	AMI	4+	4+	4+	4+	520	0	0	76–95	0

(0): negative; (–): information not available; AMI: acute myocardial infarction; C: cyclophosphamide; CA: coronary artery; CR: cardiorespiratory; CSA: cross-sectional area narrowing; HW: heart weight; IL2: interleukin 2; LAK: lymphokine-activated killer cells; LV: left ventricle, RV: right ventricle; TIL: tumor infiltrating lymphocytes.

* Hypotension: 1+ = hypotension not requiring therapy, 2+ = hypotension responding to fluid therapy, 3+ = hypotension requiring and responsive to pressors, 4+ = hypotension unresponsive to pressors.

† Ischemia: 2+ = nonspecific electrocardiographic changes, elevated CK, 3+ = angina, ischemic changes on electrocardiogram, elevated MB band, 4+ = AMI.

‡ Atrial arrhythmias: 1+ = sinus tachycardia > 110 beats/min, 2+ = premature atrial complexes, 3+ = atrial fibrillation or sinus tacchycardia > 150 beats/min, 4+ = atrial arrhythmia with hypotension.

§ Ventricular arrhythmias: 1+ = unifocal ventricular premature complexes, 2+ = multifocal ventricular premature complexes, bigeminy, trigeminy, 3+ = nonsustained ventricular tachycardia (VT), 4+ = sustained VT.

addition to IL-2, the immunotherapy regimens of three of the patients included lymphokine-activated killer (LAK) cells and two included tumor-infiltrating lymphocytes and cyclophosphamide.

The immediate cause of death varied. Severe combined cardiorespiratory failure immediately following an infusion of LAK cells occurred in two patients. Patient 1 (Table 1) had extensive plugging of pulmonary capillaries and widening of alveolar septae by lymphoid cells with early focal diffuse alveolar damage, and patient 5 (Table 1) had extensive intra-alveolar hemorrhage and early diffuse alveolar damage. Both patients also had a noninfectious myocarditis at necropsy. Patient 7 (Fig. 1) was found dead in bed following LAK therapy; the extent of metastatic disease was not considered sufficient to account for her death, but the left anterior descending coronary artery was narrowed greater than 75% in cross-sectional area by atherosclerotic plaque and a lymphocytic myocarditis also was present. Patient 8 had an acute myocardial infarction while on therapy. The remaining four patients died of consequences of bacterial sepsis, including one with severe renal failure (patient 4).

The heart weight was increased (> 350 g in women and > 400 g in men) in four patients. Two patients with cardiomegaly had coronary artery disease with more than 75% cross-sectional area narrowing by plaque of at least one of the four major epicardial coronary arteries. In one of these two (patient 8, Table 1), gross and microscopic examination of the heart showed transmural myocardial necrosis histologically compatible with a 24-hour-old infarct. Of the remaining seven patients, six had evidence of a diffuse, patchy myocarditis (Fig. 1). In four patients (1, 3, 6, and 7 [Table 1]), the inflammatory infiltrate was predominately lymphocytic; in one (patient 5), the infiltrate was composed of a mixture of eosinophils and lymphocytes; and in one (patient 2), it was composed of a mixture of polymorphonuclear leukocytes, lymphocytes, and eosinophils with microabscess formation. Only in this last patient was the etiology of the myocarditis believed to be infectious: colonies of organisms were identified within the abscesses. In all six of these patients, there was myofiber degeneration and scattered foci of myocyte necrosis. In the two patients dying with severe cardiorespiratory failure and in the one case of sudden death due to myocarditis, the myocarditis was of greater severity than in the other two cases of noninfectious myocarditis.

In no patient was there grossly visible right or left ventricular fibrosis. Microscopic examination of hematoxylin and eosin stained sections disclosed mild interstitial fibrosis in three cases (patients 2, 4, and 6). Foci of contraction-band necrosis were noted in several cases, including one (patient 2) in whom the final resuscitative measures were prolonged and had included open cardiac massage.

Discussion

While death associated with high-dose IL-2 therapy is rare (1.5% in 652 consecutive patients treated with high-dose IL-2-based immunotherapy),[6] we found cardiac morphologic abnormalities in seven of our eight patients who died within 4 days of therapy. These abnormalities

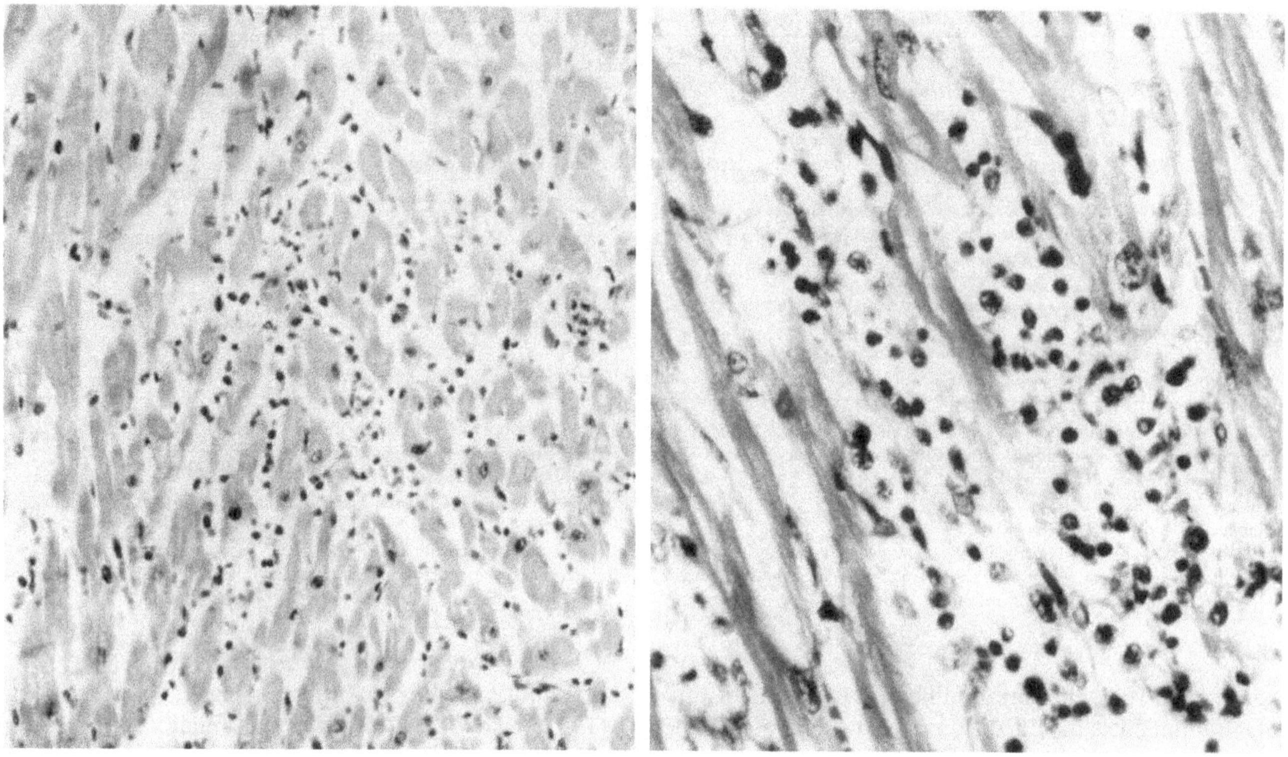

FIG. 1. Hematoxylin and eosin stained sections of left ventricular myocardium showing an interstitial lymphocytic infiltrate with degeneration and necrosis of myocytes. These sections were taken from patient 7, a 53-year-old woman who was found dead in bed, unexpectedly, 1 day after receiving her last dose of IL-2 (left, ×250; right, ×500).

included acute myocardial infarction associated with severe atherosclerotic coronary artery disease in one patient, noninfectious myocarditis in five patients, and bacterial myocarditis in one patient.

Clinical evidence of angina pectoris and acute myocardial infarction has been reported previously in patients receiving IL-2-based immunotherapy for cancer.[2,4–6] In addition to the patient described in this report in whom acute myocardial infarction was associated with severe atherosclerotic coronary artery disease and whose death occurred within 4 days of cessation of IL-2-based therapy, we have seen two additional cases at necropsy in which acute myocardial infarction occurred during therapy in the absence of atherosclerotic coronary artery disease but in whom death did not occur until later. The first patient[8] was a 53-year-old man who died 71 days after cessation of therapy, and necropsy disclosed cardiomegaly, biventricular dilatation, and a large transmural left ventricular circumferential infarct extending from apex to base. The second patient was a 20-year-old woman who died 21 days after therapy was stopped, and necropsy disclosed transmural left ventricular necrosis. In both of these cases, the epicardial coronary arteries were virtually devoid of atherosclerotic plaque. Thus, it appears that the profound hypotension associated with IL-2 therapy can precipitate ischemic myocardial injury even in the absence of underlying atherosclerotic coronary artery disease.

Noninfectious myocarditis associated with IL-2-based immunotherapy has been described previously.[7,8] It is likely that myocarditis is responsible, at least in part, for the arrhythmias and decreased ejection fractions in patients receiving this therapy. The exact role that IL-2 plays in the development of myocarditis, however, is unknown.

The presence of a direct effect of IL-2 on myocardial function has not been identified in humans. Changes in myocyte contractility in response to IL-2, however, have been observed in rat myocyte cell cultures.[9] In addition, interleukin-1 and tumor necrosis factor, whose production may be stimulated by IL-2-based immunotherapy, decrease myocardial contractility in cell culture in response to β-adrenergic stimulation.[10]

We have not observed noninfectious myocarditis in other patients who died at intervals longer than 7 days after the cessation of therapy.[8] This observation suggests that it is either a transient phenomenon or that it occurs in patients who may have an increased susceptibility to IL-2 toxicity and subsequently die shortly after therapy. Because of the high frequency of myocarditis observed in our study and the potential for ischemic myocardial damage, patients receiving IL-2 should be monitored for the development of cardiac arrhythmias and cardiac failure during IL-2-based therapy.

REFERENCES

1. Gaynor ER, Vitek L, Sticklin L *et al.* The hemodynamic effects of treatment with interleukin-2 and lymphokine-activated killer cells. *Ann Intern Med* 1988; 109:953–958.

2. Nora R, Abrams JS, Tait NS, Hiponia DJ, Silverman HJ. Myocardial toxic effects during recombinant interleukin-2 therapy. *J Natl Cancer Inst* 1989; 81:59–63.

3. Lee RE, Lotze MT, Skibber JM *et al.* Cardiorespiratory effects of immunotherapy with interleukin-2. *J Clin Oncol* 1989; 7:7–20.

4. Rosenberg SA, Lotze MT, Muul LM *et al.* A progress report on the treatment of 157 patients with advanced cancer using lymphokine-activated killer cells and interleukin-2 or high dose interleukin-2 alone. *N Engl J Med* 1987; 316:889–897.

5. Fisher RI, Coltman CA, Doroshow JH *et al.* Metastatic renal cancer treated with interleukin-2 and lymphokine-activated killer cells. A phase II clinical trial. *Ann Intern Med* 1988; 108:518–523.

6. Rosenberg SA, Lotze MT, Yang JC *et al.* Experience with the use of high dose interleukin-2 in the treatment of 652 patients with cancer. *Ann Surg* 1989;210:474–485.

7. Samlowski WE, Ward JH, Craven CM, Freedman RA. Severe myocarditis following high dose interleukin-2 administration. *Arch Pathol Lab Med* 1989; 113:838–841.

8. Kragel AH, Travis WD, Feinberg L *et al.* Pathologic findings associated with interleukin-2 based immunotherapy for cancer: A postmortem study of 19 patients. *Hum Pathol* 1990;21:493–502.

9. Fink S, Finiasz M, Sterin-Borda L, Borda E, de Bracco MM. Interleukin 2 stimulates heart contractility in the presence of exogenous arachidonate or the calcium ionophore A 23187. *Immunol Lett* 1988; 17:183–188.

10. Gulick T, Chung MK, Pieper SJ, Lange LG, Schreiner GF. Interleukin 1 and tumor necrosis factor inhibit cardiac myocyte β-adrenergic responsiveness. *Proc Natl Acad Sci* 1989; 86:6753–6757.

Gross and Semiquantitative Histologic Findings in Mononuclear Cell Myocarditis Causing Sudden Death, and Implications for Endomyocardial Biopsy

Jamshid Shirani, MD,* Lawrence J. Freant, MD, and William C. Roberts, MD†

The distribution of gross myocardial lesions and the relative density of the inflammatory cells in various myocardial locations (subepicardial and subendocardial halves of the left ventricular free wall, right ventricular and left ventricular halves of the ventricular septum, and the right ventricular free wall) were studied in 14 patients (11 male [79%], 8 black [57%], aged 7 months to 65 years [median 16 years]) who died suddenly of acute mononuclear-cell myocarditis. Grossly visible myocardial lesions were present in 8 patients, and preferentially involved the subepicardial regions of the left ventricular free wall. The highest mean number of mononuclear cells were seen in the subepicardial regions of the left ventricular free wall (193 cells per high-power field) and the lowest in the right ventricular one half of the ventricular septum (92 cells per high-power field, p <0.001). Thus the predominant location of the gross myocardial lesions in acute mononuclear-cell myocarditis is the subepicardial region of the left ventricular free wall. A relatively low density of mononuclear cells are found in the right ventricular half of the ventricular septum, the main location of endomyocardial biopsies.

(Am J Cardiol 1993;72:952–957)

From the Pathology Branch, National Heart, Lung, and Blood Institute, National Institutes of Health, Bethesda, Maryland. Manuscript received and accepted on June 4, 1993. This manuscript was reviewed and declined by another cardiology journal. The few specific suggestions from each of the 2 reviewers were responded to by making appropriate changes in the present manuscript.

*Present address: Medical College of Virginia, Department of Medicine, Division of Cardiology, MCV Station, Box 128, Richmond, Virginia 23298-0128.

†Present address: Baylor Cardiovascular Institute, Baylor University Medical Center, 3500 Gaston Avenue, Dallas, Texas 75246.

Although several reports have described clinical, epidemiologic, and histopathologic features of isolated mononuclear-cell myocarditis,[1–11] gross cardiac morphologic features of the disease and the quantity of inflammatory cells in the myocardial walls have not been described. This study examines both gross and semiquantitative histologic features of patients dying suddenly with isolated mononuclear-cell myocarditis. The quantity of myocardial inflammatory cells in the various portions of ventricular septum and left ventricular free wall at necropsy provides information pertinent to endomyocardial biopsy during life.

METHODS

Sources of patients: The files of the Pathology Branch, National Heart, Lung, and Blood Institute, National Institutes of Health, contain 82 patients coded as having had "myocarditis." Giant-cell (34 patients), bacterial (9 patients), fungal (3 patients), rheumatic (2 patients), eosinophilic (1 patient), and parasitic (1 patient) myocarditis accounted for 49 patients, and the remaining 32 patients had mononuclear-cell myocarditis. Among the latter 32 patients, 14 died suddenly and they are the subjects of this study. The hearts of these 14 patients were submitted to the Pathology Branch from 8 different medical centers in the Washington, D.C., area (9 patients) and elsewhere (5 patients). In all patients, clinical records submitted from the consulting medical center, photographs of the heart and histologic slides (9 patients) or photomicrographs (5 patients) were available for examination.

Definitions: *Mononuclear-cell myocarditis* was defined as focal, albeit extensive, myocardial inflammatory infiltrates, in ventricular walls, predominantly by mononuclear cells associated with myocyte necrosis and in the absence of other infiltrative (such as leukemia or lymphoma) or ischemic (atherosclerotic coronary artery disease) diseases.

Sudden death was defined as fatal cardiac arrest outside a hospital or shortly after admission to a hospital before any specific therapy had been given. In all 14 patients, the diagnosis of myocarditis was first made at necropsy.

Subepicardial lesion was defined as a lesion involving predominantly the subepicardial one half of the left ventricular free wall.

Histologic examination: In 9 patients histologic slides of ventricular myocardium were available for review. The left ventricular myocardial sections were di-

TABLE I Certain Clinical and Cardiac Morphologic Findings in 14 Patients with Mononuclear-Cell Myocarditis Who Died Suddenly

				Time of Death			Illness Before Death				Myocardial Lesions									Dilated (0–3+)	
											Subepicardial			Transmural							
Patient	Age (years)	Race	Sex	Year	Season	Place of Death	Fever	Other Symptoms	Duration (Days)	HW (g)	P	L	A	P	L	A	VS	RV 1/2 VS	RV	RV	LV
1	0.6	O	M	1975	Winter	ER†	0	Diarrhea	2	75	+	+	0	0	0	0	+	0	+	+++	+++
2	0.8	W	M	1968	Summer	ER†	0	Dyspnea	1	80	+	+	+	0	0	0	0	0	0	+++	+++
3	3	B	M	1992	Spring	ER†	+	Sore throat	6	70	0	0	0	0	0	0	0	0	0	++	+++
4	7	B	F	1982	Fall	ER†	+	Sore throat	3	200	0	0	0	0	0	0	0	0	0	+	++
5	12	W	M	1978	Winter	Ambulance	0	Back pain	1	125	0	0	0	0	0	0	0	0	0	++	0
6	13	B	M	1979	Fall	Home	+	Myalgia	3	300	+	+	+	0	0	0	+	+	+	+	++
7	14	B	M	1992	Spring	Home	0	Chest pain	1	275	+	+	+	0	0	0	0	+	+	++	+
8	17	B	M	1982	Winter	Home	0	Palpitation	1	420	+	0	+	0	0	+	0	0	0	0	0
9	17	W	M	1974	Spring	Car	0	0	0	390	0	0	0	0	0	0	0	0	0	+++	+++
10	24	B	M	1992	Fall	Office	0	Chest pain	1	360	+	+	0	+	+	0	0	0	+	++	+
11	28	B	F	1991	Summer	Church	0	0	0	340	+	0	+	0	0	+	+	+	+	+	0
12	33	W	M	1979	Summer	Home	+	Cough	3	360	0	0	0	0	0	0	0	0	0	0	0
13	53	B	M	1980	Winter	Home	+	Cough	5	335	0	0	0	0	0	0	+	+	+	0	0
14	65	W	F	1975	Summer	ER†	0	Weakness	7	800	0	0	0	0	0	0	0	0	0	+++	+++
Totals (mean or median*)	(16)*	8B (57%)	11M (79%)				5		(2)	(320)*	7	5	5	1	1	2	4	4	6	11 (79%)	9 (64%)

*Median.
†Fatal cardiac arrest occurred in emergency room before any treatment was initiated.
A = anterior; B = black; ER = emergency room; F = female; HW = heart weight; L = lateral; LV = left ventricle; M = male; O = oriental; P = posterior; RV = right ventricle; VS = ventricular septum; W = white.

vided into subepicardial and subendocardial halves and the ventricular septal sections were divided into right ventricular and left ventricular halves. In each case, the number of infiltrating mononuclear cells were counted in 10 consecutive high-power fields at a magnification of 400 × in both halves of the left ventricular free wall, in both halves of the ventricular septum, and in the right ventricular wall. In each microscopic field of study, the number of eosinophils, and the degree of fibrosis and myocyte necrosis also were recorded. Myocardial fibrosis was graded as 0 (absent), 1+ (perivascular), 2+ (interstitial) or 3+ (replacement). The percent myocyte necrosis was calculated by dividing the number of necrotic or degenerated muscle cells by the total number of myocytes seen in each field. The histologic data were recorded without knowledge of the gross myocardial findings.

Statistics: For each continuous variable range and median or mean ± SD, and for each noncontinuous variable, frequency and percentage were reported. Student's *t* test was used to calculate the significance of the difference between the mean number of mononuclear cells in various myocardial locations. Differences were considered significant when $p < 0.05$.

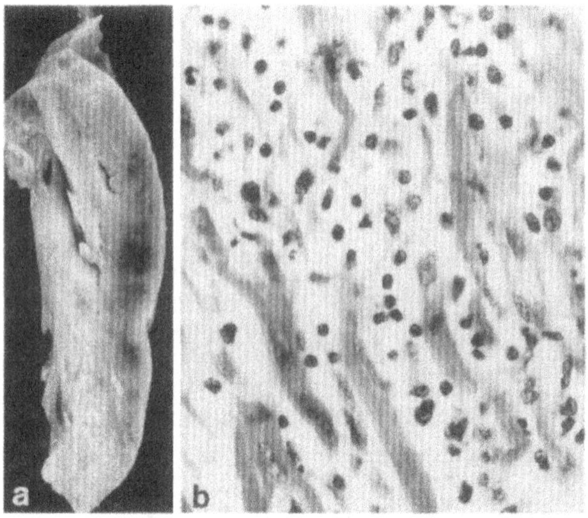

FIGURE 1. Patient 1, Table I. The heart of a 7-month-old Vietnamese boy (GT# 75A-40) who died on arrival to emergency room. He was treated for staphylococcal skin infection and shigellosis 5 weeks before death. Following antibiotic therapy, he was well for 3 weeks until diarrhea started 2 days before death. *a*, longitudinal section of the left ventricular lateral wall and the anterolateral papillary muscle showing myocardial lesions; *b*, photomicrograph of a section of a portion of left ventricular free wall showing mononuclear cellular infiltrates and degenerated muscle fibers. (Hematoxylin-eosin stain, × 630 *(b)*, reduced 37%.)

RESULTS

Clinical and gross morphologic findings (Table I and Figures 1 to 6): The patients ranged in age from 7 months to 65 years (median 16 years), and 11 (79%) were males. Eight patients (57%) were black. Death occurred outside a hospital in 9 patients (64%) and in the emergency room in 5. Twelve of the 14 patients had

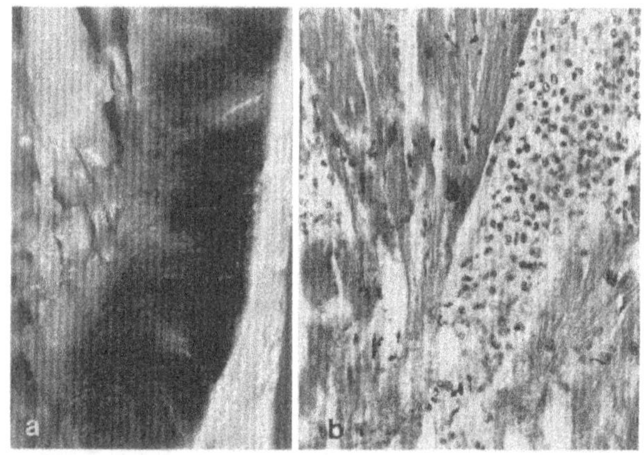

FIGURE 2. Patient 6. The heart of a 13-year-old black boy (DCMEO# 79-12-901) who was found dead at home. He had fever and generalized myalgia for 3 days before death. *a*, longitudinal section of the left ventricular free wall and the anterolateral papillary muscle showing extensive myocardial lesions but sparing the innermost subendocardial regions. *b*, photomicrograph of a section of the left ventricular free wall showing mononuclear cellular infiltrates and necrotic muscle fibers. (Hematoxylin-eosin stain, × 200 *(b)*, reduced 38%.)

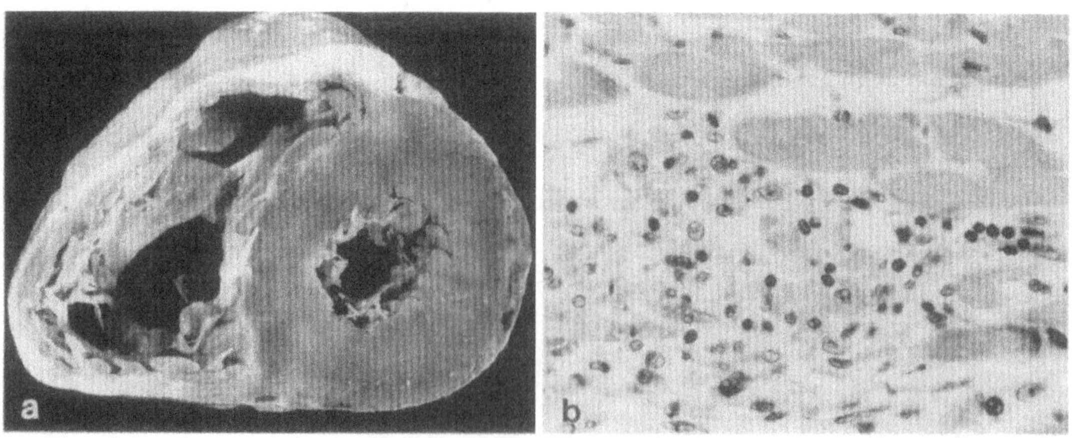

FIGURE 3. Patient 7. The heart of a 14-year-old black boy (DCMEO# 92-4-402) who died suddenly at home while dressing. He had complained of chest discomfort the day before death. *a*, transverse section through the basal portion of the cardiac ventricles showing subepicardial lesions of myocarditis in the lateral posterior left ventricular wall. *b*, photomicrograph of a section of the left ventricular myocardium showing mononuclear cellular infiltrates and necrotic muscle fibers. (Hematoxylin-eosin stain, × 630 *(b)*, reduced 32%.)

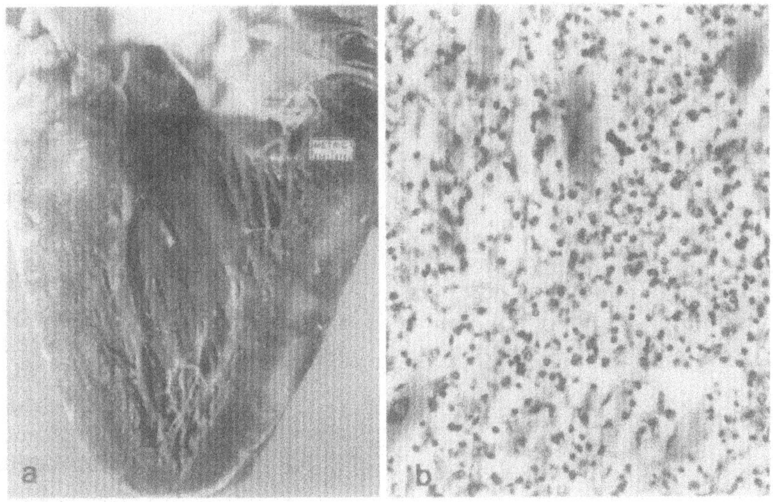

FIGURE 4. Patient 8. Heart of a 17-year-old black boy (DCMEO# 82-3-298) who was found dead in bed at home. Since the day before death he had complained of headache and palpitations. *a*, saggital section of the left ventricular wall showing predominantly subepicardial lesions in the posterior and anterior wall. *b*, photomicrograph of a section of a portion of left ventricular wall showing mononuclear cell infiltrates and destroyed muscle fibers. (Hematoxylin-eosin stain, × 400 *(b)*, reduced 39%.)

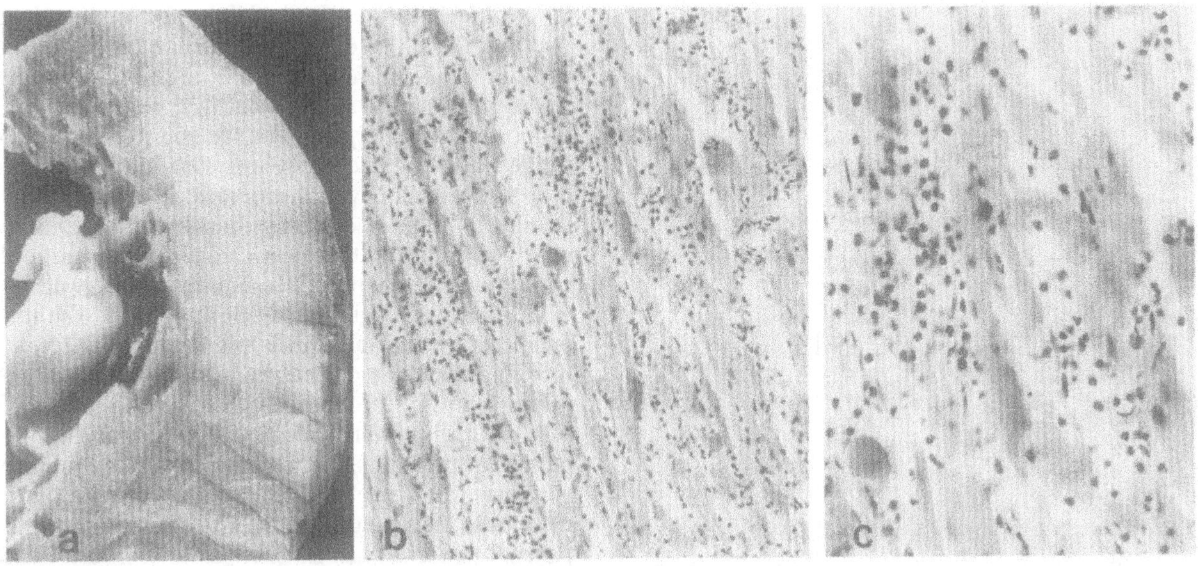

FIGURE 5. Patient 10. Heart of a 24-year-old black man (Alabama MEO# 92A-1) who died suddenly at work. He had complained of chest discomfort the day before death. *a*, transverse section of the left ventricular lateral wall showing a large transmural lesion. *b*, photomicrograph of a section of the left ventricular wall showing extensive mononuclear cellular infiltrates and necrotic muscle fibers. *c*, higher power microscopic view of the myocardium showing eosinophils. (Hematoxylin-eosin stain, × 100 *(b)* and × 200 *(c)*, reduced 29%.)

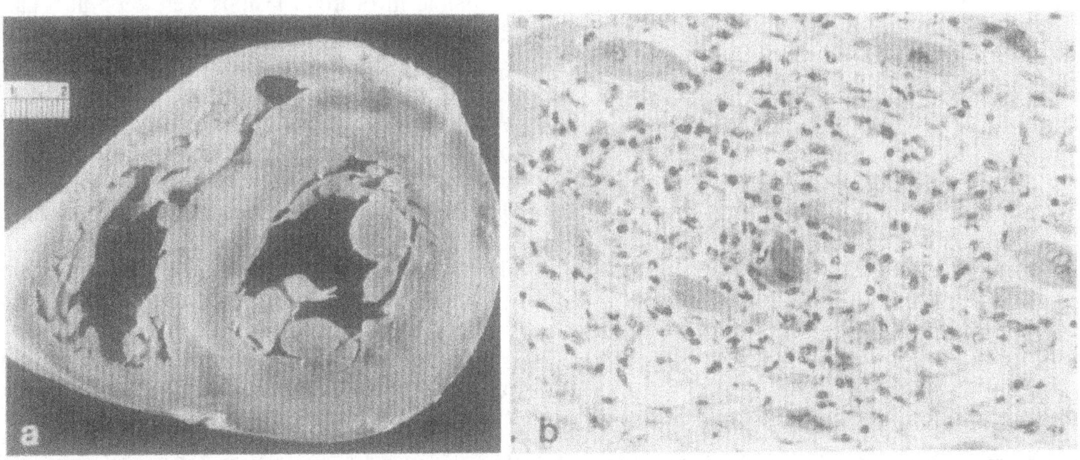

FIGURE 6. Patient 11. Heart of a 28-year-old black woman (DCMEO# 91-7-735) who died suddenly at church. She had no symptoms of any illness before death. *a*, transverse section of the cardiac ventricles showing predominantly subepicardial myocardial lesions in the anterior, lateral and posterior segments of the left ventricular wall. *b*, photomicrograph of a section of the left ventricular myocardium showing mononuclear cellular infiltrates and degenerated myocytes. (Hematoxylin-eosin stain, × 400 *(b)*, reduced 27%.)

TABLE II Quantitative Histologic Analysis of Myocardial Sections in 9 Patients Who Died Suddenly of Mononuclear-Cell Myocarditis

	Number of Myocardial Sections Examined				Number of HPFs	Number of Mononuclear Cells Counted/10 HPF: RV		RV 1/2 of VS		LV 1/2 of VS		LV Epicardial 1/2		LV Endocardial 1/2		Eosinophils		Fibrosis	Myocyte Mecrosis
Patient	RV	VS	LV	Total	Examined	Range	(mean ± SD)	Range	(mean ± SD)	Range	(mean ± SD)	Range	(mean ± SD)	Range	(mean ± SD)	Range	(mean)	(0–3+)	(mean %)
1	1	0	2	3	30	90–210	(154 ± 40)	—	—	—	—	200–285	(246 ± 25)	130–188	(169 ± 19)	0		0	50 ± 23
3	1	2	2	5	50	140–287	(215 ± 57)	101–206	(127 ± 33)	120–205	(156 ± 27)	108–212	(177 ± 32)	140–264	(199 ± 45)	0		0	54 ± 9
4	1	0	2	3	30	105–485	(320 ± 134)	—	—	—	—	180–460	(318 ± 99)	212–280	(251 ± 22)	0		0	32 ± 7
6	1	0	2	3	30	3–29	(18 ± 9)	—	—	—	—	60–116	(96 ± 16)	12–120	(54 ± 30)	0		0	5 ± 4
7	1	2	2	5	50	4–20	(13 ± 5)	12–27	(19 ± 4)	3–39	(28 ± 13)	12–112	(45 ± 30)	40–96	(62 ± 19)	0		+++	10 ± 3
8	1	2	2	5	50	36–115	(71 ± 23)	48–100	(77 ± 15)	60–140	(81 ± 22)	160–500	(390 ± 143)	40–105	(59 ± 22)	1–90	(18)	+	31 ± 22
10	0	2	2	4	40	—	—	9–80	(32 ± 20)	93–210	(131 ± 33)	110–250	(147 ± 37)	9–40	(17 ± 9)	2–11	(5)	0	26 ± 24
11	1	2	2	5	50	110–260	(176 ± 52)	146–250	(194 ± 34)	145–500	(292 ± 115)	110–310	(226 ± 55)	125–205	(172 ± 28)	4–14	(8)	+	78 ± 12
13	1	2	2	5	50	88–118	(96 ± 14)	80–125	(100 ± 16)	78–138	(117 ± 16)	50–140	(94 ± 25)	64–140	(113 ± 24)	0		0	38 ± 6
Total or (mean)	8	12	18	38	380 (42)		(133 ± 98)		(92 ± 59)		(134 ± 81)		(193 ± 106)		(122 ± 75)	0–90	(3)	3	5–78% (36 ± 21%)
p value										<0.01				<0.01					

HPF = high-power field (400 ×); LV = left ventricular; RV = right ventricular; SD = standard deviation; VS = ventricular septum.

symptoms including chest pain, cough or sore throat (2 patients each), dyspnea, palpitation, weakness, myalgia, back pain or diarrhea (1 patient each) from 1 to 7 days (mean 2) before death. At least 5 patients were febrile.

The epicardium was grossly normal in all cases. The hearts weighed from 75 to 800 g (median 317). Grossly visible myocardial lesions were present in 8 patients. The left ventricular myocardial lesions involved preferentially the subepicardial regions; the left ventricular subendocardial areas tended to be spared in 5 of the 8 patients. Myocardial lesions involved the ventricular septum in 4 patients and the right ventricular wall in 6 patients. By visual inspection, the left (9 patients) and right (11 patients) ventricular cavities were dilated. One patient (patient 13) had endocardial petechiae.

Histopathologic findings (Table II): A total of 38 histologic sections of myocardium were available for review in 9 patients (8 from the right ventricle, 12 from the ventricular septum and 18 from the left ventricular free wall). The range and mean number of mononuclear cells found in each of the 5 myocardial locations (right ventricular wall, right and left ventricular halves of the ventricular septum, and the epicardial and endocardial halves of the left ventricular free wall) for 10 consecutive high-power microscopic fields (400 ×) are detailed in Table II. The mean number of mononuclear cells was higher in the subepicardial region than in the subendocardial region of the left ventricular wall (193 vs 122 cells per high-power field [$p < 0.01$]). The mean number of mononuclear cells was significantly lower in the right ventricular one half compared with the left ventricular one half of the ventricular septum (92 vs 134 cells per high-power field [$p < 0.01$]). Eosinophils were present in myocardial sections of 3 patients. The mean percentage of necrotic or degenerated myocytes in all myocardial sites ranged from 5 to 78% (mean 36). One patient (number 7) had extensive areas of myocardial replacement fibrosis, particularly in the subepicardial regions of the left ventricular free wall.

DISCUSSION

Summary of the clinicopathologic findings: Grossly visible myocardial lesions were seen in 8 patients. In the left ventricular free wall these lesions tended to be extensive and involved the subepicardial regions preferentially. The basal portion of the ventricular septum tended to have more grossly visible lesions than were present in the apical portion. Grossly visible lesions were present in the right ventricular wall in 6 patients. The mean number of mononuclear cells in the left ventricular free wall was higher in the subepicardial regions than in the subendocardial regions, the opposite of what occurs in atherosclerotic coronary artery disease. The number of mononuclear cells was lowest in the right ventricular half of the ventricular septum, and this is the area most commonly sampled for endomyocardial biopsy.

Previously published study: Hauk and colleagues[11] obtained 10 endomyocardial biopsy specimens at necropsy from either side of the ventricular septum in each of 38 patients with lymphocytic myocarditis. Of the 380 samples from the right ventricular side of the ventricular septum, 66 (17%) showed myocarditis, allowing a diagnosis of myocarditis in 24 of the 38 patients (63%). Of the 380 samples taken from the left ventricular side of the ventricular septum, 76 (20%) showed myocarditis, allowing diagnosis of myocarditis in 21 of the 38 patients (55%). Sections of the left ventricular wall from endocardium to epicardium and the ventricular septum from endocardium to endocardium also were examined in the same study.[11] Myocarditis was present in 84 of the 114 sections (74%) of the left ventricular free wall and in 26 of the 38 sections (68%) of the septum. Foci of myocarditis were slightly more common in the subepicardial half than the subendocardial half of the left ventricular free wall (54 vs 47%). More foci of myocarditis also were seen in the middle third (58%) of the ventricular septum than in the right ventricular or left ventricular thirds (58 vs 24% and 26%). In our 9 patients, the left ventricular free wall sections were divided into subepicardial and subendocardial halves, the ventricular septum was divided into right and left ventricular halves, and we quantitated the number of mononuclear cells in each location rather than counting the number of foci of myocarditis. Compared with the mean number in the 2 halves of the left ventricular free wall and with the left ventricular half of the ventricular septum, the mean number of mononuclear cells in our study was lower in the right ventricular half of the ventricular septum, the site where endomyocardial biopsy samples are most often taken.

1. Lambert EC, Menon VA, Wagner HR, Vlad P. Sudden unexpected death from cardiovascular disease in children. A cooperative international study. *Am J Cardiol* 1974;34:89–96.

2. Noren GR, Staley NA, Bandt CM, Kaplan EL. Occurrence of myocarditis in sudden death in children. *J Forensic Sci* 1976;22:188–196.

3. Wentworth P, Jentz LA, Croal AE. Analysis of sudden unexpected death in southern Ontario, with emphasis on myocarditis. *Can Med Assoc J* 1979;120: 676–680.

4. Molander N. Sudden natural death in later childhood and adolescence. *Arch Dis Child* 1982;57:572–576.

5. Topaz O, Edwards JE. Pathologic features of sudden death in children, adolescents, and young adults. *Chest* 1985;87:476–482.

6. Neuspiel DR, Kuller LH. Sudden and unexpected natural death in childhood and adolescence. *JAMA* 1985;254:1321–1325.

7. Phillips M, Robinowitz M, Higgins JR, Boran KJ, Reed T, Virmani R. Sudden cardiac death in Air Force recruits. A 20-year review. *JAMA* 1986;256:2696–2699.

8. Okuni M, Sumitomo N. Sudden death of school children in Japan. *Jpn Circ J* 1987;51:1397–1399.

9. Driscoll DJ, Edwards WD. Sudden unexpected death in children and adolescents. *J Am Coll Cardiol* 1985;5:118B–121B.

10. Corby C. Isolated myocarditis as a cause of sudden obscure death. *J Forensic Sci* 1960;5:23–40.

11. Hauk AJ, Kearney DL, Edwards WD. Evaluation of postmortem endomyocardial biopsy specimens from 38 patients with lymphocytic myocarditis: implications for role of sampling error. *Mayo Clin Proc* 1989;64:1235–1245.

Effectiveness of Cardiac Transplantation for Primary (AL) Cardiac Amyloidosis

Frank Pelosi, Jr., MD, John Capehart, MD, and William C. Roberts, MD

From 1968 to April 1996, according to the United Network for Organ Sharing, cardiac transplantation (CT) was performed in nearly 36,000 persons. Although most patients underwent this procedure because of ischemic cardiomyopathy or idiopathic dilated cardiomyopathy, at least 44 had CT because of cardiac amyloidosis. Follow-up information on these 44 patients, however, is not available to us. At least 7 patients having CT for cardiac amyloidosis and followed to death have been reported (Table I).[1–6] The present report was prompted by studying a patient who also had CT for cardiac AL amyloidosis and survived 69 months without again developing cardiac dysfunction. This report describes the latter patient and summarizes findings in those previously reported patients having CT for cardiac amyloidosis. The question asked is: Is CT worthwhile in patients with life-threatening cardiac dysfunction from cardiac amyloidosis?

• • •

A.C., a 66-year-old white man who was born on September 14, 1928, and died on July 3, 1995, had been well until June 1985 (51 months before CT) when he noted pedal edema. In January 1987, he noted the onset of exertional dyspnea which progressively worsened. Evaluation in June 1987 disclosed his blood pressure to be 135/85 mm Hg (Figure 1). Pitting ankle edema was present. No abdominal organs were palpable. The electrocardiogram disclosed complete left bundle branch block. Cardiac catheterization was performed and the data are tabulated in Table II.

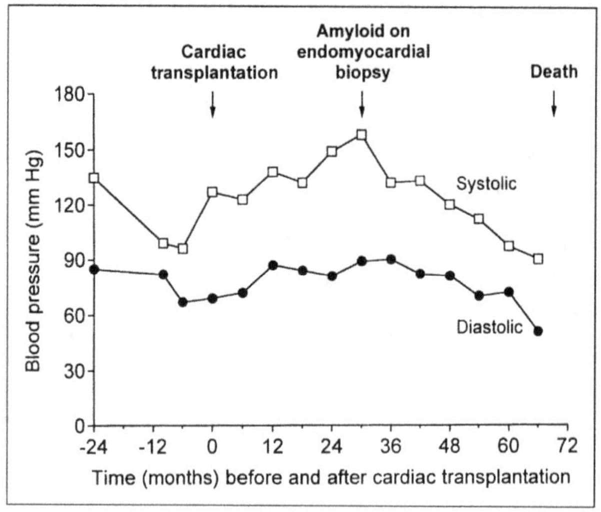

FIGURE 1. Indirect systemic arterial systolic and diastolic blood pressures before and after cardiac transplantation.

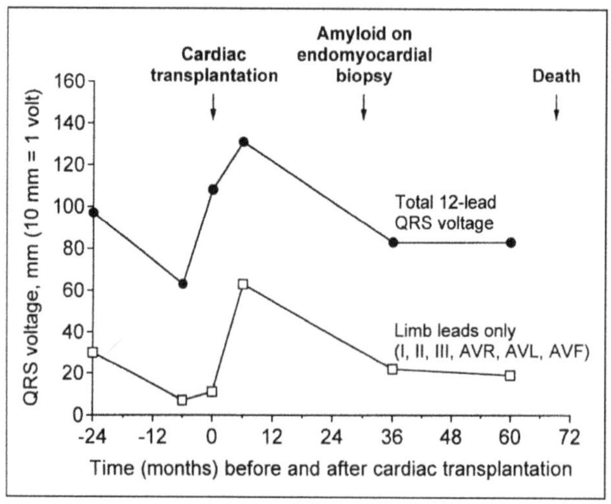

FIGURE 2. Total and limb-lead QRS voltage at various time periods before and after cardiac transplantations in patient A.C.

In May 1989, he was hospitalized again because of worsening congestive cardiac failure. Blood pressure was 95/65 mm Hg, heart rate 120 beats/min, and respiratory rate, 26 breaths/min. He now had diminished heart sounds, an S_3 gallop, diffuse pulmonary rales, hepatosplenomegaly, ascites, and massive subcutaneous pitting edema. With diuretic therapy, he lost 26 pounds. M-mode and 2-dimensional echocardiograms revealed normal-sized ventricular chambers, and decreased ventricular wall motion. Endomyocardial biopsy revealed amyloid. Monoclonal gammopathy was absent by serum and urine protein electrophoresis, and plasma cell dyscrasia was absent on bone marrow biopsy. Liver biopsy showed no amyloid. Orthotopic CT was performed on October 7, 1989; the donor was a 32-year-old man. The

From the Departments of Medicine (Cardiology Division), Cardiothoracic Surgery and Pathology, Baylor University Medical Center, Dallas, Texas. Dr. Roberts' address is: Baylor Cardiovascular Institute, Baylor University Medical Center, 3500 Gaston Avenue, Dallas, Texas 75246. Manuscript received July 31, 1996; revised manuscript received and accepted September 17, 1996.

explanted heart (excludes most of the atrial walls) weighed 485 g and extensive amyloid was present in the intramyocardial blood vessels without amyloid in the myocardial interstitium. After CT, evidence of heart failure vanished. Posttransplant cardiac catheterizations (Table I) and biopsies were performed and disclosed no abnormalities until April 1992 when endomyocardial biopsy revealed amyloid by light microscopy. Bence-Jones protein also was found in the urine protein electrophoresis. After onset of dysphagia in August 1992, esophageal and pre-pyloric biopsies showed amyloid. Two-dimensional and Doppler echocardiography in April 1995 revealed no evidence of cardiac dysfunction. Renal biopsy for declining renal function showed no amyloid. The serum albumin was 2.7 g/dl. He died suddenly at home while watching television on July 3, 1995, 69 months after CT.

At necropsy, the heart weighed 505 g. Comparison of the cardiac amyloid findings in the native and donor hearts are summarized in Table III. Amyloid was present in large and roughly equal amounts in the walls of the intramural and small epicardial vessels in the native heart and in the donor heart, and was absent from myocardial interstitium in both. Amyloid also was present in the small arteries in the liver (1,000 g) and kidney but, as in the native and donor hearts, it was limited to the walls of the small vessels. Furthermore, although amyloid was found in the tongue, pancreas, stomach, colon, spleen (275 g), skin, and adrenal glands, the deposits were limited to the the small vessels in these structures. In the lung the deposits also were present primarily in the small vessels but some deposits were found in alveolar septa. Amyloid deposits were present in large quantities in the interstitium, as well as in the walls of the small blood vessels, in the esophagus.

• • •

The hitherto described patient had CT for extensive primary cardiac amyloidosis and died suddenly at home 69 months later. During the post-CT period, he never developed evidence of cardiac dysfunction even though amyloid was found in a myocardial biopsy 3 years before his death.

The presently described patient is the only one with cardiac amyloid among 179 CT recipients at Baylor University Medical Center. Follow-up information from CT to death is available in at least 7 previously reported patients (Table I) who had CT for cardiac amyloidosis. Connor and associates[1] first reported CT for cardiac amyloidosis, and their 48-year-old man lived 46 months after CT. Valentine and Billingham's[2] 30-year-old woman died 13 months after CT. Hosenpud and colleagues[3] described 2 patients who had CT for cardiac amyloidosis: 1 died in the early postoperative period and the other lived 30 months. Deng and colleagues[4] described a 53-year-old woman who died 6 months after CT (from infection). The longest survivor is Dr. Reginald Hall who, in a unique report,[5] described his own illness. He underwent CT for cardiac amyloidosis and reported the first 112 months of his post-CT course. At 36 months after CT, endomyocardial biopsy disclosed amyloid and chemotherapy was instituted. The quantity of amyloid at myocardial biopsy appeared to be reduced by this therapy. We have recently learned that Dr. Hall died 118 months after CT from sepsis and that he never had clinical evidence of cardiac amyloidosis after CT (personal communication, P.N. Hawkins, MD, July 22, 1996). Dubrey et al[6] described a 54-year-old woman who survived 47 months after CT. If the patient who died early postoperatively is eliminated, the other 6 survived 6 to 118 months (median 46) after CT: 4 died from consequences of noncardiac amyloidosis and 2 from superimposed infection. In addition to the reported data and that from our patient, Dubrey (personal communication, July 11, 1996) has informed us that CT has been performed for cardiac amyloidosis in at least 4 other patients followed in his amyloid clinic: 3 died at 10,

TABLE I Certain Data in Seven Previously Reported Patients Having Cardiac Transplantation for Cardiac Amyloidosis and Follow-Up to Death Plus Our Presently Described Patient

Case	Publication Year	First Author (reference)	Age (yr) at CT	Gender	Duration (mo) Symptoms Before CT	Interval CT to Death (mo)	Extracardiac Amyloid Before CT	Signs of Cardiac Dysfunction After CT	Amyloid Found in Transplanted Heart After CT (mo)	Death Secondary to CHF	Death Secondary to Noncardiac Amyloid	Chemotherapy Before or After CT	Weight of Transplanted Heart (g)
1.	1988	Conner[1]	48	M	48	46	+	0	0	0	+	0	—
2.	1989	Valentine[2]	30	F	4	13	+	+	+	0	+	0	—
3.	1991	Hosenpud[3]	—	—	—	<1	—	0	—	0	0	0	—
4.	—	—	—	—	—	30	—	—	—	—	—	—	—
5.	1992	Deng[4]	53	F	24	6	0	0	+ (6)	0	0	0	—
6.	1994	Hall[5]	53	M	72	118	0	+	+ (36)	0	0	+	—
7.	1995	Dubrey[6]	54	F	13	47	0	+	+ (36)	+	0	+	540
8.	1997	Pelosi	60	M	52	69	0	0	+ (30)	0*	0	0	504

* Death was sudden at home, but congestive heart failure was never present after cardiac transplantation.
+ = present or positive; 0 = absent or negative; — = no information available.
CHF = congestive heart failure; CT = cardiac transplantation.

Interval (mo) Before (−) and After (+) CT	RA* (mean)	RV* (s/d)	PA* (s/d)	PAW* (mean)	LV* (s/d)	Aorta* (s/d)	CO (L/min)	Amyloid in Myocardial Biopsy
−24	15	36/8	42/20	20	100/6	110/60	3.4	−
−4	18	43/8	45/25	26	97/30	97/68	2.7	+†
CARDIAC TRANSPLANT OCTOBER 1989								
+12	7	25/7	28/9	8	99/11	101/61	5	0
+24	3	30/8	32/10	12	119/9	118/67	4.3	0
+30	−	−/−	−/−	−	−/−	−/−	−	+†
+66	7	27/7	30/14	13	−/−	−/−	−	+†
+69	DIED SUDDENLY AT HOME JULY 1995							

* In mm Hg.
† In walls of intramural vessels and their lumens only.
CO = cardiac output; CT = cardiac transplantation; LV = left ventricle; PA = pulmonary artery; PAW = pulmonary artery wedge; RA = right atrium; RV = right ventricle; s/d = peak systole/end-diastole; − = not done; + = present or positive; 0 = absent or negative.

TABLE III Morphologic Cardiac Findings

Location of Amyloid by Light Microscopy	Native Heart	Donor Heart
Myocardial Interstitium (0–4+)	0	0
Intramural coronary arteries (0–4+)		
Walls	++++	++++
Lumens	+++	+++
Epicardium (0–4+)		
Walls of small coronary vessels	++++	++++
Lumens of small coronary vessels	+	+
Perivascular regions	+++	+++
Parietal pericardium	−	+++*

* Of native heart.

14, and 15 months, respectively, after CT of noncardiac amyloidosis and 1 is still alive 49 months after CT.

Our patient had amyloid in both native and donor hearts limited to the walls of intramural coronary vessels often narrowing their lumens without amyloid deposits in myocardial interstitium. Nevertheless, there was evidence of cardiac dysfunction, i.e., heart failure before the CT but never afterwards. Our patient never had evidence of angina pectoris, something that has been observed with cardiac amyloidosis limited to intramyocardial vessels,[7] but he did die suddenly at home with documented ventricular fibrillation. At necropsy, none of the lumens of the major epicardial coronary arteries were significantly narrowed. It therefore appears reasonable to attribute his sudden unexpected death to the focal but extensive luminal narrowing by amyloid of numerous intramural coronary arteries.

Cardiac transplantation in cardiac amyloidosis, of course, provides the opportunity to compare cardiac function both before and after heart replacement (Table II). His indirect systemic arterial blood pressure fell progressively before CT, rose immediately thereafter, and fell again approximately at a time corresponding to cardiac endomyocardial biopsies showing amyloid in the walls of intramural coronary vessels (Figure 1). Furthermore, total 12-lead QRS voltage[8] fell to 63 mm (10 mm = 1 mV) just before CT, rose shortly after CT to a peak of 130 mm (>100% increase) and fell after amyloid was again found in endomyocardial biopsy, to 84 mm (Figure 2).

Now to the question posed in the introduction: Is CT worthwhile in patients with cardiac amyloidosis causing severe cardiac dysfunction? At the moment, the answer remains uncertain. Some persons benefit enormously, Dr. Hall, our patient, for example. Dr. Hall, who lived 118 months after CT, developed angina pectoris during his last several years of life. Our patient, who lived 69 months after CT, died suddenly without significant epicardial coronary artery disease. Our patient, however, had severe narrowing of numerous intramural coronary arteries and Dr. Hall did as well (personal communication, P.N. Hawkins, MD, July 30, 1996): neither had amyloid in the myocardial interstitium. It may be that CT will prove to be worthwhile if cardiac amyloid deposits are limited to the walls and lumina of intramural coronary arteries, but not worthwhile if myocardial interstitium is the major location of the amyloid deposits.

In summary, a patient is described who developed severe cardiac dysfunction from amyloid deposited entirely in the walls and lumens of intramural coronary arteries, underwent CT, survived another 69 months, died suddenly, and at necropsy had amyloid again limited to the walls and lumens of the intramyocardial coronary arteries in the donor heart. The rather lengthy survival in this patient and the 118-month survival in a similar previously reported patient suggests that CT may be an appropriate procedure for some patients with cardiac amyloidosis.

1. Conner R, Hosenpud JD, Norman DJ, Pantely GA, Cobanoglu MA, Starr A. Heart transplantation

Transplant 1988;7:165–167.
2. Valentine HA, Billingham ME. Recurrence of amyloid in a cardiac allograft four months after transplantation. *J Heart Transplant* 1989;8:337–341.
3. Hosenpud JD, DeMarco T, Frazier H, Griffith BP, Uretsky BF, Menkis AH, O'Connell JB, Olivari M-T, Valentine HA. Progression of systemic disease and reduced long-term survival in patients with cardiac amyloidosis undergoing heart 338–III-343.
4. Deng M, Park J-W, Roy-Chowdury R, Knieriem H-J, Reinhard U, Heinrich KW. Heart transplantation for restrictive cardiomyopathy: development of cardiac amyloidosis in preexisting monoclonal gammopathy. *J Heart Lung Transplant* 1992; 11:139–141.
5. Hall R, Hawkins PN. Cardiac transplantation for AL amyloidosis. *Br Med J* 1994;309:1135–1137.
planted heart with four-year survival. *Am J Cardiol* 1995;76:739–741.
7. Saffitz JE, Sazama K, Roberts WC. Amyloidosis limited to small arteries causing angina pectoris and sudden death. *Am J Cardiol* 1983;51:1234–1235.
8. Roberts WC, Waller BF. Cardiac amyloidosis causing cardiac dysfunction: analysis of 54 necropsy patients. *Am J Cardiol* 1983; 52:137–146.

Acute Myocarditis (Predominately Lymphocytic) Causing Sudden Death Without Heart Failure

Kevin P. Theleman, MD, Johannes J. Kuiper, MD, and William C. Roberts, MD

Acute myocarditis is an uncommon cause of sudden death. Such was the case of the patient described herein.

• • •

R.G., a 37-year-old white woman, a self-employed interior decorator, a wife, and the mother of 2 daughters aged 6 and 9 years, was well until 6 weeks before death when she developed severe diarrhea (8 to 10 defecations daily), nausea, and myalgias lasting several days. Four weeks before death the diarrhea and myalgias returned along with probable fever, and 2 episodes of emesis. These manifestations led to evaluation at Baylor University Medical Center 23 days before her death. She had had seasonal allergies for years but took no medications regularly. Her father had died of colon cancer at about age 65. She did not smoke. She drank wine on social occasions. Blood pressure was 105/70 mm Hg, and heart rate was 120 beats/min while standing, 110/75 and 112 while sitting, and 110/75 and 98 when supine. The temperature was 99.6° Fahrenheit. Her body mass index was 20 kg/m^2. She was alert and oriented. Her mucous membranes were dry. The neck veins were flat. There was no thyromegaly or adenopathy. Precordial examination disclosed a regular tachycardia but no murmurs, rubs, or gallops. Abdominal examination disclosed no abnormalities. There was no subcutaneous edema anywhere. Neurologic examination disclosed no abnormalities. Some laboratory data are listed in Table 1. Abdominal radiographs were unremarkable except for a paucity of intraintestinal gas. She was hydrated with intravenous fluids and the diarrhea was eliminated after loperamide therapy. Blood, urine, and stool were cultured and they were all negative (no growth). By the third hospital day, her leukocyte count decreased to 5.2 K/μl (15.4 K/μl on admission), her acidosis was nearly resolved as her serum bicarbonate increased to 20 mEq/L (10 mEq/L on admission), and she was able to eat and drink without nausea or emesis, and she was discharged. The etiology of the diarrhea, nausea, and myalgias was unclear, but a viral syndrome was suspected.

Nine days later (12 days before death), the patient returned to the emergency room at 16:32 complaining of a single episode of constant, midsternal, nonradiating "pressure pain" that was first noted at approximately 06:30 when she awoke. The pain was unassociated with nausea, dyspnea, orthopnea, or diaphoresis, and was not relieved by acetaminophen or ibuprofen. The day before she had been moving furniture with her husband without difficulty. The temperature was 97.6° Fahrenheit, blood pressure 110/75 mm Hg, and pulse 64 beats/min. Peripheral oxygen saturation was 97% on room air. She was ill appearing. There were no changes in physical findings from previous admission except for mild tenderness on palpation of the left anterior chest wall and no evidence of dehydration. There was still no subcutaneous edema. The electrocardiogram at 16:42 showed sinus ventricular bigeminy (Figure 1), at 19:50 sinus

TABLE 1 Laboratory Data

	Days Before Death					
	23	22	21	12	11	10
Leukocyte (k/μl)	15.4	7.3	5.2	5.9	4.8	
Lymphocyte (%)	1	12	19	18	19	
Monocyte (%)	0	9	8	12	12	
Neutrophil (%)	99	79	71	68	67	
Band (%)	10	0	0	0	0	
Semented (%)	89	79	71	68	67	
Eosinophil (%)	0	0	1	1	2	
Hemoglobin (g/dl)	14.8	11.3	11.2	12.3	11.5	
Hematocrit (%)	44	33.6	32.1	36.2	34	
Platelet (k/μl)	234	155	121	239	230	
Glucose (mg/dl)	96	90	108	124	105	
Sodium (mEq/L)	139	141	141	138	140	
Potassium (mEq/L)	4.5	4	3.2	4.2	4.1	
Chloride (mEq/L)	99	115	110	101	104	
Bicarbonate (mEq/L)	10	13	20	27	28	
Urea nitrogen (mg/dl)	7	4	2	5	4	
Creatinine (mg/dl)	0.8	0.8	0.5	0.6	0.7	
Total bilirubin (mg/dl)	0.9			0.4	0.5	
Alkaline phosphatase (U/L)	79			54	49	
Serum glutamic oxalacetic transaminase (U/L)	101			114	176	
Serum glutamic pyruvic transaminase (U/L)	41			28	29	
Lactate dehydrogenase (U/L)				460		
Creatinine phosphokinase (U/L)				420	555	
Creatinine phosphokinase-MB (ng/ml)				60.1	73.1	
Troponin-I (ng/ml)				20.6	22.1	18.5

From the Departments of Medicine and Pathology and the Baylor Heart and Vascular Center, Baylor University Medical Center, Dallas, Texas. Dr. Roberts' address is: Baylor Heart & Vascular Center, Baylor University Medical Center, 3500 Gaston Avenue, Dallas, Texas 75246. Manuscript received April 30, 2001; revised manuscript received and accepted June 21, 2001.

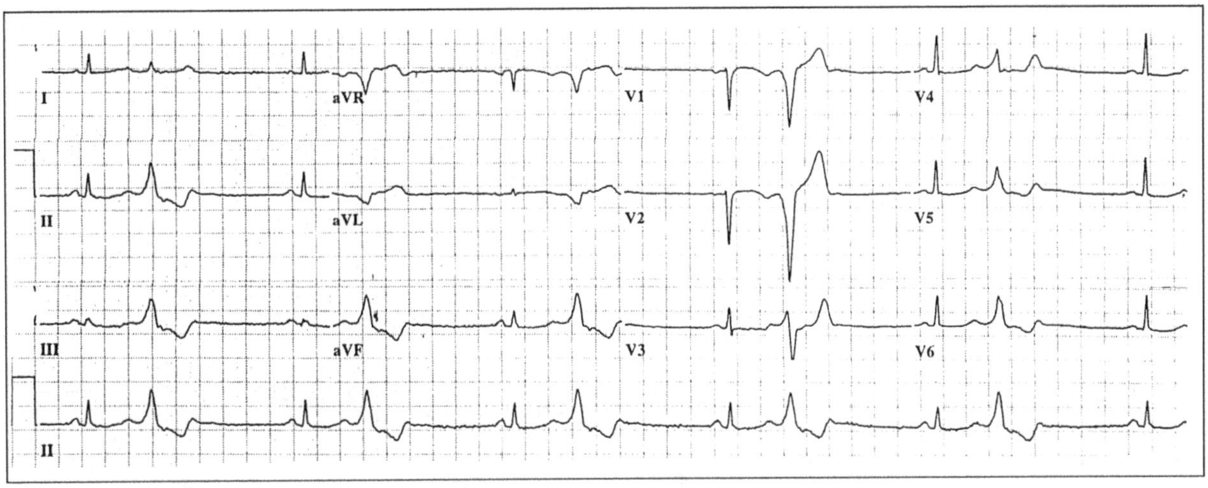

FIGURE 1. Electrocardiogram recorded 12 days before death showing sinus rhythm and ventricular bigeminy.

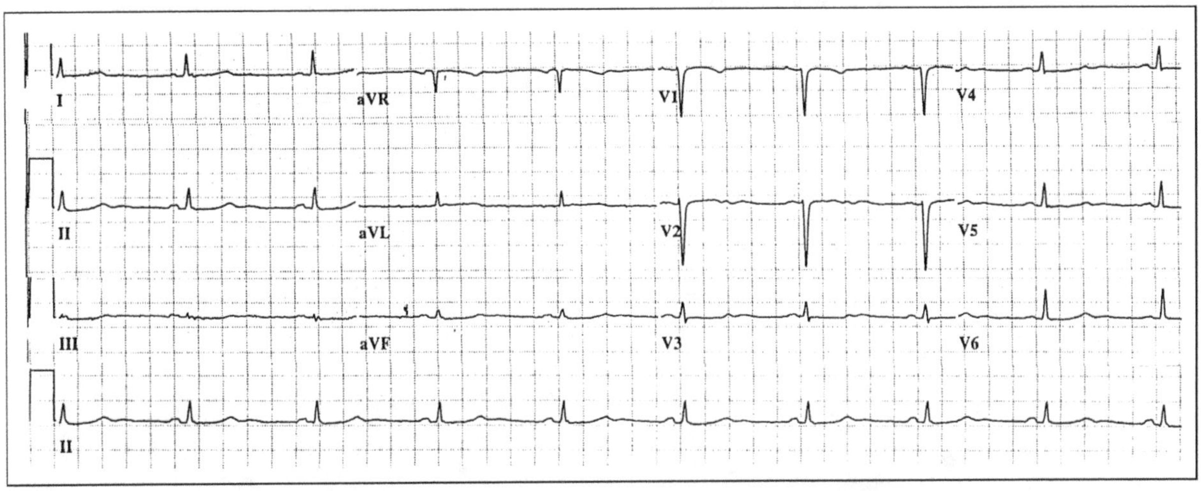

FIGURE 2. Electrocardiogram recorded approximately 3 hours after the one shown in Figure 1. The ST segments and T waves are now normal. The total 12-lead QRS voltage was only 54 ml.

rhythm was present with a rate of 59 beats/min without ST-segment or T-wave changes, and a low total QRS voltage (total 12-lead QRS voltage was 54 mm [normal 80 to 180 mm[1]) (Figure 2). Serum creatinine phosphokinase was 420 U/L (normal 30 to 135) and creatinine kinase-MB was 60.1 ng/ml (normal 0 to 7.0) (Table 1). Troponin-I was 20.6 ng/ml (normal 0 to 0.4)]. Aspartate transaminase (serum glutamic oxalacetic transaminase) was 114 U/L (normal 15 to 46); alanine transaminase (serum glutamic pyruvic transaminase) was 28 U/L (normal 9 to 52). The alkaline phosphatase was 54 U/L (normal 38 to 126) and the total bilirubin was 0.4 mg/dl (normal .2 to 1.3).

The patient was given acetylsalicylic acid (325 mg) and morphine sulfate (2 mg) intravenously. Her chest pain lessened but it was not completely resolved until the third hospital day. A transthoracic echocardiogram showed normal chamber sizes, an estimated left ventricular ejection fraction of 60%, trace mitral regurgitation, trace tricuspid regurgitation, and no pericardial effusion. Telemetry disclosed episodes of bigeminy and runs of nonsustained ventricular tachycardia up to 11 consecutive beats (Figure 3). Serum creatinine phosphokinase was 420, 555, and 541 U/L (normal 30 to 135), respectively; creatinine kinase-MB was 60.1, 73.1, and 67.4 ng/ml (normal 0 to 7.0), and troponin-I was 20.6, 22.1, 21.6, and 18.5 ng/ml (normal 0 to 0.4), respectively. Aspartate transaminase, which was 114 U/L on admission, increased to 176 U/L (normal 15 to 46). Antinuclear antibody titer was <1:40 (normal <1:40). Erythrocyte sedimentation rate was 6 mm/hour (normal 0 to 20). Quantitative immunoglobulin (Ig)G, IgA, and IgM were within normal limits. The patient was treated with a single 2-g/kg dose of intravenous immunoglobulin and started on ramipril (10 mg/day). The ramipril dose was decreased to 2.5 mg/day after hypotension (range 72/46 to 108/72 mm Hg) appeared. On the third hospital day (10 days before death), the patient was discharged after complete resolution of chest pain. Serologic studies for coxsackie B virus, enterovirus, mumps virus, and cytomegalovirus were negative for acute infection.

During the next 9 days, the pa-

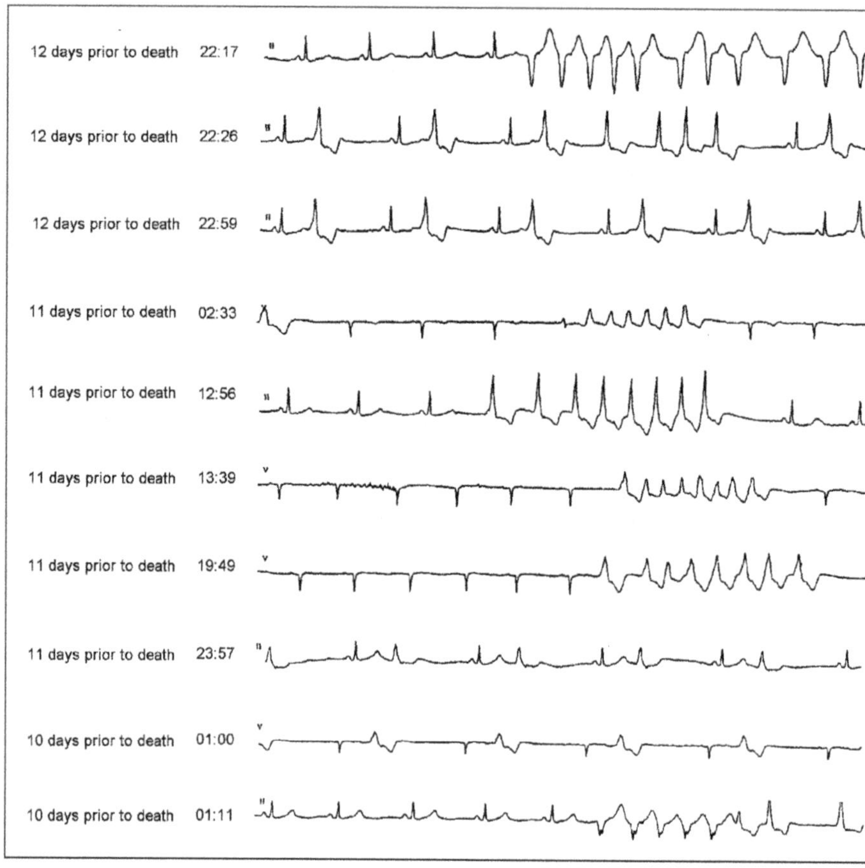

FIGURE 3. These rhythm strips were recorded from 12 to 10 days before death.

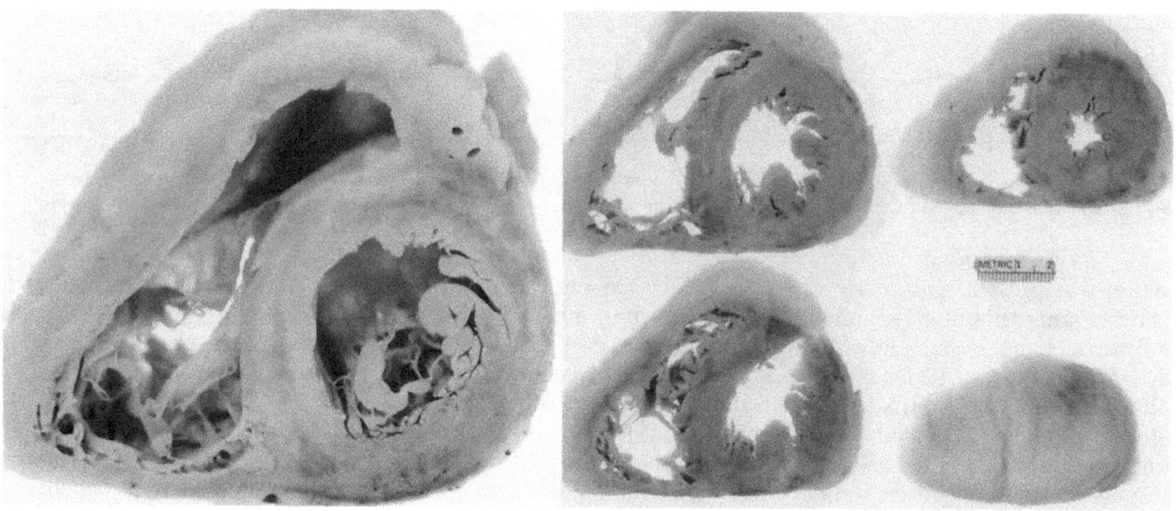

FIGURE 4. The heart in the patient described. *Left,* view of both ventricles, each of which is dilated. The left ventricular free wall and the ventricular septum contain many lesions, some of which are mainly subepicardial and others (ventricular septum, e.g.) are central. The coronary arteries are free of plaque. *Right,* "Breadloaf" slides of the cardiac ventricles showing dilatation of cavities and many left ventricular and septal lesions.

tient was at home and was asymptomatic except for low-grade fevers 2 days after discharge (attributed to the immunoglobulin infusion) and periodic, unsustained palpitations without dizziness. The day before death she was seen in her private physician's office. No evidence of heart failure was observed. At approximately 2:00 A.M. the next morning, her husband was awakened by his wife's gasping for breath. The paramedics were called but resuscitation efforts were unsuccessful.

At necropsy (limited to heart and lungs), the heart weighed 320 g (Figure 4). The right ventricular cavity was considerably dilated (3+/4+) and the left ventricular cavity was mildly dilated (1+/4+) (Figure 5). Subepicardial and midwall lesions were present focally in the left ventricular free

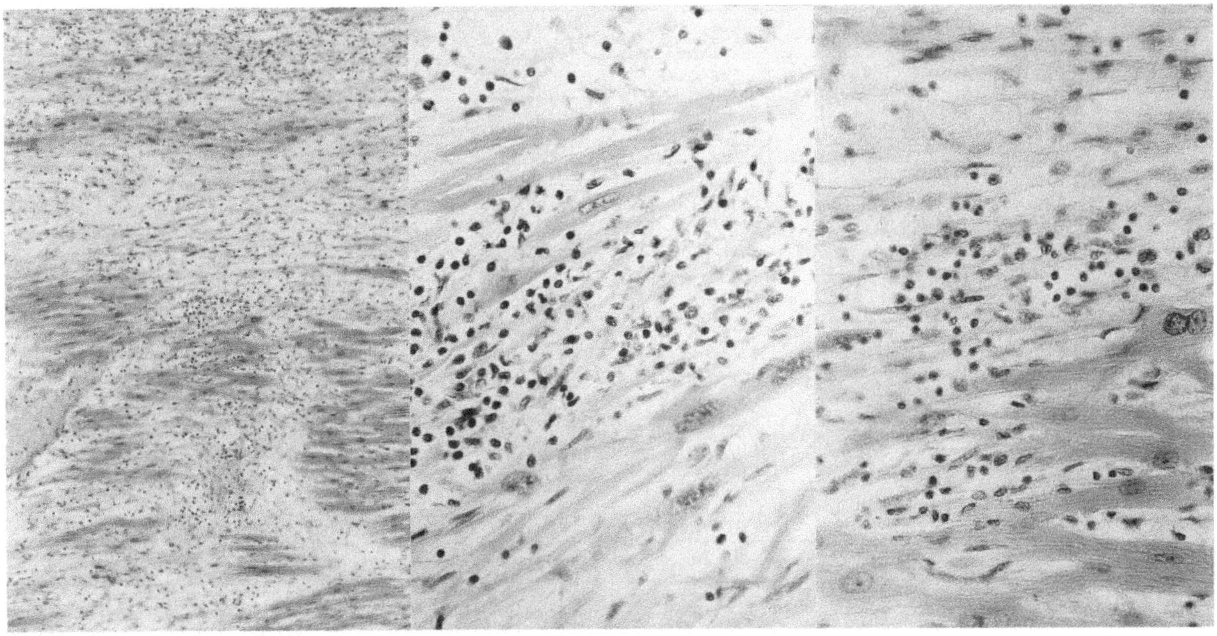

FIGURE 5. Photomicrographs of various portions of the left ventricular free wall. *Left,* there is marked loss of myofibers with infiltration with inflammatory cells magnified × 40. *Middle and right,* close-up views showing the inflammatory cells which are mainly lymphocytes. Lipochrome pigment is visible *(right)* in areas of destroyed myocardium. Each magnified × 400. All are hematoxilyn-eosin stains, reduced by 46%.

TABLE 2 Certain Clinical Data in 32 Previously Reported Necropsy Cases Dying Suddenly of Lymphocytic Myocarditis

Case	Year of Publication	First Author (R)	Age (yrs) at Death	Race	Sex	Previous S + S	Place of Death	Length of Illness (d)	Heart Weight (g)	SD During Exertion
1	1982	Molander[2]	5	-	F	0	Ambulance	0	-	0
2	1982	Molander	1.7	-	M	0	Crib	0	-	0
3	1982	Molander	6	-	F	0	-	0	-	0
4	1982	Molander	6	-	M	0	Bed	0	-	0
5	1986	Phillips[3]	19	W	M	+(URI)	Outside	14	500	+
6	1986	Phillips	22	B	M	0	Outside	0	360	+
7	1986	Phillips	18	W	M	0	Outside	0	340	+
8	1986	Phillips	20	W	M	0	Outside	0	430	+
9	1986	Phillips	19	W	M	0	-	0	385	0
10	1990	Brampton[4]	35	-	F	0	RR	0	-	0
11	1993	Shirani[5]	0.6	A	M	+(D)	ER	2	75	0
12	1993	Shirani	0.8	W	M	+(Dy)	ER	1	80	0
13	1993	Shirani	3	B	M	+(ST)	ER	6	70	0
14	1993	Shirani	7	B	F	+(ST)	ER	3	200	0
15	1993	Shirani	12	W	M	+(CP)	Ambulance	1	125	0
16	1993	Shirani	13	B	M	+(My)	Home	3	300	0
17	1993	Shirani	14	B	M	+(CP)	Home	1	275	0
18	1993	Shirani	17	B	M	+(P)	Home	1	420	0
19	1993	Shirani	17	W	M	0	Car	0	390	0
20	1993	Shirani	24	B	M	+(CP)	Office	1	360	0
21	1993	Shirani	28	B	F	0	Church	0	340	0
22	1993	Shirani	33	W	M	+(C)	Home	3	360	0
23	1993	Shirani	53	B	M	+(C)	Home	5	335	0
24	1993	Shirani	65	W	F	+(We)	ER	7	800	0
25	1995	Shen[6]	36	-	F	-	Home	0	-	0
26	1995	Shen	37	-	F	-	-	0	-	0
27	1995	Shen	37	-	M	-	-	0	-	0
28	1995	Shen	25	-	M	-	-	0	-	0
29	1996	Wesslén[7]	26	-	M	0	Outside	0	-	+
30	1996	Wesslén	27	-	M	0	-	0	-	0
31	1996	Wesslén	20	-	M	0	Outside	0	-	+
32	1996	Wesslén	27	-	M	0	Outside	0	-	+

A = Asian; B = black; C = cough; CP = chest pain; D = diarrhea; Dy = dyspnea; ER = emergency room; F = female; M = male; My = myalgias; P = palpitations; R = reference number; RR = recovery room; SD = sudden death; S & S = signs and symptoms; ST = sore throat; URI = upper respiratory infection; W = white; We = weakness.

TABLE 3 Reported Frequency of Acute Myocarditis Among Necropsy Cases of Nonviolent Sudden Death at Age <45 Years

						Causes of Sudden Death				
First Author	Year of Publication	Country of Patients	Definition of Sudden Death (h)	Age Range (mean) (yrs)	Sudden Death Cases	Cardiac (nonmyocarditis)	Cardiac (myocarditis)	Vascular (noncardiac)	Noncardiac Nonvascular	Cause Uncertain
Molander[2]	1982	Sweden	-	1–20 (11)	31	5 (16%)	4 (13%)	0	18	4
Topaz[8]	1985	USA (MN)	≤6	7–35	50	39 (78%)	3 (6%)*	1	5	2
Driscoll[9]	1985	USA (MN)	≤24	3–20 (13)	12	3 (25%)	1 (8%)	1	1	6
Neuspiel[10]	1985	USA (PA)	≤24	1–22	207†	34 (15%)	14 (6%)*	23	124	29
Raymond[11]	1988	USA (NC)	1	18–45	83	41 (49%)	0 (0%)	5	31	6
Drory[12]	1991	Israel	≤24	9–39	162	92 (57%)	26 (16%)*	10	15	19
Corrado[13]	1994	Italy	1	≤35	200	139 (74%)	12 (6%)	27	10	12
Anderson[14]	1994	USA (NM)	≤24	5–39	650	153 (24%)	9 (1%)	12	435	41
Shen[6]	1995	USA (MN)	1	20–40	54	28 (52%)	4 (7%)	7	8	7
Steinberger[15]	1996	USA (MN)	≤24	1–21 (13)	50	26 (52%)	14 (28%)	0‡	0‡	10
Maron[16]	1996	USA	-	12–40 (17)	158§	127 (80%)	4 (3%)*	7	17	3
Wren[17]	2000	UK	≤24	1–20	270	46 (17%)	5 (2%)	15	163	41
Morentin[18]	2000	Spain	≤6	1–19	34	9 (26%)	1 (3%)	3	10	11
TOTALS					1961†	742 (38%)	97 (5%)	111 (5%)	837 (42%)	191 (10%)

*Definition of myocarditis provided; †Seventeen patients had 2 causes of death; ‡These patients were excluded from the study; §Competitive athletes only.

wall and histologic study disclosed them to be areas of cytomyolysis with mononuclear cell infiltrates (Figure 5). Other smaller areas of mononuclear cell infiltrates associated with myofiber necrosis also were seen in areas of the left ventricular wall, which appeared grossly normal. Histologic study also disclosed a few areas of interstitial fibrosis.

• • •

The hitherto described 37-year old woman had a 6-week illness characterized by diarrhea, myalgias, nausea and vomiting, palpitations, runs of ventricular tachycardia, marked elevation of certain hepatic enzymes, extreme low voltage on the electrocardiogram, and ending by sudden death while sleeping. Never was there evidence of heart failure. Necropsy disclosed dilated cardiac ventricular cavities and many grossly visible left ventricular and ventricular septal lesions that histologically proved to be large areas of myocytolysis with inflammatory cell infiltrates, predominantly lymphocytes.

At least 32 other patients have been reported with necropsy-proved lymphocytic myocarditis and sudden nonviolent (natural) death[2–7] (Table 2). Most patients were young. Excluding the 8 who died before reaching 10 years of age, the average age at death in the other 24 patients was 25 years. Of the 32 patients, 24 (75%) were male, 8 (25%) were female. Thirteen of the 28 patients (46%) for whom information was available had some symptoms (suggestive of a viral illness) before their sudden death. The symptoms existed from 1 to 14 days (mean 4) previously. The heart mass was increased in 4 (21%) of the 19 in whom the heart weight was provided.

Among patients dying suddenly from natural causes, lymphocytic or mononuclear myocarditis is an uncommon cause of death. Table 3 summarizes reports of sudden nonviolent death among necropsy patients ≤45 years of age with lymphocytic myocarditis.[2,6,8–18] Of the 1,961 total patients, 97 (5%) had lymphocytic myocarditis at necropsy.

Although hepatic enzyme determinations were not reported in the previously described necropsy patients with fatal lymphocytic myocarditis until the present report, elevated serum creatinine phosphokinase and the MB fraction have been described in several live patients with biopsy-proved lymphocytic myocarditis.[19]

An unexpected finding in our patient was the extreme low voltage on the electrocardiogram in the absence of evidence of pericardial effusion. The total 12-lead QRS voltage in our patient 23 days before death was only 54 mm (5.4 mV), and the patient was at ideal body weight (body mass index = 20 kg/m^2). The explanation is unclear but presumably is related to the extensive extent of the left ventricular and ventricular septal lesions. In 7 patients with biopsy-proved myocarditis, Nakashima et al[20] described a decrease in the total QRS amplitude in the acute stage compared with prior electrocardiograms obtained for health screening (limb lead 4.7 vs 2.8 mV, chest lead 11.9 vs 7.7 mV), and electrocardiograms obtained during the convalescent stage (limb lead 3.0 vs 3.9 mV, chest lead 7.8 vs 9.2 mV).

In summary, a 37-year-old previously healthy woman with a 6-week illness died suddenly at home, and necropsy disclosed extensive myocarditis. Cardiac enzymes were elevated and electrocardiograms showed severe low voltage and episodic ventricular tachycardia. Insertion of a cardiodefibrillator should be considered in the setting of acute myocarditis associated with episodic ventricular tachycardia.

1. Odom H, II, Davis JL, Dinh H, Baker BJ, Roberts WC, Murphy ML. QRS voltage measurements in autopsied men free of cardiopulmonary disease: a basis for evaluating total QRS voltage as an index of left ventricular hypertrophy. *Am J Cardiol* 1986;58:801–804.
2. Molander N. Sudden natural death in later childhood and adolescence. *Arch Dis Child* 1982;57:572–576.

3. Phillips M, Robinowitz M, Higgins JR, Boran KJ, Reed T, Virmani R. Sudden cardiac death Air Force recruits: 20-year review. *JAMA* 1986;256:2696–2699.
4. Brampton WJ, Jago RH. Acute viral myocarditis: A death associated with anaesthesia. *Anesthesia* 1990;45:215–217.
5. Shirani J, Freant LJ, Roberts WC. Gross and semiquantitative histologic findings in mononuclear cell myocarditits causing sudden death, and implications for endomyocardial biopsy. *Am J Cardiol* 1993;72:952–957.
6. Shen WK, Edwards WD, Hammill SC, Bailey KR, Ballard DJ, Gersh BJ. Sudden unexpected nontraumatic death in 54 young adults: a 30-year population-based study. *Am J Cardiol* 1995;76:148–152.
7. Wesslén L, Påhlson C, Lindquist O, Hjelm E, Gnarpe J, Larsson E, Baandrup U, Eriksson L, Fohlman J, Engstrand L, Linglöf T, Nyström-Rosander C, Gnarpe H, Magnius L, Rolf C, Friman G. An increase in sudden unexpected cardiac deaths among young Swedish orienteers during 1979–1992. *Eur Heart J* 1996;17:902–910.
8. Topaz O, Edwards JE. Pathologic features of sudden death in children, adolescents, and young adults. *Chest* 1985;87:476–482.
9. Driscoll DJ, Edwards WD. Sudden unexpected death in children and adolescents. *J Am Coll Cardiol* 1985;5:118B–121B.
10. Neuspiel DR, Kuller LH. Sudden and unexpected natural death in childhood and adolescence. *JAMA* 1985;254:1321–1325.
11. Raymond JR, van den Berg EK, Knapp MJ. Nontraumatic prehospital sudden death in young adults. *Arch Intern Med* 1988;148:303–308.
12. Drory Y, Turetz Y, Hiss Y, Lev B, Fisman EZ, Pines A, Kramer MR. Sudden unexpected death in persons <40 years of age. *Am J Cardiol* 1991;68:1388–1392.
13. Corrado D, Basso C, Poletti A, Angelini A, Valente M, Thiene G. Sudden death in the young: is acute coronary thrombosis the major precipitating factor? *Circulation* 1994;90:2315–2323.
14. Anderson RE, Hill RB, Broudy DW, Key CR, Pathak D. A population-based autopsy study of sudden, unexpected deaths from natural causes among persons 5 to 39 years old during a 12-year period. *Hum Pathol* 1994;25:1332–1340.
15. Steinberger J, Lucas RV Jr, Edwards JE, Titus JL. Causes of sudden unexpected cardiac death in the first two decades of life. *Am J Cardiol* 1996;77:992–995.
16. Maron BJ, Shirani J, Poliac LC, Mathenge R, Roberts WC, Mueller FO. Sudden death in young competitive athletes: clinical, demographic, and pathological profiles. *JAMA* 1996;276:199–204.
17. Wren C, O'Sullivan JJ, Wright C. Sudden death in children and adolescents. *Heart* 2000;83:410–413.
18. Morentin B, Aguilera B, Garamendi PM, Suarez-Mier MP. Sudden unexpected non-violent death between 1 and 19 years in north Spain. *Arch Dis Child* 2000;82:456–461.
19. Dec GW Jr, Waldman H, Southern J, Fallon JT, Hutter AM Jr, Palacios I. Viral myocarditis mimicking acute myocardial infarction. *J Am Coll Cardiol* 1992;20:85–89.
20. Nakashima H, Honda Y, Katayama T. Serial electrocardiographic findings in acute myocarditis. *Int Med* 1994;33:659–666.

Lymphocytic myocarditis as a cause of fulminant fatal heart failure

William Lance Garner, MD, MS, Cherry Starling, MD, Johannes Jacob Kuiper, MD, and William Clifford Roberts, MD

A 63-year-old Hispanic woman with prior systemic hypertension was well until 39 days before death when she fainted in her kitchen and was hospitalized. An electrocardiogram and telemetry monitoring disclosed sinus bradycardia (50 beats per minute) with first-degree atrioventricular block, left bundle branch block, frequent atrial and ventricular premature complexes, and sinus pauses up to 8 seconds. An echocardiogram showed mitral regurgitation (2+/4+) and an ejection fraction of 60%. An angiogram disclosed normal coronary arteries. The left ventricular and aortic pressures were normal. During her 3 days in the hospital, she had recurrent sinus pauses with associated syncope, and a permanent atrioventricular sequential pacemaker was implanted.

Thereafter, she felt well and was active until 22 days before she died, when exertional dyspnea appeared and progressed, prompting rehospitalization 20 days before death. Her blood pressure was 120/75 mm Hg, her paced heart rate was 80 beats per minute, and her temperature was normal. A grade 2/6 apical systolic ejection murmur and a third heart sound were audible. She had diffuse pulmonary rales and decreased breath sounds at both lung bases. A chest radiograph showed pulmonary vascular congestion, cardiomegaly, and bilateral pulmonary effusions. An electrocardiogram disclosed atrioventricular sequentially paced rhythm with no ST-T changes. Her serum troponin I level was 6.6 ng/mL, and her creatine phosphokinase level was 189 U/L with an MB fraction of 39 ng/mL. Her brain natriuretic peptide level was 2570 ng/L, and her white blood cell count was $10.7 \times 10^3/\text{mm}^3$. An echocardiogram showed severe global hypokinesis with an ejection fraction of 35%.

Over the subsequent 19 days in the hospital, the patient's status progressively deteriorated, requiring intravenous inotropic support, mechanical ventilation, and continuous veno-venous hemodialysis. She also developed hemodynamically unstable

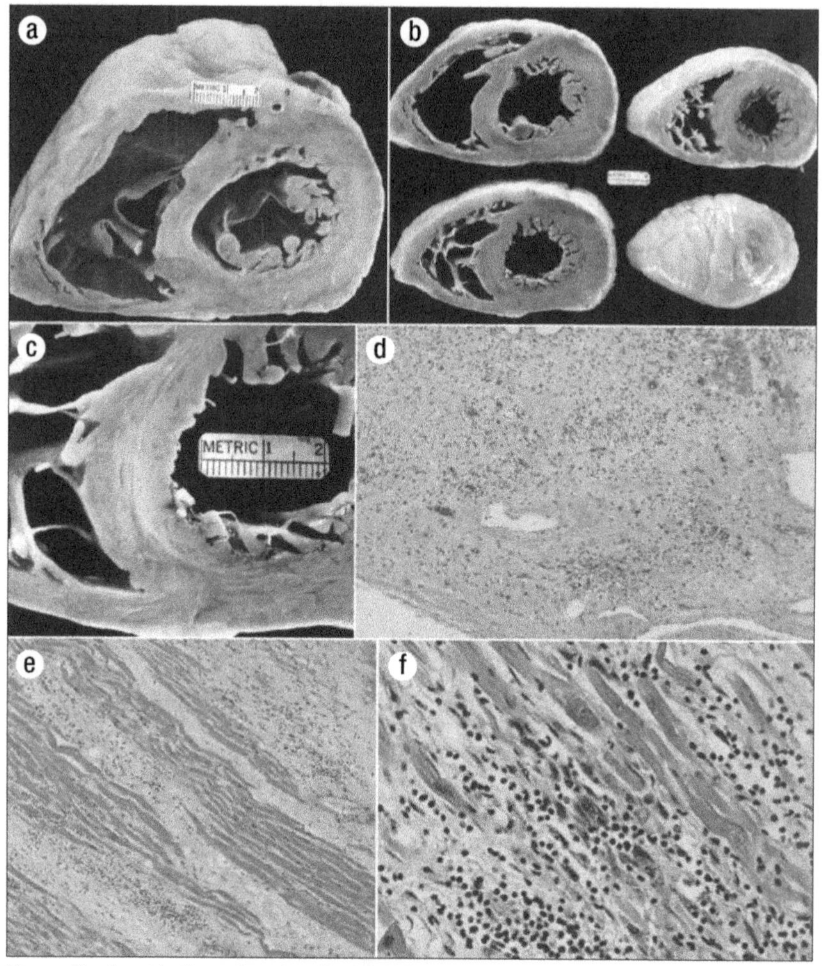

Figure. The heart in the patient described. **(a)** View of dilated right and left ventricles just caudal to the atrioventricular valves. **(b)** Transverse cuts of the cardiac ventricles. **(c)** Close-up view of the ventricular septum and right and left ventricular walls. Linear scars are present in the septum and in the posterior wall of the left ventricle. **(d)** Low-power view of foci of lymphocytes in an area of scar. **(e)** Low-power view of collections of lymphocytes in areas of scar between muscle bundles. **(f)** Higher-power view of lymphocytes associated with myofiber necrosis. Hematoxylin and eosin stains. (Photographs by Jong Mi Ko.)

From the Division of Cardiology, Department of Internal Medicine (Garner, Kuiper, Roberts) and Department of Pathology (Starling, Roberts), Baylor Heart and Vascular Institute and Baylor University Medical Center, Dallas, Texas.

Corresponding author: William C. Roberts, MD, Baylor Heart and Vascular Institute, 621 North Hall Street, Dallas, Texas 75226 (e-mail: wc.roberts@BaylorHealth.edu).

atrial fibrillation and had multiple electrical cardioversions. Right-sided heart catheterization a day before death showed the following pressures (in mm Hg): right atrial mean, 15; right ventricle, 25/10; pulmonary artery, 30/20. The cardiac output was 2.1 L/min and the cardiac index, 1.1 L/min/m^2. She was transferred to Baylor University Medical Center 12 hours before death, which resulted from inadequate perfusion of multiple body organs.

At necropsy, the heart weighed 470 grams. The quantity of subepicardial adipose tissue was increased. The coronary arteries were widely patent with no identifiable plaques. All 4 cardiac chambers were dilated *(Figure)*. The 4 valves were anatomically normal. Multiple myocardial lesions were present grossly in the left ventricular wall and ventricular septum, and histologically numerous foci of lymphocytic infiltrates were present with associated myocardial cell necrosis and foci of replacement fibrosis (Figure).

Table. Data in 9 previous necropsy reports of patients with lymphocytic myocarditis and fatal heart failure

Case	First author, year (reference)	Age at death (years)	Sex	Previous signs and symptoms	Months of illness before death	Prior conduction defect (type)	Heart weight (grams)
1	Kawai, 1988 (10)	18	F	URI, dyspnea, palpitations	11	0	370
2	Kawai, 1988 (10)	28	M	URI, dyspnea, edema	78	0	660
3	Okabe, 1992 (11)	54	F	Chest pain	74	+ (3°)	480
4	Okabe, 1992 (11)	56	F	Dyspnea	36	+ (IVCD)	530
5	Okabe, 1992 (11)	52	F	Dyspnea	36	+ (IVCD)	430
6	Morimoto, 1992 (12)	31	F	URI	12	+ (IVCD)	510
7	Morimoto, 1992 (12)	40	M	Dyspnea, edema, fever	21	0	940
8	Morimoto, 1992 (12)	7	F	Abdominal pain, dyspnea, fever	6	+ (2°)	280
9	Itoh, 1997 (13)	47	F	Fever, nausea	0.7	+ (3°)	NA

URI indicates upper respiratory infection; IVCD, intraventricular conduction delay; 2°, type II second-degree heart block; 3°, third-degree heart block; NA, not available.

• • •

This patient had a clinical course of about 40 days, and it was characterized initially by syncope, presumably the result of prolonged sinus pauses without electrocardiographic evidence of myocardial damage. Her final 20 days were characterized by progressive and finally fatal heart failure. Cardiac studies during her final days disclosed angiographically normal coronary arteries but generalized inadequate cardiac function. This short clinical course suggests, of course, an acute myocarditis that would be characterized by the presence of numerous polymorphonuclear leukocytes in the myocardial walls. What was observed histologically, however, was the presence of numerous lymphocytes in the ventricular walls and associated microventricular scars compatible with her 40-day course. No polymorphonuclear leukocytes were seen in the myocardial walls.

Such cases appear unusual. One of us (WCR) has previously studied at necropsy 14 patients who had died suddenly out of the hospital from lymphocytic myocarditis without evidence of congestive heart failure (1, 2), and others have described similar cases (3–9). The present case of lymphocytic myocarditis with clinical evidence of heart failure is the first seen by one of us (WCR). A search of previous publications disclosed only 9 previously reported patients with fatal heart failure from lymphocytic myocarditis *(Table)* (10–13). Why patients with lymphocytic myocarditis appear to present more frequently with sudden arrhythmia—either fatal or nonfatal—than with heart failure is unclear. Such, however, is the uniqueness of the patient described here.

1. Shirani J, Freant LJ, Roberts WC. Gross and semiquantitative histologic findings in mononuclear cell myocarditis causing sudden death, and implications for endomyocardial biopsy. *Am J Cardiol* 1993;72(12):952–957.
2. Theleman KP, Kuiper JJ, Roberts WC. Acute myocarditis (predominately lymphocytic) causing sudden death without heart failure. *Am J Cardiol* 2001;88(9):1078–1083.
3. Molander N. Sudden natural death in later childhood and adolescence. *Arch Dis Child* 1982;57(8):572–576.
4. Phillips M, Robinowitz M, Higgins JR, Boran KJ, Reed T, Virmani R. Sudden cardiac death in Air Force recruits. A 20-year review. *JAMA* 1986;256(19):2696–2699.
5. Brampton WJ, Jago RH. Acute viral myocarditis. A death associated with anaesthesia. *Anaesthesia* 1990;45(3):215–217.
6. Shen WK, Edwards WD, Hammill SC, Bailey KR, Ballard DJ, Gersh BJ. Sudden unexpected nontraumatic death in 54 young adults: a 30-year population-based study. *Am J Cardiol* 1995;76(3):148–152.
7. Wesslén L, Pahlson C, Lindquist O, Hjelm E, Gnarpe J, Larsson E, Baandrup U, Eriksson L, Fohlman J, Engstrand L, Linglof T, Nystrom-Rosander C, Gnarpe H, Magnius L, Rolf C, Friman G. An increase in sudden unexpected cardiac deaths among young Swedish orienteers during 1979–1992. *Eur Heart J* 1996;17(6):902–910.
8. Basso C, Corrado D, Rossi L, Thiene G. Ventricular preexcitation in children and young adults: atrial myocarditis as a possible trigger of sudden death. *Circulation* 2001;103(2):269–275.
9. Corrado D, Basso C, Thiene G. Sudden cardiac death in young people with apparently normal heart. *Cardiovasc Res* 2001;50(2):399–408.
10. Kawai S, Kasuya H, Shimizu M, Okada R, Yamauchi T, Uruga K, Yamamoto S, Kobayashi T. Three autopsied cases of postmyocarditic cardiomegaly. Comparison with dilated cardiomyopathy. *Jpn Heart J* 1988;29(6):809–821.
11. Okabe M, Fukuda K, Nakashima Y, Hiroki T, Arakawa K, Kikuchi M. Lymphocytic active myocarditis characterized by numerous clusters of lymphocytes: a chronic variant of myocarditis? *Am Heart J* 1992;123(1):128–136.
12. Morimoto S, Hiramitsu S, Yamada K, Uemura A, Kubo N, Kimura K, Mizuno Y, Nishikawa T, Hasumi M, Sekiguchi M. Clinical and pathologic features of chronic myocarditis: four autopsy cases presenting as dilated cardiomyopathy in life. *Am J Cardiovasc Pathol* 1992;4(2):181–191.
13. Itoh E, Saitoh H, Miida T, Oda H, Toeda T, Higuma N, Okazaki E. An autopsied case of acute myocarditis with myocardial calcification. *Jpn Circ J* 1997;61(9):798–802.

Cardiac Transplantation for Cardiac Sarcoidosis With Initial Diagnosis by Examination of the Left Ventricular Apical "Core" Excised for Insertion of a Left Ventricular Assist Device for Severe Chronic Heart Failure

William Clifford Roberts, MD[a,b,d,*], Travis James Vowels[d], Jong Mi Ko, BA[d], John Edward Capehart, MD[c], and Shelley Anne Hall, MD[a,d]

Three quinquagenarians who underwent insertion of a left ventricular assist device (LVAD) because of severe heart failure and for whom histologic examination of the left ventricular apical "core" (removed to insert the device) showed noncaseating giant cell granulomas typical of sarcoidosis are described. Later, cardiac transplantation showed widespread sarcoid granulomas in the walls of the right and left ventricles and ventricular septum in 2 patients and extensive scarring in the third patient in the absence of coronary narrowing. Previously, 11 patients who underwent cardiac transplantation because of cardiac sarcoidosis had been reported, and in 1 of these patients, diagnosis was also initially made by examination of the left ventricular core excised at the time of insertion of an LVAD. In conclusion, excision of a portion of left ventricular wall to enable insertion of a therapeutic device (LVAD) can also serve as the means of definitive diagnosis of the underlying cardiac condition. **(Am J Cardiol 2009;103:110–114)**

Although it may involve virtually any body organ, sarcoidosis infrequently involved the heart, and when it did, it usually did not cause dysfunction of ≥1 noncardiac organ.[1] Cardiac sarcoidosis was usually not diagnosed until percutaneous cardiac biopsy or at necropsy. Earlier, we reported a patient who underwent cardiac transplantation for severe heart failure and diagnosis of cardiac sarcoidosis was not made until morphologic examination of the recipient heart.[2] We found sarcoid granulomas in the left ventricular apical "core" in 3 patients who had a left ventricular assist device (LVAD) inserted because of severe heart failure. Initial diagnosis of cardiac sarcoidosis by this means is most unusual and prompted this report.

Methods and Results

Pertinent findings in each of the 3 patients are listed in Table 1. All were aged in their 50s and 2 were men. All were mildly overweight (body mass indexes 27.0, 26.5, and 27.0 kg/m^2). Chronic heart failure before cardiac transplantation had been present for 3, 4, and 5 years, respectively. Two patients had transient runs of ventricular tachycardia, including 1 with documented ventricular fibrillation. Two had complete branch bundle block and 1 had complete heart block. All had cardioverter defibrillators implanted and 2 had pacemakers implanted. Coronary angiograms showed the epicardial coronary arteries to be either normal (2 patients) or narrowed <50% in diameter (patient 3; Table 1). All 3 had indirect systemic peak systolic blood pressures ≤100 mm Hg. Two were anemic. Only 1 (patient 2) underwent a percutaneous myocardial biopsy, which was negative for sarcoid. Patient 2 also had biopsy-proven sarcoidosis of the lung 16 years earlier (age 36 years) and had been treated with prednisone (10 mg/day) during all 16 years. Spirometry 3 months before cardiac transplantation showed forced vital capacity to be 2.76 L (59% of predicted), forced expiratory volume in 1 second was 1.78 L (49% of predicted), total lung capacity was 76% of predicted value, and diffusing capacity was 57% of predicted value. Times from insertion of the LVAD to cardiac transplantation were 11, 53, and 522 days. Patients 1 and 3 had never been treated with prednisone or other type of corticosteroid, and diagnosis of sarcoid had not been made before the left ventricular apical core had been examined histologically.

Examination of the surgically excised recipient heart showed 2 to have increased cardiac mass. Both ventricular cavities were dilated in all 3 hearts (Figures 1 to 4). (On pretransplantation echocardiograms in patients 1 and 3, right ventricular cavities were 2.6 and 2.3 cm and left ventricular cavities were 9.4 and 5.7 cm, respectively.) All 3 had extensive scarring in the ventricular walls and 2 had numerous noncaseating granulomas.[3] The patient without noncaseating granulomas (patient 1) in the ventricular walls on examination after cardiac transplantation had extensive scarring and foci of lymphocytes in the areas of scarring.

Cardiac transplantation was performed in patient 1 on January 14, 2005; in patient 2, on July 9, 2005; and in

Departments of [a]Internal Medicine, (Division of Cardiology), [b]Pathology, and [c]Cardiothoracic Surgery and the [d]Baylor Heart and Vascular Institute; and Baylor University Medical Center, Dallas, Texas. Manuscript received August 26, 2008; accepted August 27, 2008.

*Corresponding author: Tel: 214-820-7911; Fax: 214-820-7533.

E-mail address: wc.roberts@baylorhealth.edu (W.C. Roberts).

Table 1
Clinical and cardiac morphologic findings in 3 patients with cardiac sarcoidosis diagnosed for the first time by histologic examination of the left ventricular apical core excised for insertion of left ventricular assist device for severe heart failure

Patient No.	Age at Heart Transplantation	Race	Sex	AF	VT	VF	Heart Block	Hct (%)	Pressures (mm Hg)				CI (L/min/m^2)	EF (%)	ICD	PM	Heart Weight (g)	Location of Sarcoid			Cavity (cm)	
									LV	RV	PA	PAW mean						RV	VS	LV	RV	LV
1	50	W	M	+	+	+	+ (LBBB)	38	127/33	81/19	81/40	51	1.0	10	+	0	604	0*	0*	+*	8.0	7.0
2	52	W	M	+	0	0	+ (RBBB)	26	N/A	N/A	51/23	24	1.6	15	+	+	480	+	+	+	5.2	4.2
3	59	B	F	0	+	0	+ (CHB)	42	N/A	33/11	35/16	24	1.3	25	+	+	371	+	+	+	7.5	5.0

* Sarcoid granulomas present in the left ventricular apical core removed for insertion of the LVAD. The walls of the left ventricle, ventricular septum, and right ventricle in the excised native heart (at transplantation) had extensive scarring, but no granulomas. Focal collections of lymphocytes were present in the scarred ventricular walls.

AF = atrial fibrillation; B = black; CHB = complete heart block; CI = cardiac index; EF = ejection fraction; Hct = hematocrit; ICD = implantable cardioverter-defibrillator; LBBB = left bundle branch block; LV = left ventricle; PA = pulmonary artery; PAW = pulmonary artery wedge; PM = pacemaker; RBBB = right bundle branch block; RV = right ventricle; VF = ventricular fibrillation; VS = ventricular septum; VT = ventricular tachycardia; W = white.

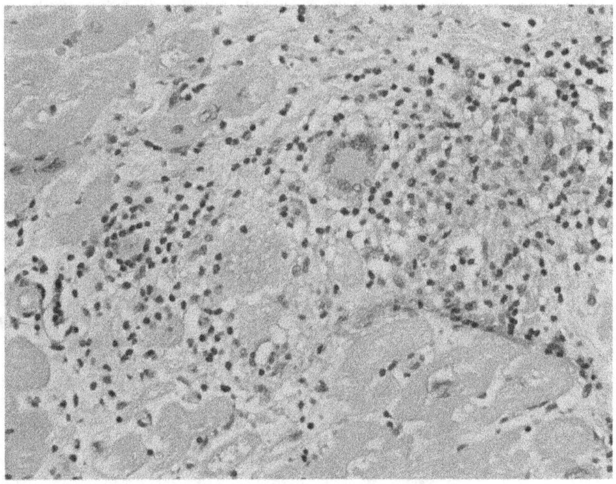

Figure 1. Patient 1. Photomicrograph of sarcoid granuloma in the left ventricular apical core removed 11 days before cardiac transplantation. (Hematoxylin-eosin stain; original magnification ×400.)

patient 3, on July 10, 2006. All 3 patients are alive and active as of August 15, 2008.

The Baylor University Medical Center, Dallas, Texas, Internal Review Board approved the study.

Discussion

The unique feature of the 3 cases briefly described in this report is the initial diagnosis of cardiac sarcoidosis by histologic examination of the left ventricular apical core excised at the time of insertion of a LVAD for severe heart failure of unclear cause. One other patient with a similar diagnostic scenario was reported previously.[4]

We found 11 previously published case reports of patients who underwent cardiac transplantation for severe heart failure (10 patients) or recurring refractory ventricular arrhythmias (1 patient) secondary to cardiac sarcoidosis (Table 2).[2,4–11] Right-sided intracardiac biopsies after cardiac transplantation were reported later in 7 of these 11 patients, and in 2, noncaseating granulomas were found, indicating recurrence of cardiac sarcoidosis, but this time in the donor heart. The positive biopsies were performed 6 and 19 months after transplantation. Biopsies in 5 other patients were negative for sarcoid 6 to 96 months (mean 29) after transplantation. The other 2 patients died 6 days and 42 months after transplantation. Each of the 3 patients described in this report had right-sided biopsies 15, 24, and 14 months performed after cardiac transplantation and none had noncaseating granulomas in the excised cardiac specimens.

Although not performed for cardiac sarcoidosis, Bartram et al[12] reported findings in a 9-year-old boy who developed systemic sarcoidosis (unclear whether the heart was involved) nearly 9 years after orthotopic heart transplantation for Shone syndrome (supravalvular mitral ring, mitral valve stenosis, valvular and supravalvular aortic stenosis, and aortic coarctation).

Zaidi et al[13] reviewed the United Network for Organ Sharing database to assess survival of patients with sar-

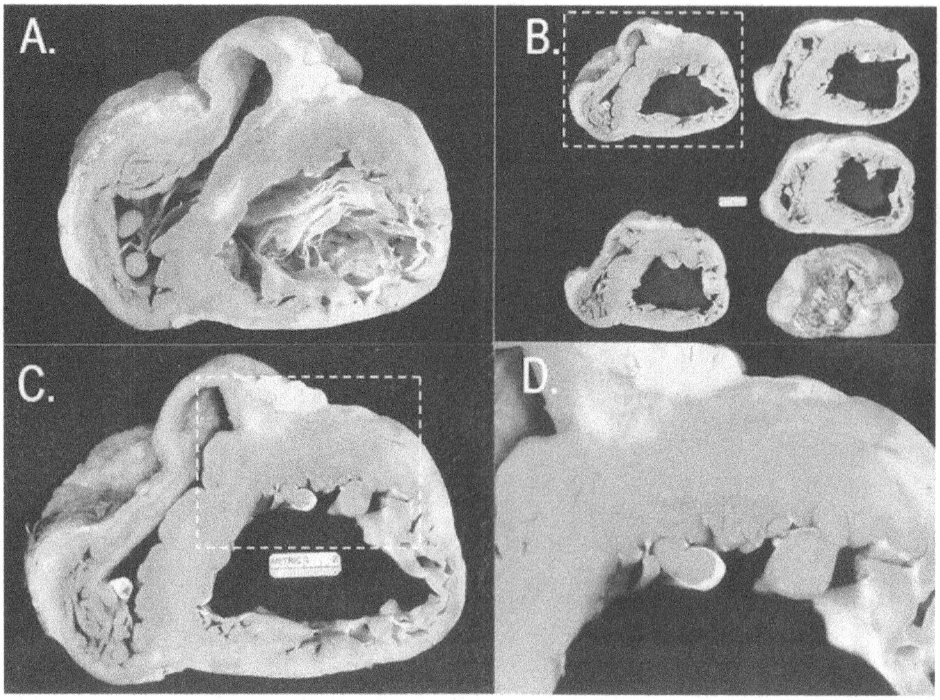

Figure 2. Patient 1. Explanted heart. *(A)* Base shows extensive lateral wall left ventricular scarring and focal ventricular septal scarring by sarcoidosis. Both ventricular cavities are dilated. *(B)* One-centimeter thick slices of the ventricular walls show that scarring extends from base to apex. *(C)* Close-up of 1 ventricular slice shown in *B*. *(D)* Close-up of subepicardial scar in the anterior portion of the ventricular septum shown in *C*.

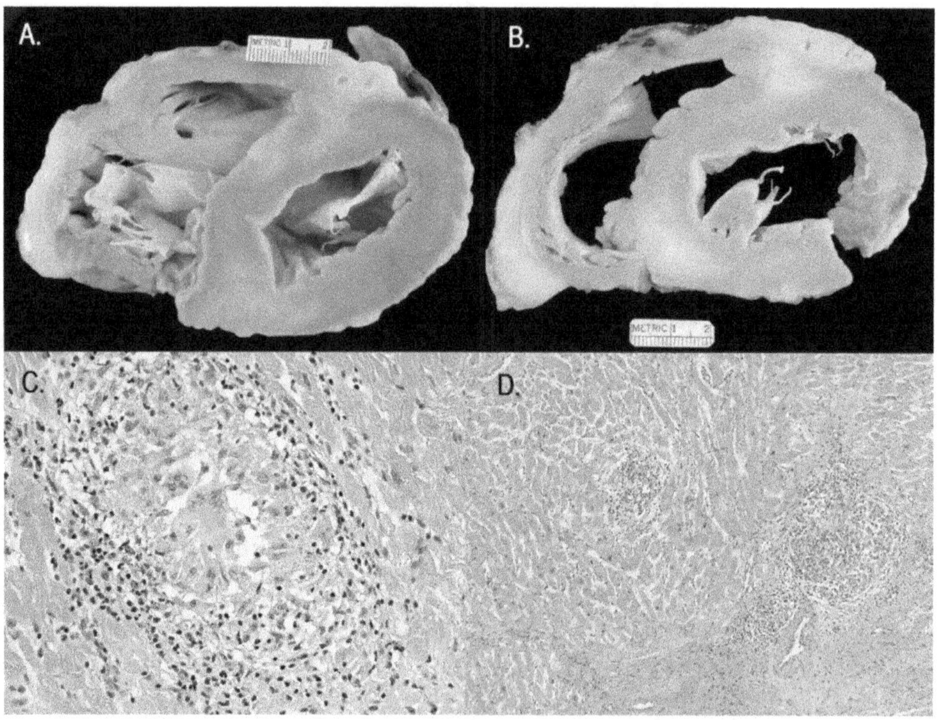

Figure 3. Patient 2. *(A)* Base of heart and *(B)* 1 slice of ventricular walls caudal to the base. Scars are present in the ventricular septum and posterior left ventricular walls. Both cavities are dilated. *(C)* Photomicrograph of a sarcoid granuloma in the left ventricular core removed to insert the LVAD. *(D)* Photomicrograph of portion of explanted heart shows 2 sarcoid granulomas. (Hematoxylin-eosin stain; original magnification *[C]* ×400, *[D]* ×100.)

coidosis treated using heart transplantation. During an 18-year period, 65 patients (40 men, 25 women) with sarcoidosis underwent orthotopic heart transplantation. There were 4 operative deaths and 12 late deaths at a mean follow-up of 40 months. One-year posttransplantation, survival was better for patients with sarcoid undergoing orthotopic transplantation compared with patients undergoing transplantation for nonsarcoid conditions

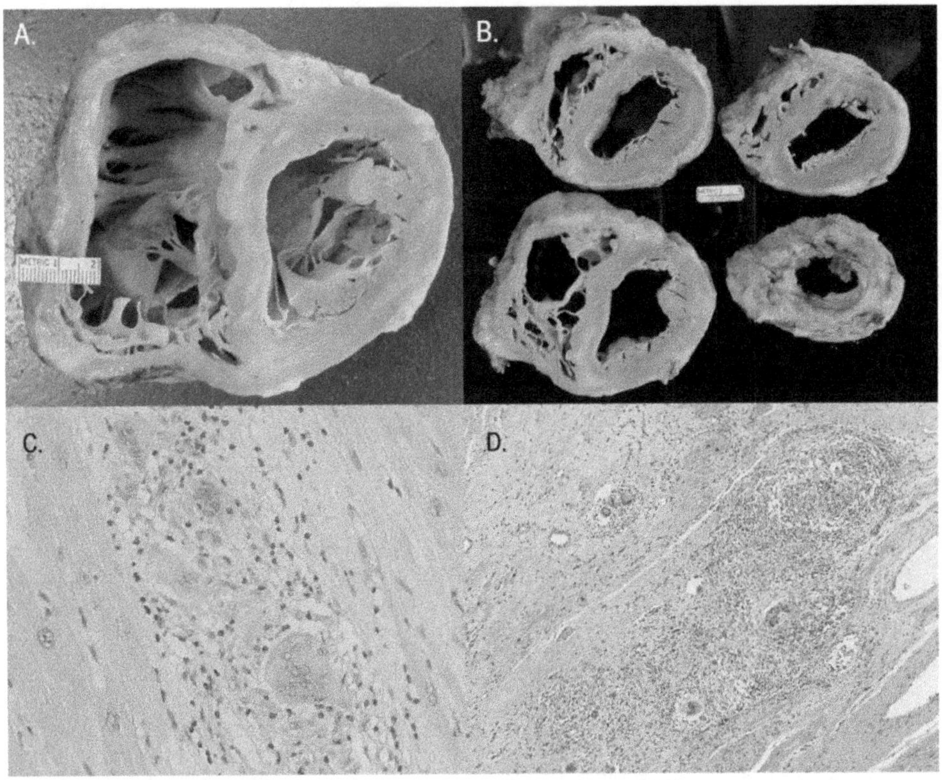

Figure 4. Patient 3. *(A)* Base of heart shows very dilated ventricular cavities and patchy scars in the ventricular septum and left ventricular free wall. *(B)* Slices of ventricular walls caudal to the base again show focal scars. *(C)* Photomicrograph shows sarcoid granuloma in the left ventricular core excised at time of placement of the LVAD. *(D)* Photomicrograph of sarcoid granulomas in the explanted heart. (Hematoxylin-eosin stain; original magnification *[C]* ×400, *[D]* ×100.)

(88% vs 85%; p = 0.03). The investigators concluded that diagnosis of sarcoidosis should not disqualify potential transplantation candidates.

1. Roberts WC, McAllister HA Jr, Ferrans VJ. Sarcoidosis of the heart. A clinicopathologic study of 35 necropsy patients (group I) and review of 78 previously described necropsy patients (group II). *Am J Med* 1977;63:86–108.
2. Donsky AS, Escobar J, Capehart J, Roberts WC. Heart transplantation for undiagnosed cardiac sarcoidosis. *Am J Cardiol* 2002;89:1447–1449.
3. Shirani J, Roberts WC. Subepicardial myocardial lesions. *Am Heart J* 1993;125:1346–1352.
4. Yagar JE, Hernandez AF, Steenbergen C, Persing B, Russell SD, Milano C, Felker GM. Recurrence of cardiac sarcoidosis in a heart transplant recipient. *J Heart Lung Transplant* 2005;24:1988–1990.
5. Gokel JM, Reichart B, Struck E. Human cardiac transplantation—evaluation of morphologic changes in serial endomyocardial biopsies. *Path Res Pract* 1985;79:354–365.
6. Valantine HA, Tazelaar HD, Macoviak J, Mullin AV, Hunt SA, Fowler MB, Billingham ME, Schroeder JS. Cardiac sarcoidosis: response to steroids and transplantation. *J Heart Transplant* 1987;6:244–250.
7. Oni AA, Hershberger RE, Norman DJ, Ray J, Hovaguimian H, Cobanoglu AM, Hosenpud JD. Recurrence of sarcoidosis in a cardiac allograft: control with augmented corticosteroids. *J Heart Lung Transplant* 1992;11:367–369.
8. Ankersmit HJ, Wieselthaler GA, Moser B, Taghavi S, Grimm M, Roth G, Gorlitzer M, Tschernich H, Horvat R, Wolner E. Automated implantable cardiac defibrillator and biventricular thoratec assist device as bridge to transplantation in a patient with sarcoidosis. *J Thorac Cardiovasc Surg* 2001;121:1198–1199.
9. Treaba DO, Benson MD, Assad LW, Dainauskas JR. Sarcoidosis and immunoglobulin lambda II light-chain amyloidosis diagnosed after orthotopic heart transplantation: a case report and review of the literature. *Mod Pathol* 2005;18:451–455.
10. Halushka MK, Yuh DD, Russell SD. Right ventricle-dominant cardiac sarcoidosis with sparing of the left ventricle. *J Heart Lung Transplant* 2006;25:479–482.
11. Greif M, Petrakopoulou P, Weiss M, Reithmann C, Reichart B, Nabauer M, Steinbeck G. Cardiac sarcoidosis concealed by arrhythmogenic right ventricular dysplasia/cardiomyopathy. *Nat Clin Pract Cardiovasc Med* 2008;5:231–236.
12. Bartram U, Thul J, Bauer J, Wössmann W, Schranz D. Systemic sarcoidosis after cardiac transplantation in a 9-year-old child. *J Heart Lung Transplant* 2006;25:1263–1267.
13. Zaidi AR, Zaidi A, Vaitkus PT. Outcome of heart transplantation in patients with sarcoid cardiomyopathy. *J Heart Lung Transplant* 2007;26:714–717.

Clinical and morphologic cardiac data in previously reported case reports of patients undergoing cardiac transplantation for cardiac sarcoidosis

Case	Reference	Year Published	Age at HT (yrs)	Race	Sex	Pre-HT Dx of Sarcoid	Reason for HT	Native Heart Weight (g)	Location of Granulomas			Dilated		BBB	CHB	VT	PR >0.20 s	Died (mo after HT)	Recurrence of Cardiac Sarcoid After HT
									RV	VS	LV	RV	LV						
1	Gokel et al[5]	1985	37	N/A	M	+ (Bx)	HF	N/A	–	–	–	–	–	–	–	–	–	+ (8)	–
2	Valantine et al[6]	1987	46	W	M	0	VT	630	+	+	+	0	0	+ [R]	0	+	+	+ (42)	0 (A)
3	Valantine et al[6]	1987	47	B	M	+ (Bx)	HF	420	"Widespread"			0	+	0	0	+	+	0 (16+)	0 (Bx)
4	Valantine et al[6]	1987	51	W	F	0	HF	400	0	+	+	–	–	+ [R]	0	0	+	0 (20+)	0 (Bx)
5	Oni et al[7]	1992	34	N/A	M	+ (Bx)	HF	N/A	–	–	–	+	+	0	0	+	0	0 (13+)	+ (Bx)
6	Ankersmit et al[8]	2001	30	N/A	M	+ (Bx)	HF	N/A	–	–	–	+	+	0	0	+	0	0 (1+)	–
7	Donsky et al[2]	2002	53	W	M	0	HF	510	+	+	+	+	+	+ [L]	0	+	+	0 (105+)	0 (Bx)
8	Yager et al[4]	2005	26	B	M	+ (LVAD)	HF	N/A	–	–	–	–	–	0	0	0	0	0 (24+)	+ (Bx)
9	Treaba et al[9]	2005	53	B	M	0	HF	N/A	+	+	+	–	–	0	+	0	0	+ (0.2)	0 (A)
10	Halushka et al[10]	2006	53	W	M	+ (Bx)	HF	380	+	+	+	+	0	0	0	+	0	0 (6+)	0 (Bx)
11	Greif et al[11]	2008	37	N/A	M	0	HF	N/A	+	+	+	+	0	+ [L]	0	+	0	0 (8+)	0 (Bx)

A = autopsy; B = black; BBB = bundle branch block; Bx = biopsy of myocardium; CHB = complete heart block; Dx = diagnosis; HF = heart failure; HT = heart transplantation; L = left; LV = left ventricle; R = right; RV = right ventricle; VS = ventricular septum; VT = ventricular tachycardia; W = white.

Diagnosing cardiac sarcoidosis clinically without tissue confirmation

Poonam S. Sharma, MD, Jordon G. Lubahn, MD, Alan S. Donsky, MD, Anthony Dong H. Yoon, MD, Melissa M. Carry, MD, Paul A. Grayburn, MD, Prescilla Barrientos Wood, MD, Jong Mi Ko, BA, Elizabeth C. Burton, MD, and William Clifford Roberts, MD

A 52-year-old woman is described in whom cardiac sarcoidosis was diagnosed clinically on the basis of high-grade heart block, recurring ventricular tachyarrhythmias, and acute cardiac decompensation. Confirmation of sarcoidosis was not determined until necropsy. When it causes cardiac dysfunction, sarcoidosis rarely causes dysfunction of another body organ, although small sarcoid granulomas may also be present in noncardiac organs or tissues. In the present patient, neurosarcoidosis accompanied the cardiac sarcoidosis, but it was the latter that produced the life-threatening symptoms and was fatal.

Sarcoidosis is characterized by the presence of noncaseating giant-cell granulomas in more than one body organ. Although these granulomas may be present in virtually any organ, most commonly they occur in the lungs and in adjacent lymph nodes (1), but they are rare in the spinal cord. Symptoms usually appear gradually. Diagnosis often is made by chest radiograph showing hilar adenopathy with or without pulmonary parenchymal lesions before appearance of symptoms. Occasionally, sarcoidosis presents with symptoms related to the heart, and in such circumstances the manifestations usually are acute, consisting of a ventricular arrhythmia or a high grade of heart block or symptoms of heart failure (2). When sarcoidosis causes cardiac dysfunction, infrequently is there dysfunction of another body organ (2). To emphasize the fact that patients with cardiac sarcoidosis severe enough to cause cardiac dysfunction rarely have more than minimal involvement of noncardiac body organs, we describe the following case.

DESCRIPTION OF PATIENT

A 52-year-old nonsmoking, overweight African American female bus driver, who was born in February 1956, had been well until November 2007 when she noted right-sided mid back pain and, in December 2007, impaired vision in the right eye. The right optic disc was swollen and pale. The back pain made it difficult for her to dress herself, it was burning and shooting in nature, and it radiated to her right arm and breast. The impaired vision in the right eye caused blurriness and occasional double vision and was associated with pain with eye movement. Magnetic resonance imaging in January 2008 disclosed multiple small thoracic spine neural foramen tumors and abnormal contrast enhancement in the right retrobulbar fat and along the right optic nerve sheath, and a 15-mm "low-density" lesion in the left lower lobe of the lung was detected by computed tomography. The hilar and mediastinal structures were normal. Treadmill stress echocardiogram disclosed intermittent right bundle branch block throughout exercise and sinus bradycardia at rest, but no ST changes. A four-beat run of atrial tachycardia with aberrant conduction occurred during exercise. No wall-motion abnormalities were seen. Because of the eye problem, she was started on prednisone 80 mg daily and tapered to 10 mg for 7 months. She was off prednisone for the last 5 months of her life. Her vision improved in the right eye from 20/400 to 20/40 as a consequence of treatment.

Repeat chest radiograph in July 2008 disclosed no abnormalities. Echocardiogram disclosed normal-sized ventricular cavities and hyperdynamic left ventricular systolic function. Left ventricular diastolic function, however, was abnormal.

The eye problem cleared and, except for continued periodic right-sided back pain, occasional leg numbness, and some difficulty walking up stairs, she was active and continued working as a bus driver until December 26, 2008, when severe dyspnea appeared. She was found to have complete heart block, and a pacemaker was inserted. The dyspnea, however, persisted and within a week was accompanied by severe substernal chest pain radiating to both arms, dizziness, and worsening dyspnea. She was rehospitalized on January 6, 2009. The erythrocyte sedimentation rate was 76 mm in 1 hour; hematocrit, 31%; troponin, 2.92 ng/mL; and B-type natriuretic peptide, 1183 pg/mL. At cardiac catheterization, the epicardial coronary arteries were normal. The left ventricular ejection fraction was about 55%. Pressures (in mm Hg) were as follows: pulmonary artery, 45/26; pulmonary wedge a wave, 28, v wave, 33, and mean, 26; right atrial a wave, 18, v wave, 23, and mean, 15; left ventricle, 105/14; and aorta, 109/64. A left ventricular angiogram showed a mildly hypokinetic posterobasal wall

From the Department of Internal Medicine (Sharma, Lubahn), Division of Cardiology (Donsky, Yoon, Carry, Grayburn, Roberts), Department of Pathology (Wood, Burton, Roberts), and the Baylor Heart and Vascular Institute (Grayburn, Ko, Roberts), Baylor University Medical Center, Dallas, Texas.

Corresponding author: William C. Roberts, MD, Baylor Heart and Vascular Institute, Baylor University Medical Center, 3500 Gaston Avenue, Dallas, Texas 75246 (e-mail: wc.roberts@BaylorHealth.edu).

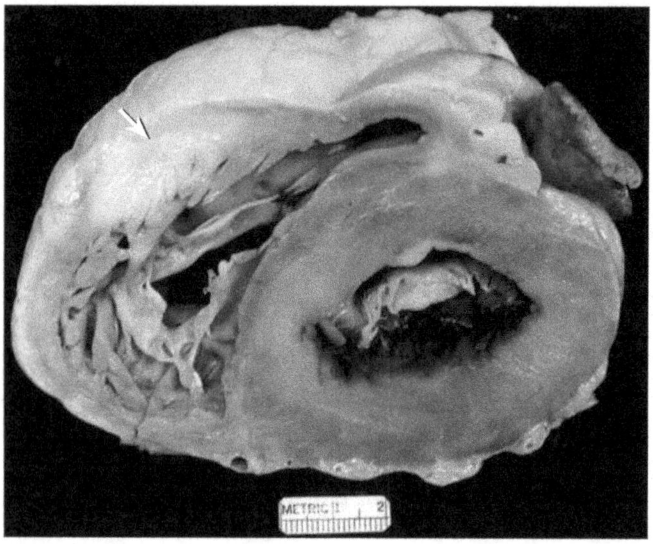

Figure 1. The base of the heart, showing a large sarcoid nodule in the right ventricular free wall anteriorly (arrow).

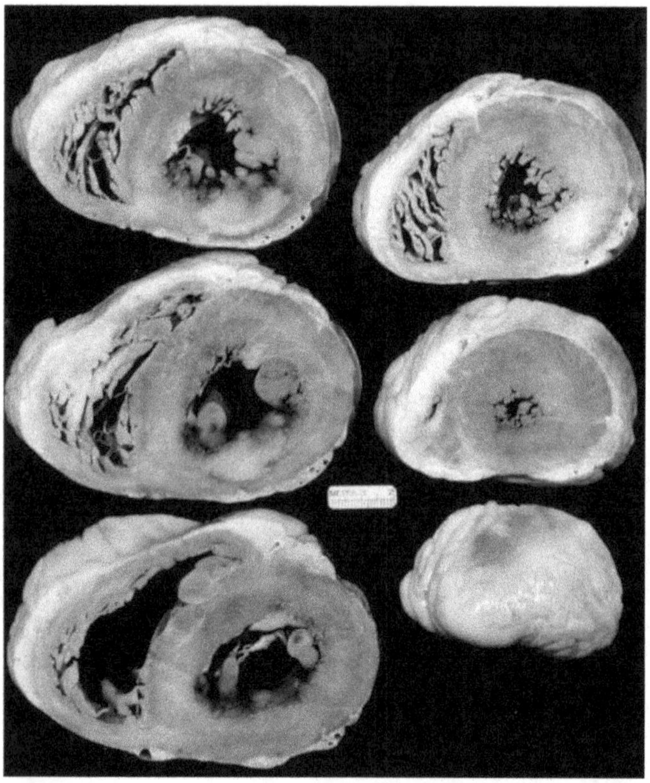

Figure 2. Cross-sections of the ventricular walls and cavities showing multiple sarcoid granulomas. One sarcoid focus involves a portion of the posteromedial papillary muscle of the left ventricle, and this deposit may have played a role in causing the mitral regurgitation.

and 2+/4+ mitral regurgitation. Ventricular tachycardia occurred during the procedure. An echocardiogram on January 16 showed depressed right and left ventricular systolic function (ejection fraction 45%), a restrictive left ventricular diastolic filling pattern, and severe mitral regurgitation. The heart failure progressively worsened, the blood pressure dropped, and ventricular tachycardia refractory to cardioversion occurred followed subsequently by fatal ventricular fibrillation on January 22, 2009.

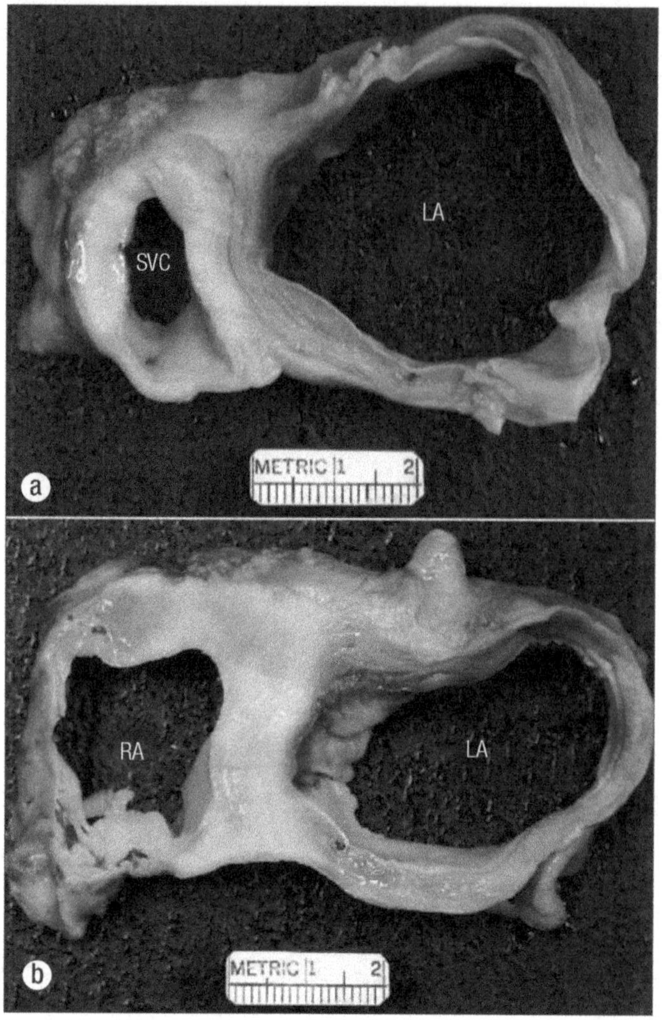

Figure 3. **(a)** The superior vena cava (SVC) entering the right atrium (RA), with the wall of this large vein replaced by sarcoid granulomas. **(b)** The more caudal portion of the RA and left atrium (LA), showing sarcoid granuloma in the right atrial wall posteriorly and in the atrial septum.

At necropsy, the heart weighed 485 g. The epicardial coronary arteries were normal. Multiple lesions were present in the right and left ventricular free walls and in the ventricular septum *(Figures 1 and 2)*. Additionally, the wall of the superior vena cava as it entered the right atrium and portions of the right atrial wall and atrial septum were infiltrated by similar lesions, which histologically were noncaseating giant-cell granulomas *(Figure 3)*. Sarcoid granulomas in the right ventricular wall are shown in *Figure 4* and in the left ventricular wall in *Figure 5*. The four cardiac valves were anatomically normal.

The lung parenchyma was normal grossly except for one lesion in the lower lobe of the left lung, and it too was a sarcoid granuloma *(Figures 6 and 7)*. At least two hilar lymph nodes were infiltrated by similar granulomas: one was normal sized, and one about 4 times larger than normal (Figure 7a).

The spinal cord tumors, seen by magnetic resonance, proved to be sarcoid granulomas *(Figure 8)*. Similar granulomas were present in the single kidney (one had been removed earlier for donation to a family member for renal transplantation).

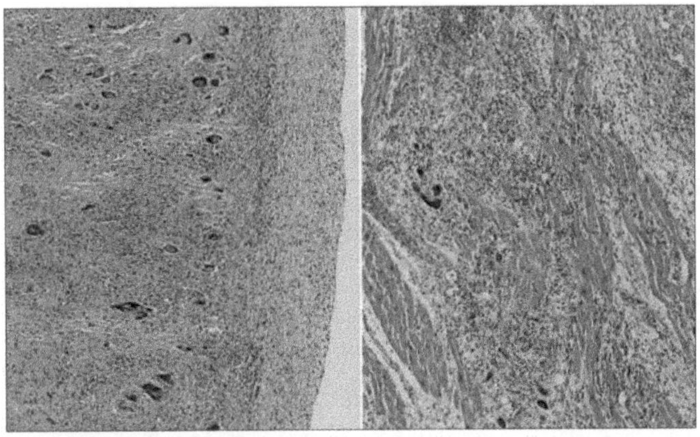

Figure 4. Granulomas in the right ventricular wall. Hematoxylin and eosin stains, each ×100. Stains for fungi and acid-fast organisms were negative.

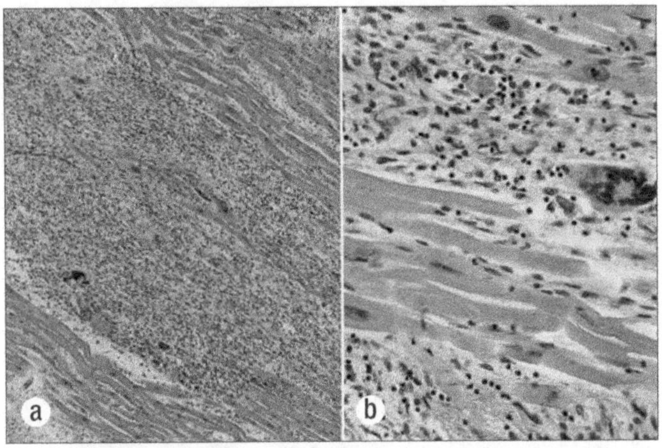

Figure 5. Sarcoid myocarditis in the left ventricular wall. Hematoxylin and eosin stains, **(a)** ×100, **(b)** ×400.

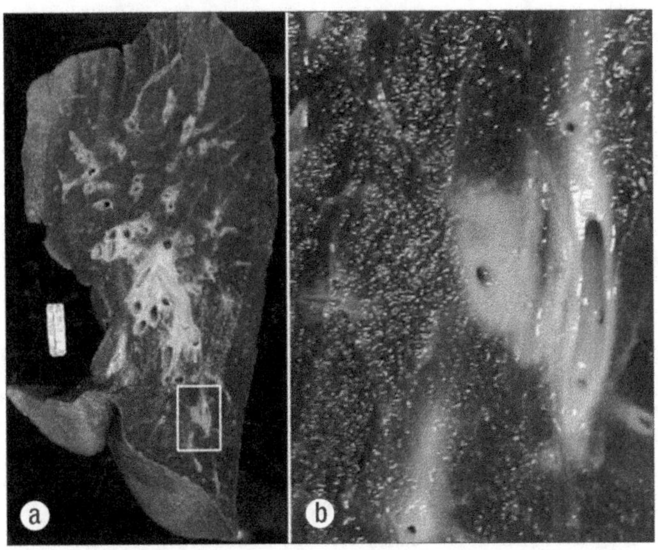

Figure 6. (a) Longitudinal section of the lung showing a single sarcoid granuloma. **(b)** A close-up of the area in the square.

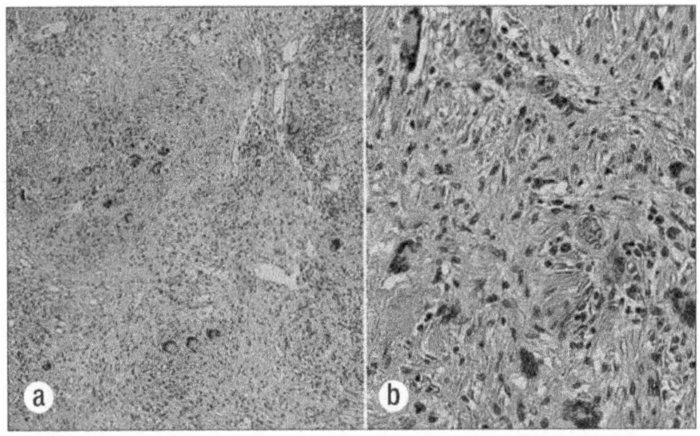

Figure 7. Sarcoid granulomas in the **(a)** hilar lymph node and **(b)** lung. Hematoxylin and eosin stains, ×100 (a), ×400 (b).

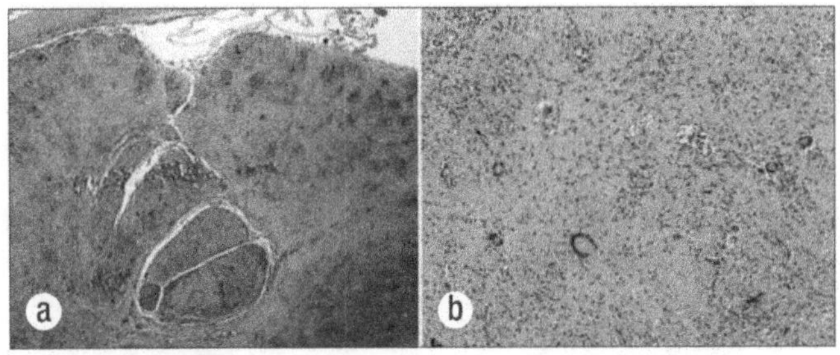

Figure 8. Sarcoid granulomas in the thoracic spinal cord. Hematoxylin and eosin stains, **(a)** ×2, **(b)** ×100.

DISCUSSION

The patient described had classic features of cardiac sarcoidosis, namely a high degree of heart block (third degree), recurring ventricular arrhythmias, and both systolic and diastolic cardiac dysfunction resulting in severe heart failure. Because of this triad of cardiac manifestations, cardiac sarcoidosis was diagnosed clinically. Necropsy confirmed the diagnosis of sarcoidosis, which involved extensively the heart, thoracic spinal cord, and hilar lymph nodes (only one of which was enlarged), and minimally the lung and kidney. The cause of her back pain was sarcoid granulomas within the spinal cord. Although its cause about a year before death was never definitely determined, the visual disturbance prompted the initiation of prednisone therapy, which eliminated the eye problem and obviously is the treatment of choice for sarcoidosis.

A very unusual feature of the present case is the occurrence of sarcoid granulomas in the spinal cord, which led to some nonlimiting symptoms. Others also have reported neurosarcoid involvement in patients with cardiac sarcoidosis (3, 4). Saleh and colleagues (3) reviewed 172 patients with spinal cord sarcoidosis, and 7 (4%) had cardiac involvement. Perry and Vuitch (4), however, found no cases of neurosarcoidosis among 14 autopsied patients with fatal cardiac sarcoidosis.

1. Crystal RG, Roberts WC, Hunninghake GW, Gadek JE, Fulmer JD, Line BR. Pulmonary sarcoidosis: a disease characterized and perpetuated by activated lung T-lymphocytes. *Ann Intern Med* 1981;94(1):73–94.
2. Roberts WC, McAllister HA Jr, Ferrans VJ. Sarcoidosis of the heart. A clinicopathologic study of 35 necropsy patients (group I) and review of 78 previously described necropsy patients (group II). *Am J Med* 1977;63(1):86–108.
3. Saleh S, Saw C, Marzouk K, Sharma O. Sarcoidosis of the spinal cord: literature review and report of eight cases. *J Natl Med Assoc* 2006;98(6):965–976.
4. Perry A, Vuitch F. Causes of death in patients with sarcoidosis. A morphologic study of 38 autopsies with clinicopathologic correlations. *Arch Pathol Lab Med* 1995;119(2):167–172.

Alcohol Ablation or Ventricular Septal Myotomy/Myectomy for Severe Obstructive Hypertrophic Cardiomyopathy?

Moderated by **William Roberts, MD**[1]
Discussants: **Joseph Dearani, MD**[2] and **Barry Maron, MD**[3]

The following Expert Roundtable Discussion was held on March 12, 2010. Dr. William Roberts from the Baylor Heart and Vasclar Institute moderated the topic "Alcohol Ablation or Ventricular Septal Myotomy/Myectomy for Severe Obstructive Hypertrophic Cardiomyopathy?" with Drs. Joseph Dearani from the Mayo Clinic and Barry Maron from the Hypertrophic Cardiomyopathy Center at the Minneapolis Heart Institute participating.

The discussion focused primarily on: (1) hypertrophic cardiomyopathy (HC) and prevalence of left ventricular outflow obstruction, (2) therapeutic plan for patients with HC, including beta blocker therapy, alcohol ablation and surgical myectomy, (3) gradients for determining suitability for surgery, (4) technique of performing surgical myectomy, (5) post-surgical follow-up patient care, (5) effectiveness of myectomy surgery on patient quality of life, (6) considerations for using alcohol septal ablation, and (7) probability of installing an ICD post surgery. (*Med Roundtable Cardiovasc Ed.* 2010;1(2):128–133) ©2010 FoxP2 Media, LLC

From the Baylor Heart and Vascular Institute, Dallas, TX[1]; the Hypertrophic Cardiomyopathy Center, Minneapolis Heart Institute Foundation, Minneapolis, MN[2]; and the Mayo Clinic, Rochester, MN[3]
Address for correspondence: William Roberts, MD, Baylor Heart and Vascular Institute, 600 Gaston Avenue, Dallas, Texas 75246
E-mail: wc.roberts@baylorhealth.edu
Published online: www.themedicalroundtable.com • Search for ID: CV0032

DR. ROBERTS: Although several case reports and very small series of cases had been reported earlier, hypertrophic cardiomyopathy (HC) was really put on the screen 50 years ago when Braunwald and Morrow reported their first experiences. At the time obstruction to left ventricular outflow was believed to be universal in the condition, and they called it IHSS, or idiopathic hypertrophic subaortic stenosis. Morrow in 1960 devised the ventricular septal myotomy-myectomy procedure, and it proved quite successful in most patients. In 1995, another procedure to reduce or eliminate the outflow gradient was introduced, namely alcohol septal ablation, and it has been employed in hundreds of patients in the last 15 years.

Today we will discuss both of these gradient-reducing procedures, the advantages and disadvantages of each. I'm William C. Roberts, and I'm the Executive Director of the Baylor Heart and Vascular Institute at Baylor University Medical Center in Dallas, Texas. With me are Dr. Barry Maron, who is Director of the Hypertrophic Cardiomyopathy Center in Minneapolis at the Minneapolis Heart Institute Foundation, and Dr. Joseph A. Dearani, who is a cardiovascular surgeon at the Mayo Clinic in Rochester, Minnesota, and the person there who does most of the HC myectomy operations. May we start with you, Dr. Maron? How often do patients with HC have left ventricular outflow obstruction either at rest or with exercise?

DR. MARON: Left ventricular outflow tract obstruction is very common in the overall disease. If you combine those patients with obstruction at rest with those who have obstruction only with physiologic provocation such as exercise, then the percentage could be as high as 75%. Therefore, hypertrophic cardiomyopathy can be regarded as a predominantly obstructive disease which comes full circle, of course, back to the original descriptions of IHSS by Dr. Braunwald that you mentioned.

DR. ROBERTS: You follow a large number of patients with HC. What is your general plan? What percent of these individuals do you send to surgery to do a ventricular septal myotomy-myectomy? Do you send any patients to have alcohol septal ablation? What is the effect of medical therapy alone on the outflow gradient?

DR. MARON: Medical therapy is not usually effective in reducing the outflow gradient. Neither beta blockers nor verapamil have proven to be of value in reducing resting obstruction. The only exception to that would be the possibility that beta blocker therapy can minimize or reduce physiologically provocable outflow tract obstruction with exercise. The concept of reducing the gradient to reduce symptoms continues to require invasive intervention. We call this *septal reduction* to encompass both surgical myectomy, which is a gold standard, and the alternative in very select patients, which is alcohol septal ablation.

The overall percentage of patients who are referred to surgery, of course, depends some on the referral patterns that are operative, but it is a very small percentage of the overall HC patient population who become eligible. These would be those patients who progress in terms of heart failure, usually to New York Heart Association functional class 3 or 4. We are talking about a patient subset here, which is characterized by severe exertional dyspnea. Putting this into real-life terms, it is a patient who cannot walk comfortably for one block on level ground or one flight of stairs.

If patients meet that symptomatic threshold—that is, no longer benefit from and are refractory to drug therapy (which can include beta blockers, verapamil, possibly disopyramide or diuretics), then they become candidates to have the mechanical obstruction or impedance to left ventricular outflow reversed. Obstructive HC is a reversible form of heart failure because it is due to mechanical obstruction, i.e., systolic anterior motion of the mitral valve, and mitral septal contact. So the concept of surgical myectomy—which goes back, as you alluded, to 1960 and Andrew G. Morrow at the National Institutes of Health—is a procedure which removes obstruction and normalizes left ventricular pressures. That dramatically reduces the level of symptoms which patients incur, and it very often returns them to normal activity.

DR. ROBERTS: You do not refer a patient for the operative procedure unless they are quite symptomatic, New York Heart Association 3 or 4?

DR. MARON: Right, the only exception to this would be in children. The principle of the New York Heart Association functional class III doesn't hold as well for them because young children are rarely allowed to progress to that level of limitation. In that age group, surgery is often performed much earlier. Whether it should be performed in asymptomatic children or not is controversial, but it is a question that arises in some young patients because most cardiac surgery for congenital heart disease is, of course, in asymptomatic patients.

DR. ROBERTS: What if the patient has a very high gradient on provocation only, and no gradient at rest, but is quite symptomatic?

DR. MARON: That patient is an operative candidate as well, because the symptoms of heart failure that patients experience occur during exertion. Placing that patient on the treadmill (the Bruce protocol) and eliciting a gradient as well as symptoms during exercise, makes a reasonable connection between the gradient with exercise and external symptoms. Traditionally, those patients have benefitted in a similar fashion as the larger group of patients with rest obstruction.

DR. ROBERTS: What if the patient has a 90 mm peak systolic pressure gradient between the left ventricle and aorta and is asymptomatic?

DR. MARON: It is a subgroup that has always been difficult to manage or make decisions for. I'll put it in a historical context. When myectomy surgery was associated with a higher operative mortality, (5%-8%), which takes us back maybe 25 years, then there was a bias, of course, against operating on asymptomatic or mildly symptomatic patients. Operative mortality today is quite different than 5 decades ago. At centers experienced with the myectomy operation, as Dr. Dearani will be able to tell us, 30-day mortality following surgery is now <1%. It has been more than a decade, for example, at the Mayo Clinic since a patient undergoing a surgical septal myectomy has died as a result of the surgery.

Myectomy has become one of the safest open-heart operations. The question that is sometimes debated now is whether that fact should alter the level of symptoms that would justify surgical myectomy. However, clinical practice at this time is still to reserve surgery for severely symptomatic obstructive patients, because cardiac surgery is always associated with an unpredictable small risk.

DR. ROBERTS: When I was at NIH with you, Barry, Glen Morrow told me he did 299 myotomy-myectomy procedures for patients with HC. As you indicated, the operative mortality at that time over 25 years ago was about 8%, and a few of those patients developed ventricular septal defects. When you say the operative mortality for this procedure now is <1%, you're talking about the operative mortality by a surgeon like Dr. Dearani, who does this procedure many times a year, not once a year as happens it seems to me in many parts of the country. Dr. Dearani, how do you do this procedure, and how do you get such a low mortality and presumably morbidity from the procedure?

DR. DEARANI: Before I answer that I'd like to make a brief comment about the two issues that you just described that are important to me as a surgeon when I'm seeing a patient and discussing the risks and benefits of myectomy. You made a comment about rest gradient versus provocable gradient. For me as a surgeon, there are many patients whom I operate on that have minimal or no pressure gradient between the LV and the aorta at rest, but a substantial gradient with provocation. A thorough echocardiogram should include a rest gradient and some provocative maneuver (amylnitrate or Valsalva) to see what the gradient is with the provocation since this is such a dynamic problem that is dependent on their hydration status, their medical program, etc. At any point in time you can change the echo findings depending upon these variables. It is important to me to know what the provocative gradient is since this usually correlates with exertion. There are many patients who have surgery who have a minimal gradient at rest, but have a considerable gradient with provocation.

The second issue that you commented on was the asymptomatic patient. It should be pointed out that asymptomatic may not mean asymptomatic if they have an abnormal exercise test. Many patients will tell you that they do not have any symptoms, but on exercise, they often have markedly reduced exercise capacity. To me that's not an asymptomatic patient. If they have normal exercise tolerance and report no symptoms, then this is a truly asymptomatic patient. Since many of these patients live a very limited lifestyle, they may appear to be asymptomatic, but with exercise examination they perform poorly indicating that they are not really asymptomatic.

With regard to the operation, the cardiac surgical community has the impression that septal myectomy is not a terribly difficult operation and that many cardiac surgeons can do it. I would say is that it's a hard operation to do well. There is an increasing number of patients being considered for repeat myectomy, and it's usually because the first myectomy was an inadequate myectomy. Looking down the aortic root and carving out the inside of the left ventricle can be quite an intimidating endeavor for a surgeon who's not used to doing it. The risk of aortic valve injury, the risk of mitral valve injury, the risk of ventricular septal defect or heart block is a very real problem for somebody who is not used to doing it.

In addition, the myectomy that we do now is different than the myectomy that Dr. Morrow described some 50 years ago where the myectomy was more limited. We've learned over the last 20 years that the myectomy needs to be much broader, particularly as you get further into the ventricle. This issue of ventricular septal defect that you touched on in the early days resulted from this notion that it was important to focus the myectomy and thinning of the septum right at the base of the heart. This would increase your risk of ventricular septal defect (VSD), and you would just move the point of obstruction a little further into the ventricle. The focus in the current era of myectomy surgery is to make the myectomy wider as you go further in the ventricle.

It is important for the myectomy to be comprehensive opposite the mitral valve and the subvalvular apparatus, including resection of muscle opposite the papillary muscles, opposite the chordae, and opposite the anterior leaflet of the mitral valve. In addition, the extended version of the myectomy also involves limited resection of muscle along the left ventricular free wall extending around toward the anterior mitral valve leaflet. This is very different than what Dr. Morrow discussed many years ago where the myectomy was confined to the basal septum. Now, the extended myectomy includes removing muscle along the left ventricular free wall and a broader resection at the midventricular level.

> ***"It is very common for these patients to report New York Heart Association functional class 1 after myectomy—that is, they can do virtually anything..."***
>
> *- Barry Maron, MD*

Thus, in the current era, the myectomy is a much more comprehensive myectomy than was done in the early years, and the mortality is reportedly low in the hands of surgeons and experienced centers that take care of many patients with hypertrophic cardiomyopathy. It's not an everyday operation for the vast majority of busy cardiac surgeons. The learning curve is steep. And to put it in perspective, it is very difficult for me to teach a resident how to do this operation. In fact, I find it to be one of the hardest operations to teach a resident because you can't see what's being done by the person you are helping. The only person who can see is the person who's holding the knife and performing the myectomy. It's very difficult to coach somebody through it because you can't see at the same time they're doing it to help him/her them navigate where the knife should be going. For all of these reasons, it's an operation that I think is vulnerable to problems when it gets in inexperienced hands. In experienced hands, like everything else, you get good at it, and the mortality and morbidity gets to be quite low.

DR. ROBERTS: How many of these operations do you do a year?

DR. DEARANI: There are two of us at the Mayo Clinic (Dr. Hartzell Schaff and me) who routinely perform the myectomies, and we do between 150 and 200 a year. We each do approximately 75 to 100 cases annually. Our total experience now approaches 2000 cases. Of course, my mentor and predecessor, Dr. Gordon Danielson, was also largely involved with this operation. He helped introduce some of the extended resection maneuvers.

DR. ROBERTS: When I was at the NIH, I saw the portions of ventricular septum that Dr. Morrow would excise in patients with HC. Early on (in the 1960s and 1970s) he excised as much as 15 grams or so, but toward the end of his career, he would take out only about 2 grams. Also, I think toward the end of his career he did more myotomy than myectomy. I would agree that the thickest portion of the ventricular septum is not just below the aortic valve, but is indeed about halfway between the aortic valve and the apex of the left ventricle. How much myocardium do you excise, Dr. Dearani, in your HC patients?

DR. DEARANI: That question is asked by both physicians and patients. It depends on the thickness of the ventricular septum. When the septum is 3–5 cm thick, the amount of muscular resection is substantial. Many grams can come out. In contrast, those with a septum 1.5 cm thick have small amounts of septum excised. In fact, our approach here has been that if they have dynamic left ventricular outflow tract obstruction, which is sort of one of the principle findings with this diagnosis, we always do a myectomy. The magnitude of the myectomy is lessened if the septum is thin. Somebody with a 1.5 cm septum may not have even a gram of muscle excised, whereas somebody who has a septum that's up to 5 cm or more will have multiple grams of muscle excised.

In general, I like to have the remaining septum, particularly at the base of the heart, to be anywhere from 0.5 to 1 cm in thickness.

DR. ROBERTS: Dr. Dearani, when you say you take out some of the muscle of the left ventricular free wall, what do you mean?

DR. DEARANI: It's the posterolateral wall. It's the segment of lateral free wall that is between the anterior leaflet of the mitral valve and the commissure between the left and the right coronary cusps. I begin the myectomy in the middle of the noncoronary cusp, maybe just slightly to the right, being careful of the conduction tissue. Once moving beyond the commissure between the left and the right cusps, this becomes the lateral free wall of the left ventricle and it is not ventricular septum anymore. In many of these patients, as you know, the hypertrophy involves more than just the ventricular septum. If the free wall is also quite hypertrophied, there is an opportunity to enlarge the outflow tract by resecting muscle in this area as well.

DR. ROBERTS: You see these patients after operation for about 30 days and then send them back to their cardiologist.

DR. DEARANI: In our practice at the Mayo Clinic, we have many out of town patients. In general, they're in the hospital about five days, and when they get discharged, many of them will stay in town for a few days and we will see them prior to their departure from Rochester. When they get

> ***"...myotomy-myectomy is the gold standard, but there are a lot of cardiologists around the world now who love injecting alcohol into those septal arteries."***
>
> *– William Roberts, MD*

home they usually follow up with their home medical physician within a week or two. If somebody lives within driving distance of the Mayo Clinic, they usually come back for a followup visit within that first 4-6 weeks.

We keep track of them in our database, and all patients who have had cardiac surgery here, not just the myectomy patients. It's the exception rather than the rule that I would see most of the patients 30-days postoperatively. Many of them are back home by then, and if it's far away they don't make a trip back here for a follow-up visit unless there's a concern that needs to be addressed.

DR. ROBERTS: Dr. Maron, what happens to these patients after ventricular myotomy-myectomy? How many lose their symptoms? How many have the outflow gradient completely obliterated? I remember at NIH virtually all of the patients had left bundle branch block immediately after the procedure. What happens to these patients? You follow them all.

DR. MARON: Surgical myectomy is the gold standard based on the consensus in the cardiovascular community. In other words, it is the primary treatment option. The reason that consensus has been reached is surgical myectomy has proven over this considerable period of time to be highly beneficial in improving the quality of life of patients. Relief of the mechanical impedance to left ventricular outflow normalizes left ventricular systolic pressures and returns these patients to normal or near-normal functional capacity. Very often, as Dr. Dearani will tell you, it is very common for these patients to report New York Heart Association functional class 1 after myectomy—that is, they can do virtually anything, and it makes sense if one understands the basic effect of surgical myectomy.

The second benefit in addition to improvement in quality of life has to do with survival. We published a paper based on the Mayo Clinic operative experience with Dr. Dearani in which Steve Ommen is the first author, showing that many years after surgical myectomy patients had a survival that was equivalent to and did not differ significantly from the general US population. A control group—and I should indicate this was not a randomized study—of patients who had obstruction to left ventricular outflow and were not operated on had a total mortality that was very different. The percentages for total mortality were 83% for the operated patients and 61% for the nonoperated patients. For cardiovascular mortality only, the operated patients (after more than a decade on the average post-myectomy) had a cardiovascular survival rate of 93%. We've learned a lot about long-term effects of surgery that we didn't know before, and the myectomy operation improves quality of life as well as survival, and may allow patients with obstructive HCM who have had surgical myectomy to achieve normal or near-normal longevity.

DR. ROBERTS: Dr. Maron, patients go on the Internet a lot now, and I'm sure some of your patients read about alcohol septal ablation. You talk to them about that alternative procedure. What is your view on alcohol septal ablation? You have stressed that myotomy-myectomy is the gold standard, but there are a lot of cardiologists around the world now who love injecting that alcohol into septal arteries.

DR. MARON: The interventional community has aggressively promoted alcohol septal ablation as a treatment option over the last 15 years. I think Dr. Dearani and I have similar views, and that is that we're we are pleased that there is an alternative to surgical myectomy for those very few patients who require it. The alcohol ablation has been shown to reduce the outflow gradient, and any technique that reduces gradient will probably reduce heart failure symptoms in obstructive HC.

However, the key issue is, are these equivalent procedures? I believe the evidence is that they are not. That argument begins with the principle that alcohol ablation produces a transmural myocardial infarct (intentionally) which occupies 10% on average of the left ventricular wall and as much as 30% of ventricular septum. This is not a small matter. Alcohol ablation is an unusual technique, which has to be considered as such because it is highly destructive to myocardial tissue.

The controversy, which at this time is not completely resolved, has to do with the potential for lethal ventricular tachyarrhythmia that would emanate from that alcohol induced transmural scar. About 10% of patients after alcohol ablation have life-threatening ventricular tachyarrhythmias, which may trigger sudden death. The scar can be arrhythmogenic, at least in some patients. This is one of the reasons that surgical myectomy is regarded as the primary treatment option for most severely symptomatic patients with obstruction.

Now, the exceptions to that could be, for example, patients of advanced age, who, for one reason or another, would not be good operative candidates. For example, any patient who has a morbid fear of open-heart surgery could benefit from the alternative alcohol ablation because no surgeon or cardiologist would want to refer a patient to myectomy who looked upon the operation in that way. Patients with associated diseases, particularly those that elevate the potential risk to surgery could be candidates for alcohol ablation.

> ***"The strategy of, we can use surgery as plan B if plan A, septal alcohol ablation, doesn't work out is really not a good one"***
>
> *- Joseph Dearani, MD*

But the primary issue is age, because if the infarct potentially promotes risk for sudden death and arrhythmia, then patients who are older would be preferred, since they have shorter risk periods. The idea of alcohol ablation in young patients, and this procedure has been performed in patients as young as age 4, doesn't make a lot of sense to many of us who take care of patients with hypertrophic cardiomyopathy.

DR. DEARANI: Another point should be made about the issue of septal alcohol ablation, which I think the patient community and the medical community oftentimes don't realize. There are many patients sent for ventricular septal myotomy/myectomy who have already had a septal alcohol ablation. The rationale is, let's begin with this less invasive technique, and if it doesn't work out, we can then consider surgery. There are a couple of major problems with that strategy. The first is that the risk of myectomy after septal alcohol ablation is not less than 1%. It is definitely higher.

The second issue relates to the comment made earlier about a left bundle branch block with septal myectomy. We haven't mentioned this except in passing, but if the septal myectomy is extended as we do it in the current era, most patients will end up with a left bundle branch block. Importantly, with septal alcohol ablation, many patients will get a right bundle branch block, or they will get complete heart block right after that procedure. Consequently, if myectomy is performed after septal alcohol ablation, many of those patients will require a pacemaker after surgery (if they do not already have one). Also, many of those patients will end up needing a defibrillator because of the preexisting presence of an infarct.

The strategy of, we can use surgery as plan B if plan A, septal alcohol ablation, doesn't work out is really not a good one, since the operative risk is increased and the need for an ICD after surgery increases substantially. In our experience more than 50% will require a device, but in many cases it can approach 90% or more depending upon the nature of the preoperative rhythm.

DR. ROBERTS: Good point. Barry. What about dual chamber pacing? Does anybody do that anymore to lessen the gradient?

DR. MARON: Virtually no one, although I must say it's still popular in Japan, so there are pockets of interest in dual chamber pacing because perhaps other treatments such as surgery or alcohol ablation are not popular in a culture.

I wanted to make one other point; Joe would agree with this. Another limitation of alcohol ablation in addition to the consequence of the scar has to do with ablation and myectomy not providing the same exposure to left ventricular outflow tract anatomy. Alcohol ablation is limited, of course, to the course of the septal perforator that is chosen by the operator for injection.

As we all agree, and Dr. Dearani has described this in some detail, the anatomy of the left ventricular outflow tract is complex in hypertrophic cardiomyopathy, particularly in certain patients, and the extended myectomy that he described has the obvious advantage of direct operative visualization to take into account that structural diversity. The alcohol ablation doesn't have that capability or advantage because, as I have mentioned, it is performed based on the course and distribution of the artery chosen to inject the alcohol. I guess the bottom line to all of this is that these are not at all equal or equivalent procedures.

DR. DEARANI: Another comment worth making about septal alcohol ablation has to do with the anatomy of the outflow tract. There are two anatomic issues that are extremely important and can help guide management. Approximately 5% and at times up to 8% of patients who are referred to the HC clinic at the Mayo Clinic do not have HC, but fixed subaortic stenosis which can only be treated with surgery. Septal alcohol ablation will not treat subaortic stenosis because of the fibrous membrane in the outflow tract.

The second issue regarding anatomy is that there are frequently concomitant abnormalities with the mitral valve, myxomatous abnormalities that would require mitral valve repair, and, other anatomical abnormalities such as, direct insertions of papillary muscles into the anterior leaflet of the mitral valve, accessory papillary muscles, and abnormal chordal attachments into the left ventricular outflow tract. A cardiologist that is thinking about these anatomical issues when an echocardiogram is being performed on a patient with a presumed diagnosis of HC has a responsibility to identify these findings. Importantly, if they are found to be present, then people are not candidates for septal alcohol ablation. They can only be properly treated with surgery so that these other anatomic abnormalities can be addressed at the same time. Of course, if there is myxomatous or ruptured chordae of the mitral valve, then it would need to be addressed at the time of surgery in addition to the myectomy.

DR. ROBERTS: You mean replacing the mitral valve?

DR. DEARANI: No, repairing the mitral valve. The role of mitral valve replacement in the current era is limited to complex mitral valve disease which would include rheumatic mitral valve stenosis and/or stenosis regurgitation where successful mitral valve repair would be unlikely. In this situation, it would be preferable to replace the valve, treating both the problem of outflow tract obstruction and mitral pathology. In this country rheumatic valvular heart disease is not common. Consequently, in an experienced center, the need to resort to mitral valve replacement is going to be less than 2% of the time to treat obstructive hypertrophic cardiomyopathy.

DR. ROBERTS: Dr. Maron has described insertion of one papillary muscle directly into the anterior mitral leaflet, and that does occur in an occasional HC patient. Also, these patients have an increased frequency of infective endocarditis that can tear up the mitral valve. It seems to me that possibly those patients might be candidates for mitral replacement.

DR. DEARANI: Yes.

DR. ROBERTS: Gentlemen, I think we've done it. The conclusion is that the ventricular myotomy-myectomy operation remains the gold standard assuming that the surgery is done by someone who is a student of HC and does a lot of these procedures, not the occasional cardiac surgeon. You would both agree with that, I presume?

DR. MARON AND DR. DEARANI: Yes.

Continue the Discussion:
www.TheMedicalRoundtable.com/Discuss

Some Previously Neglected Examples of Arrhythmogenic Right Ventricular Dysplasia/Cardiomyopathy and Frequency of Its Various Reported Manifestations

William Clifford Roberts, MD[a,b,c,*], Jong Mi Ko, BA[c], Johannes Jacob Kuiper, MD[d], Shelley Anne Hall, MD[d], and Dan Marshall Meyer, MD[d,e]

Four patients are described with either parchment-like thinning or partial but extensive myocyte depletion with severe fatty or fibrofatty infiltration of the free wall of the right ventricle in its outflow tract, including 2 previously reported patients who also had focal parchment-like thinning of the left ventricular free wall. Three had documented ventricular tachycardia, and the remaining patient had sudden death as his first and only manifestation of heart disease. Three patients had severe heart failure: in 1, it was fatal, and the other 2 underwent cardiac transplantation. Necropsy cases of parchment-heart syndrome before 1980 are reviewed, as well as large series of cases with arrhythmogenic right ventricular dysplasia (ARVD) reported subsequently. It is suggested that ARVD is not an ideal name for this condition, because malignant ventricular arrhythmias are not universal, the left ventricular free wall and/or ventricular septum are sometimes involved, and the name "ARVD" neglects the fact that severe heart failure may be prominent in these patients. The right ventricular wall can be thin or parchment-like, or it may not be thinned but consist mainly of adipose tissue with or without focal fibrous tissue and a few islands of myocytes. Nevertheless, because the name "ARVD" has been commonly used and recognized for >30 years, it is probably best retained for this condition. **(Am J Cardiol 2010;106:268–274)**

In 1905, Osler[1] reported a man in his 40s who had died suddenly and unexpectedly while walking up a hill, and necropsy disclosed "parchment-like" thinning of portions of the right and left ventricular free walls in the absence of coronary narrowing or apparent cardiac valve dysfunction. In 1950, Segall[2] described in more detail the patient briefly reported by Osler.[1] The second patient reported (in 1952) to have a parchment-like heart was a 23-year-old woman who had chronic, eventually fatal heart failure and focal thinning of the walls of both ventricles.[3] The third patient, a 7-year-old girl with severe right-sided heart failure and severe thinning of much of the right ventricular free wall, was described by Uhl,[4] also in 1952. Thereafter, through 1980, ≥23 additional patients with parchment-like thinning of the right ventricular wall were reported (Table 1).[5–22] Except for the initial patient reported by Osler[1] and later by Segall[2] and 2 patients reported by Waller et al[23] in 1980, all had myocardial wall thinning limited to the wall of the right ventricle. The 1 patient reported by Osler[1] and later by Segall,[2] the 1 patient reported by Castleman and Sprague,[3] and the 2 patients reported by Waller et al[23] all had congenital hypoplasia of portions of the right and left ventricular free walls in the absence of associated coronary or valvular heart disease. The term "arrhythmogenic right ventricular dysplasia" (ARVD) was first proposed by Fontaine et al[24] in 1977 in a book chapter describing 6 patients with sustained ventricular tachycardia without heart failure and was put on the popular screen by Marcus et al in 1982.[25] Since that time, numerous publications have appeared describing its clinical, radiographic, electrocardiographic, and hemodynamic features. The present report briefly describes again the 2 cases reported by Waller et al[23] in 1980 and describes 2 additional patients, neither diagnosed clinically, with this syndrome treated by cardiac transplantation.

Patients Studied

Pertinent clinical and morphologic features of the 4 patients are listed in Table 2 and illustrated in Figures 1 to 6. One of the 2 earlier cases (patient 1) had severe, eventually fatal heart failure, and in the other (patient 2), sudden death was the first and only manifestation of his cardiac disease.[23] Patients 3 and 4 had severe intractable heart failure and as a consequence underwent cardiac transplantation. Patient 2's mother and sister had pacemakers. Patient 3 had ventricular tachycardia at 12 years of age treated by an ablation procedure, without recurrence thereafter. Patient 4 also had runs of ventricular tachycardia, and patients 3 and 4 underwent intracardiac defibrillator device insertion.

Comments

Described and illustrated herein are 4 patients with clinical and morphologic features of ARVD. Three patients had severe heart failure, 1 fatal and 2 severe enough to warrant

[a]Department of Internal Medicine, Division of Cardiology, [b]Department of Pathology, [c]Baylor Heart and Vascular Institute, [d]Baylor Regional Transplant Institute, and the [e]Department of Cardiothoracic Surgery, Baylor University Medical Center, Dallas, Texas. Manuscript received December 2, 2009; revised manuscript received and accepted March 4, 2010.

*Corresponding author: Tel: 214-820-7911; fax: 214-820-7533.

E-mail address: wc.roberts@baylorhealth.edu (W.C. Roberts).

Table 1
Clinical and morphologic observations in necropsy patients with parchment hearts reported from 1905 to 1979

Study	Age at Death	Gender	HF	Symptom Duration (months)	CE (X-Ray)	Abnormal Results on ECG	Mode of Death	HW (g)	Location of Thinned Ventricular Myocardium			
									RV			LV
									I	A	O	
Patients aged ≤5 years												
Haworth et al (1975)[5]	1 day	M	+	1/30	+	+	HF	—	+	+	0	—
Diaz et al (1973)[6]	4 mo	M	+	4	+	+	HF	—	+	0	0	0
Novak et al (1957)[7]	5 mo	M	+	5	+	+	HF	—	+	+	0	0
Arcilla et al (1961)[8]	6 mo	M	+	6	+	+	HF	—	+	+	+	0
Uhl (1952)[4]	7 mo	F	+	4	+	+	HF	—	+	+	0	0
Cumming et al (1965)[9]	7 mo	F	+	4	+	+	PO	48	0	+	0	0
Aherne (1973)[10]	7 mo	F	+	3	+	+	HF	—	+	+	+	0
Perrin and Mehrizi (1965)[11]	10 mo	M	+	7	+	+	HF	—	0	+	0	0
Sherman (1963)[12]	15 mo	F	+	12	+	+	HF	—	+	+	+	0
Kinare et al (1969)[13]	60 mo	F	+	60	+	+	HF	130	+	+	+	0
Patients aged >15 years												
Abe et al (1973)[14]	17 yrs	F	+	48	+	+	PO	400	0	+	+	0
Murata et al (1976)[15]	18 yrs	F	+	12	+	+	HF	400	0	+	+	0
Froment et al (1968)[16]	19 yrs	M	+	—	+	—	HF	350	0	+	0	—
Vecht et al (1979)[17]	19 yrs	M	+	132	+	+	PO	435	+	0	0	—
Castleman and Sprague (1952)[3]	24 yrs	F	+	12	+	+	HF	300	+	+	+	0
Froment et al (1968)[16]	26 yrs	M	+	—	+	—	HF	430	0	+	0	—
Bharati et al (1978)[18]	29 yrs	F	+	108	+	+	HF+CHB	545	+	+	+	0
Osler (1905)[1] (Segall [1950][2])	40 s	M	—	—	—	—	SD	168	+	+	+	+
Reeve and MacDonald (1964)[19]	47 yrs	F	+	432	+	+	CVA	290	+	0	0	0
Forssman and Bjorkman (1972)[20]	47 yrs	M	0	—	—	+	SD	—	0	+	0	—
Gould et al (1967)[21]	66 yrs	M	0	0	0	0	L	600	+	+	0	0
Sugiura et al (1970)[22]	84 yrs	F	0	0	0	0	AP	220	0	0	+	0

Modified with permission from *Am J Cardiol.*[23]

A = ventricular apex; AP = acute pneumonia; CE = cardiac enlargement; CHB = complete heart block; CVA = cerebrovascular accident; ECG = electrocardiography; HF = heart failure; HW = heart weight; I = inflow tract; L = leukemia; LV = left ventricle; O = outflow tract; PO = early postoperatively; RV = right ventricle; SD = sudden death; — = no information available; + = present or positive; 0 = negative or absent.

Table 2
Clinical and morphologic features in the 4 patients described with arrhythmogenic right ventricular dysplasia

Variable	Patient			
	1	2	3	4
Age (years) at death or CT	61	55	26	44
Gender	Male	Female	Male	Male
Age at symptom onset (years)	61	53	12	42
Heart failure, chronic	0	++++	++++	++++
Ventricular arrhythmia	—	+	+	+
Bundle branch block	—	+	+	+
Body mass index (kg/m^2)	—	17	24	22
Diagnosis of ARVD clinically	0	0	0	0
Clinical diagnosis	SD	Pericardial disease	IDC	HC
Intracardiac defibrillator implanted	0	0	+	+ (2004)
Indirect blood pressure (mm Hg)	130/70	115/80*	100/60	90/60
4-chamber dilatation	0	0	+	+
Pulmonary arterial pressure (mm Hg) (s/d)	—	28/20*	50/30 (mean 38)	19/12 (mean 14)
Cardiac index (L/min/m^2)	—	—	0.8	1.9
Ejection fraction (%)	—	65*	15	25
Heart weight (g)	350	320	595	323

* Cardiac catheterization was performed 21 months before death, and heart failure at that time was purely right sided.

CT = cardiac transplantation; HC = hypertrophic cardiomyopathy; IDC = idiopathic dilated cardiomyopathy; s/d = peak systole/end diastole. Other abbreviations as in Table 1.

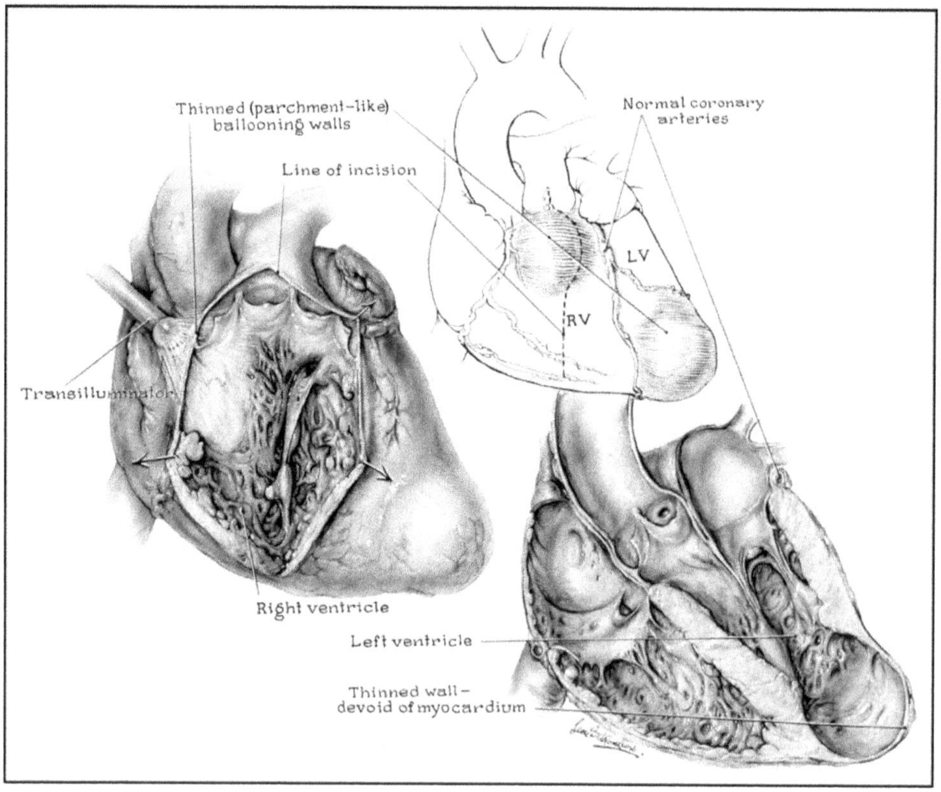

Figure 1. Case 1: drawing of the heart showing the thinned portions of walls of the right ventricle (RV) and left ventricle (LV). Reproduced with permission from *Am J Cardiol*.[23]

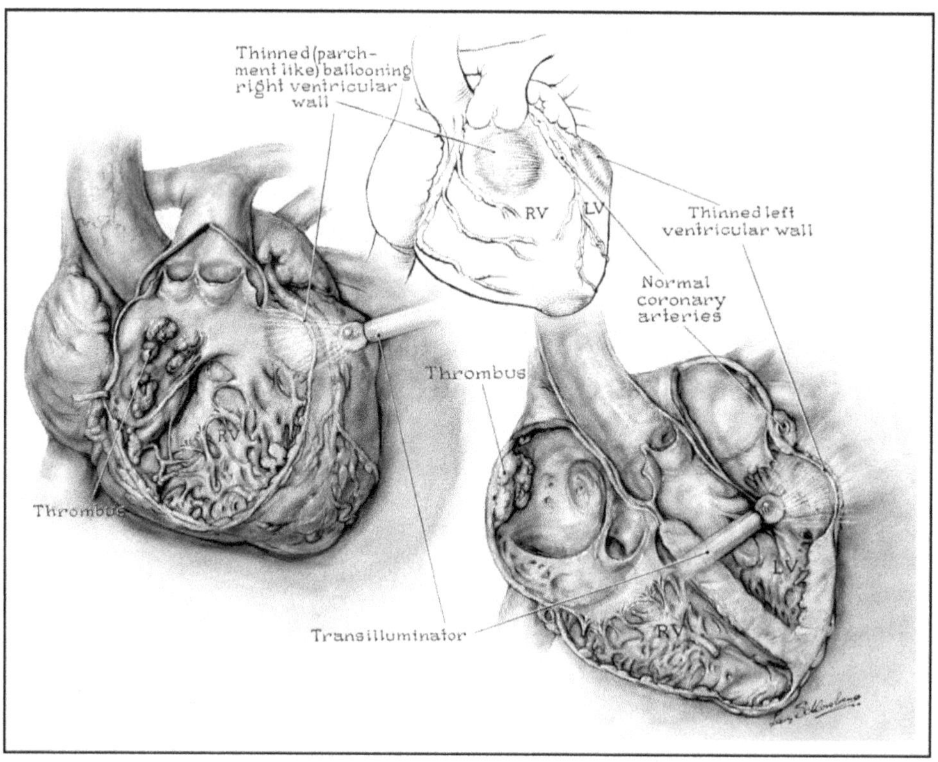

Figure 2. Case 2: drawings of the heart showing thinned portions of the walls of the right ventricle (RV) and left ventricle (LV). Thrombi were present in the right ventricular and right atrial cavities. Reproduced with permission from *Am J Cardiol*.[23]

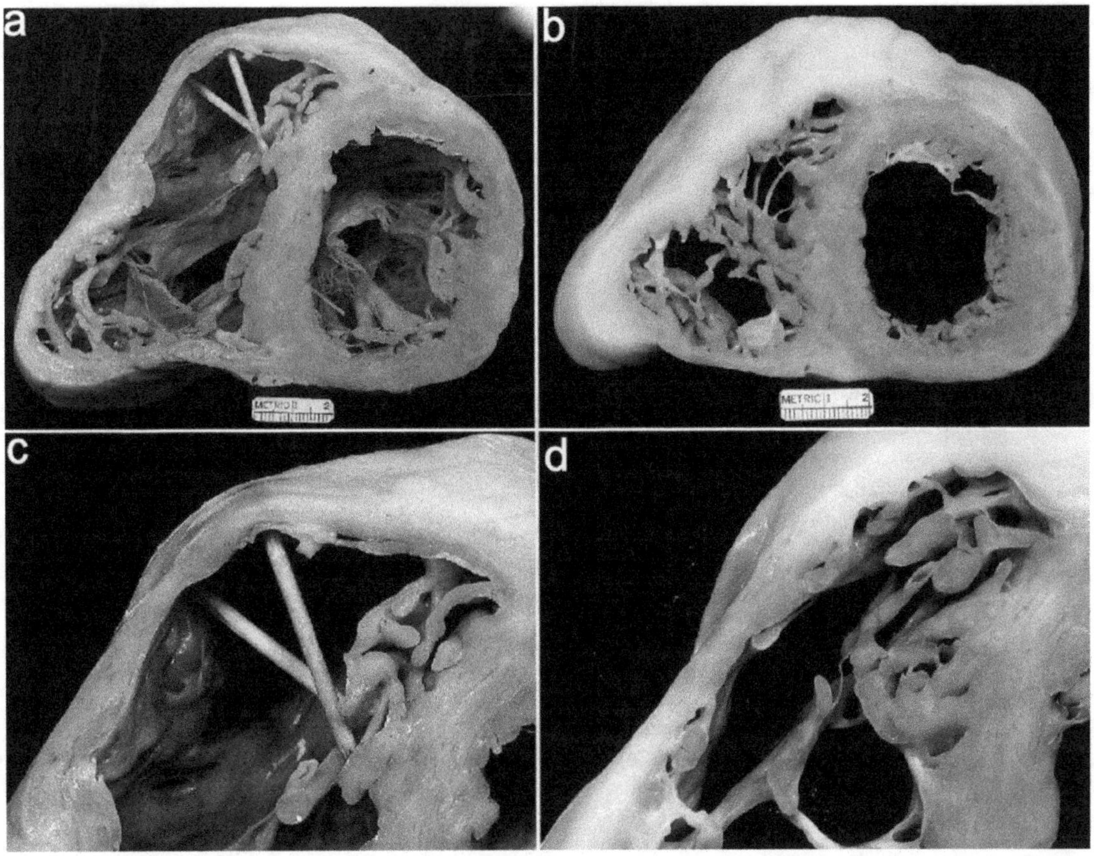

Figure 3. Case 3: cardiac ventricular walls and cavities showing marked dilatation of both cavities *(a,b)* and thinning of the wall in the right ventricular outflow tract *(c,d)*. The amount of subepicardial adipose tissue is excessive.

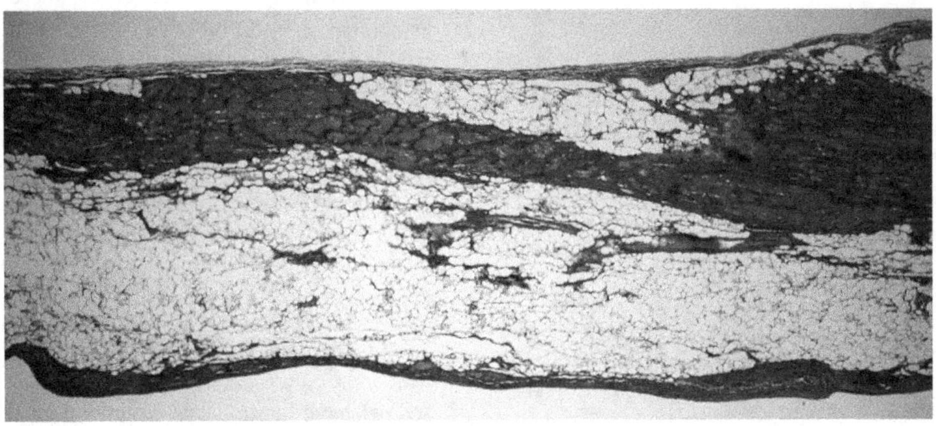

Figure 4. Case 3: photomicrograph (Masson stain, 20×) of the right ventricular wall in its outflow tract. Most of the wall consists of adipose tissue. A thin band of myocardium *(red)* with excessive interstitial fibrous tissue *(blue)* is present.

cardiac transplantation. The other patient died suddenly and unexpectedly, and sudden death was his first manifestation of cardiac disease. Two patients had parchment-like thinning of the right ventricular wall in its outflow portion, and both also had similar thinning in the left ventricular free wall: at its apex in 1 and at its posterobasal portion in the other (Figures 1 and 2). Patients 3 and 4 had fatty infiltrations and partial but severe myocyte depletion in the right ventricular outflow tract. None of the 4 patients had coronary arterial or valvular heart disease. Three had documented ventricular tachycardia, and the 1 who died suddenly while walking presumably also had a "malignant" ventricular arrhythmia.

Table 3 lists selected studies of patients reported with ARVD and the frequency in them of ventricular tachycardia, sudden death, chronic heart failure, left ventricular "dysplasia," and cardiac transplantation.[25–45] Ventricular tachycardia was the most frequent manifestation, but the accuracy of this percentage is unclear. The patients included in the first few studies were referred because of the ventricular arrhythmia, and the necropsy studies had few data on the frequency of these arrhythmias. Sudden, unexpected

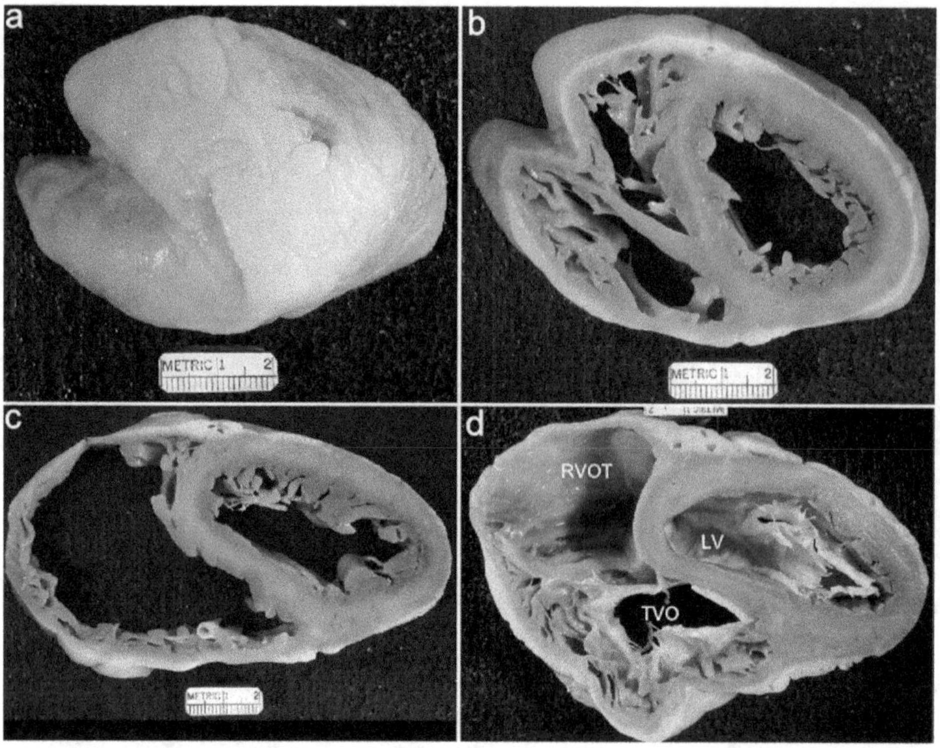

Figure 5. Case 4: heart. *(a)* View from the cardiac apex showing excessive subepicardial adipose tissue and a V-shaped indentation in the right ventricular wall. *(b)* Transverse cut showing the cavities and walls of both cardiac ventricles. The indentation of the right ventricular free wall was caused by the "pull" of a moderator and extending from the right ventricular aspect of the ventricular septum to the right ventricular free wall. *(c)* A more basal view of both ventricles showing the marked dilatation of both cavities, the right greater than the left. *(d)* View showing the very dilated and thin-walled right ventricular outflow tract. LV = left ventricular cavity; RVOT = right ventricular outflow tract; TVO = tricuspid valve orifice.

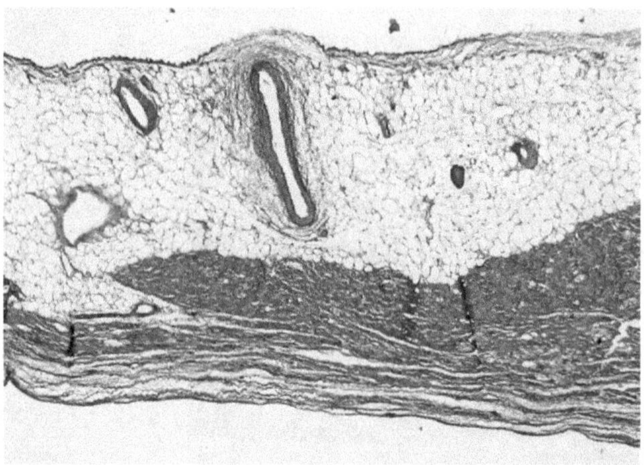

Figure 6. Case 4: photomicrograph (Masson stain, 40×) of the wall of the right ventricle in its outflow portion showing the wall to consist mainly of adipose tissue and scarred *(blue)* myocardium *(red)*.

death was the next most frequent manifestation. Chronic heart failure, as occurred in 3 of our 4 patients, was far less common. Some type of left ventricular dysfunction or wall motion abnormality was mentioned in a number of reports. Relatively few patients underwent cardiac transplantation.

Gerlis et al[46] distinguished between Uhl's anomaly and ARVD but suggested, as we do, that the term "Uhl's anomaly" has frequently been used to describe cases that should be considered examples of ARVD. From a study of 5 patients (2 with Uhl's anomaly and 3 with ARVD) and review of many published cases, these investigators proposed that "Uhl's anomaly" might best be limited to cases in which there is a paper-thin right ventricular free wall, with complete absence of myocardium and "apposition of the endocardial and epicardial layers," and that ARVD be characterized by cases with localized fibrofatty tissue replacement of the right ventricular free wall.

Although most clinicians now call this condition ARVD, that term does not recognize that the only common denominator of this condition is marked focal thinning of the right ventricular free wall or infiltration of that wall by adipose tissue with or without fibrous tissue. Similar focal thinning or fatty or fibrous replacement of the left ventricular free wall may also occur.[23,43,47–53] Although no reports of ARVD have included patients without focal right ventricular free wall thinning or virtual fatty replacement, it is possible that patients with isolated focal left ventricular free wall thinning—diverticuli or left ventricular aneurysm in the absence of coronary arterial narrowing or sarcoidosis—may also be a part of ARVD. Recently, Coats et al[54] described such a case. That heart failure may be its most prominent feature and that it may occur in the absence of a malignant ventricular arrhythmia is not suggested by the term "ARVD." Nevertheless, the phrase is probably here to stay.

1. Osler W. The Principles and Practice of Medicine. 6th ed. New York: Appleton Century Crofts, 1905:820.
2. Segall HN. Parchment heart (Osler). *Am Heart J* 1950;40:948–950.

Table 3
Patients reported with arrhythmic right ventricular dysplasia from 1982 to 2005

Study	Number of Patients	M	F	Age (years) Range (Mean)	VT	SD	HF	LVD	CT	Follow–up (Years) Range (Mean)	Death
				Mainly clinical studies							
Marcus et al (1982)[25]	24	16	8	17–65 (39)	22	0	0	1	0	0.1–12.7 (3)	2*
Reiter et al (1983)[26]	7	4	3	13–69 (39)	7	1	0	0	0	—	0
Manyari et al (1983)[27]	6	4	2	21–60 (41)	6	0	0	5[†]	0	—	0
Blomström-Lundqvist et al (1987)[28]	15	10	5	7–50 (27)	14	2	3	3	0	1.5–28 (9)	3
Marcus et al[‡] (1989)[29]	6	5	1	26–41 (34)	4	0	0	0	0	1–20	
Lemery et al (1989)[30]	12	—	—	21–54 (33)	12	0	0	2	0	2.5–15 (8)	1
Pinamonti et al (1995)[31]	45	27	18	0.33–59 (32)	14	3	6	10	1	1–23 (8.2)	8
Kullo et al (1995)[32]	20	8	12	3–60 (30)	9	2	5	10	2	2–17 (7)	4
Hulot et al (2004)[33]	130	100	30	10–73 (—)	102	7	8	13	0	8 ± 8	24
Dalal et al (2005)[34]	100[§]	51	49	2–70 (—)	47/69	31	5	0	2	0–37 (median 6)	34
Tops et al (2009)[35]	52	22	30	41 ± 12	14	0	0	0	0	—	0
Marcus et al (2009)[36]	95	35	60	38 ± 14	72	0	6	0	0	1.3 ± 1.1	0
				Mainly morphologic studies							
Basso et al (1996)[38]	30[‖]	20	10	15–65 (28)	15/19	24	3	14	3	—	27
Corrado et al (1997)[40]	42	27	15	9–65 (30)	17	34	8	32[¶]	4	—	38
Burke et al (1998)[41]	25	20	5	13–72 (31)	10**	23	2	16	0	—	25
Fornes et al (1998)[42]	20	9	11	17–80 (41)	—	20	0	8	0	—	20
Lobo et al (1999)[43]	26[††]	14	3	16–60 (—)	—	15	—	17/22	2		15
D'Amati et al (2001)[44]	27	16	11	12–66 (—)	9/22[‡‡]	11/12	15	15	15	—	12
Tabib et al (2003)[45]	200	108	92	1–65 (33)	4	158	0	8	0	—	200

* Five more patients died as described in Marcus et al's[29] 1989 follow-up study. Seven of the 25 patients subsequently developed chronic HF.
[†] Left ventricular wall motion abnormalities.
[‡] This study provides follow-up in 20 of the 22 patients initially alive when reported by Marcus et al[25] in 1982; it adds 6 new patients studied by Marcus et al and provides follow-up for the 7 patients reported by Reiter et al[26] in 1983.
[§] These patients were also included in Jain R, Dalal D, Daly A, Tichnell C, James C, Evenson A, Jain R, Abraham T, Tan BY, Tandri H, Russell SD, Judge D, Calkins H. Electrocardiographic features of arrhythmogenic right ventricular dysplasia. *Circulation* 2009;120:477–487.
[‖] These 30 patients include the 12 previously reported by Thiene et al[37] in 1988. Only 4 of these 30 had the diagnosis of arrhythmogenic right ventricular cardiomyopathy made during life. This number was 36 in Corrado D, Basso C, Thiene G. Sudden cardiac death in young people with apparently normal heart. *Cardiovasc Res* 2001;50:399–408.
[¶] Observed histologically only in 15 and both grossly and histologically in 17.
** "Arrhythmic or syncope."
[††] Gender not given for 9 patients.
[‡‡] Included only patients with electrocardiograms.
CT = cardiac transplantation; F = female; HF = heart failure; LVD = left ventricular dysplasia; M = men; SD = sudden death; VT = ventricular tachycardia.

3. Castleman B, Sprague HB. Case records of the Massachusetts General Hospital. Weekly clinicopathological exercises. *N Engl J Med* 1952; 246:785–790.
4. Uhl HS. A previously undescribed congenital malformation of the heart: almost total absence of the myocardium of the right ventricle. *Bull Johns Hopkins Hosp* 1952;91:197–209.
5. Haworth SG, Shinebourne EA, Miller GAH. Right to left interatrial shunting with normal right ventricular pressure. *Br Heart J* 1975;37: 386–391.
6. Diaz LP, Jimenez MQ, Granados FM, Martinez VP, Batres GM. Congenital absence of myocardium of right ventricle: Uhl's anomaly. *Br Heart J* 1973;35:570–572.
7. Novak G, Szanto PB, Gasul B, Dillon E. Congenital aplasia of the myocardium of the right ventricle. *Proc Inst Med Chic* 1957;21:334–339.
8. Arcilia RA, Gasul BM. Congenital aplasia or marked hypoplasia of the myocardium. *J Pediatr* 1961;58:381–388.
9. Cumming GR, Bowman JM, Whytehead L. Congenital aplasia of the myocardium of the right ventricle (Uhl's anomaly). *Am Heart J* 1965; 70:671–676.
10. Aherne WA. Uhl's anomaly [abstract]. *Arch Dis Child* 1973;48:160.
11. Perrin EV, Mehrizi A. Isolated free-wall hypoplasia of the right ventricle. *Am J Dis Child* 1965;109:558–566.
12. Sherman FE. An Atlas of Congenital Heart Disease. Philadelphia: Lea & Febiger, 1963:270, 290–291.
13. Kinare SG, Panday SR, Deshmukh SM. Congenital aplasia of the right ventricular myocardium (Uhl's anomaly). *Chest* 1969;55:429–431.
14. Abe T, Kuribayashi R, Sato M, Nieda S, Abe S. Congenital hypoplasia of the right ventricular myocardium (Uhl's anomaly). A case report and review of literature. *J Cardiovasc Surg* 1973;14:431–438.
15. Murata K, Matsuo H, Yoshitake Y, Ishizawa Y, Shigiya R, Okamato K. Functionally atrialized parchment-like right ventricle with extensive myocardial fibrosis of left ventricle. *Jpn Heart J* 1976;17:428–435.
16. Froment R, Perrin A, Loire R, Dalloz CJ. Ventricule droit papyrace du jeune adultre par dystrophie congenitale. *Arch Mal Coeur* 1968;61: 477–503.
17. Vecht RJ, Carmichael JS, Gopal R, Philip G. Uhl's anomaly. *Br Heart J* 1979;41:676–682.
18. Bharati S, Ciraulo DA, Bilitch M, Rosen KM, Lev M. Inexcitable right ventricle and bilateral bundle branch block in Uhl's disease. *Circulation* 1978;57:636–644.
19. Reeve R, MacDonald D. Partial absence of the right ventricular musculature—partial parchment heart. *Am J Cardiol* 1964;14:415–419.
20. Forssman O, Bjorkman G. Absence of the solid part of the right ventricular musculature. *Acta Pathol Microbiol Scand[A]* 1972;80: 263–270.

21. Gould K, Guttman AB, Carrasco J, Lyon AF. Partial absence of the right ventricular musculature. A congenital lesion. *Am J Med* 1967; 42:636–641.
22. Sugiura M, Hayashi T, Ueno K. Partial absence of the right ventricular muscle in an aged. *Jpn Heart J* 1970;11:582–585.
23. Waller BF, Smith ER, Blackbourne BD, Arce FP, Sarkar NN, Roberts WC. Congenital hypoplasia of portions of both right and left ventricular myocardial walls. Clinical and necropsy observations in two patients with parchment heart syndrome. *Am J Cardiol* 1980;46:885–891.
24. Fontaine G, Guiraudon G, Frank R, Vedel J, Grosgogeat Y, Cabrol C, Facquet J. Stimulation studies and epicardial mapping in ventricular tachycardia: study of mechanism and selection for surgery. In: Kulbertus H, ed. Reentrant Arrhythmias, Mechanism and Treatment. Lancaster, Pennsylvania: MTP Publishing, 1977:334.
25. Marcus FI, Fontaine GH, Guiraudon G, Frank R, Laurenceau JL, Malergue C, Grosgogeat Y. Right ventricular dysplasia: a report of 24 adult cases. *Circulation* 1982;65:384–398.
26. Reiter MJ, Smith WM, Gallagher JJ. Clinical spectrum morphology. *Am J Cardiol* 1983;51:113–121.
27. Manyari DE, Klein GJ, Gulamhusein S, Boughner D, Guiraudon GM, Wyse G, Mitchell B, Kostuk WJ. Arrhythmogenic right ventricular dysplasia: a generalized cardiomyopathy? *Circulation* 1983;68:251–257.
28. Blomström-Lundqvist C, Sabel KG, Olsson SB. A long term follow-up of 15 patients with Arrhythmogenic right ventricular dysplasia. *Br Heart J* 1987;58:477–488.
29. Marcus FI, Fontaine GH, Frank R, Gallagher JJ, Reiter MJ. Long-term follow-up in patients with arrhythmogenic right ventricular disease. *Eur Heart J* 1989;10(suppl):68–73.
30. Lemery R, Brugada P, Janssen J, Cheriex E, Dugernier T, Wellens HJJ. Nonischemic sustained ventricular tachycardia: clinical outcome in 12 patients with arrhythmogenic right ventricular dysplasia. *J Am Coll Cardiol* 1989;14:96–105.
31. Pinamonti B, Di Lenarda A, Sinagra G, Silvestri F, Bussani R, Camerini F. Long-term evolution of right ventricular dysplasia-cardiomyopathy. *Am Heart J* 1995;129:412–415.
32. Kullo IJ, Edwards WD, Seward JB. Right ventricular dysplasia: the Mayo Clinic experience. *Mayo Clin Proc* 1995;70:541–548.
33. Hulot JS, Jouven X, Empana JP, Frank R, Fontaine G. Natural history and risk stratification of arrhythmogenic right ventricular dysplasia/cardiomyopathy. *Circulation* 2004;110:1879–1884.
34. Dalal D, Nasir K, Bomma C, Prakasa K, Tandri H, Piccini J, Roguin A, Tichnell C, James C, Russell SD, Judge DP, Abraham T, Spevak PJ, Bluemke DA, Calkins H. Arrhythmogenic right ventricular dysplasia. A United States experience. *Circulation* 2005;112:3823–3832.
35. Tops LF, Prakasa K, Tandri H, Dalal D, Jain R, Dimaano VL, Dombroski D, James C, Tichnell C, Daly A, Marcus F, Schalij MJ, Bax JJ, Bluemke D, Calkins H, Abraham TP. Prevalence and pathophysiologic attributes of ventricular dyssynchrony in arrhythmogenic right ventricular dysplasia/cardiomyopathy. *J Am Coll Cardiol* 2009;54:445–451.
36. Marcus GM, Glidden DV, Polonsky B, Zareba W, Smith LM, Cannom D, Estes NAM III, Marcus F, Scheinman MM. Efficacy of antiarrhythmic drugs in arrhythmogenic right ventricular cardiomyopathy. A report from the North American ARVC registry. *J Am Coll Cardiol* 2009;54:609–615.
37. Thiene G, Nava A, Corrado D, Rossi L, Pennelli N. Right ventricular cardiomyopathy and sudden death in young people. *N Engl J Med* 1988;318:129–133.
38. Basso C, Thiene G, Corrado D, Angelini A, Nava A, Valente M. Arrhythmogenic right ventricular cardiomyopathy. *Circulation* 1996; 94:983–991.
39. Basso C, Corrado D, Marcus F. Arrhythmogenic right ventricular cardiomyopathy. *Lancet* 2009;373:1289–1300.
40. Corrado D, Basso C, Thiene G, McKenna WJ, Davies M, Fontaliran F, Nava A, Silvestri F, Blomström-Lundqvist C, Wlodarska EK. Spectrum of clinicopathologic manifestations of arrhythmogenic right ventricular cardiomyopathy/dysplasia: a multicenter study. *J Am Coll Cardiol* 1997;30:1512–1520.
41. Burke AP, Farb A, Tashko G, Virmani R. Arrhythmogenic right ventricular cardiomyopathy and fatty replacement of the right ventricular myocardium. Are they different diseases? *Circulation* 1998;97: 1571–1580.
42. Fornes P, Ratel S, Lecomte D. Pathology of arrhythmogenic right ventricular cardiomyopathy/dysplasia-an autopsy study of 20 forensic cases. *J Forensic Sci* 1998;43:777–783.
43. Lobo FV, Silver MD, Butany J, Heggtveit HA. Left ventricular involvement in right ventricular dysplasia/cardiomyopathy. *Can J Cardiol* 1999;15:1239–1247.
44. D'Amati G, Leone O, Di Gioia CRT, Magelli C, Arpesella G, Grillo P, Marino B, Fiore F, Gallo P. Arrhythmogenic right ventricular cardiomyopathy: clinicopathologic correlation based on a revised definition of pathologic patterns. *Hum Pathol* 2001;32:1078–1086.
45. Tabib A, Loire R, Chalabreysse L, Meyronnet D, Miras A, Malicier D, Thivolet F, Chevalier P, Bouvagnet P. Circumstances of death and gross and microscopic observations in a series of 200 cases of sudden death associated with arrhythmogenic right ventricular cardiomyopathy and/or dysplasia. *Circulation* 2003;108:3000–3005.
46. Gerlis LM, Schmidt-Ott SC, Ho SY, Anderson RH. Dysplastic conditions of the right ventricular myocardium: Uhl's anomaly v arrhythmogenic right ventricular dysplasia. *Br Heart J* 1993;69:142–150.
47. Webb JG, Kerr CR, Huckell VF, Mizgala HF, Ricci DR. Left ventricular abnormalities in arrhythmogenic right ventricular dysplasia. *Am J Cardiol* 58;1986:568–570.
48. Horimoto M, Funayama N, Satoh M, Igarashi T, Sekiguchi M. Histological evidence of left ventricular involvement in arrhythmogenic right ventricular dysplasia. *Jpn Circ J* 1989;53:1530–1534.
49. Nishikawa H, Kasai A, Ono N, Unno M, Kakuta Y, Nishimura S, Nishiyama S, Nakanishi S, Seki A, Nakano T. Two cases of biventricular dysplasia associated with ventricular tachycardia and familial occurrence of sudden death. *J Cardiol* 1991;21:735–747.
50. Shoji T, Kaneko M, Onodera K, Konnno A, Hasegawa T, Ikeda T, Minase T, Uchiyama S, Iwamoto M. Arrhythmogenic right ventricular dysplasia with massive involvement of the left ventricle. *Can J Cardiol* 1991;7:303–307.
51. Pinamonti B, Sinagra G, Salvi A, Di Lenarda A, Morgera T, Silvestri F, Bussani R, Camerini F. Left ventricular involvement in right ventricular dysplasia. *Am Heart J* 1992;123:711–724.
52. Gallo P, D'Amati G, Pelliccia F. Pathologic evidence of extensive left ventricular involvement in arrhythmogenic right ventricular cardiomyopathy. *Hum Pathol* 1992;23:948–952.
53. Sugrue DD, Edwards WD, Olney BA. Histolgic abnormalities of the left ventricle in a patient with arrhythmogenic right ventricular dysplasia. *Heart Vessels* 1958;1:179–181.
54. Coats CJ, Quarta G, Flett AS, Pantazis AA, McKenna WJ, Moon JC. Arrhythmogenic left ventricular cardiomyopathy. *Circulation* 2009; 120:2613–2614.

Examination of Isolated Ventricular Noncompaction (Hypertrabeculation) as a Distinct Entity in Adults

William Clifford Roberts, MD[a,b,d,*], Sumit Jagdish Karia, MD[a], Jong Mi Ko, BA[d], Paul Arthur Grayburn, MD[a,d], Betsy Ann George, MD[a], Shelley Anne Hall, MD[a], Johannes Jacob Kuiper, MD[a,d], and Dan Marshall Meyer, MD[c,e]

Three patients (2 women) 36, 45, and 49 years of age underwent cardiac transplantation for what was diagnosed clinically as nonischemic dilated cardiomyopathy. Examination of the transthoracic echocardiogram and explanted heart in each disclosed marked hypertrabeculation involving the free wall of the very dilated left ventricle, a finding consistent with what has been termed "isolated ventricular noncompaction" (IVNC). Although these 3 cases anatomically fulfilled the echocardiographic definition of IVNC, review of previous publications containing gross photographs of the heart suggests that IVNC is overdiagnosed at least morphologically. **(Am J Cardiol 2011;108:747–752)**

Although newborns with aortic valve atresia unassociated with mitral valve atresia have true sinusoids from the endocardium that burrow into the myocardium, the endocardium is smooth and devoid of trabeculations.[1] Therefore, it is not proper in our view to consider the left ventricle in aortic valve atresia unassociated with mitral valve atresia an example of ventricular noncompaction as has been done. The first description of what later came to be termed "isolated ventricular noncompaction" (IVNC) in an adult was by Engberding and Bender[2] who described a 33-year-old woman with heart failure, left bundle branch block, marked left ventricular dilatation, and echocardiographically demonstrated large trabeculations (called "sinusoids" by the investigators) within the left ventricular cavity. Subsequently, numerous reports have appeared describing—mainly by echocardiogram—features of IVNC.[3–36] The present report describes morphologic features of hearts in 3 adults who underwent cardiac transplantation and the explanted hearts were characteristic of IVNC. In addition, previous published reports illustrating the heart at necropsy or after cardiac transplantation are reviewed to determine if IVNC is overdiagnosed at least morphologically.

Methods

Pertinent clinical and morphologic features in each of the 3 patients are presented in Table 1, and transthoracic echocardiographic and morphologic features are illustrated in Figures 1 through 6. All 3 patients had evidence of chronic heart failure for 7, 10, and 12 years before cardiac transplantation at 36, 45, and 49 years of age, respectively. Three had episodes of ventricular tachycardia, and patient 2 had ventricular tachycardia ablation procedures on >1 occasion. All 3 had elevated pulmonary arterial pressures, low systemic arterial pressures, low cardiac indices, and very low left ventricular ejection fractions. All 3 by angiography had normal epicardial coronary arteries. None had a neuromuscular disorder. Examination of explanted hearts from all patients disclosed increased cardiac weight and hugely dilated left ventricular cavities with noncompacted portions of left ventricular free walls ≥2 times as thick as the compacted portions of these walls. Patient 1 had an organizing thrombus in the apex of the left ventricle. Patient 3 had an episode typical of transient ischemic attack. Patients 2 and 3 each had small transmural left ventricular free wall scars. Histologically, myofibers in each were hypertrophied, inflammatory cells were absent, and interstitial fibrous tissue was focally increased in the ventricular walls.

Comments

Each of the 3 patients described had excessive ventricular trabeculations in very dilated left ventricles, bundle branch block, periodic ventricular tachycardia, severe heart failure, and finally cardiac transplantation.

What is IVNC in adults? Is it really a distinctive entity? Oechslin et al[6] from Zurich described 34 adults with IVNC and stated that ". . . the characteristic discriminating feature . . . [of IVNC is a] . . . two layered myocardial wall structure with both a thin epicardial compacted zone and an extremely thickened endocardial non-compacted zone with deep recesses filled with blood from the ventricular cavity." In 2006 alone, 3 reports described 61, 53, and 57 patients, respectively, >15 years of age with IVNC, each from sep-

Departments of [a]Internal Medicine, [b]Pathology, and [c]Cardiothoracic Surgery, and the [d]Baylor Heart and Vascular Institute, Baylor University Medical Center, Dallas, Texas; [e]Department of Thoracic and Cardiovascular Surgery, University of Texas Southwestern Medical Center, Dallas, Texas. Manuscript received February 22, 2011; revised manuscript received and accepted April 24, 2011.

*Corresponding author: Tel: 214-820-7911; fax: 214-820-7533.

E-mail address: wc.roberts@baylorhealth.edu (W.C. Roberts)

Table 1
Features of the three patients described

Variable	Patient 1	Patient 2	Patient 3
Age (years) at cardiac transplantation	36	45	49
Month and year of cardiac transplantation	October 2008	March 2011	May 2011
Gender	Woman	Man	Woman
Age (years) at onset of signs and symptoms of cardiac dysfunction	26	33	42
Chronic heart failure	+	+	+
Atrial fibrillation	+	0	+
Ventricular tachycardia	+	+	+
Intracardiac pressures (mm Hg)			
Mean pulmonary arterial wedge	29	35	25*
Pulmonary artery (peak systolic pressure/end-diastolic pressure)	60/30	55/27	54/22*
Right ventricle (peak systolic pressure/end-diastolic pressure)	60/5	55/18	54/17*
Right atrium (mean)	14	8	14*
Aorta (peak systolic pressure/end-diastolic pressure)	90/60†	90/50†	100/80*
Cardiac index (L/min/m²)	1.8	1.8	2.0*
Left ventricular ejection fraction (%)	10	15	5
Automatic implantable cardioverter–defibrillator cardiac resynchronizing therapy	+	+	+
Left bundle branch block	+	+	0
Total cholesterol (mg/dl)	110	160	147
Body mass index (kg/m²)	19.6	26.6	22.1
Heart weight (g)	420	530	360
Maximal left ventricular cavity (cm)	7.0	7.0	8.0
Scar, left ventricular wall	0	+	+

* Recorded 14 months before heart transplantation.
† Indirect pressure.

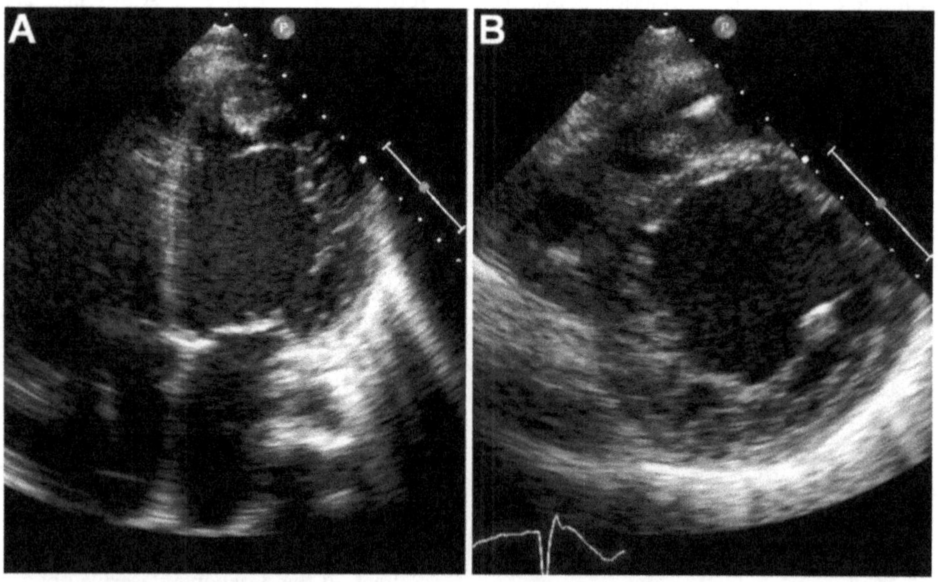

Figure 1. Patient 1. Echocardiogram. *(A)* Four-chamber view shows a dilated left ventricular cavity with excessive trabeculations and a thrombus in the apex. *(B)* Short-axis view demonstrates trabeculations better than in the 4-chamber view.

arate single medical centers.[13,21,22] In 2007 another 65 adults were reported,[23] in 2008 another 60 adults were reported,[33] and in 2010, 140 more adults were reported, each study from single medical centers.[22] In addition, many other case studies and small series of patients have been described.

In the many publications on IVNC, most from Europe, we found 18 gross photographs of the heart in adults in peer-reviewed journals.[3–20] Of these, in the view of 1 of the authors (W.C.R.), only 7 of the 18 cases represent clear examples of IVNC (hypertrabeculation).[3,4,7,8,11,13] Burke et al[11] were the only investigators to report and illustrate morphologically 2 adults with IVNC. One was an 18-year-old man who underwent cardiac transplantation for chronic heart failure. The second was a 30-year-old man who died suddenly and had a nondilated left ventricular cavity. (A beautiful example of IVNC was a heart prepared by Dr. William D. Edwards and published in an *Up-to-Date* piece in 2011 authored by Dr. H.M. Connolly and Dr. C.H.A. Jost.) The photograph shown of

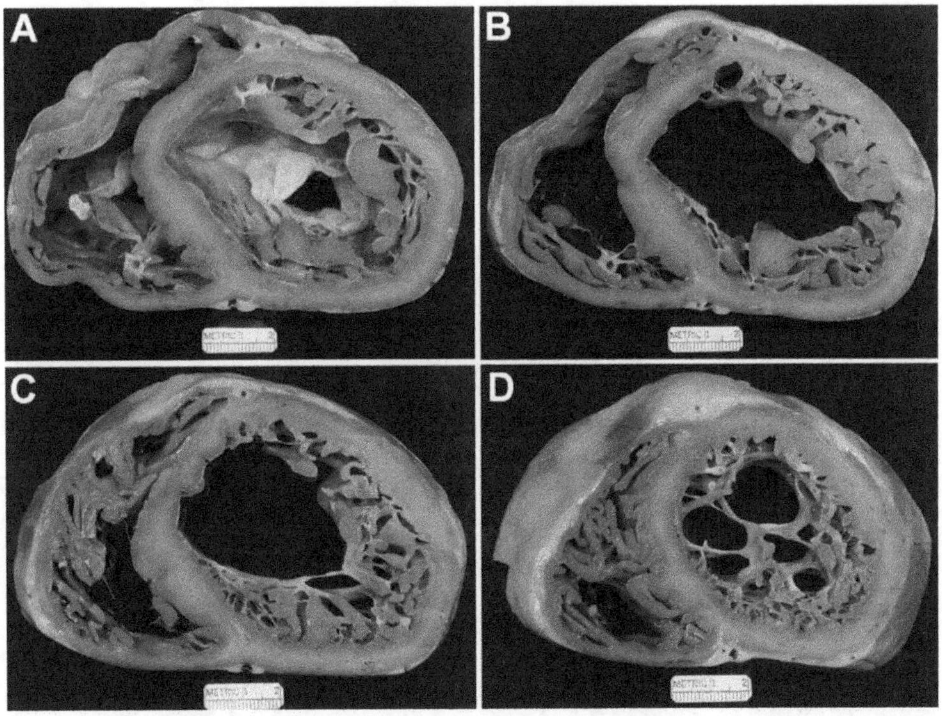

Figure 2. Patient 1. Explanted heart. Views of the right and left ventricles at 4 different levels: *(A)* near the base exposing the tricuspid and mitral valves, *(B, C)* intermediate levels, and *(D)* near the apex. The noncompacted portion of the free wall of the left ventricle is thicker than the compacted portion of the wall.

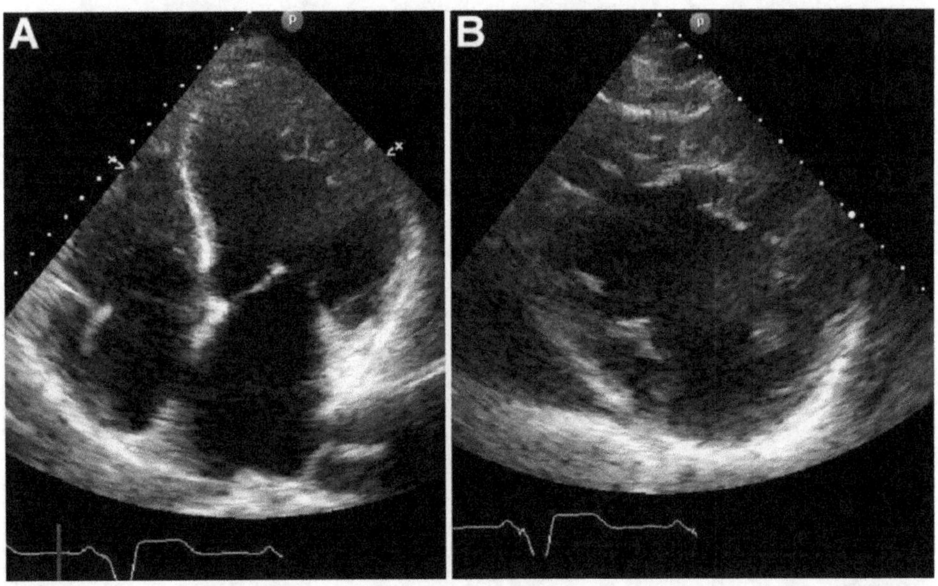

Figure 3. Patient 2. Echocardiogram. *(A)* Four-chamber view shows a dilated left ventricular cavity with excessive trabeculations. *(B)* Short-axis view demonstrates trabeculations better than in the 4-chamber view.

the heart in 1 report appears to be a classic example of cor pulmonale.[6] Most published illustrated hearts were opened when fresh by cuts according to the flow of blood. These cuts result in flattened cardiac chambers and then comparison of the thickness of the compacted to that of the noncompacted portions of the cardiac ventricles is more difficult to discern. Cuts of the ventricles made parallel to the posterior atrioventricular sulcus after fixation appears to provide the best opportunity of demonstrating ventricular hypertrabeculation if present.

In Table 2 we attempt to show various characteristics of patients with 4 different types of cardiomyopathies. The various clinical features of IVNC and idiopathic dilated cardiomyopathy are virtually identical. Clearly, hypertrophic cardiomyopathy is the most distinctive. Whether IVNC deserves a special characterization is debatable.

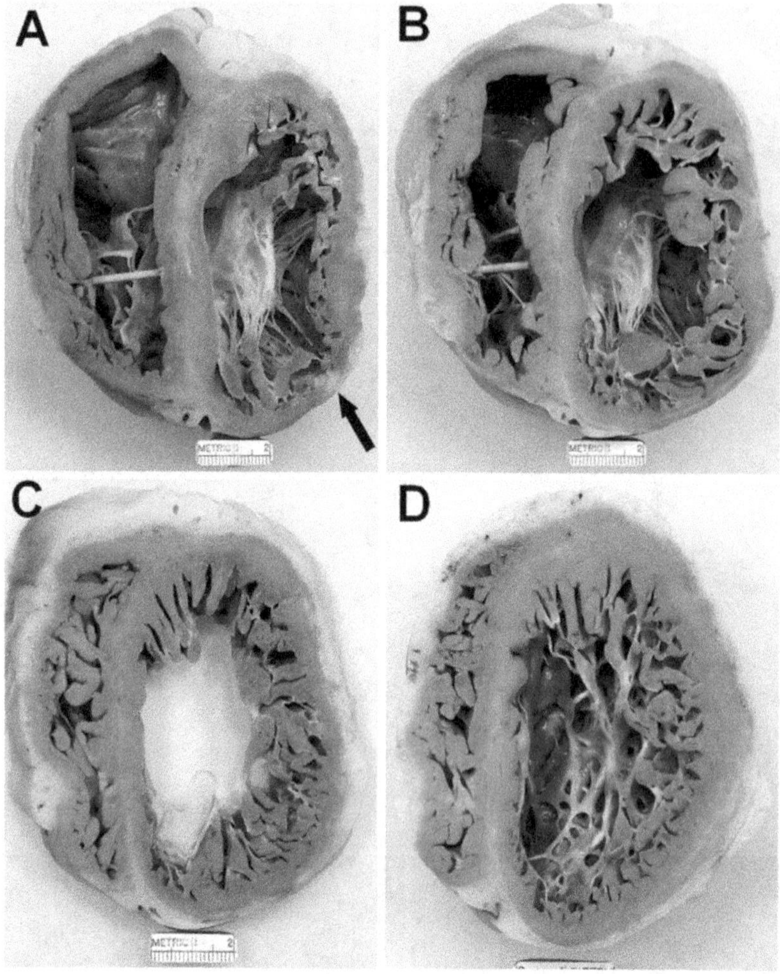

Figure 4. Patient 2. Views of the right and left ventricles at 4 different levels: *(A)* near the base exposing the tricuspid and mitral valves, *(B, C)* intermediate levels, and *(D)* near the apex. A small scar *(arrow)* is present in the left ventricular wall. The noncompacted portion of the left ventricular free wall is thicker than the compacted portion, which is especially thin in the basilar portion *(A, B)*.

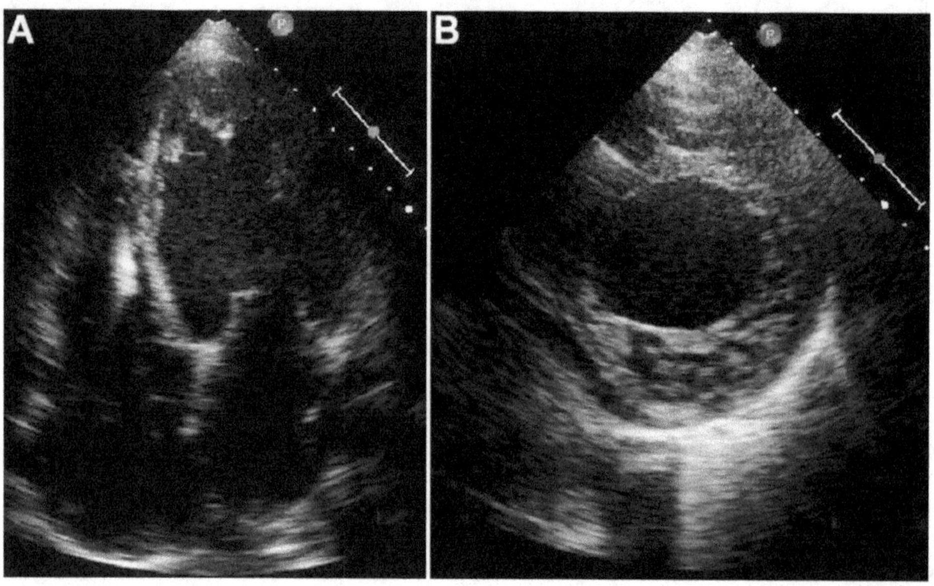

Figure 5. Patient 3. Echocardiogram. *(A)* Four-chamber view shows a dilated left ventricular cavity with excessive trabeculations. *(B)* Short-axis view demonstrates excessive trabeculations in the left ventricular cavity.

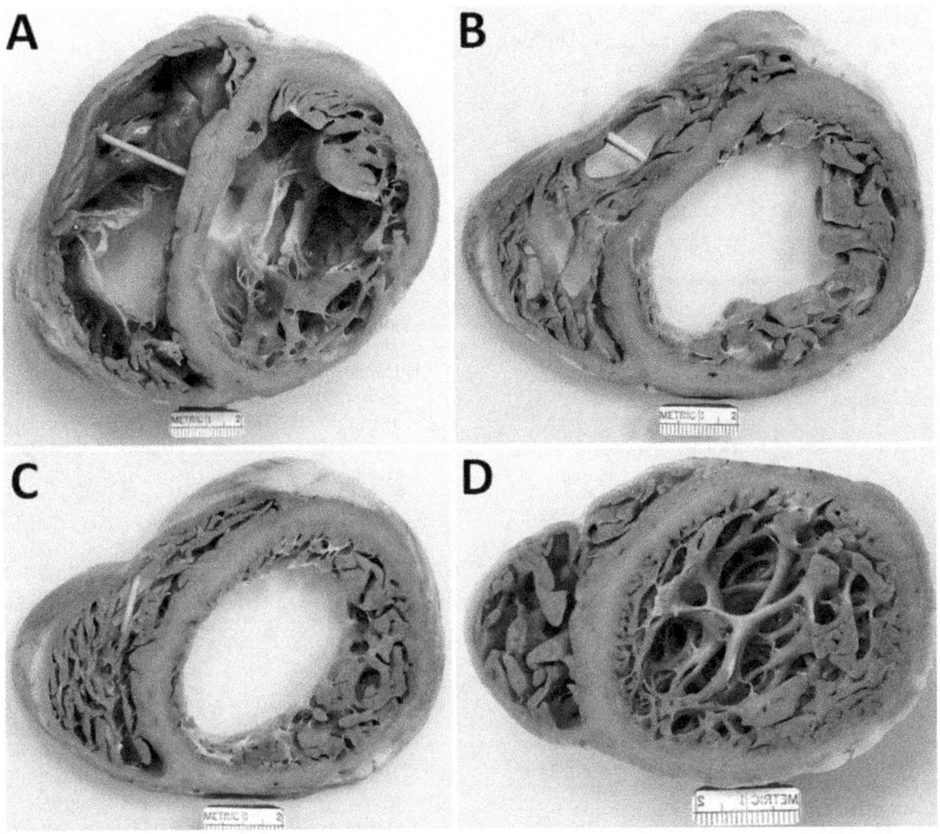

Figure 6. Patient 3. Views of the right and left ventricles at 4 different levels: *(A)* near the base exposing the tricuspid and mitral valves, *(B, C)* intermediate levels, and *(D)* near the apex. *C* corresponds almost precisely with the echocardiogram shown in Figure 5B. The noncompacted portion of the left ventricular free wall is thicker than the compacted portion, which is particularly thin in the basilar portion *(A)*.

Table 2
Clinical features of four major cardiomyopathies

Variable	IVNC	IDC	ARVD	HC
Ages	All	All	All	All
Men	+++	+++	+++	+++
Women	+	+	+	+
Heart failure	+++	+++	++	++
Atrial arrhythmias	++	+++	+++	+
Ventricular arrhythmias	+++	+++	+++	+++
Bundle branch block	+++	++	+++	+
Heart block	+	+	+++	+
Epsilon waves	0	0	+	0
Right + left ventricular dilatation	+++	+++	+++	0
Atrial dilatation	++	++	++	+++
Sudden death	+	+	++	+++
Heart failure death	+++	+++	++	+
Left ventricular scars	+	+	+	++
Tricuspid and/or mitral regurgitation	++	++	++	+++
Familial	+	+	+++	+++
Heart weight	↑↑	↑↑	↑↑	↑↑↑
Ejection fraction	↓↓↓	↓↓↓	↓↓	↑

ARVD = arrhythmogenic right ventricular dysplasia; HC = hypertrophic cardiomyopathy; IDC = idiopathic dilated cardiomyopathy; IVNC = isolated ventricular noncompaction; + = positive or present; ↑ = increased; ↓ = decreased.

1. Roberts WC, Perry LW, Chandra RS, Myers GE, Shapiro SR, Scott LP. Aortic valve atresia: a new classification based on necropsy study of 73 cases. *Am J Cardiol* 1976;37:753–756.
2. Engberding R, Bender F. Identification of a rare congenital anomaly of the myocardium by two-dimensional echocardiography: persistence of isolated myocardial sinusoids. *Am J Cardiol* 1984;53:1733–1734.
3. Jenni R, Goebel N, Tartini R, Schneider J, Arbenz U, Oelz O. Persisting myocardial sinusoids of both ventricles as an isolated anomaly: echocardiographic, angiographic, and pathologic anatomical findings. *Cardiovasc Interv Radiol* 1986;9:127–131.
4. Steiner I, Hrubecký J, Pleskot J, Kokštejn Z. Persistence of spongy myocardium with embryonic blood supply in an adult. *Cardiovasc Pathol* 1996;5:47–53.
5. Ritter M, Oechslin E, Sütsch G, Attenhofer C, Schneider J, Jenni R. Isolated noncompaction of the myocardium in adults. *Mayo Clin Proc* 1997;72:26–31.
6. Oechslin EN, Jost CH, Rojas JR, Kaufmann PA, Jenni R. Long-term follow-up of 34 adults with isolated left ventricular noncompaction: a distinct cardiomyopathy with poor prognosis. *J Am Coll Cardiol* 2000; 36:493–500.
7. Jenni R, Oechslin E, Schneider J, Attenhofer Jost C, Kaufmann PA. Echocardiographic and pathoanatomical characteristics of isolated left ventricular non-compaction: a step towards classification as a distinct cardiomyopathy. *Heart* 2001;86:666–671.
8. Zambrano E, Marshalko SJ, Jaffe CC, Hui P. Isolated noncompaction of the ventricular myocardium: clinical and molecular aspects of a rare cardiomyopathy. *Lab Invest* 2002;82:117–122.
9. Finsterer J, Stöllberger C, Feichtinger H. Histological appearance of left ventricular hypertrabeculation/noncompaction. *Cardiology* 2002; 98:162–164.
10. Hughes SE, McKenna WJ. New insights into the pathology of inherited cardiomyopathy. *Heart* 2005;91:257–264.
11. Burke A, Mont E, Kutys R, Virmani R. Left ventricular noncompaction: a pathological study of 14 cases. *Hum Pathol* 2005;36:403–411.
12. Pujadas S, Bordes R, Bayes-Genis A. Ventricular non-compaction cardiomyopathy: CMR and pathology findings. *Heart* 2005;91:582.

13. Biagini E, Ragni L, Ferlito M, Pasquale F, Lofiego C, Leone O, Rocchi G, Perugini E, Zagnoni S, Branzi A, Picchio FM, Rapezzi C. Different types of cardiomyopathy associated with isolated ventricular noncompaction. *Am J Cardiol* 2006;98:821–824.
14. Engberding R, Yelbuz TM, Breithardt G. Isolated noncompaction of the left ventricular myocardium—a review of the literature two decades after the initial case description. *Clin Res Cardiol* 2007;96:481–488.
15. Finsterer J, Stöllberger C, Feichtinger H. Noncompaction in Duchenne muscular dystrophy: frustrated attempt to create a compensatory left ventricle? *Cardiology* 2006;105:223–225.
16. Finsterer J, Stöllberger C, Feichtinger H. Noncompaction and endocarditis in suspected mitochondrial disorder. *Int J Cardiol* 2008; 123(suppl):e45–e47.
17. Karner J, Keller H, Stöllberger C, Feichtinger H, Finsterer J. Deficiency of mannose-binding lectin, myopathy, calcified endomyocardial fibrosis, and left ventricular noncompaction. *Heart Lung* 2008;37: 476–478.
18. Finsterer J, Stöllberger C, Bonner E. Left ventricular hypertrabeculation/noncompaction associated with coronary heart disease and myopathy. *Int J Cardiol* 2011;148:e53–e55.
19. Stöllberger C, Ormin V, Finsterer J. Fatal outcome of aortic-valve endocarditis in noncompaction/hypertrabeculation. *Int J Cardiol* 2009 [Epub ahead of print].
20. Stöllberger C, Finsterer J, Sodeck GH, Grassberger M, Zimpfer D. Stroke from noncompaction overlooked by echocardiography. *Int J Cardiol* 2011;148:357–358.
21. Espinola-Zavaleta N, Soto ME, Castellanos LM, Játiva-Chávez S, Keirns C. Non-compacted cardiomyopathy: clinical–echocardiographic study. *Cardiovasc Ultrasound* 2006;4:35.
22. Aras D, Tufekcioglu O, Ergun K, Ozeke O, Yildiz A, Topaloglu S, Deveci B, Sahin O, Kisacik HL, Korkmaz S. Clinical features of isolated ventricular noncompaction in adults long-term clinical course, echocardiographic properties, and predictors of left ventricular failure. *J Card Fail* 2006;12:726–733.
23. Lofiego C, Biagini E, Pasquale F, Ferlito M, Rocchi G, Perugini E, Bacchi-Reggiani L, Boriani G, Leone O, Caliskan K, ten Cate FJ, Picchio FM, Branzi A, Rapezzi C. Wide spectrum of presentation and variable outcomes of isolated left ventricular non-compaction. *Heart* 2007;93:65–71.
24. Stöllberger C, Blazek G, Wegner C, Winkler-Dworak M, Finsterer J. Neuromuscular and cardiac comorbidity determines survival in 140 patients with left ventricular hypertrabeculation/noncompaction. *Int J Cardiol* 2010 [Epub ahead of print].
25. Conces DJ Jr, Ryan T, Tarver RD. Noncompaction of ventricular myocardium: CT appearance. *AJR Am J Roentgenol* 1991;156:717–718.
26. Agmon Y, Connolly HM, Olson LJ, Khandheria BK, Seward JB. Noncompaction of the ventricular myocardium. *J Am Soc Echocardiogr* 1999;12:859–863.
27. Hamamichi Y, Ichida F, Hashimoto I, Uese KH, Miyawaki T, Tsukano S, Ono Y, Echigo S, Kamiya T. Isolated noncompaction of the ventricular myocardium: ultrafast computer tomography and magnetic resonance imaging. *Int J Cardiovasc Imaging* 2001;17:305–314.
28. Koo BK, Choi D, Ha JW, Kang SM, Chung N, Cho SY. Isolated noncompaction of the ventricular myocardium: contrast echocardiographic findings and review of the literature. *Echocardiography* 2002; 19:153–156.
29. Daimon Y, Watanabe S, Takeda S, Hijikata Y, Komuro I. Two-layered appearance of noncompaction of the ventricular myocardium on magnetic resonance imaging. *Circ J* 2002;66:619–621.
30. Stöllberger C, Finsterer J, Blazek G. Left ventricular hypertrabeculation/noncompaction and association with additional cardiac abnormalities and neuromuscular disorders. *Am J Cardiol* 2002;90:899–902.
31. de Groot-de Laat LE, Krenning BJ, ten Cate FJ, Roelandt JR. Usefulness of contrast echocardiography for diagnosis of left ventricular noncompaction. *Am J Cardiol* 2005;95:1131–1134.
32. Murphy RT, Thaman R, Blanes JG, Ward D, Sevdalis E, Papra E, Kiotsekoglou A, Tome MT, Pellerin D, McKenna WJ, Elliott PM. Natural history and familial characteristics of isolated left ventricular non-compaction. *Eur Heart J* 2005;26:187–192.
33. Belanger AR, Miller MA, Donthireddi UR, Najovits AJ, Goldman ME. New classification scheme of left ventricular noncompaction and correlation with ventricular performance. *Am J Cardiol* 2008; 102:92–96.
34. Ichida F, Tsubata S, Bowles KR, Haneda N, Uese K, Miyawaki T, Dreyer WJ, Messina J, Li H, Bowles NE, Towbin JA. Novel gene mutations in patients with left ventricular noncompaction or Barth syndrome. *Circulation* 2001;103:1256–1263.
35. Jenni R, Wyss CA, Oechslin EN, Kaufmann PA. Isolated ventricular noncompaction is associated with coronary microcirculatory dysfunction. *J Am Coll Cardiol* 2002;39:450–454.
36. Bozić I, Fabijanić D, Carević V, Polić S. Echocardiography in the diagnosis and management of isolated left ventricular noncompaction: case reports and review of the literature. *J Clin Ultrasound* 2006;34: 416–421.

Isolated atrial amyloidosis and the importance of molecular classification

Varsha Podduturi, MD, Danielle R. Armstrong, DO, Michael A. Hitchcock, MD, William C. Roberts, MD, and Joseph M. Guileyardo, MD

Amyloid is identified microscopically as an amorphous extracellular hyaline material that exhibits "apple-green" birefringence with Congo red stains. Amyloid is not a chemically distinct entity, and currently available molecular methods are capable of identifying over 20 amyloidogenic precursor proteins. Some of the more common diseases associated with amyloidosis include plasma cell dyscrasias, chronic inflammatory disorders, hereditary-familial mutations involving transthyretin, Alzheimer's disease, and so-called "senile" or age-related amyloidosis. The amyloid deposits in these various diseases may be isolated to a single organ such as the heart or brain, or the amyloidosis may be systemic. The senile types of cardiac amyloidosis can result from overproduction of atrial natriuretic factor or from accumulation of otherwise normal or wild-type transthyretin. We present the case of an 83-year-old hospitalized woman with known atrial fibrillation and previous pacemaker implantation who had cardiac arrest unresponsive to attempted resuscitation. Autopsy disclosed prominent amyloidosis involving the left atrium, and subsequent molecular studies identified the amyloidogenic material as alpha atrial natriuretic factor. Since the clinical management and genetic implications of the various diseases associated with amyloidosis are markedly different, we stress the importance of molecular classification whenever possible.

Although identified microscopically as an extracellular amorphous eosinophilic material with "apple-green" birefringence by Congo red staining, amyloid is not a chemically distinct entity (1). Furthermore, the tissue distribution of amyloid among the various subtypes may be systemic or isolated to a single organ such as the heart or brain, producing completely different clinical syndromes. The more common disorders associated with amyloid deposition include immunocyte or plasma cell dyscrasias, chronic inflammatory disorders, genetic (familial) disorders, Alzheimer's dementia, and so-called "senile" or age-related amyloid deposition. Also, within the "senile" amyloidosis category, involvement may be systemic or isolated to the heart, and two distinct subtypes of senile cardiac amyloidosis have been described. In isolated atrial amyloidosis (IAA), amyloid accumulates due to an overproduction of alpha-atrial natriuretic factor or protein (alpha-ANF, alpha-ANP) (2), whereas in senile systemic amyloidosis, the amyloid is derived from native or wild-type transthyretin, a transport protein produced by the liver (3). Since amyloidosis may cause abnormal cardiac function, including restrictive heart disease, conduction disorders, arrhythmias, and death, the clinical diagnosis and pathologic identification of this disorder are important (1). Furthermore, amyloid subtyping may inform therapy, and molecular typing may have profound implications for family members (4).

CASE STUDY

An 83-year-old woman was admitted to Baylor University Medical Center at Dallas with new-onset dyspnea and bilateral pulmonary infiltrates on chest radiograph. In the past a pacemaker had been implanted for "permanent" atrial fibrillation, and she was on warfarin with a recorded international normalized ratio of 4.4. Also, she was a long-term rehabilitation facility resident, and her problems included osteoarthritis, a hip fracture a year earlier, and poor mobility. On examination there was lower-extremity edema and muscle weakness, and she fatigued quickly. Her body mass index was 21.4 kg/m^2.

The patient was admitted to the telemetry floor and given diuretics. The night of admission, acute hypercapnic respiratory failure prompted admission to the intensive care unit, and bilevel positive airway pressure support was initiated. Her blood pressure was 130/70 mm Hg; heart rate, 75 beats/minute; and respiratory rate, 34 breaths per minute. A grade 2/6 holosystolic murmur was audible at the cardiac apex. Computed tomographic examination of the chest disclosed right atrial enlargement, biapical pulmonary opacities (pneumonia versus edema), and pleural effusions (left > right). A brain natriuretic peptide was 314 pg/mL (normal ≤100 pg/mL), and an alanine transaminase was 67 U/L (normal 9–60 U/L). Troponin I was 0.03 ng/mL (normal <0.05 ng/mL). Transthoracic echocardiogram disclosed a normal left ventricular cavity size and normal systolic function with an ejection fraction of 55%; a dilated right atrium and right ventricle with preserved right ventricular systolic function; mild to moderate tricuspid regurgitation; an estimated right ventricular systolic pressure of 46 mm Hg; a dilated left atrium; mild aortic regurgitation; and a small pericardial effusion.

From the Department of Pathology, Baylor University Medical Center at Dallas.

Corresponding author: Joseph M. Guileyardo, MD, Department of Pathology, Baylor University Medical Center at Dallas, 3500 Gaston Avenue, Dallas, TX 75246 (e-mail: Joseph.Guileyardo@BaylorHealth.edu).

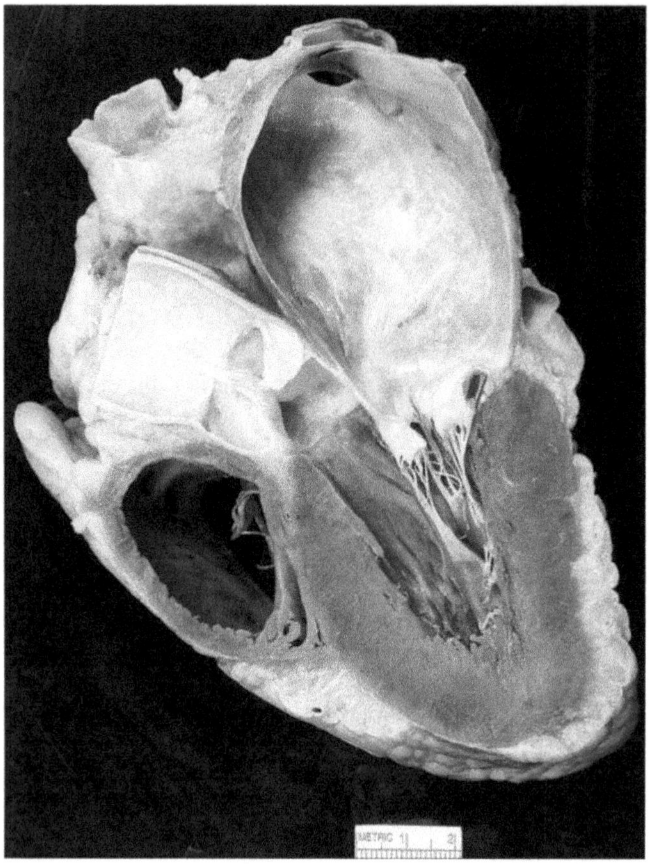

Figure 1. Sagittal section of the heart showing a markedly dilated left atrium with brown endocardial discolorations.

Shortly after intubation and placement of a central line, she developed ventricular fibrillation and pulseless electrical activity and died.

At necropsy, the pericardial sac contained 100 mL of clear fluid. The pacemaker leads were well seated. The heart weighed 460 g. The subepicardial adipose tissue was markedly increased, causing flotation of the heart in formalin. The epicardial surface was smooth and devoid of adhesions. The heart was examined through parasagittal incisions after fixation. The left atrial appendage was markedly dilated. Both atrial cavities were quite large and roughly dilated to similar degrees. Brown discolorations were present in the left atrial endocardium *(Figure 1)*. The right ventricular cavity and the coronary sinus were dilated.

Microscopically, there were amyloid deposits within the walls of both atria (confirmed by Congo red stains), but these deposits were much more prominent within the left atrial wall *(Figure 2)*. Congo red stains of the ventricular walls were negative.

CD138 immunostain and kappa and lambda in situ hybridization studies of the spinal bone marrow did not reveal plasmacytosis or cellular clonality. Postmortem serum immunofixation electrophoresis was also negative for monoclonal peaks.

To further characterize the amyloid deposits, paraffin blocks were submitted to the Mayo Clinic Laboratories, where molecular amyloid subtyping by liquid chromatography-tandem mass spectrometry was performed on peptides extracted from Congo red–positive/microdissected areas of paraffin-embedded left atrial tissue. The resultant diagnosis was amyloidosis, atrial natriuretic factor type, in the left atrium of the heart.

The remainder of the autopsy revealed moderate cerebral and aortic atherosclerosis, centrilobular hepatic congestion, mild arteriolar nephrosclerosis with prominent medullary congestion, and a previous right thyroidectomy with residual left lobe nodular goiter. A small leiomyoma was present at the gastroesophageal junction, and several small gastrointestinal stromal tumors of the stomach wall were seen. Acute and chronic bronchitis was present microscopically, but there was no bronchopneumonia.

DISCUSSION

Although more than 20 amyloidogenic precursor proteins have been identified by current molecular methods (5), some forms are more common than others. Furthermore, the subtypes of amyloidosis have markedly different clinical implications. For example, AL amyloidosis, a common systemic form, is due to overproduction of immunoglobulin components associated with immunocyte dyscrasias, and effective treatment may require chemotherapy. AA amyloidosis, in contrast, may be associated with chronic inflammatory disorders, and therapy involves control of the underlying condition. Hereditary-familial forms of amyloidosis may be associated with mutations involving production of an abnormal form of transthyretin (prealbumin), and

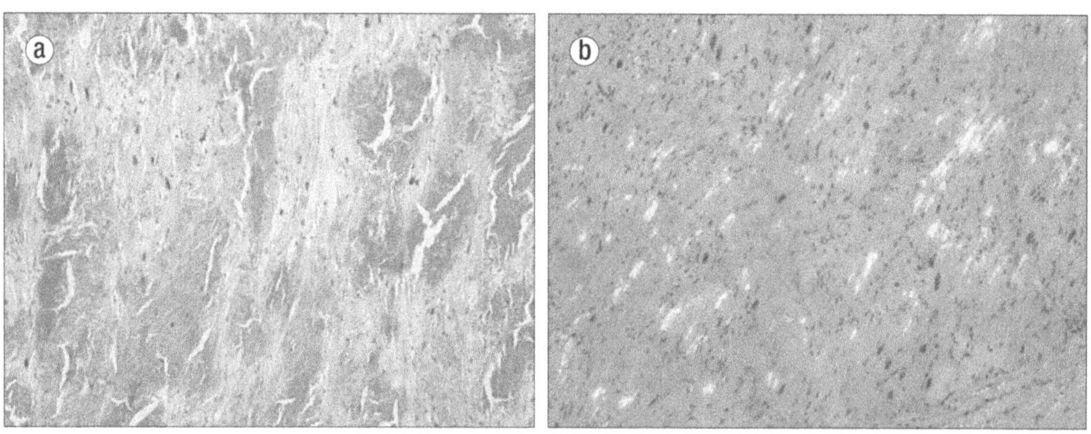

Figure 2. The left atrium showing heavy amyloid deposits. **(a)** Congo red stain, ×100. **(b)** "Apple-green" birefringence apparent on Congo red stain (polarized), ×100.

management may include genetic counseling and consideration for liver and heart transplantation.

The so-called senile or age-related forms of cardiac amyloidosis can be further divided into two major groups. In one form an otherwise normal or wild type of transthyretin molecule accumulates to form amyloid deposits for generally unknown reasons (6). In so-called IAA, amyloid deposition is limited to the cardiac atria (predominantly the left) as a result of overproduction of atrial natriuretic factor. This subtype of amyloidosis has been cited as one of the most common forms of amyloidosis. The clinical implications of this disorder remain controversial. IAA is frequently associated with atrial fibrillation, but whether this accumulation is its cause is not known. One theory postulates a vicious circle in which atrial dilatation and fibrillation lead to overproduction of atrial natriuretic factor and amyloid deposition, which further exacerbates fibrillation and dilatation (7).

Overall, cardiac amyloidosis remains the primary determinant of prognosis in patients with systemic amyloidosis (3). However, regardless of the subtype of cardiac amyloidosis, this diagnosis may be clinically elusive, and management of these patients may be difficult. The gold standard for diagnosis of cardiac amyloidosis remains endocardial biopsy, but indirect evidence for diagnosis includes echocardiographic evidence of amyloidosis and histologic confirmation of amyloid in noncardiac tissues.

Diagnostic efforts can be rewarding, as shown by the case above, since a diagnosis of amyloidosis may help explain functional cardiac disturbances and a patient's failure to respond to therapeutic and supportive measures, even if amyloid is only one contributor to the problem. Furthermore, as previously stated, the clinical implications and management of the various subtypes of amyloidosis are profoundly different; therefore, we encourage molecular subtyping of these disorders whenever possible. Fortunately, such testing is now reasonably available; however, research is still needed in order to improve our understanding of the clinical implications and optimal management of the various forms of cardiac and systemic amyloidosis as we proceed into this era of precision medicine. Furthermore, this case illustrates, once again, the relevance of traditional autopsy, especially when combined with modern and precise molecular tools to elucidate the true nature of a patient's disease.

Acknowledgment

We thank Jong M. (Jamie) Ko, BA, for photographic and technical assistance.

1. Kumar V, Abbas A, Fausto N, Aster J. *Robbins and Cotran Pathologic Basis of Disease,* 8th ed. Philadelphia: Saunders/Elsevier, 2010.
2. Steiner I, Hájková P. Patterns of isolated atrial amyloid: a study of 100 hearts on autopsy. *Cardiovasc Pathol* 2006;15(5):287–290.
3. Kapoor P, Thenappan T, Singh E, Kumar S, Greipp PR. Cardiac amyloidosis: a practical approach to diagnosis and management. *Am J Med* 2011;124(11):1006–1015.
4. Gertz MA. The classification and typing of amyloid deposits. *Am J Clin Pathol* 2004;121(6):787–789.
5. Loo D, Mollee PN, Renaut P, Hill MM. Proteomics in molecular diagnosis: typing of amyloidosis. *J Biomed Biotechnol* 2011;2011:754109.
6. Picken M, Dogan A, Herrera G. *Amyloid and Related Disorders, Surgical Pathology and Clinical Correlations.* New York: Humana Press, 2012.
7. Goette A, Röcken C. Atrial amyloidosis and atrial fibrillation: a gender-dependent "arrhythmogenic substrate"? *Eur Heart J* 2004;25(14):1185–1186.

Morphologic Features of Cardiac Sarcoidosis in Native Hearts of Patients Having Cardiac Transplantation

William C. Roberts, MD[a,b,c,*], Monica S. Chung, MS[a], Jong Mi Ko, BA[a], John E. Capehart, MD[d], and Shelley A. Hall, MD[c]

Described herein are 10 patients who underwent cardiac transplantation (CT) for severe chronic systolic heart failure resulting from cardiac sarcoidosis. None had the diagnosis of sarcoidosis established before CT except for the 3 patients who earlier had had a portion of left ventricular wall excised for insertion of a left ventricular assist device and non-caseating granulomas were present in the removed myocardium. Although none of the 10 patients had significant narrowing of any of the epicardial coronary arteries, all had focal scarring of the walls of the left and right ventricles and ventricular septum and all had dilated ventricular cavities. The patients with the most ventricular wall scarring tended to have the fewest sarcoid granulomas in the ventricular walls. Two patients had no sarcoid granulomas in the excised heart although one did have typical sarcoid granulomas in the portion of left ventricular wall excised to insert a left ventricular assist device. Patients with cardiac sarcoidosis severe enough to warrant CT had characteristic cardiac ventricular morphologic findings, and no dysfunction of other non-cardiac organs, making clinical diagnosis of cardiac sarcoidosis rather difficult. **(Am J Cardiol 2014;113:706–712)**

Although sarcoidosis of the heart has been recognized for over 70 years, most reports have appeared in the last 30 years. The condition continues to fascinate physicians because of its multiple modes of presentation—ventricular arrhythmias with or without cardiac arrest, various forms of heart block, heart failure, mitral regurgitation, left ventricular aneurysm—and its difficulty in diagnosis.[1–4] Single case reports on the topic continue to appear as well as frequent reviews.[5–12] In the last 2 decades a number of patients with cardiac sarcoidosis have undergone cardiac transplantation (CT) and few of them have had the condition diagnosed before CT or at least before cardiac biopsy (including the histologic examination of a portion of the left ventricular wall excised for insertion of a left ventricular assist device) (Table 1).[13–19] Since 1993, we have studied the hearts of 10 patients who underwent CT for severe chronic heart failure found to be the result of cardiac sarcoidosis. Our purpose was to subjectively quantify the relative density of the cardiac non-caseating granulomas in the myocardium and the extent and characteristics of the resulting scarring in the walls of the cardiac ventricles.

[a]Baylor Heart and Vascular Institute, [b]Department of Pathology, [c]Division of Cardiology, Department of Internal Medicine, and [d]Department of Cardiothoracic Surgery, Baylor University Medical Center, Dallas, Texas. Manuscript received October 15, 2013; revised manuscript received and accepted November 9, 2013.

Monica S. Chung is a second-year medical student at Texas Tech University Health Science Center, Paul L. Foster School of Medicine, El Paso, Texas.

See page 712 for disclosure information.

*Corresponding author: Tel: (214) 820-7911; fax: (214) 820-7533.

E-mail address: wc.roberts@baylorhealth.edu (W.C. Roberts).

Methods

The explanted hearts were sent to the surgical pathology division of the Baylor University Medical Center department of pathology. All hearts were examined and described by WCR and, after "cleaning" and fixation in formalin, weighed, and opened by him. At least 5 sections from the walls of the cardiac ventricles (endocardium through to epicardium) were processed, stained, and examined. From each paraffin block, 2 sections were cut: one was stained by both hematoxylin/eosin and the other by Masson, and each was examined by WCR. The medical records were then examined by MSC, JMK, and WCR.

The quantity of scarring in the left ventricular free wall, ventricular septum, and right ventricular free wall was graded subjectively by WCR on a scale of zero to 4+. Likewise, the density of sarcoid granulomas in the ventricular myocardium was graded zero (none seen) to 4+ (granulomas present in virtually all microscopic fields magnified ×40).

Results

From January 1993 through June 2013, a total of 346 isolated CTs were performed at Baylor University Medical Center. Of them, examination of the explanted hearts disclosed that 10 (3%) had cardiac sarcoidosis. Pertinent clinical and cardiac morphologic findings in them are summarized in Table 2. Their ages at the time of CT ranged from 38 to 55 years (mean 48); 6 were women and 4 were men; 4 of 6 women were black and all 4 men were white. Symptoms of cardiac dysfunction in the 10 patients were present from 1 to 15 years (mean 7). Of the 10 patients, electrocardiograms before CT were available to examine in 9; of the 5 without a pacemaker, total 12-lead QRS voltage varied from 74 to 168 mm (1 mm = 1 millivolt) (mean 132)[20] (Table 2). Body mass index (10 patients) ranged from 19.0 to 32.0 kg/m^2

Table 1
Reported frequency of cardiac sarcoidosis among patients having cardiac transplantation (CT)

First Author (Reference)	Year of Publication	Total CT (Years of CT)	No. (%) With Sarcoidosis	Ages of S Patients (Years)	F/M	W/B	Dx S Before CT	Extra Cardiac Sarcoid	Died	Cardiac Sarcoid Recurrence
Zaidi[13]	2007	38,230 (1987–2005)	65 (0.2%)	4–71 (m 45)	25/40	44/19	—	—	16	—
Miliman[14]	2008	250 (1990–2006)	4 (2%)	25–57	3/1	4/0	1	0	2	0
Luk[15]	2009	296 (1987–2006)	6 (2%)	—	—	—	1	—	—	—
Chang[16]	2012	411 (2003–2011)	5 (1%)	31–40	1/4	—	1	0	0	0
Akashi[17]	2012	825 (1997–2010)	14 (2%)	42–67	7/7	5/7	6	7*	6	2
Totals		40,012	94 (2.3%)	4–67	36/52	53/26	9/1,782	7	24/88 (27%)	2/23 (9%)

B = black; Dx = diagnosis; F = female; M = male; S = sarcoidosis; W = white; — = no information.
* Lungs in all 7.

(mean 25.3). The lowest left ventricular ejection fractions ranged from 10% to 20% (mean 16). Three patients at the time of CT had a left ventricular assist device (Nos 6, 7, and 8, Table 2).

The weights in the hearts in the 4 men ranged from 440 to 605 g (mean 506) and in the 6 women, from 370 to 600 g (mean 476). The maximal internal dimension of the left ventricular cavity ranged from 5.0 to 9.0 cm (mean 6.3); the maximal internal diameter of the right ventricular cavity (right ventricular free wall to ventricular septum at posterior wall at the base) ranged from 2.0 to 9.0 cm (mean 4.5).

Grossly visible scars were present in the left and right ventricular free walls and in the ventricular septum in all 10 patients (Figures 1 to 4) and none of the 10 patients had narrowing of any significant degrees in any of the epicardial coronary arteries. The left ventricular scars were most often transmural but often were also or only subepicardial (outer one-half of the myocardial wall). Scars in the right ventricular free wall were transmural (full thickness scarring). Scars in the ventricular septum also varied in extent: some were transmural and when not were often centrally located in the septum or in the right ventricular half rather than the left ventricular half of the septum. No grossly visible scars or other lesions were observed in the walls of either the right atrium or left atrium, but much of these walls were retained in the recipient to connect to the donor heart. No patient had sarcoid lesions in the cardiac valves, coronary arteries or subepicardial adipose tissue.

The numbers of or density of the sarcoid granulomas in the ventricular walls varied considerably. Some patients had granulomas in virtually every microscopic field magnified ×40 (graded 4+). On the other extreme, 2 patients (#5 and #7, Table 2) had no granulomas in multiple sections of the explanted heart although one of them had typical sarcoid granulomas in the portion of left ventricular free wall excised for insertion of a left ventricular assist device. The patient (#5) in whom granulomas were never observed in the heart had ventricular wall scarring similar to that in the other patients with cardiac granulomas.

An attempt was made to correlate the amount of ventricular wall scarring to the density of giant-cell granulomas in the myocardium. In the 2 patients (#5 and #7, Table 2) without granulomas in the explanted heart each had severe and extensive ventricular wall scarring (grade 4+). Two others (#2 and #10, Table 2) had nearly as extensive ventricular wall scarring (grade 3+) and few (grade 1+) sarcoid granulomas in the heart. Patient #4 (Table 2, Figure 6) had 4+ ventricular wall scarring and 3+ density of sarcoid granulomas in the ventricular walls. The correlation between ventricular wall scarring and the density of cardiac granulomas was less clear in the other 6 patients.

No meaningful correlation was found between the duration of symptoms of heart failure and the extent of left ventricular scarring.

Discussion

All 10 patients included in this study underwent CT for chronic systolic heart failure. In none was the diagnosis of cardiac sarcoidosis made clinically although all 3 patients who underwent insertion of a left ventricular assist device had non-caseating granulomas in the portion of left ventricular wall excised to insert the device. The amount of ventricular wall scarring was considerable in all 10 patients but the number of granulomas in the ventricular myocardium varied considerably in them. Two of the 10 patients had no granulomas in the operatively excised native heart although one of them did have classic sarcoid granulomas in the left ventricular wall removed to insert the left ventricular assist device. One might reasonably question how the other patient without cardiac granulomas was included in the study. The answer is that the quantity of and distribution of the ventricular fibrous tissue in this patient (#5, Table 2) was similar to that in the other 9 patients, none of whom had significant coronary narrowing. The scarring often preferentially involved the subepicardial portions of left ventricular free wall, and also the ventricular septum. Portions of right ventricular free wall were usually involved. We know of no other condition which produces such a distinctive type and distribution of ventricular scarring.

Would diagnosis of cardiac sarcoidosis before CT in these patients with severe systolic heart failure been beneficial to the patient? The answer has not been determined because this diagnosis has been so infrequent before CT.[13–17] Some patients with cardiac sarcoidosis have been benefited by corticosteroid therapy and pre-CT diagnosis would allow a trial of this therapy. Is corticosteroid therapy beneficial after CT for cardiac sarcoidosis? The answer has not been determined. Recurrence of sarcoid in the donor heart has occurred and therefore the answer may be "yes."[21,22]

One feature of cardiac sarcoidosis is clear. Although patients with cardiac sarcoidosis may have non-caseating

Table 2
Pertinent data in the 10 patients having cardiac transplantation (CT) for sarcoidosis

Patient	Age at CT (Years)	Race	Age at Onset of Symptoms (Years)	Duration of Symptoms (Years)	Total 12-lead QRS Voltage (ECG)	ECG Date	BMI (kg/m^2)	Pressures (mm Hg)					CI (L/min/m^2)	Lowest LVEF (%)	LV AD	Date of CT	HW (g)	Largest Diameter (cm)		Grossly Visible Scar (0–4+)			Density Of LV Sarcoid Granulomas (0–4+)	Figure Number
								PA (s/d)	RV (s/d)	RA (Mean)	LV (s/d)	Aorta (s/d)						LV	RV	LV	VS	RV		
										WOMEN														
1	50	B	38	12	113*	10/05/2008	27.0	—	43/—†	10†	—	—	—	20	0	1/28/2012	440	7.5	4.0	3+	2+	1+	4+	1
2	52	B	48	4	—	—	28.7	59/28	59/15	9	115/34	115/79	1.7	20	0	9/4/2010	440	5.5	2.0	3+	2+	1+	1+	2
3	56	W	55	1	—	—	25.7	—	—	—	109/33	104/79	—	15	0	10/30/2009	445	5.5	3.5	4+	4+	4+	4+	
4	58	W	54	4	74	3/10/2012	26.4	20/11	—	8	—	—	2.2	20	0	3/10/2012	560	5.0	2.5	4+	4+	2+	3+	3,6
5	62	B	49	13	168	2/18/2013	19.0	36/14	62/—†	20†	—	—	2.6	10	0	3/16/2013	600	7.5	6.0	4+	0	2+	0	4
6	59‡	B	55	4	—	—	20.8	44/21	—	—	—	—	1.8	20	+	7/9/2006	370	5.0	7.5	2+	2+	0	4+	6
										MEN														
7	50‡,§	W	47	3	147	1/02/2005	24.7	97/45	92/15	11	—	—	1.7	10	+	1/14/2005	605	7.0	2.5	4+	1+	0	0‖	
8	52‡,§	W	48	4	158*	11/22/2002	21.6	51/23	49/6	6	—	—	1.6	20	+	7/8/2005	440	5.0	3.5	2+	2+	0	4+	
9	54¶	W	41	13	—	—	27.5	32/14	32/12	8	—	—	2.1	10	0	9/5/1999	510	9.0	9.0	1+	1+	1+	4+	
10	63	W	48	15	—	—	32	23/8	24/7	−1	—	—	1.6	15	0	1/6/2013	470	6.0	4.0	3+	1+	4+	1+	5

B = black; BMI = body mass index; CI = cardiac index; ECG = electrocardiogram; HW = heart weight; IC = ischemic cardiomyopathy; LV = left ventricular; LVAD = left ventricular assist device; LVEF = left ventricular ejection fraction; PA = pulmonary artery; RA = right atrial; RV = right ventricular; S = sarcoidosis; VS = ventricular septum; W = white.

* Electrocardiogram recorded 3 or 4 years before CT.

† Values from echocardiogram.

‡ These 3 patients were included in a previous report (*Am J Cardiol* 2009;103:110–114)[19].

§ Diagnosis of cardiac sarcoid made from histologic study of "left ventricular core" excised for insertion of a left ventricular device.

‖ Sarcoid granulomas present in the left ventricular "core" but not in the excised native heart.

¶ Case previously published (*Am J Cardiol* 2002;89:1447–1450)[18].

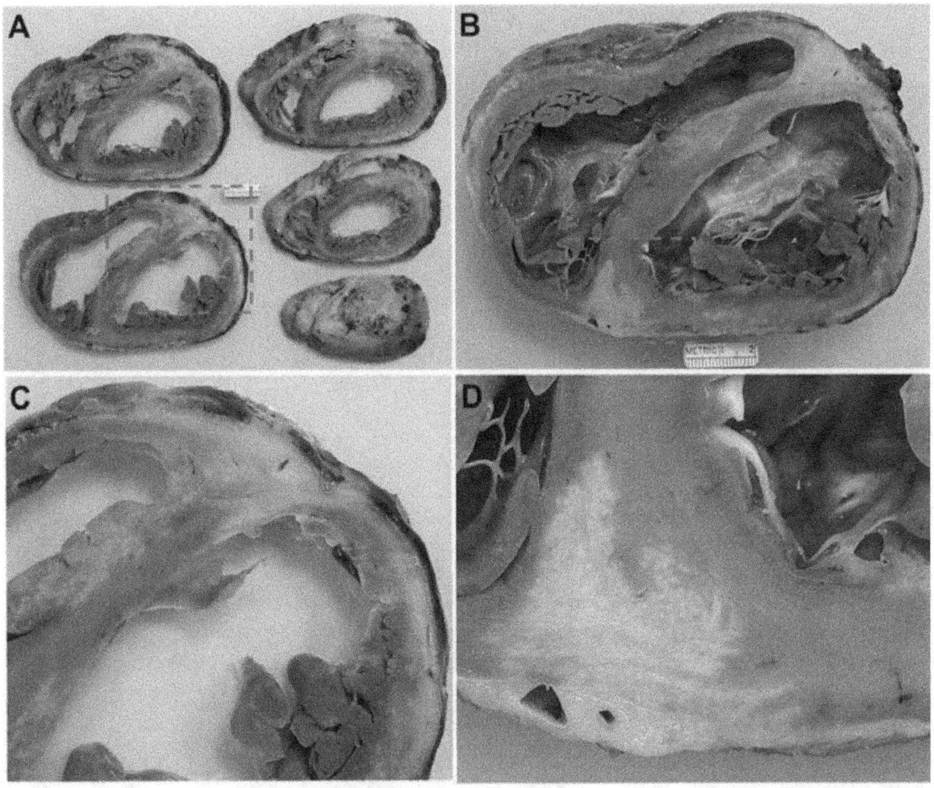

Figure 1. Patient 1, Table 1. Heart in a 50-year-old man who had had symptoms of heart failure for approximately 12 years. *(A)* Sections of the ventricles approximately 1 cm in thickness showing lesions in the right ventricular wall and pectinate muscles, ventricular septum and left ventricular free wall. Some of the scarring, as in the lower left figure of the left ventricular free wall, is subepicardial only. *(B)* Section of the base of the heart exposing the tricuspid and mitral valves, again showing the extensive scarring in the ventricular septum and left ventricular free wall. The anterior descending coronary artery is wide open. *(C)* Close-up view of the anterior wall of left ventricle, right ventricle, and ventricular septum. *(D)* Close-up of the posterior left ventricular free wall showing a large sarcoid granulomatous lesion in the ventricular septum posteriorly.

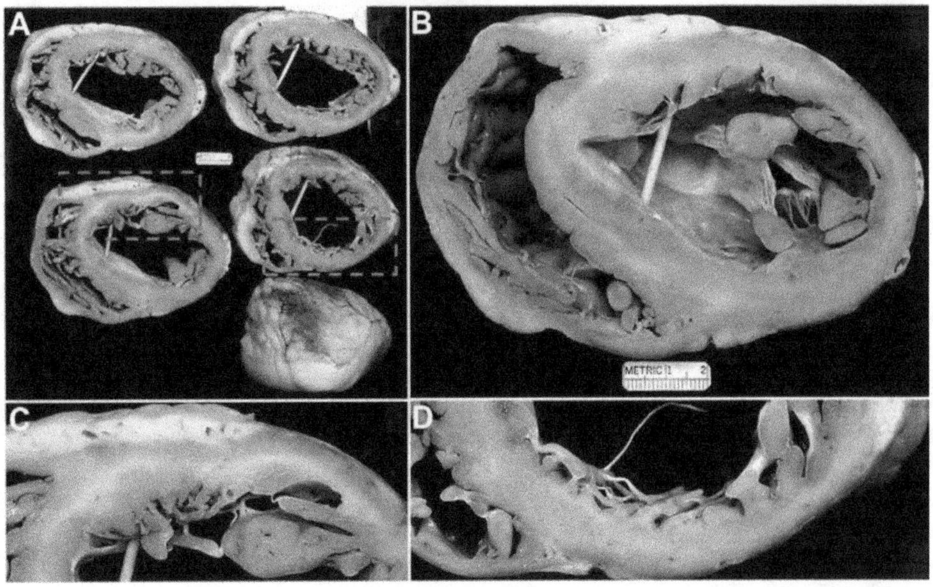

Figure 2. Patient 2, Table 1. *(A)* Views of the various ventricular slices, each about a cm in thickness. Extensive scarring is seen in the left ventricular free wall and ventricular septum anteriorly. *(B)* Close-up of the basal portion showing the mitral valve and the scarring in the ventricular septum and left ventricular free wall. *(C)* Close-up of the anterior left ventricular free wall. The coronary arteries are wide open. *(D)* Close-up view of the posterior wall of left ventricle shown in the brackets in *(A)*. The scarring is mainly subepicardial with relative sparing of the subendocardial portion.

granulomas in other body organs (always in lymph nodes[1]), dysfunction of the involved non-cardiac organ is uncommon. Thus, patients with severe pulmonary sarcoidosis or ocular sarcoid, infrequently have cardiac dysfunction, although an occasional granuloma may be present in myocardium. In other words, patients with sarcoidosis either

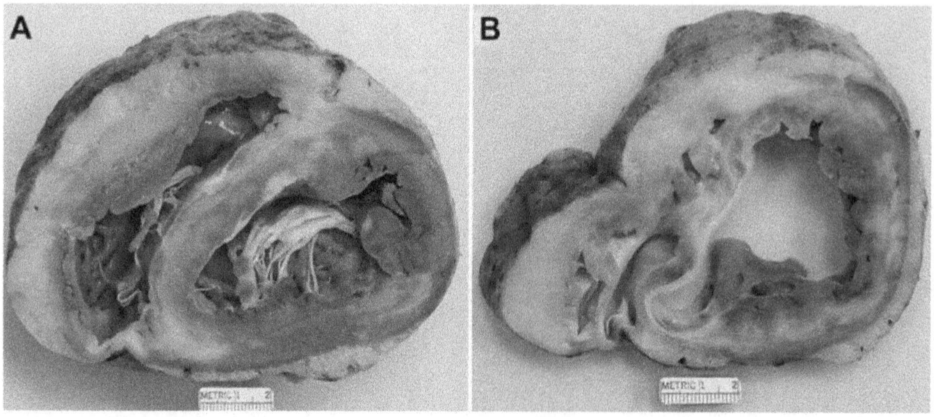

Figure 3. Patient 4, Table 1. *(A)* View of the base of the heart showing extensive scarring in the ventricular septum and also in the left ventricular and right ventricular free walls. Both tricuspid and mitral leaflets are visible. The quantity of subadipose tissue is such that the heart floated in a container of formaldehyde. *(B)* Close-up of a transverse section in the more apical portion, showing an internal aneurysm at the posterior portion of the ventricular septum and left ventricular free wall. The left ventricular free wall scarring is more subepicardial than subendocardial. The scarring in the ventricular septum is transmural.

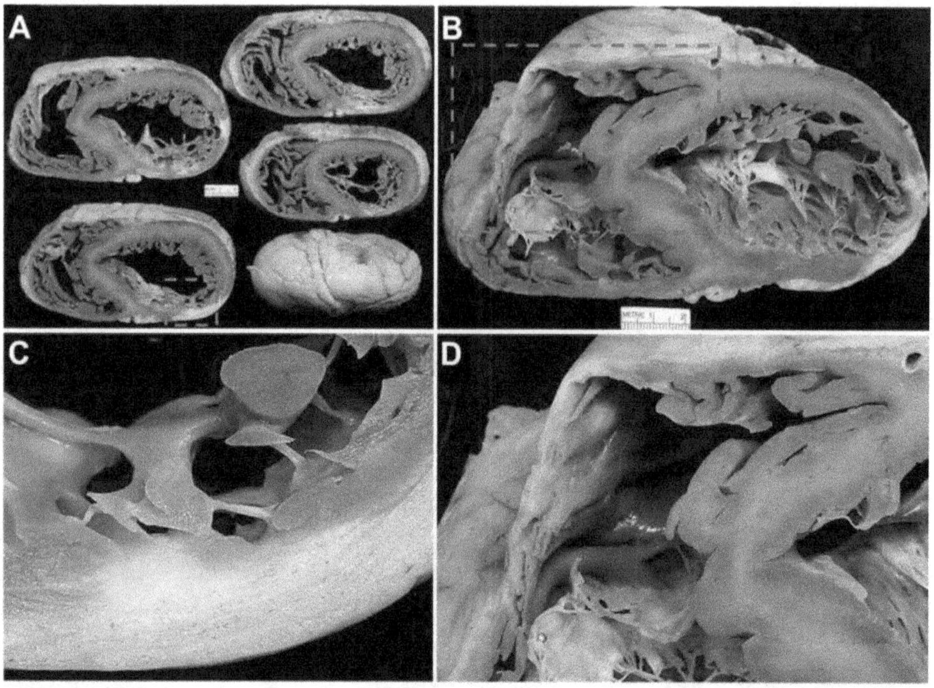

Figure 4. Patient 5, Table 1. *(A)* Transverse sections of the cardiac ventricles showing scarring in the right ventricular anterior wall and left ventricle posterior wall. *(B)* Close-up view of the base showing the tricuspid and mitral valves. The right ventricular free wall is made quite thin by the scarring as is the scarring in the lateral wall of left ventricle. *(C)* Close-up view of the left ventricular free wall showing the scarring to be much greater in the subepicardial region than in the subendocardial region. *(D)* Close-up of the right ventricular free wall showing marked thinning in its anterior lateral portion.

travel the clinical cardiac road or the clinical non-cardiac road, with little to no crossing of the two.

Why is diagnosis of cardiac sarcoidosis so difficult clinically? First, there is nothing specific about the electrocardiogram, echocardiogram, or cardiac catheterization findings. Magnetic resonance imaging and positron emission tomography may be suggestive but biopsy is the only definitive procedure.[23–25] Electrophysiological mapping may be helpful in those patients with ventricular tachycardia.[26] Biopsy of the ventricular septum via the right side of the heart may be negative because the granulomas are focal and can be missed by the biocap. The condition can mimic arrhythmogenic right ventricular dysplasia as demonstrated in our patient #10 (Figure 5) and as reported by others.[27–30]

The positive feature of the present study is the detailed morphologic description and illustrations of the scarring observed in the ventricular walls of these patients with cardiac sarcoidosis. A deficiency is the subjective characterization of the density of sarcoid granulomas and the degree of scarring in the ventricular walls.

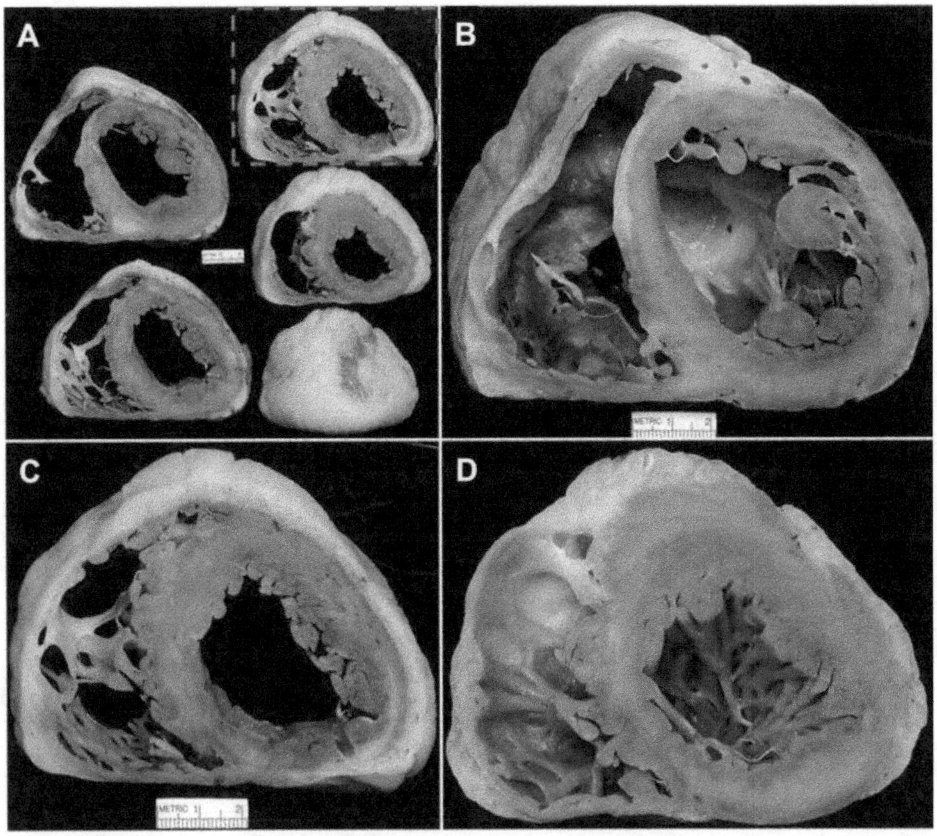

Figure 5. Patient 10, Table 1. *(A)* Close-up views of the various slices of the cardiac ventricles showing extensive scarring in the right ventricular free wall and ventricular septum, and less in the left ventricular free wall. *(B)* Close-up of the cardiac base showing severe scarring of the right ventricular free wall and portions of the ventricular septum and left ventricular free wall. *(C)* Close-up view showing the scarring in the left ventricular free wall to be mainly sub-epicardial. The scarring in the right ventricular free wall and papillary muscle is transmural. *(D)* View showing the severe thinning of the right ventricular free wall anteriorly such that it would assimilate arrhythmogenic right ventricular cardiomyopathy.

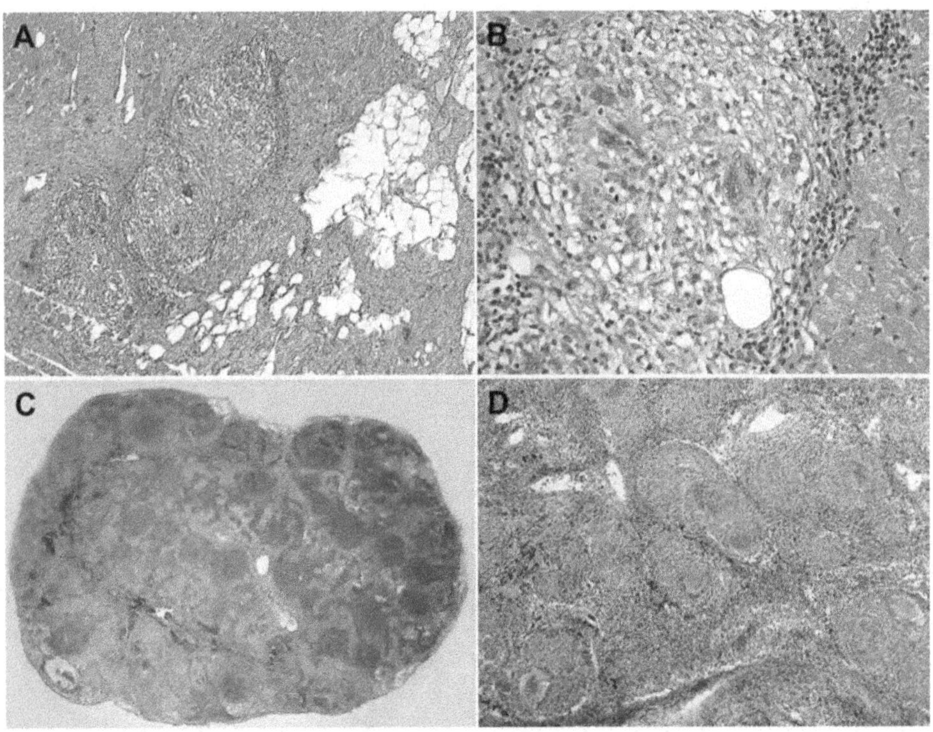

Figure 6. Photomicrographs of cardiac sarcoid granulomas *(A* and *B)* in patient #4 (Table 2) and of lymph node *(C* and *D)* in patient #6 (Table 2). Hematoxylin-eosin stains: *(A)* ×100; *(B)* ×400; *(C)* ×20, and *(D)* ×100. Patient #6 had a mediastinal lymph node excised at the time of CT, the only patient of the 10 to have a lymph node to examine. Giant-cell granulomas typical of sarcoidosis are present in the node.

Disclosures

The authors have no conflicts of interest to disclose.

1. Roberts WC, McAllister HA Jr, Ferrans VJ. Sarcoidosis of the heart: a clinicopathologic study of 35 necropsy patients (group I) and review of 78 previously described necropsy patients (group II). *Am J Med* 1977;63:86–108.
2. Virmani R, Bures JC, Roberts WC. Cardiac sarcoidosis: a major cause of sudden death in young individuals. *Chest* 1980;77:423–428.
3. Sharma PS, Lubahn JG, Donsky AS, Yoon AD, Carry MM, Grayburn PA, Wood PB, Ko JM, Burton EC, Roberts WC. Diagnosing cardiac sarcoidosis clinically without tissue confirmation. *Proc (Bayl Univ Med Cent)* 2009;22:236–238.
4. Tavora F, Cresswell N, Li L, Ripple M, Solomon C, Burke A. Comparison of necropsy findings in patients with sarcoidosis dying suddenly from cardiac sarcoidosis versus dying suddenly from other causes. *Am J Cardiol* 2009;104:571–577.
5. Kim JS, Judson MA, Donnino R, Gold M, Cooper LT Jr, Prystowsky EN, Prystowsky S. Cardiac sarcoidosis. *Am Heart J* 2009;157:9–21.
6. Lagana SM, Parwani AV, Nichols LC. Cardiac sarcoidosis: a pathology-focused review. *Arch Pathol Lab Med* 2010;134:1039–1046.
7. Dubrey SW, Falk RH. Diagnosis and management of cardiac sarcoidosis. *Prog Cardiovasc Dis* 2010;52:336–346.
8. Yeboah J, Lee C, Sharma OP. Cardiac sarcoidosis: a review 2011. *Curr Opin Pulm Med* 2011;17:308–315.
9. Mantini N, Williams B Jr, Stewart J, Rubinsztain L, Kacharava A. Cardiac sarcoid: a clinician's review on how to approach the patient with cardiac sarcoid. *Clin Cardiol* 2012;35:410–415.
10. Saidha S, Sotirchos ES, Eckstein C. Etiology of sarcoidosis: does infection play a role? *Yale J Biol Med* 2012;85:133–141.
11. Hamzeh NY, Wamboldt FS, Weinberger HD. Management of cardiac sarcoidosis in the United States: a Delphi study. *Chest* 2012;141:154–162.
12. Mitropoulos FA, Floudas CS, Kanakis MA, Vaiopoulos GA. Cardiac sarcoidosis. *Thorac Cardiovasc Surg* 2009;57:187–190.
13. Zaidi AR, Zaidi A, Vaitkus PT. Outcome of heart transplantation in patients with sarcoid cardiomyopathy. *J Heart Lung Transplant* 2007;26:714–717.
14. Milman N, Andersen CB, Mortensen SA, Sander K. Cardiac sarcoidosis and heart transplantation: a report of four consecutive patients. *Sarcoidosis Vasc Diffuse Lung Dis* 2008;25:51–59.
15. Luk A, Metawee M, Ahn E, Gustafsson F, Ross H, Butany J. Do clinical diagnoses correlate with pathological diagnoses in cardiac transplant patients? The importance of endomyocardial biopsy. *Can J Cardiol* 2009;25:e48–e54.
16. Chang TI, Chi NH, Chou NK, Tsao CI, Yu HY, Chen YS, Wang SS. Isolated cardiac sarcoidosis in heart transplantation. *Transplant Proc* 2012;44:903–906.
17. Akashi H, Kato TS, Takayama H, Naka Y, Farr M, Mancini D, Schulze PC. Outcome of patients with cardiac sarcoidosis undergoing cardiac transplantation—single-center retrospective analysis. *J Cardiol* 2012;60:407–410.
18. Donsky AS, Escobar J, Capehart J, Roberts WC. Heart transplantation for undiagnosed cardiac sarcoidosis. *Am J Cardiol* 2002;89:1447–1450.
19. Roberts WC, Vowels TJ, Ko JM, Capehart JE, Hall SA. Cardiac transplantation for cardiac sarcoidosis with initial diagnosis by examination of the left ventricular apical "core" excised for insertion of a left ventricular assist device for severe chronic heart failure. *Am J Cardiol* 2009;103:110–114.
20. Roberts WC, Filardo G, Ko JM, Siegel RJ, Dollar AL, Ross EM, Shirani J. Comparison of total 12-lead QRS voltage in a variety of cardiac conditions and its usefulness in predicting increased cardiac mass. *Am J Cardiol* 2013;112:904–909.
21. Yager JE, Hernandez AF, Steenbergen C, Persing B, Russell SD, Milano C, Felker GM. Recurrence of cardiac sarcoidosis in a heart transplant recipient. *J Heart Lung Transplant* 2005;24:1988–1990.
22. Luk A, Lee A, Ahn E, Soor GS, Ross HJ, Butany J. Cardiac sarcoidosis: recurrent disease in a heart transplant patient following pulmonary tuberculosis infection. *Can J Cardiol* 2010;26:e273–e275.
23. Ichinose A, Otani H, Oikawa M, Takase K, Saito H, Shimokawa H, Takahashi S. MRI of cardiac sarcoidosis: basal and subepicardial localization of myocardial lesions and their effect on left ventricular function. *Am J Roentgenol* 2008;191:862–869.
24. Greulich S, Deluigi CC, Gloekler S, Wahl A, Zürn C, Kramer U, Nothnagel D, Bültel H, Schumm J, Grün S, Ong P, Wagner A, Schneider S, Nassenstein K, Gawaz M, Sechtem U, Bruder O, Mahrholdt H. CMR imaging predicts death and other adverse events in suspected cardiac sarcoidosis. *JACC Cardiovasc Imaging* 2013;6:501–511.
25. Khan R, Tweedie EJ, Pflugfelder PW, White JA. Cardiac sarcoid in a heart transplant recipient: detection with cardiac magnetic resonance imaging. *Transplant Proc* 2010;42:1976–1978.
26. Koplan BA, Soejima K, Baughman K, Epstein LM, Stevenson WG. Refractory ventricular tachycardia secondary to cardiac sarcoid: electrophysiologic characteristics, mapping, and ablation. *Heart Rhythm* 2006;3:924–929.
27. Vasaiwala SC, Finn C, Delpriore J, Leya F, Gagermeier J, Akar JG, Santucci P, Dajani K, Bova D, Picken MM, Basso C, Marcus F, Wilber DJ. Prospective study of cardiac sarcoid mimicking arrhythmogenic right ventricular dysplasia. *J Cardiovasc Electrophysiol* 2009;20:473–476.
28. Corrado D, Thiene G. Cardiac sarcoidosis mimicking arrhythmogenic right ventricular cardiomyopathy/dysplasia: the renaissance of endomyocardial biopsy? *J Cardiovasc Electrophysiol* 2009;20:477–479.
29. Chia PL, Subbiah RN, Kuchar D, Walker B. Cardiac sarcoidosis masquerading as arrhythmogenic right ventricular cardiomyopathy. *Heart Lung Circ* 2012;21:42–45.
30. Barbou F, Lahutte M, Gontier E. Cardiac sarcoidosis presenting as an arrhythmogenic right ventricular cardiomyopathy. *Heart* 2012;98:1753–1754.

Cardiac Restriction Secondary to Massive Calcific Deposits in the Left Ventricular Cavity

William C. Roberts, MD[a,b,c,*], Randall L. Rosenblatt, MD[d], Jong Mi Ko, BA[a], Paul A. Grayburn, MD[a,c], Johannes J. Kuiper, MD[c], and Joseph M. Guileyardo, MD[b]

Described herein are clinical and necropsy findings in a 61-year-old woman with fatal left ventricular diastolic failure secondary to massive calcific deposits primarily within the left ventricular cavity. At age 3, an isthmic aortic coarctation was resected, and at age 44, a stenotic congenitally bicuspid aortic valve was replaced. The cause of the intracavitary calcific deposits remains unclear, but surgical resection of the deposits has been an effective form of therapy. **(Am J Cardiol 2014;113:1442–1446)**

Calcific deposits are common in the heart particularly in older individuals and especially in atherosclerotic plaques in coronary arteries, in aortic valve cusps, and in the mitral annulus.[1] These deposits may also occur but far less commonly in other areas of the heart. In 1984, Silver et al[2] described clinical and necropsy findings in a 56-year-old woman with numerous calcific deposits in the left ventricular cavity causing severe impairment to left ventricular filling. This report describes clinical and necropsy findings in a similar patient and reviews other reported cases of large, mainly intracavitary, left ventricular calcific deposits.

Case Report

This 61-year-old white woman had resection of an aortic isthmic coarctation at age 3. At age 44, she underwent an aortic valve replacement with a bileaflet mechanical prosthesis for a stenotic congenitally bicuspid aortic valve. At age 54 (2006), she experienced her first episode of acute pulmonary edema requiring mechanical ventilator. Coronary angiography showed significant narrowing of the left circumflex coronary artery and a stent was inserted. A year later (age 55), another acute episode of heart failure occurred. Repeat angiography disclosed that the lumen of the stent in the left circumflex coronary artery was partially thrombosed, the clot was extracted, and angioplasty was performed. Echocardiogram disclosed a left ventricular ejection fraction of about 30%, but the prosthesis in the aortic valve position was functioning well. She had another episode of acute pulmonary edema 1 year later.

Because of increasing fatigue and periodic evidence of worsening heart failure, she was admitted to the Baylor University Medical Center, Dallas, for the first time at age 59 (February 2011). An echocardiogram, at that time, disclosed severe left ventricular endocardial thickening with numerous intracavitary calcific deposits, a restrictive left ventricular filling pattern without respiratory variation, normal-sized right and left ventricular cavities, and a normally functioning aortic valve prosthesis. The cavitary calcific deposits were also seen by chest radiographs and by chest computed tomography. Right-sided cardiac catheterization showed the following pressures in mm Hg: pulmonary arterial wedge mean 20, a wave 26, v-wave 40, pulmonary artery 72/24, and right ventricle 78/15. The cardiac index was 2.25 L/min/m^2.

Over the next 2 years, the heart failure gradually worsened. Her body mass index was 17 kg/m^2. The pulmonary arterial pressure rose to 99/29, the right ventricular pressure to 99/0, and the pulmonary arterial wedge pressure to mean 30, a wave 38, and v wave 33 mm Hg. Echocardiogram (Figure 1) revealed findings similar to the one performed 2 years earlier. Repeat chest radiograph showed more left ventricular intracavitary calcific deposits (Figure 2) than had been seen 5 years earlier. Computed tomography (Figure 3) showed the calcific deposits filling the left ventricular cavity. An electrocardiogram a month before death is shown in Figure 4. Cardiopulmonary transplantation was deemed inappropriate and she died of heart failure in August 2013 at age 61.

Numerous serum calcium levels were available between June 2007 and August 2013 and ranged from 8.1 to 9.5 mg/dl. Several serum phosphorous levels in February 2008 ranged from 2.4 to 3.6 mg/dl.

At necropsy, the heart weighed 440 g. Huge calcific deposits were present in the left ventricular cavity from apex to base (Figures 5 and 6). The right ventricular and left ventricular walls and the ventricular septum were of similar thicknesses and free of grossly visible myocardial lesions, and neither ventricular cavity was dilated. Histologically, sections of the myocardium were normal except for enlargement of the myofibers. The discs of the mechanical prosthesis (St. Jude Medical) in the aortic valve position appeared to move properly without interference. Metallic stents were present in the left circumflex coronary artery (Figure 3). The right and left anterior descending coronary

[a]Baylor Heart and Vascular Institute, [b]Department of Pathology, and Divisions of [c]Cardiology and [d]Pulmonology, Department of Internal Medicine, Baylor University Medical Center, Dallas, Texas. Manuscript received December 19, 2013; revised manuscript received and accepted December 26, 2013.

The study was funded by the Baylor Health Care System Foundation, Dallas, Texas.

See page 1446 for disclosure information.

*Corresponding author: Tel: (214) 820-7911; fax: (214) 820-7533.

E-mail address: wc.roberts@baylorhealth.edu or ajc@baylorhealth.edu (W.C. Roberts).

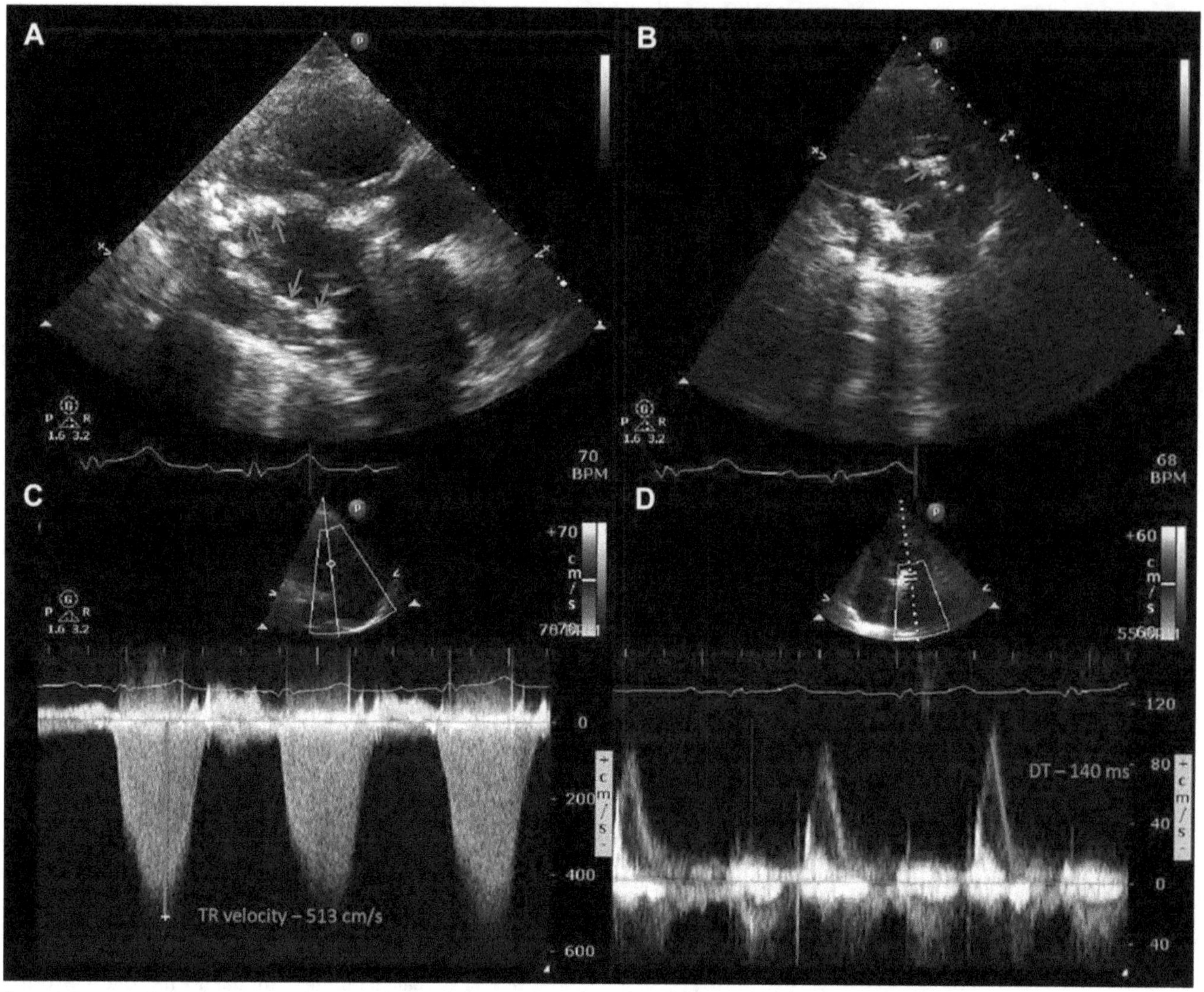

Figure 1. End-systolic frames *(A)* from parasternal long-axis view and *(B)* from short-axis view. *Arrows* point to dense endocardial calcium, which is bright white. *(C)* Continuous-wave Doppler profile from tricuspid regurgitation shows a peak velocity of 513 m/s, consistent with systemic pulmonary artery pressure. *(D)* Mitral inflow pattern exhibits a short deceleration time of 140 ms, consistent with restrictive filling.

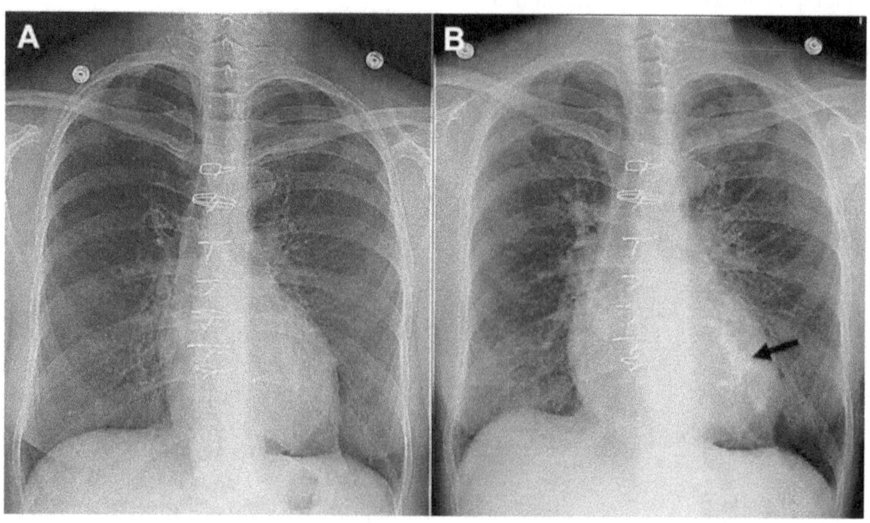

Figure 2. Chest radiographs. *(A)* Taken 5 years before death and *(B)* taken 4 months before death. The left ventricular intracavitary calcific deposits are visible in both, but they are larger *(arrow)* in the latest radiograph.

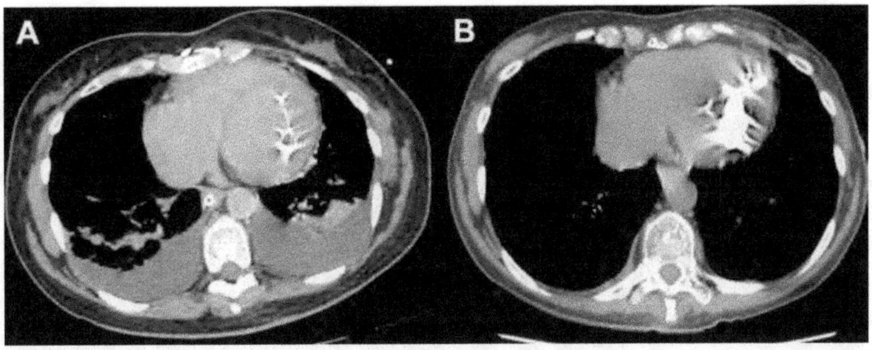

Figure 3. Computed tomographic studies. *(A)* Taken 6 years before death and *(B)* taken 4 months before death.

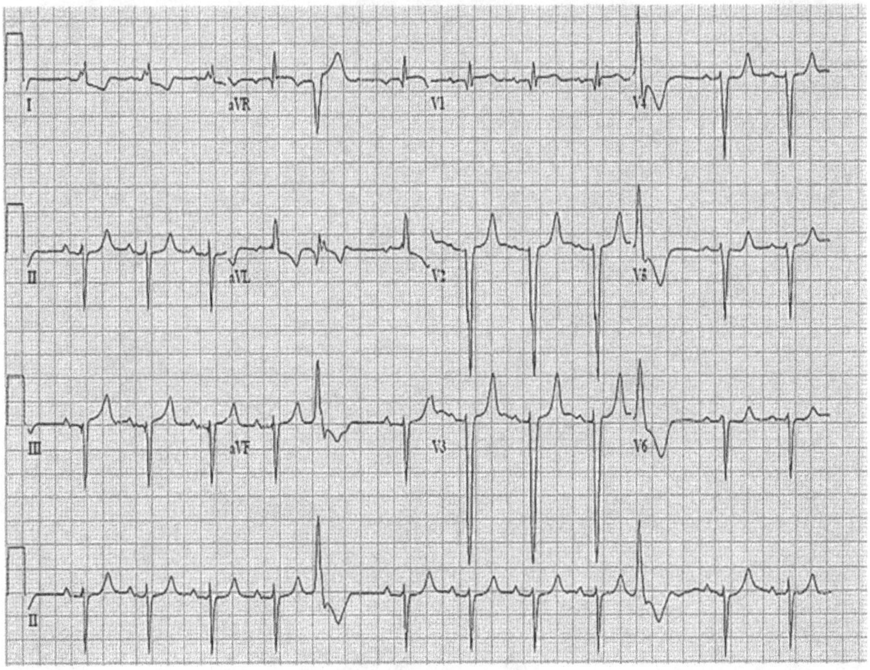

Figure 4. Electrocardiogram, recorded 3 months before death, showing changes of marked right ventricular hypertrophy and frequent ventricular premature complexes.

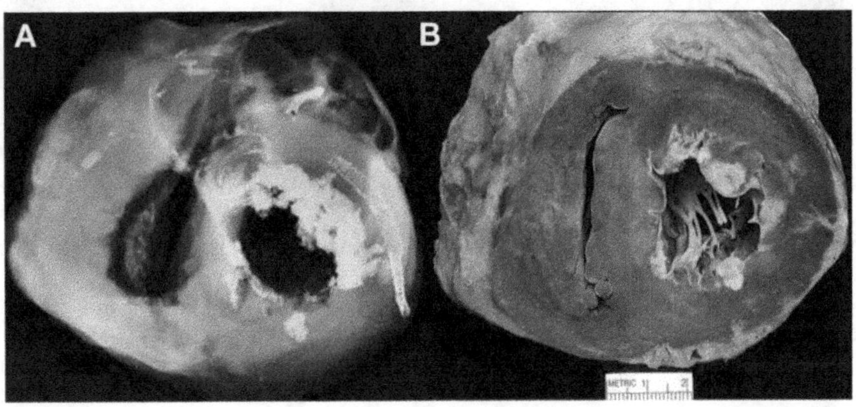

Figure 5. *(A)* Radiograph and *(B)* photograph of transverse section of the heart at the base showing extensive left ventricular endocardial calcific deposits and severe thickening of the right ventricular free wall.

arteries were virtually free of atherosclerotic plaques. The right atrium was larger than the left atrium. A saccular aneurysm with a very thin wall was present at the aortic anastomotic site where the isthmic aortic coarctation had been resected.

The right pleural space contained 750 ml and the left 950 ml of serous fluid. Sections of the lungs stained by the Movat method showed that the media of the pulmonary arteries were thickened, and many had mild thickening of the intima, but no plexiform lesions were present. The

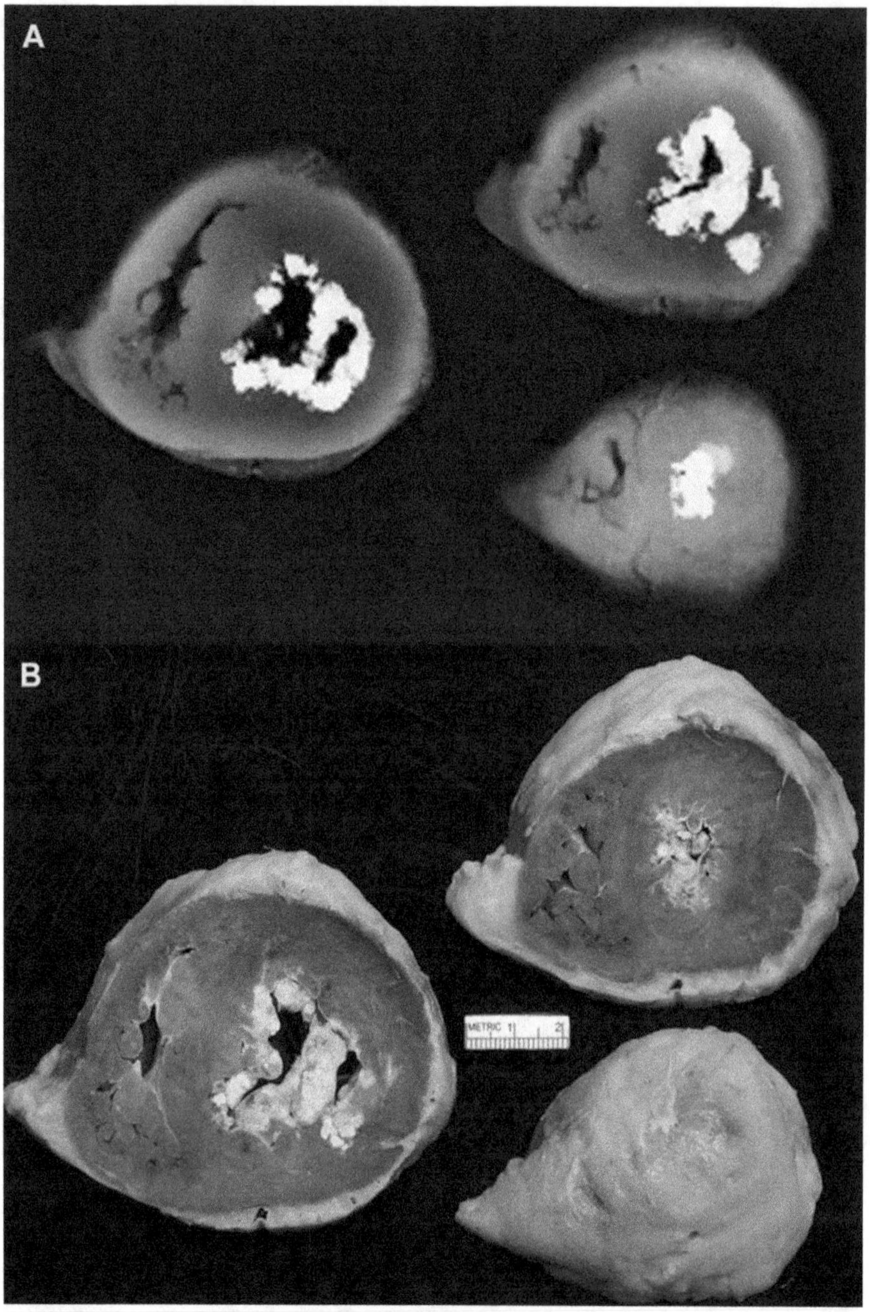

Figure 6. *(A)* Radiograph and *(B)* transverse views of the cardiac ventricles in the apical half again show the extent of the calcific deposits.

intrapulmonary pulmonary veins were dilated, the interlobular septa were thickened (Kerley B lines), and extravasated erythrocytes and hemosiderin-laden macrophages were present in some alveolar spaces. Although most were of normal thickness, some alveolar septa were thickened by fibrous tissue.

Discussion

The patient described herein is virtually identical to the one described in 1984 by Silver et al[2] with huge intracavitary left ventricular calcific deposits leading to extreme difficulty in filling the left ventricular cavity with resulting severe secondary pulmonary hypertension.

In recent years, a number of reports have appeared describing calcific deposits in 1 or more cardiac chambers.[3–20] Reynolds et al[5] in 1997 coined the phrase "calcified amorphous tumor of the heart" to characterize the cardiac calcific deposits because the individual calcific deposits are held together by an "amorphous material," mainly fibrous tissue. In our patient, the intracavitary calcific deposits were essentially "glued" together and to the mural endocardium by the "amorphous" material that prevented the left ventricular cavity from expanding much during ventricular diastole. Similar huge calcific deposits within the left ventricular and ventricular septal walls unassociated with similar intracavitary calcific deposits can result in similar restriction of left ventricular diastolic filling. A list of reported cases of left ventricular wall

Table 1
Previously reported patients with large left ventricular intracavitary calcific deposits

	First Author	Publication Year	Reference Number	Age (yrs)	Sex	Method of Diagnosis	ESRD	DM
1	Silver	1984	2	56	F	Necropsy	0	0
2	Reynolds	1997	5	30	M	Operation	0	0
3	Tom	2006	6	36	F	CT	+*	+
4	Ho	2008	9	44	M	CT	0	0
5	Kubota	2010	12	64	F	E	+	+
				44	M	CT†	+‡	0
6	Habib	2010	14	58	F	E	0	0
7	van Kruijsdijk	2011	15	56	M	CT	0	0
8	Segura	2011	18	20	M	CT§	0	0
9	Mana	2012	18	55	F	E	0	0
10	Nasli*	2013	19	54	F	CT†	0	0

CT = computed tomography; DM = diabetes mellitus; E = echocardiogram; ESRD = end-stage renal disease; F = female; M = male.
* Secondary hyperparathyroidism.
† The calcific deposits were successfully excised at operation.
‡ Patient had systemic lupus erythematosus.
§ Patient underwent successful cardiac transplantation.

and/or intracavitary huge calcific deposits is listed in Table 1. The calcific deposits in each of these patients were clearly visible by echocardiographic and/or computed tomographic studies. Cases in which the calcific deposits involved cardiac valves were excluded from the list.

The cause of "calcified amorphous tumor of the heart" unassociated with heavy calcific deposits involving 1 or more cardiac valves is unclear. At least 4 of the 10 patients listed in Table 1 had chronic renal disease with chronic hemodialysis and at least 1 had secondary hyperparathyroidism. The serum calcium levels in these patients were nearly always normal.

What is the proper management of patients with left ventricular diastolic heart failure secondary to huge intracavitary calcific deposits? The answer appears to be operative excision of the calcific deposits. Both Reynolds et al[5] and Kubota et al[12] have reported operative success by this procedure leading to complete resolution of the left ventricular diastolic heart failure. Cardiac transplantation has been also successful.[18]

Disclosures

The authors have no conflicts of interest to disclose.

1. Roberts WC. The senile cardiac calcification syndrome. *Am J Cardiol* 1986;58:572–574.
2. Silver MA, Bonow RO, Deglin SM, Maron BJ, Cannon RO III, Roberts WC. Acquired left ventricular endocardial constriction from massive mural calcific deposits: a newly recognized cause of impairment to left ventricular filling. *Am J Cardiol* 1984;53:1468–1470.
3. Dean DC, Pamukcoglu T, Roberts WC. Rocks in the right ventricle. A complication of congenital right ventricular infundibular obstruction associated with chronic pulmonary parenchymal disease. *Am J Cardiol* 1969;23:744–747.
4. Waller BF, Maron BJ, Morrow AG, Roberts WC. Hypertrophic cardiomyopathy mimicking pericardial constriction or myocardial restriction. *Am J Cardiol* 1981;102:790–792.
5. Reynolds C, Tazelaar HD, Edwards WD. Calcified amorphous tumor of the heart (cardiac CAT). *Hum Pathol* 1997;28:601–606.
6. Tom CW, Talreja DR. Heart of stone. *Mayo Clin Proc* 2006;81:335.
7. Lewin M, Nazarian S, Marine JE, Yuh DD, Argani P, Halushka MK. Fatal outcome of a calcified amorphous tumor of the heart (cardiac CAT). *Cardiovasc Pathol* 2006;15:299–302.
8. Fealey ME, Edwards WD, Reynolds CA, Pellikka PA, Dearani JA. Recurrent cardiac calcific amorphous tumor: the CAT had a kitten. *Cardiovasc Pathol* 2007;16:115–118.
9. Ho HH, Min JK, Lin F, Wong SC, Bergman G. Images in cardiovascular medicine. Calcified amorphous tumor of the heart. *Circulation* 2008;117:e171–e172.
10. Gutiérrez-Barrios A, Muriel-Cueto P, Lancho-Novillo C, Sancho-Jaldón M. Calcified amorphous tumor of the heart. *Rev Esp Cardiol* 2008;61:892–893.
11. Vaideeswar P, Karunamurthy A, Patwardhan AM, Hira P, Raut AR. Cardiac calcified amorphous tumor. *J Card Surg* 2010;25:32–35.
12. Kubota H, Fujioka Y, Yoshino H, Koji H, Yoshihara K, Tonari K, Endo H, Tsuchiya H, Mera H, Soga Y, Taniai S, Sakata K, Sudo K. Cardiac swinging calcified amorphous tumors in end-stage renal failure patients. *Ann Thorac Surg* 2010;90:1692–1694.
13. Gupta R, Hote M, Ray R. Calcified amorphous tumor of the heart in an adult female: a case report. *J Med Case Rep* 2010;4:278.
14. Habib A, Friedman PA, Cooper LT, Suleiman M, Asirvatham SJ. Cardiac calcified amorphous tumor in a patient presenting for ventricular tachycardia ablation: intracardiac echocardiogram diagnosis and management. *J Interv Card Electrophysiol* 2010;29:175–178.
15. van Kruijsdijk RC, van der Heijden JJ, Uijlings R, Otterspoor LC. Sepsis-related myocardial calcification. *Circ Heart Fail* 2011;4:e16–e18.
16. Greaney L, Chaubey S, Pomplun S, St Joseph E, Monaghan M, Wendler O. Calcified amorphous tumour of the heart: presentation of a rare case operated using minimal access cardiac surgery. *BMJ Case Rep* 2011. http://dx.doi.org/10.1136/bcr.02.2011.3882.
17. Vlasseros I, Katsi V, Tousoulis D, Tsiachris D, Bousiotou A, Souretis G, Stefanadis C, Kallikazaros I. Visual loss due to cardiac calcified amorphous tumor: a case report and brief review of the literature. *Int J Cardiol* 2011;152:e56–e57.
18. Segura AM, Radovancevic R, Connelly JH, Loyalka P, Gregoric ID, Buja LM. Endomyocardial nodular calcification as a cause of heart failure. *Cardiovasc Pathol* 2011;20:e185–e188.
19. Mana M, Sanguineti F, Unterseeh T, Bouvier E, Garot J. Petrified myocardium: the age of stone? *Circulation* 2012;126:1139–1142.
20. Nazli Y, Colak N, Atar IA, Alpay MF, Haltas H, Eryonucu B, Cakir O. Sudden unilateral vision loss arising from calcified amorphous tumor of the left ventricle. *Tex Heart Inst J* 2013;40:453–458.

Morphologic Features of the Recipient Heart in Patients Having Cardiac Transplantation and Analysis of the Congruence or Incongruence Between the Clinical and Morphologic Diagnoses

William C. Roberts, MD, Carey Camille Roberts, BS, Jong Mi Ko, BA, Giovanni Filardo, PhD, John Edward Capehart, MD, and Shelley Anne Hall, MD

Abstract: Cardiac transplantation (CT) has been one of the great medical advances of the last nearly 50 years. We studied the explanted hearts of 314 patients having CT at Baylor University Medical Center Dallas from 1993 to 2012, and compared the morphologic diagnoses to the clinical diagnoses before CT. Among the 314 patients the morphologic and clinical diagnoses were congruent in 272 (87%) and incongruent in 42 (13%). Most of the incongruity occurred among the 166 patients with non-ischemic cardiomyopathy (non-IC) (36/166 [22%]), and of that group the major incongruity occurred among the patients with hypertrophic cardiomyopathy (7/17 [41%]), non-compaction left ventricular cardiomyopathy (NCLVC) (3/3 [100%]), mononuclear myocarditis (3/3 [100%]), arrhythmogenic right ventricular cardiomyopathy (ARVC) (4/4 [100%]), and cardiac sarcoidosis (8/8 [100%]). The phrase "non-IC" is a general term that includes several subsets of cardiac diseases and simply means "insignificant narrowing of 1 or more of the epicardial coronary arteries," but it does not specify the specific cause of the heart failure leading to CT. A number of cardiac illustrations are provided to demonstrate the morphologic variability occurring among the patients with IC and non-IC.

(*Medicine* 2014;93: 211–235)

Abbreviations: ARVC = arrhythmogenic right ventricular cardiomyopathy, CT = cardiac transplantation, HC = hypertrophic cardiomyopathy, IC = ischemic cardiomyopathy, IDC = idiopathic dilated cardiomyopathy, NCLVC = non-compaction left ventricular cardiomyopathy.

INTRODUCTION

The first cardiac transplantation (CT) procedure was done in Capetown, South Africa, by Christiaan Barnard in 1967.[3] From that time through 2012, more than 90,000 CT procedures were performed worldwide, approximately 3500 a year with about 2200 of that number being performed in the United States.[30] The immediate pre-op care, the operation, and the first 6-month post-operative care cost about \$1,000,000. Although most have been performed in patients with idiopathic dilated cardiomyopathy (IDC) or ischemic cardiomyopathy (IC), CT is also performed, albeit less frequently, for a variety of other cardiac conditions. In 1998 Waller and colleagues reported clinical and morphologic findings in 92 patients who had had CT for IDC, IC, or hypertrophic cardiomyopathy (HC).[71] Of them, 57 had CT at Baylor University Medical Center (BUMC) Dallas from March 1993 through June 1997. (The remaining 35 patients had CT at other institutions and are not included in the present analysis.) Surprisingly, that clinico-pathologic study appears to have been the first to report morphologic findings in a systematic fashion in the recipient hearts in those 3 conditions. The present report was prompted by finding incongruity between the clinical and morphologic diagnoses in some patients having CT, and that incongruity led to a thorough analysis of that frequency in 314 patients who had had CT at BUMC in the past 20 years.

METHODS

The recipient hearts in each of the 314 patients were submitted to the surgical pathology division of the department of pathology of BUMC Dallas. The patients included had undergone CT at BUMC from March 1993 through June 2012. All hearts during this period were described and classified by 1 of the authors (WCR). Figure 1 displays the number of CTs done at BUMC during each of those 20 years and the 3 major reasons for CT among the 314 patients. Each heart after formalin fixation and "cleaning" was weighed carefully by WCR, opened by him, and photographed (most by JMK). Although some were opened by parasagittal cuts, especially in those patients with HC, the cardiac ventricles in most were incised by transverse cuts parallel to the posterior atrioventricular sulcus. The resulting "bread-loaf" slices were approximately 1 cm in thickness except for the most apical portion, which was about 3 cm thick. The heart was weighed after these cuts and after all extraneous tissues were removed. The left ventricular cavity was measured both from anterior to posterior and from right to left dimensions, and the largest of these cavity numbers were used as the maximal cavity dimension. The right ventricular cavity dimension was the length from the right ventricular aspect of the ventricular septum to the endocardial lining of the right ventricular free wall along the posterior wall of this chamber.

From the Departments of Internal Medicine (Division of Cardiology) (WCR, SAH), Pathology (WCR), and Cardiothoracic Surgery (JEC), and the Baylor Heart and Vascular Institute (WCR, CCR, JMK), Baylor University Medical Center, Dallas, Texas. Carey Camille Roberts is currently a freshman at Georgetown University School of Medicine, Washington, DC.
Correspondence: Dr. William C. Roberts, Baylor Heart and Vascular Institute, Baylor University Medical Center, 3500 Gaston Avenue, Dallas, TX (e-mail: wc.roberts@baylorhealth.edu).
Financial support and conflicts of interest: Support for this investigation was provided by the Baylor Health Care System Foundation. The authors have no conflicts of interest to disclose.

ISSN: 0025-7974
DOI: 10.1097/MD.0000000000000038

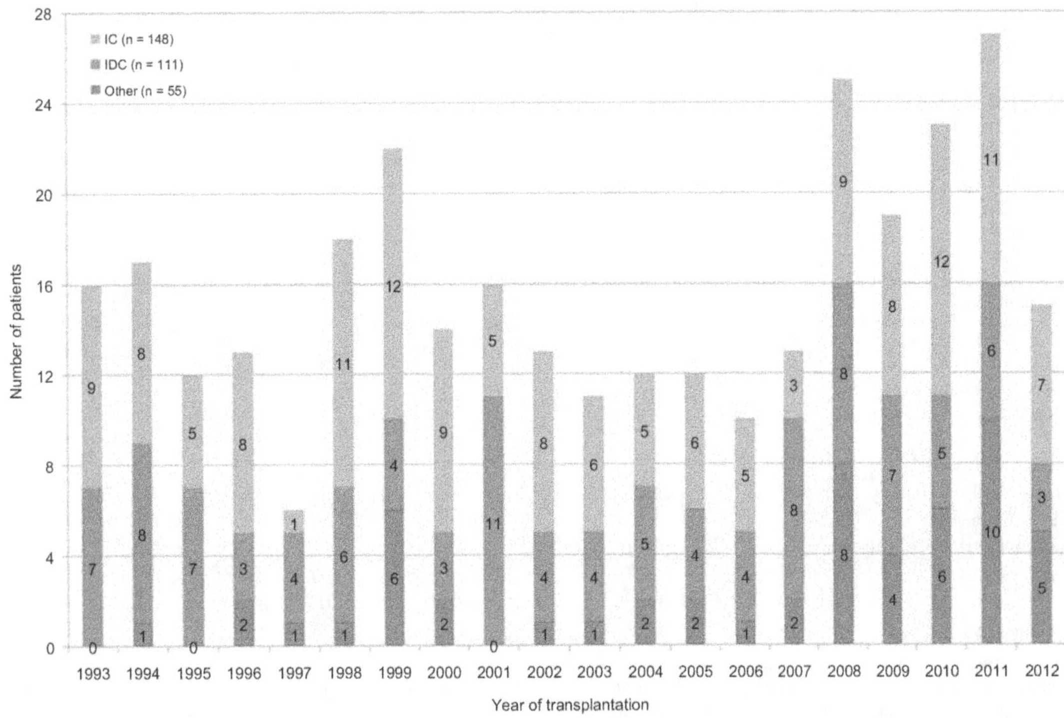

FIGURE 1. Bar graph showing the number of cardiac transplantation procedures done each year at Baylor University Medical Center 1993–2012 (through June 2012), and the 3 major reasons for the transplant (IC = ischemic cardiomyopathy [green]; IDC = idiopathic dilated cardiomyopathy [red], and other [blue]).

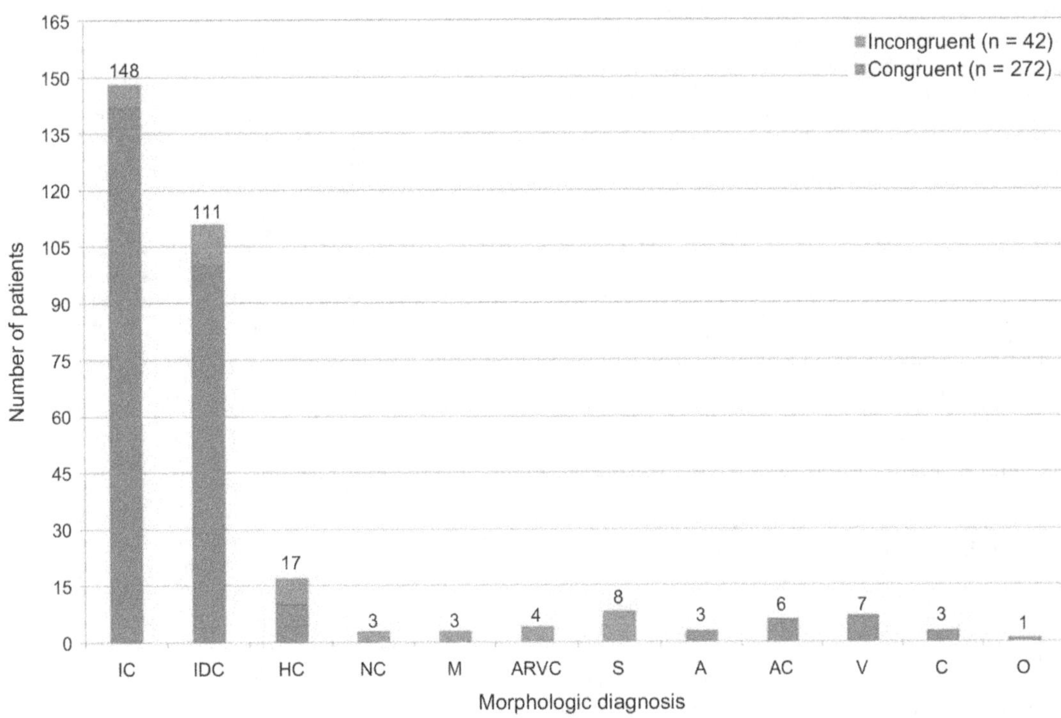

FIGURE 2. Bar graph showing frequency of congruence and incongruence among the various conditions cardiac transplantation among the 314 patients. IC = ischemic cardiomyopathy; IDC = idiopathic dilated cardiomyopathy; HC = hypertrophic cardiomyopathy; NC = non-compaction left ventricular cardiomyopathy; M = mononuclear myocarditis; ARVC = arrhythmogenic right ventricular cardiomyopathy; S = sarcoidosis; A = amyloidosis; V = valvular heart disease; C = congenital heart disease; O = other.

TABLE 1. Clinical and Morphologic Diagnoses of the 2 Basic Conditions Leading to Cardiac Transplantation: Ischemic Cardiomyopathy and Non-Ischemic Cardiomyopathy, and Incongruence Found Between the Diagnoses (Number of Patients in Each Category With the Clinical and Morphologic Diagnoses)

Condition	Clinical Diagnosis	Morphologic Diagnosis	Incongruence Between Clinical and Morphologic Diagnosis
Ischemic cardiomyopathy	142 (96%)	148	6 (4%)*
Non-ischemic cardiomyopathy	130 (78%)	166	36 (22%)
Idiopathic dilated	100	111	11[†]
Hypertrophic	10	17	7[‡]
Non-compaction left ventricular	0	3	3[‡]
Mononuclear myocarditis	0	3	3[‡]
Arrhythmogenic right ventricular	0	4	4[‡]
Cardiac sarcoidosis	0	8	8[‡]
Cardiac amyloidosis	3	3	0
Adriamycin cardiomyopathy	6	6	0
Valvular heart disease	7	7	0
Cyanotic congenital heart disease	3	3	0
Other	1	1	0
Total	272 (87%)	314	42 (13%)

*All 6 morphologically had normal or near normal coronary arteries.
[†]All 11 had severe narrowing of 1 or more epicardial coronary arteries by atherosclerotic plaques.
[‡]All 25 were diagnosed clinically as "non-ischemic cardiomyopathy."

The orifices of the right and left main coronary arteries in the aorta were carefully examined for proper location and degrees of narrowing, if any. Random cuts were made in the 4 major (right, left main, left anterior descending, and left circumflex) coronary arteries, and the arteries were probed (1.5 mm diameter probe) both anterograde and retrograde. The 2 coronary orifices in the aorta were probed to determine any resistance to movement of the probe. Additionally, all incisions into the major coronary arteries were carefully explored for atherosclerotic plaques and luminal narrowing.

Each of the 4 cardiac valves was examined for abnormality.

At least 6 sections of each heart were submitted for preparation of histology slides. They included at least 2 sections of the left ventricular free wall, 1 of ventricular septum, 1 of right ventricular free wall, and 1 each of the walls of left and right atria. If coronary artery bypass grafts were present, sections of them were also prepared. Both hematoxylin-eosin and Masson stains were prepared on all myocardial sections and Movat stains were prepared on all sections of coronary bypass conduits and/or native coronary arteries. If heavy calcific deposits were palpated in the epicardial coronary arteries or in other areas of the heart, usually a radiograph was made of the recipient heart.

The clinical, echocardiographic, hemodynamic, and operative records were sought from the patients' medical records and/or the BUMC Apollo cardiovascular database. Information regarding death of any patient was obtained from the medical records in deaths during hospitalization at the time of CT and from the Social Security Death Index for post-hospitalization deaths. Survival was assessed as March 31, 2013.

Means, standard deviations (SDs), and percentages were calculated to describe the study cohort. The Kaplan-Meier method was used to construct the survival curve for the whole population. The log-rank test statistic was computed to compare unadjusted survival curves between men and women.

The study was approved by the institutional review board at BUMC.

RESULTS

The main findings in the 314 patients are summarized in Tables 1 and 2. All patients at the time of CT were aged >18 years of age: 230 (73%) were men, and 84 (27%) were women. The patients included had CT only; there were no patients having heart/lung, heart/liver, or heart/bone marrow transplantation. Clinically, the patients were divided into 2 major groups: 1) *ischemic cardiomyopathy* (IC), 148 patients (47%); and 2) *non-ischemic cardiomyopathy* (N-IC), 166 patients (53%). The N-IC patients were subdivided into 11 groups, the 2 largest being IDC, 111 patients (66%), and HC, 17 patients (10%). The remaining 9 groups under N-IC consisted of 38 patients (23% of 166).

The frequency of congruity between the clinical and morphologic diagnoses is summarized in Table 1 and in Figure 2. Both the clinical and morphologic diagnoses were congruous in 272 (87%) of the 314 patients: in 142 (96%) of the 148 patients with IC and in 130 (78%) of the 166 patients with N-IC. Incongruity between the clinical and morphologic diagnoses was most glaring among the patients with HC (10 of 17 [59%]), non-compaction left ventricular cardiomyopathy (0 of 3); arrhythmogenic right ventricular cardiomyopathy (0 of 4), and cardiac sarcoidosis (0 of 8). Details of individual patients in the non-IC subgroups (excluding IDC) are tabulated in Tables 3–10.

Ischemic Cardiomyopathy

The 148 IC patients had hearts with dilated left ventricular cavities (>3.5 cm: range, 3.5–8.5 cm [mean 5.9]);

TABLE 2. Morphologic Findings in Patients Having Cardiac Transplantation, by Cardiac Condition (n = 314)

Variable	IC (n = 148)	IDC (n = 111)	HC (n = 17)	NCLVC (n = 3)	M (n = 3)	ARVC (n = 4)	S (n = 8)	A (n = 3)	AC (n = 6)	V (n = 7)	C (n = 3)	O (n = 1*)
Age (mean), yr												
Men	38–70 (58)	24–69 (51)	19–68 (51)	45	24, 56	21–44 (30)	50–54 (52)	57–61 (58)	30, 55	30–65 (50)	40	62
Women	30–66 (55)	26–67 (51)	35–56 (46)	36, 49	46	NA	50–59 (55)	NA	49–69 (62)	43–64 (56)	28,38	NA
Sex												
Male	129 (87%)	66 (59%)	13 (76%)	1 (33%)	2 (67%)	4 (100%)	3 (38%)	3 (100%)	2 (30%)	5 (71%)	1 (33%)	1 (100%)
Female	19 (13%)	45 (41%)	4 (24%)	2 (67%)	1 (33%)	0	5 (62%)	0	4 (60%)	2 (29%)	2 (67%)	0
Heart weight (mean), g												
Men	324–839 (531)	285–940 (544)	355–780 (547)	438	443, 545	314–686 (521)	440–604 (518)	420–550 (494)	366, 526	605–732 (651)	653	707
Women	255–726 (451)	232–660 (444)	220–424 (358)	380, 422	356	NA	371–562 (453)	NA	326–558 (446)	258–635 (388)	460,573	NA
Number of major coronary arteries narrowed >50% in cross-sectioned area												
0	0	100	13	3	2	4	7	1	5	5	3	1
1	25	5	3	0	1	0	0	2	1	0	0	0
2	30	6	0	0	0	0	1	0	0	1	0	0
3	51	0	1	0	0	0	0	0	0	0	0	0
4	42	0	0	0	0	0	0	0	0	1	0	0
LV cavity size (mean), cm	3.5–8.5 (5.9)	3–10 (6.3)	3.0–7.5 (5.5)	7.5–8 (7.5)	7–9 (8)	4.5–11 (6.6)	5–9 (6.3)	3.0–4.5 (3.8)	6–8 (6.7)	3.4–7.5 (5.4)	5.5–7 (6.1)	6
RV cavity size (mean), cm	1.0–5.0 (2.8)	0.7–9 (3.1)	1.0–4.5 (2.6)	2.5–4 (3.2)	2–2.5 (2.3)	3–6 (4.6)	2–9 (4.4)	3.0–4.0 (3.5)	2–3 (2.5)	2–5 (3.3)	3	5.5
Grossly visible LV scarring	147	5	13	1	3	1	8	0	0	5	2	1
Grossly visible foci of necrosis	2	0	0	0	0	0	0	0	0	1	0	0
Died postoperatively												
≤60 d	6	1	0	0	0	0	0	0	1	1	0	0
>60 d	25	20	3	0	1	0	1	1	0	0	0	1
Previous major cardiac operation												
Coronary artery bypass grafting	52	2	2	0	0	0	0	0	0	1	0	0

LVAD insertion	22	10	6	0	0	0	3	0	0	1	1	0
Valve operation	2†	1	0	0	0	0	0	0	0	7	3	0
Body mass index (kg/m^2)	n = 118	n = 86	n = 15	n = 3	n = 3	n = 4	n = 8	n = 3	n = 6	n = 6	n = 3	n = 1
<25.0	33 (28%)	33 (38%)	6 (40%)	2 (67%)	3 (100%)	2 (50%)	3 (38%)	1 (33%)	2 (33%)	2 (33%)	2 (66%)	0
≥25.0–30.0	62 (53%)	39 (45%)	7 (47%)	1 (33%)	0	2 (50%)	5 (62%)	0	2 (33%)	3 (50%)	1 (33%)	1 (100%)
>30.0–35.0	21 (18%)	12 (14%)	2 (13%)	0	0	0	0	2 (66%)	2 (33%)	1 (17%)	0	0
>35.0–40.0	2 (1%)	2 (2%)	0	0	0	0	0	0	0	0	0	0
>40.0	0	0	0	0	0	0	0	0	0	0	0	0

Abbreviations: A = cardiac amyloidosis, AC = Adriamycin cardiomyopathy, C = congenital heart disease, LV = left ventricular, LVAD = left ventricular assist device, M = myocarditis, NA = not applicable, O = other, RV = right ventricular, S = cardiac sarcoidosis, V = valvular heart disease.
*Previously reported.[48]
†Mitral valve repairs.

1 or more major epicardial coronary arteries narrowed >75% in cross-sectional area by atherosclerotic plaque; 1 or more grossly visible transmural (>50% of wall thickness) scars in the left ventricular free wall with or without similar scars in the ventricular septum and right ventricular free wall; normal or nearly normal cardiac valves; and absent inflammatory, giant, neoplastic cell or non-fibrous infiltrates (such as amyloid).[56] Additionally, the intramural coronary arteries were normal. Of the total 314 patients, 148 (47%) morphologically fulfilled these criteria. Of these 148 patients, 52 (35%) had had a coronary artery bypass grafting procedure previously and 22 (15%) had a left ventricular assist device. Of these 148 patients, 142 (96%) before CT were diagnosed as IC; the remaining 6 patients were diagnosed clinically as IDC because coronary angiograms, some performed several years earlier, had indicated no significant luminal narrowing, although all 6 had transmural left ventricular scars and severe (>75% cross-sectional area) narrowing of 1 or more major coronary arteries. Examples of IC are shown in Figures 3–13.

Idiopathic Dilated Cardiomyopathy

The 111 IDC patients had dilated left ventricular cavities (4.0–10.0 cm [mean 6.3]); normal or nearly normal cardiac valves; normal epicardium; no inflammatory, giant, neoplastic cells or non-fibrous interstitial infiltrates (such as amyloid) in the cardiac walls; and usually normal epicardial coronary arteries (Figures 14–17).[20,51,54,71] A few patients had some atherosclerotic plaques but the plaques had narrowed the lumen ≤50% in cross-sectional area in 1 or more of the 4 major epicardial coronary arteries. Eleven patients had narrowing of 1 or more major epicardial coronary arteries >75% in cross-sectional area by plaques, but none of them had grossly visible left ventricular or ventricular septal scars. These 11 patients do not fulfill our definition of IDC because of the coronary narrowing, but none of the 11 had 1 or more grossly visible left ventricular scars. In these patients the coronary angiogram appeared to simply underestimate the degree of coronary narrowing. Their lack of myocardial scarring prevents them from being placed in the IC group. It is likely that these 11 patients actually had IDC, but because they lived in a high-cholesterol environment (United States), their coronary arteries developed significant plaque.[55] Five patients with normal epicardial coronary arteries had grossly visible left ventricular free wall and/or ventricular septal scars. The 5 patients were diagnosed morphologically and clinically as IDC.[23]

Hypertrophic Cardiomyopathy

The 17 HC patients (Table 3) had either normal sized (<4 cm) (5 patients) or dilated (>4 cm) (12 patients) left ventricular cavities and past clinical evidence of non-dilated left ventricular cavities (Figures 18–21).[5,13,21,24,33,36,37,42,49,61] Transmural scarring involved the ventricular septum and left ventricular free walls in 13 patients (76%) with or without grossly visible scarring of portions of the right ventricular free wall. The ventricular septum at sometime in the past or presently was thicker than the left ventricular free wall; typical myofiber disorganization was present in the ventricular septum, and the intramural coronary arteries on histologic study were abnormal in all 13 patients with ventricular wall scarring.[35] None of the 17 HC patients had clinical or hemodynamic evidence of left

TABLE 3. Pertinent Data in 17 Patients Having Cardiac Transplantation for Hypertrophic Cardiomyopathy

Patient	Age at CT (yr)	Sex	Clinical Diagnosis	BMI (kg/m^2)	Lowest LVEF (%)	Year of CT	HW (g)	LV Diameter (cm)	Narrowed Coronary Arteries	Grossly Visible LV Scar*	LVAD
1	35	F	Non-IC	26.9	15	2010	367	5.0	0	+	+
2	43	F	HC	–	60	1994	220	3.7	0	+	0
3	50	F	HC	21.7	–	1999	422	3.7	0	+	0
4	56	F	Non-IC	18.4	10	2012	424	7.0	0	+	0
5	19	M	HC	16.8	58	1999	451	3.5	0	0	0
6	35	M	HC	35.5	5	2011	705	6.0	0	+	+
7	41	M	HC	27.6	27	2009	566	6.5	0	+	0
8	45	M	Non-IC	25.7	65	2010	411	3.0	0	0	0
9	48	M	Non-IC	30.6	25	2012	442	4.5	+	+	+
10	50	M	HC	–	10	1999	674	7.5	0	0	0
11	54	M	Non-IC	28.7	20	1997	637	5.5	0	+	0
12	55	M	IC†	27.3	25	1998	506	4.5	+	+	+
13	58	M	HC	–	15	1996	355	6.9	+	+	0
14	58	M	HC & IC†	29.4	35	1999	374	7.0	+	+	+
15	63	M	HC	21.7	–	2011	625	7.4	0	0	0
16	68	M	Non-IC	32.4	10	2009	780	7.5	0	+	+
17	68	M	HC	25.4	35	2010	580	3.5	0	+	0

Abbreviations: See previous tables. BMI = body mass index, CT = cardiac transplantation, HW = heart weight, LVEF = left ventricular ejection fraction.

*Excludes papillary muscles.

†Each also had coronary artery bypass grafting.

TABLE 4. Pertinent Data in 3 Patients Having Cardiac Transplantation for Non-Compaction Left Ventricular Cardiomyopathy*

Patient	Age at CT (yr)	Sex	Clinical Diagnosis	BMI (kg/m^2)	Lowest LVEF (%)	Year of CT	HW (g)	Diameter (cm)		LV Scar
								LV	RV	
1	36	F	Non-IC	22.6	15	2008	422	7.0	4.0	0
2	49	F	Non-IC	22.5	5	2011	380	7.5	3.0	0
3	45	M	Non-IC	26.1	10	2011	438	8.0	2.5	+

*None had narrowed coronary arteries or coronary artery bypass grafting or a left ventricular assist device.

TABLE 5. Pertinent Data in 3 Patients Having Cardiac Transplantation for Active or Healed Mononuclear Myocarditis*

Patient	Age at CT (yr)	Sex	Clinical Diagnosis	BMI (kg/m^2)	Lowest LVEF (%)	Year of CT	HW (g)	Diameter (cm)		Narrowed Coronary Arteries	LV Scar
								LV	RV		
1	46	F	Non-IC	24.6	20	2008	356	7.0	2.5	0	+
2	24	M	Non-IC	19.8	5	2011	545	9.0	2.0	0	+
3	56	M	IC	18.4	10	2008	443	8.0	2.5	+	+

Abbreviations: See previous tables.

*None had coronary artery bypass grafting or a left ventricular assist device.

TABLE 6. Pertinent Data in 4 Men Having Cardiac Transplantation for Arrhythmogenic Right Ventricular Cardiomyopathy*

Patient	Age at CT (yr)	Clinical Diagnosis	BMI (kg/m^2)	Lowest LVEF (%)	Year of CT	HW (g)	Diameter (cm)		LV Scar	RV Scar
							LV	RV		
1	21	Non-IC	26.5	10	2012	489	4.5	6	0	+
2	26	Non-IC	24.8	10	2009	594	6.0	5.5	0	+
3	30	Non-IC	27.6	10	2008	686	11.0	3.0	+	+
4	44	Non-IC	22.5	25	2008	314	5.0	4.0	0	+

Abbreviations: See previous tables.
*None had narrowed coronary arteries or coronary artery bypass grafting or a left ventricular assist device.

TABLE 7. Pertinent Data in 8 Patients Having Cardiac Transplantation for Cardiac Sarcoidosis*

Patient	Age at CT (yr)	Sex	Clinical Diagnosis	BMI (kg/m^2)	Lowest LVEF (%)	Year of CT	HW (g)	Diameter (cm)		Narrowed Coronary Arteries	LV Scar	LVAD
								LV	RV			
1	50	F	Non-IC	27.0	20	2012	442	7.5	4.0	0	+	0
2	52	F	Non-IC	28.7	20	2010	441	5.5	2.0	0	+	0
3	56	F	Non-IC	25.7	15	2009	447	5.5	3.5	0	+	0
4	58	F	Non-IC	26.4	20	2012	562	5.0	2.5	0	+	0
5	59	F	Non-IC	20.8	20	2006	371	5.0	7.5	+	+	+
6	50	M	Non-IC†	24.7	10	2005	604	7.0	2.5	0	+	+
7	52	M	Non-IC†	21.6	20	2005	440	—	–	0	+	+
8	54	M	Non-IC†	27.5	10	1999	511	9.0	9.0	0	+	0

Abbreviations: See previous tables.
*None had coronary artery bypass grafting.
†Diagnosis of cardiac sarcoid made from histologic study of "left ventricular core" excised for insertion of a left ventricular assist device.

TABLE 8. Pertinent Data in 3 Men Having Cardiac Transplantation for Cardiac Amyloidosis*

Patient	Age at CT (yr)	Clinical Diagnosis	BMI (kg/m^2)	Lowest LVEF (%)	Year of CT	HW (g)	Diameter (cm)		Narrowed Coronary Arteries	LV Scar
							LV	RV		
1	57	Amyloidosis	20.2	30	2004	550	4.0	3.5	0	0
2	57	Amyloidosis	32.0	20	2010	420	4.5	3.0	+†	0
3	61	Amyloidosis	30.6	46	2008	513	3.0	4.0	+	0

Abbreviations: See previous tables.
*None had coronary artery bypass grafting or a left ventricular assist device.
†Stent to the right coronary artery in October 2009.

TABLE 9. Pertinent Data in 6 Patients Having Cardiac Transplantation for Adriamycin Cardiomyopathy*

Patient	Age at CT (yr)	Sex	Clinical Diagnosis	BMI (kg/m^2)	Lowest LVEF (%)	Year of CT	HW (g)	Diameter (cm)		Narrowed Coronary Arteries	LV Scar
								LV	RV		
1	49	F	AC	–	–	2007	404	8.0	2.5	0	0
2	64	F	AC	24.6	10	2004	326	6.5	3.0	+	0
3	65	F	AC	25.7	–	2011	558	6.5	2.5	0	0
4	69	F	AC	34.3	25	2011	497	6.0	3.0	0	0
5	30	M	AC	25.9	35	2008	366	7.0	2.0	0	0
6	55	M	AC	31.6	15	2011	526	6.0	2.2	0	0

Abbreviations: See previous tables. AC=Adriamycin cardiomyopathy.
*None had coronary artery bypass grafting or a left ventricular assist device.

TABLE 10. Pertinent Data in 6 Patients Having Cardiac Transplantation for Valvular Disease

Patient	Age at CT (yr)	Sex	Clinical Valve Dysfunction	Valve Replaced	Interval (yr) AVR → CT	BMI (kg/m^2)	Lowest LVEF (%)	Year of CT	HW (g)	Diameter (cm) LV	Diameter (cm) RV	Narrowed Coronary Arteries	LV Scar	CABG	LVAD
1	30	M	AS (BAV)	Aortic	8	25	10	1999	650	5.5	2.8	0	+	0	0
2	47	M	AS (BAV)	Aortic*	–	–	–	1996	605	–	–	0	+	0	0
3	56	M	AS (BAV)	Aortic	4.7	28.3	5	2007	732	6.0	4.0	0	0	0	+
4	65	M	AS (BAV)	Aortic	5.2	18.4	20	2003	616	7.5	3.0	+	+	+†	0
5	43	F	AR‡, MR‡	Aortic, mitral	–	–	30	2002	258	3.4	2.0	0	0	0	0
6	64	F	MS, MR	Mitral (x2)	–	31.8	25	2010	635	5.5	5.0	0	+	0	0
7	60	F	MR‡	0§	–	27.1	35	2011	271	4.5	3.0	+	+	0	0

Abbreviations: See previous tables. AR = aortic regurgitation, AS = aortic stenosis, AVR = aortic valve replacement, BAV = bicuspid aortic valve, CABG = coronary artery bypass grafting, MR = mitral regurgitation, MS = mitral stenosis.

*Procedure at another hospital (non-BUMC).

†CABG done 6 yr before AVR.

‡Radiation therapy for Hodgkin disease.

§Mitral valve repair twice.

TABLE 11. Pertinent Data in 3 Patients Having Cardiac Transplantation for Congenital Heart Disease*

Patient	Age at CT (yr)	Sex	Clinical Diagnosis	BMI (kg/m^2)	Lowest LVEF (%)	Year of CT	HW (g)	LV Diameter (cm)	LV Scar	LVAD
1	28	F	TGA	19.4	10	2008	460	7.0	+	0
2	38	F	RV hypoplasia	19.6	10	2011	573	5.9	0	+
3	40	M	T of F	27.3	10	2010	653	5.5	+	0

Abbreviations: See previous tables. TGA = transposition of great arteries, T of F = tetralogy of Fallot.

*None had narrowed coronary arteries or coronary artery bypass grafting.

TABLE 12. Previously Reported Data on Congruity vs Incongruity Among 296 Patients Having Cardiac Transplantation (From Luk et al[29])

Cardiac Condition	Clinical Diagnosis (No.)	Morphologic Diagnosis (No.)
Ischemic cardiomyopathy	140	144
Idiopathic dilated cardiomyopathy	96	54
Hypertrophic cardiomyopathy	15	17
Myocarditis	8*	25†
Valvular "cardiomyopathy"	6	5
Infiltrative	5‡	4‡
Congenital	18	18
Doxorubicin	6	6
Becker's muscular dystrophy	1	1
Fabry's	1	2
Arrhythmogenic RV cardiomyopathy	0	12
Cardiac sarcoid	0	6
Mitochondrial myopathy	0	1
Iron cardiomyopathy	0	1
TOTAL	296	296

Modified and reprinted with permission from Elsevier.[29]
*"Viral myocarditis" in 6, hypersensitive/eosinophilic in 2.
†"Viral myocarditis" in 20, hypersensitive/eosinophilic in 4, and giant cell in 1.
‡Amyloid in 3.

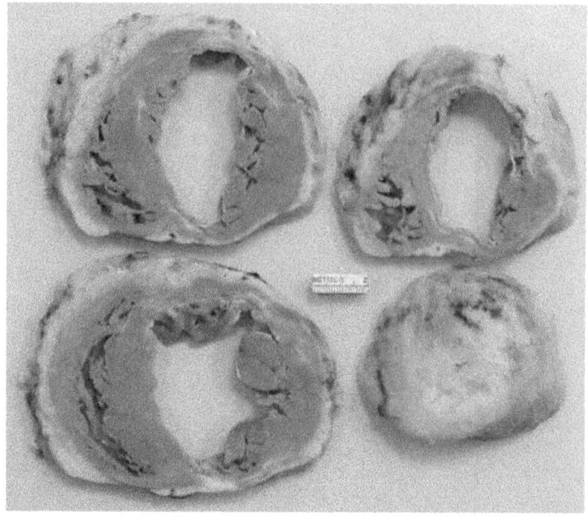

FIGURE 4. Ischemic cardiomyopathy. Photographs of sections of the cardiac ventricles caudal to the mitral valve in a 54-year-old woman who had an acute myocardial infarction when she was 33 years of age and underwent percutaneous coronary intervention at that time. At age 39 years, she had another acute myocardial infarct and underwent coronary artery bypass grafting. Cardiac catheterization 2 years later disclosed that all bypass conduits were closed. At age 42 years, she had another percutaneous coronary intervention. The left ventricular ejection fraction shortly before cardiac transplantation was 10%. These views show a healed myocardial infarct in the anterior wall of left ventricle and another in the posterior wall opposite one another. The quantity of subepicardial adipose tissue is clearly increased. The left ventricular cavity is quite dilated.

ventricular outflow obstruction just prior to CT. Four (24%) of the 17 patients also had severe narrowing of 1 or more epicardial coronary arteries, and all 4 had grossly visible left ventricular and ventricular septal scars. Nine other HC patients had left ventricular or ventricular septal scar without narrowing of the epicardial coronary arteries. The clinical diagnosis in 6 of the 17 patients was "non-IC," in 1 patient IC, and in 1 patient both HC and IC. Each of the latter 2 patients had coronary bypass grafting in the remote past before CT. Thus, the clinical and morphologic diagnosis were incongruous in 7 (41%) of these 17 patients.

Non-Compaction Left Ventricular Cardiomyopathy

Three patients had NCLVC (Table 4, Figures 22 and 23). Each had very dilated ventricular cavities with the non-compacted portion of left ventricular free wall in 1 or

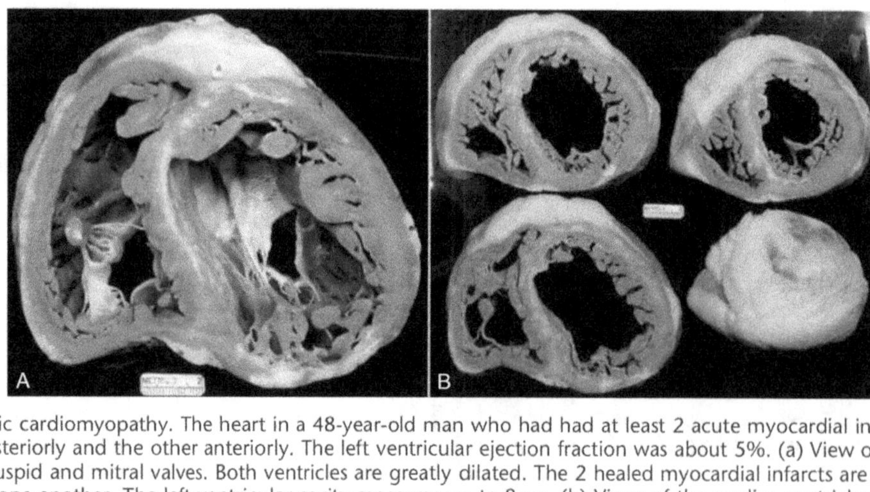

FIGURE 3. Ischemic cardiomyopathy. The heart in a 48-year-old man who had had at least 2 acute myocardial infarcts in the past. One is located posteriorly and the other anteriorly. The left ventricular ejection fraction was about 5%. (a) View of the heart showing both tricuspid and mitral valves. Both ventricles are greatly dilated. The 2 healed myocardial infarcts are clearly seen, and they are opposite one another. The left ventricular cavity measures up to 8 cm. (b) Views of the cardiac ventricles caudal to the picture shown on the left. These views show both the anterior and posterior scars are present from apex to base.

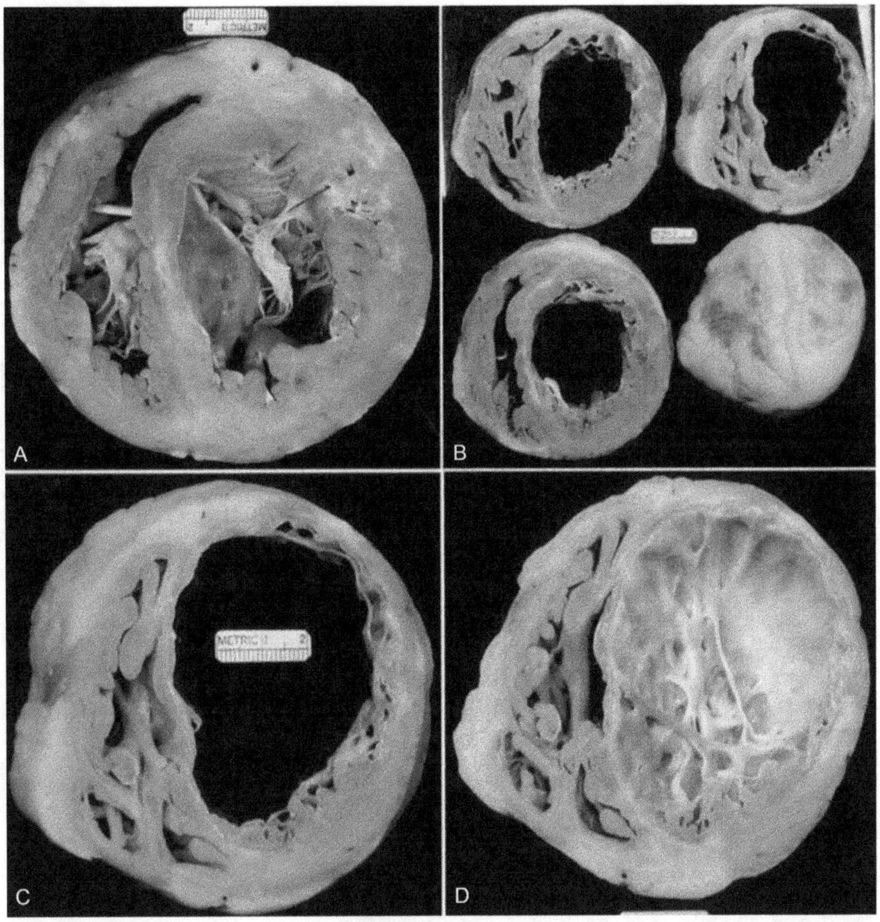

FIGURE 5. Ischemic cardiomyopathy. Heart in a 56-year-old man who had a large anterior wall acute myocardial infarct at age 46 years. Subsequently, a stent was inserted into the left anterior descending and left circumflex coronary arteries. His left ventricular ejection fraction shortly before cardiac transplantation was 10%. (a) View of the ventricular cavities at the base showing both tricuspid and mitral valves. A scar is present in the central portion of the ventricular septum and in the anterior left ventricular free wall. (b) Views of the cardiac ventricles caudal to the base showing a huge amount of scaring in the anterior wall of left ventricle with scaring of the entire ventricular septum. Less than half of the left ventricular free wall is devoid of scars. (c) A close-up view of a portion of ventricular walls showing full thickness scarring of the ventricular septum and anterior lateral left ventricular free wall. (d) View of the interior of the left ventricular apex showing the extensive septal and free wall left ventricular scaring.

more areas being >2 times the thickness of the underlying compacted portion of the wall and unassociated with narrowing of the epicardial coronary arteries.[11,45,68] Clinically, each of the 3 patients were diagnosed as "non-IC." One of the 3 patients had a small grossly visible left ventricular scar.

Mononuclear Myocarditis

Three patients had active or healed mononuclear myocarditis (Table 5, Figures 24 and 25). The key identifying mark of this condition was focal subepicardial left ventricular wall lesions.[19,25,58,60,62,65] Each had mononuclear -cell infiltrates–mainly lymphocytes–in the left ventricular free wall or subepicardial scars with or without mononuclear-cell infiltrates and without granulomas. The hearts were of increased weight (>350 g in women; >400 g in men), and the ventricular cavities were very dilated. One of the 3 patients had significant narrowing by atherosclerotic plaque of 1 or more epicardial coronary arteries. This patient clinically was diagnosed as IC, the other 2 as "non-IC."

Arrhythmogenic Right Ventricular Cardiomyopathy

Four patients had ARVC; pertinent findings for them are summarized in Table 6 and illustrated in Figure 26.[2,4,8,12,14,28,31,32,46,64,66,70,72,73] All 4 during life were diagnosed as "non-IC." All 4 had thinning of the right ventricular free wall with replacement of the myocardial wall focally by adipose tissue and/or scar tissue without focal thinning (except in 1 patient) of the left ventricular free wall. All 4 had very dilated ventricular chambers. Before CT all 4 had documented runs of ventricular tachycardia. Three had other family members with a similar cardiac disease.

Cardiac Sarcoidosis

Pertinent findings in the 8 cardiac sarcoidosis patients are summarized in Table 7 and illustrated in Figure 27.[9,15,43,47,52,62,67] All 8 were diagnosed clinically as "non-IC." Six had focal but extensive scars in the free walls of both right and left ventricles and in the ventricular septum

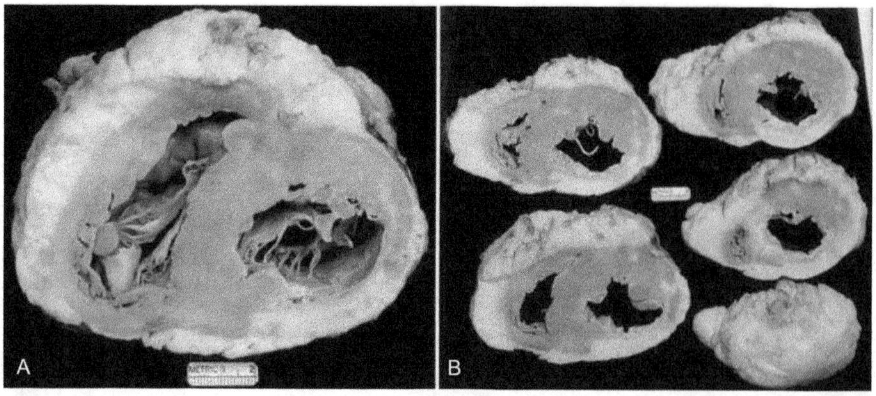

FIGURE 6. Ischemic cardiomyopathy. Heart in a 56-year-old man who at age 49 years had an acute myocardial infarction, and percutaneous coronary intervention with multiple stents was performed. Six months later he underwent coronary artery bypass grafting. Heart failure gradually progressed thereafter such that the left ventricular ejection fraction fell to 25%. (a) View of the basal portion of the heart exposing both tricuspid and mitral valves. The posterior wall of left ventricular is transmurally scarred resulting in the ventricular septum's being thicker than the left ventricular free wall. The quantity of subepicardial adipose tissue is enormous, such that the heart floated in a container of formaldehyde. (b) Views of the ventricles more caudally showing that the posterior wall infarct extends from apex to base.

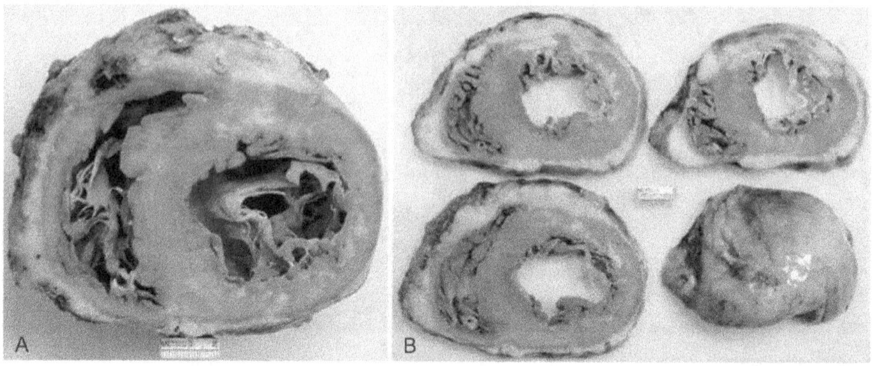

FIGURE 7. Ischemic cardiomyopathy. Views of the heart showing a transmural left ventricular scar from apex to base and a lateral and posterior walls scar which is probably not transmural in a 57-year-old man who had an acute myocardial infarct at age 48 years followed later by a coronary bypass grafting. Heart failure gradually progressed through the years, and his lowest left ventricular ejection fraction was 30%. (a) View of the base of the heart exposing both tricuspid and mitral valves. There is scarring in the anterior wall and in the posterior lateral wall. The lateral wall is much thinner than the ventricular septum. (b) Views of the ventricles more caudally showing extensive transmural anterior wall scarring. The quantity of subepicardial adipose tissue is increased.

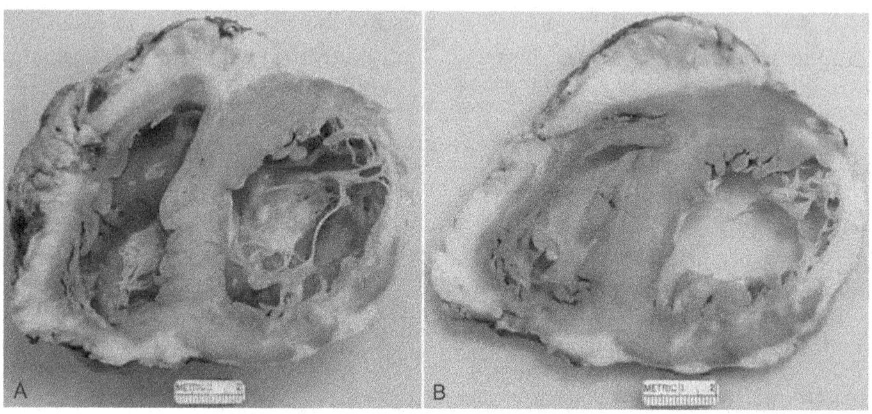

FIGURE 8. Ischemic cardiomyopathy. Heart in a 58-year-old man who had an acute myocardial infarct at age 29 years. A sibling and a parent had had myocardial infarcts at age 42 years. He clearly had heterozygous familial hypercholesterolemia. At age 30 years, he had coronary bypass grafting. His lowest left ventricular ejection fraction was 20%. (a) View of the basal portion of the heart exposing both tricuspid and mitral valves. The anterolateral wall is transmurally scarred such that the ventricular septum is thicker than the left ventricular free wall. (b) A more caudal view of the left ventricular wall showing the severe degree of scarring in the lateral wall with lesser degrees of scarring in the anterior and posterior walls. The quantity of subepicardial adipose tissue is increased.

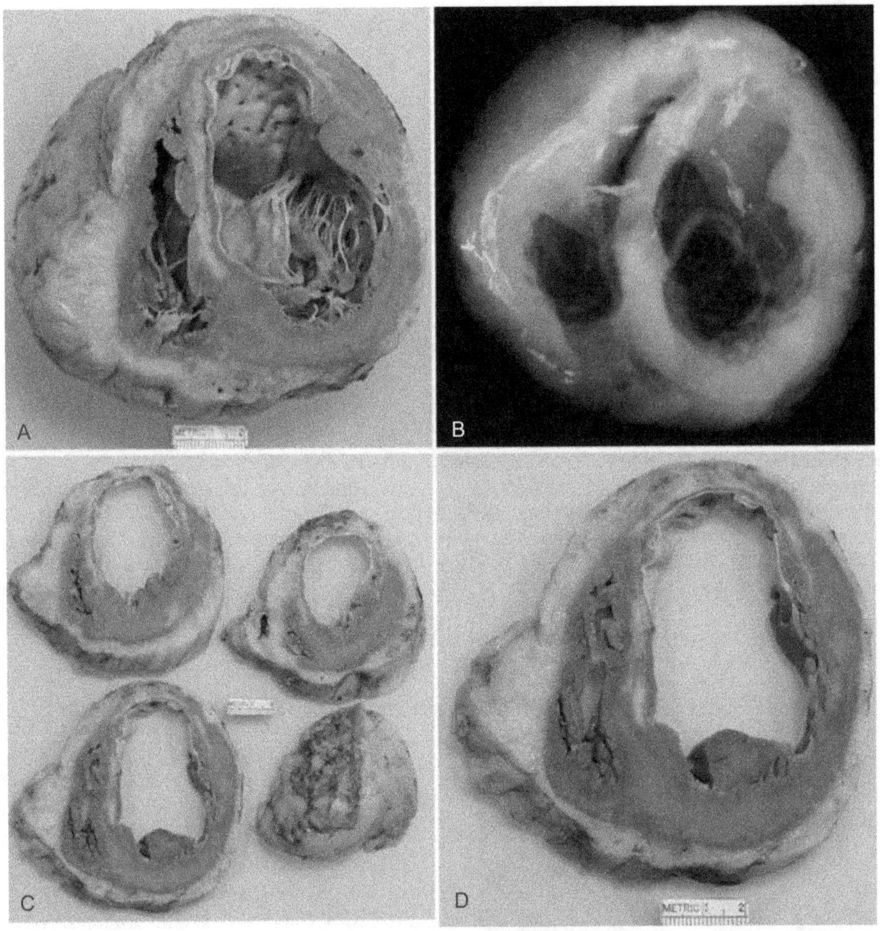

FIGURE 9. Ischemic cardiomyopathy. Heart in a 63-year-old man who had an acute myocardial infarct when he was 51 years of age. Subsequently, he underwent coronary artery bypass grafting. Percutaneous coronary intervention followed the bypass operation, and at age 58 years an implantable cardioverter defibrillator was inserted. Not long before cardiac transplantation his ejection fraction was 15%. At age 61 years, he had a stroke, and also during that year he underwent bilateral iliac stent implantation. (a) View of the basal portion of the heart exposing both tricuspid and mitral valves. Nearly the entire septum is scarred as is the anterior left ventricular free wall. The left ventricular cavity is greatly dilated. The quantity of subepicardial adipose tissue is considerably increased. (b) Radiograph of the basal portion of the heart showing a metallic stent in the right coronary artery with considerable scarring of the right and left anterior descending coronary arteries. (c) These more basal portions of the ventricular wall show that the large infarct extends to the cardiac apex. (d) View of 1 of the slices of left ventricular free wall showing marked thinning due to scar of the anterior wall.

without associated narrowing of the epicardial coronary arteries (except for 1 patient), and the scarring tended to be subepicardial. The ventricular chambers were very dilated in all 8 patients. Non-caseating giant cell granulomas were present in the ventricular walls in 7 of the 8 patients. In 1 patient the typical "hard" granulomas were present in the portion of left ventricular free wall excised to insert a left ventricular assist device but not in the recipient heart sometime later. Another patient had right and left ventricular free wall and ventricular septal scarring typical of cardiac sarcoidosis but no granulomas were found in the histologic sections of left ventricular free wall. This case we believe is an example of "burnt out" sarcoidosis.[43]

Cardiac Amyloidosis

Pertinent findings in the 3 cardiac amyloidosis patients are summarized in Table 8, and the hearts are illustrated in Figure 28.[7,10,16–18,40,53,69] The clinical and morphologic diagnoses were congruous in all 3 patients. The ventricular cavities were either not dilated or dilated to a small degree. The patients had firm—actually rubbery—myocardium, no grossly visible focal myocardial lesions but focal endocardial lesions in either the right atrium or left atrium or both and in the tricuspid valve leaflets. The presence of amyloid was confirmed by Congo-red stains of sections of the heart. Two of the 3 patients had narrowing >75% in cross-sectional area by atherosclerotic plaque, but none had grossly visible ventricular wall scars.

Adriamycin Cardiomyopathy

Pertinent findings in the 6 patients with Adriamycin cardiomyopathy are summarized in Table 9 and illustrated in Figure 29.[22,26,27,41,44] The clinical and morphologic diagnoses were congruous in each. All 6 had severely dilated ventricular chambers. All had received Adriamycin for cancer treatment.

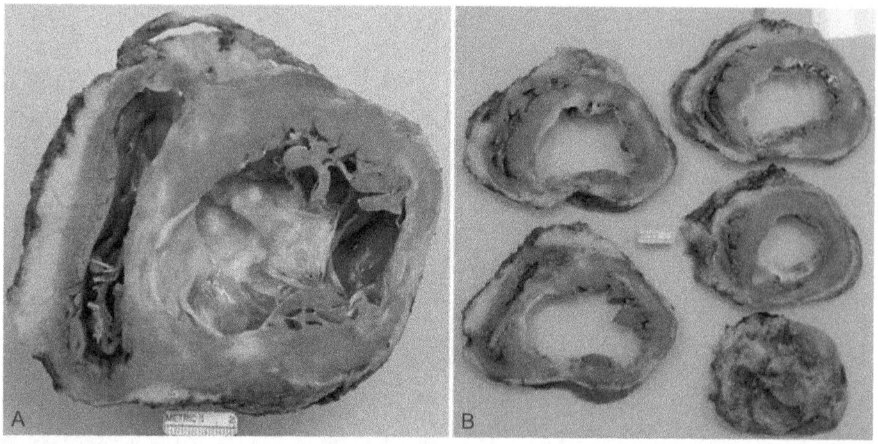

FIGURE 10. Ischemic cardiomyopathy. Heart in a 61-year-old man who had a acute myocardial infarct at age 53 years followed by a coronary artery bypass grafting. By age 59 years, his left ventricular ejection fraction was as low as 15%. An intracardiac defibrillator had been inserted also at age 54 years. (a) View of the basal portion of the heart showing a portion of tricuspid valve and a good bit of the anterior mitral leaflet. A large transmural scar is present in the lateral wall between the 2 left ventricular papillary muscles and in the ventricular septum in apposition to the lateral wall infarct. The left ventricular cavity is greatly dilated. (b) View of the more caudal portions of the ventricular wall again showing the 2 infarcts extending almost to the apex of the heart.

Valvular Heart Disease

Pertinent findings in the 7 patients with valvular heart disease are summarized in Table 10.[39,50,57] Four had aortic valve stenosis initially and repeated valve replacements; 1 had mitral valve replacements for mitral stenosis in 1 and for pure mitral regurgitation in the other. The latter patient also had severe tricuspid valve regurgitation, which had not been approached at a previous operation. The clinical and morphologic diagnoses were congruous in all 7 patients.

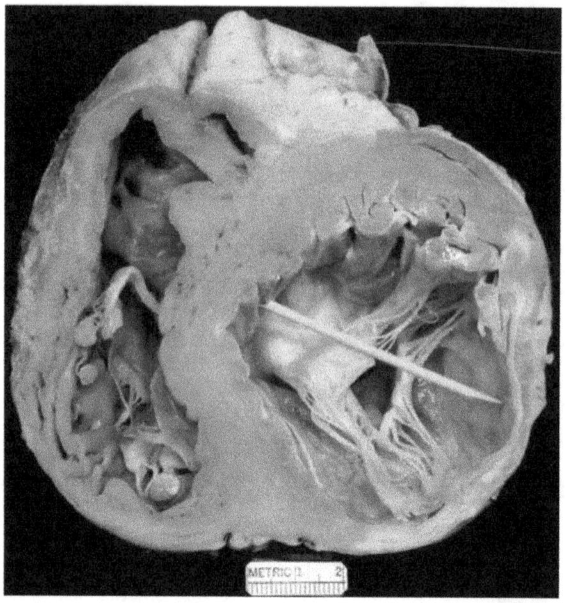

FIGURE 11. Ischemic cardiomyopathy. Heart in a 67-year-old man who had a large acute myocardial infarction at age 53 followed by coronary artery bypass grafting. At age 60, he had another bypass grafting operation. Heart failure progressed and was accompanied by several mitral regurgitation. His ejection fraction not long before cardiac transplantation was 10%. The view of the heart shows its basal portion exposing both mitral and tricuspid valves. The posterior and lateral walls of the heart are extremely thin from the extensive scarring. The posteromedial papillary muscle is flattened from the scarring and the anterolateral 1 is atrophied. The ventricular septum as a consequence is much thicker than the left ventricular free wall.

Cyanotic Congenital Heart Disease

Pertinent findings in the 3 patients with cyanotic congenital heart disease are summarized in Table 11.[38,63] One had complex complete transposition of the great arteries, 1 severe right ventricular hypoplasia, and 1 tetralogy of Fallot. All 3 had had more than 1 previous cardiac operation. The clinical and morphologic diagnosis were congruous in all 3.

Other

One patient had CT for ventricular septal defect resulting from a stab wound to the heart many years earlier. Details of this patient are described elsewhere.[48]

Outcomes

The survival probabilities for all 257 patients are shown in Figure 30. Of the 257 (of 314) patients in whom survival data are available, 66 (26%) have died: 8 (12%) within 60 days of CT and 58 (88%) at later periods. The log-rank test show no significant survival differences between men and women (log-rank = 0.479, p value = 0.4926) (Figure 30).

DISCUSSION

The present study serves 2 major functions: 1) it illustrates by gross photographs of the hearts the variability that occurs morphologically in each of the etiologic categories, and 2) it determines the frequency among the 314 patients of discrepancies between the clinical and morphologic diagnoses. Just like clinical presentations and courses are quite variable among patients with various types of cardiac diseases, the morphologic features in each type of cardiac

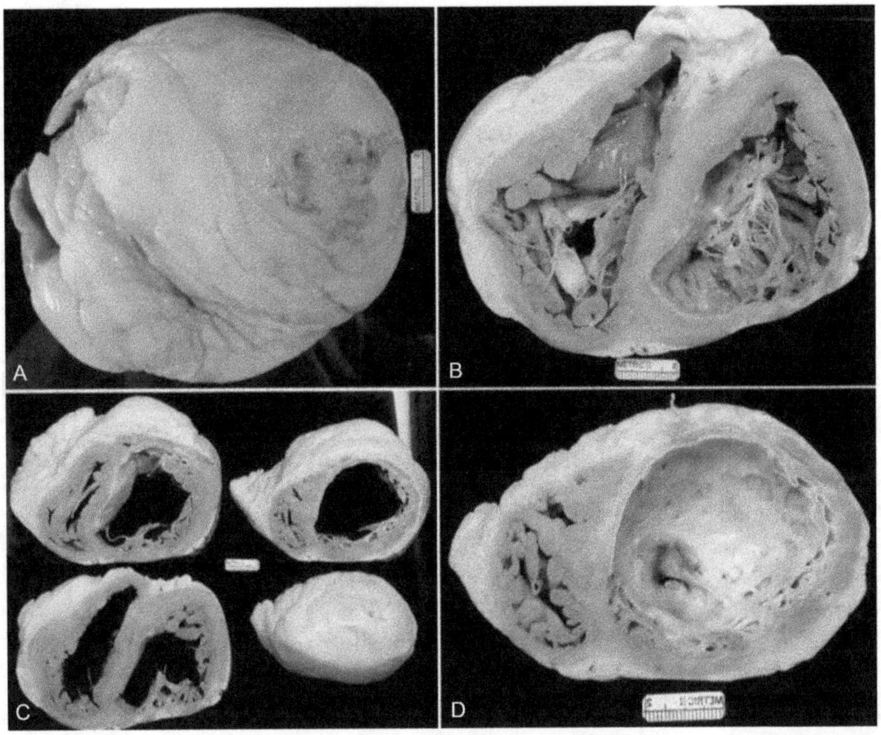

FIGURE 12. Ischemic cardiomyopathy. Heart in a 67-year-old man who had a large anterior wall infarct and another posterior wall infarct in the distant past. The exact dates of the infarcts are unclear, but radiograph of the excised heart showed calcium in the wall of the apex of the left ventricle indicating that the infarct was probably at least 10 years earlier. Heart failure had been a problem for many years. The left ventricular ejection fraction not long before cardiac transplantation was as low as 5%. (a) View of the exterior of the heart showing that most of the myocardial walls are covered by adipose tissue. (b) View of the base of the heart exposing both tricuspid and mitral valves. The posterior left ventricular free wall is thinned by scar tissue. (c) Views of the ventricles more caudally now showing both anterior and posterior wall infarcts. (d) View of the apex showing scarring in probably 300° of the 360° left ventricular wall. The heart contained so much adipose tissue that it floated in formaldehyde.

disease are also quite variable. To properly illustrate that variability a number of photographs of recipient hearts are presented.

As part of the second purpose of this report, we determined the frequency of congruity or incongruity between the clinical and morphologic diagnoses among the 314 patients. As shown in Table 1, most (96%) of the patients with IC at morphologic study had been diagnosed with that condition clinically. The discrepancy occurred when 6 patients with IC anatomically had insignificant coronary narrowing by angiography before CT, but nevertheless severe narrowing of 1 or more major epicardial coronary arteries morphologically and extensive left ventricular wall scarring. We defined IC as the presence of severe

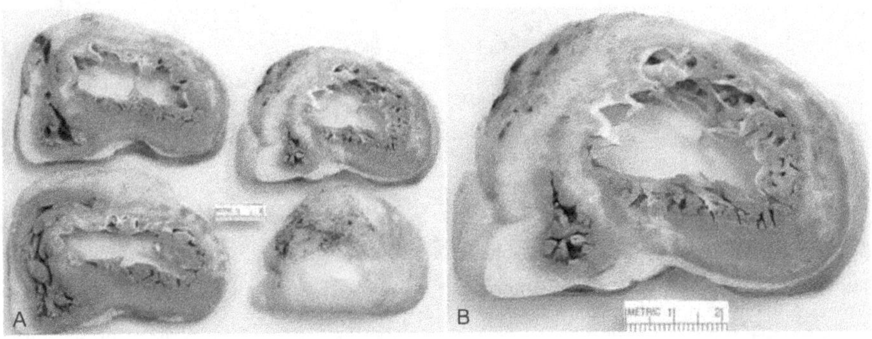

FIGURE 13. Ischemic cardiomyopathy. Heart in a 69-year-old man who had a large myocardial infarct, involving the anterior, septal, and lateral walls of the left ventricle only 4 months earlier with severe heart failure thereafter. (a) Sections of the ventricular walls caudal to the atrioventricular valves show a healed septal, anterior, and lateral wall infarct from apex to base. (b) A close-up of 1 of the slices showing the extensive scarring.

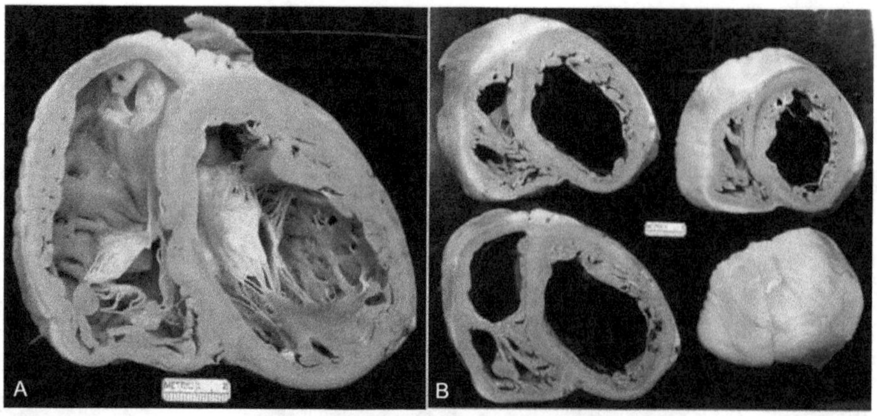

FIGURE 14. Idiopathic dilated cardiomyopathy. Heart of a 68-year-old man who had had evidence of heart failure since age 54 years. He was known to have severe hypothyroidism and was treated appropriately. He had never had chest pain. He did however have evidence of chronic obstructive lung disease and at 1 time was a habitual alcoholic. He also was known to have a fatty liver. The lowest left ventricular ejection fraction before transplantation was 5%. (a) View of the cardiac ventricles at the base exposing the tricuspid, mitral, and pulmonic valves. Both ventricular cavities are enormously dilated, and the walls of the left ventricle, ventricular septum, and right ventricle are free of foci of fibrosis and necrosis. (b) Views of the ventricles caudal to the atrioventricular valves. The moderator band is prominent in the right ventricle. The right coronary artery wall was quite calcified, and the lumen was quite narrowed. Nevertheless, the patient was classified as having idiopathic dilated cardiomyopathy because there were no lesions in the myocardial walls. It appears that this happened to be a patient who had both a narrowed coronary artery and idiopathic dilated cardiomyopathy.

(>75% in cross-sectional area) coronary narrowing accompanied by 1 or more transmural left ventricular wall scars. The reverse occurred in the case of IDC. Of the 111 patients with IDC anatomically (no left ventricular wall lesion grossly), 11 had severe narrowing of 1 or more major epicardial coronary arteries such that these patients in actuality did not fulfill our definitions for either IC or IDC. We suspect, however, that these 11 patients actually had IDC but resided in a high-cholesterol environment (United States), where coronary atherosclerosis is so prevalent.

Most of the incongruity between clinical and morphologic diagnoses occurred in the non-IC subgroups other than IDC. Thus, among the 56 patients with non-IC, excluding the patients with IDC, only 31 (55%) had congruity between the clinical and morphologic diagnoses. Specifically, among the 17 patients with HC, the 3 with NCLVC, the 3 with

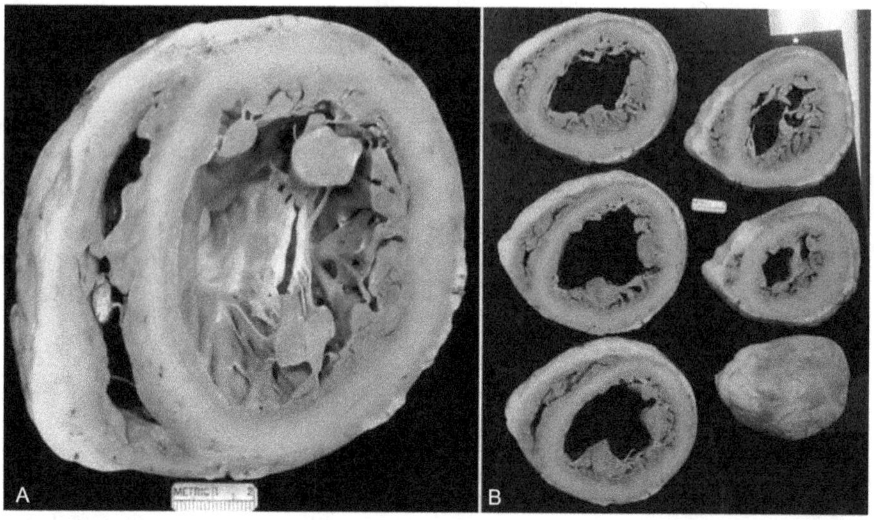

FIGURE 15. Idiopathic dilated cardiomyopathy. Views of the heart in a 61-year-old woman who had had evidence of chronic heart failure since age 51 years. She did reasonably well on medical therapy until age 59 years, when the heart failure worsened considerably and an implantable cardiac defibrillator was inserted. During the 2 years before transplant, the heart failure progressively worsened, and the left ventricular ejection fraction fell to a low of approximately 10%. She never had chest pain. Earlier in life she had had several children. (a) Basal portion of heart exposing well the mitral valve. The left ventricle is greatly enlarged measuring up to 7.5 cm. No foci of fibrosis or necrosis are seen in the ventricular walls. (b) Views of the ventricles caudal to the mitral valve, again showing considerable left ventricular cavity dilatation.

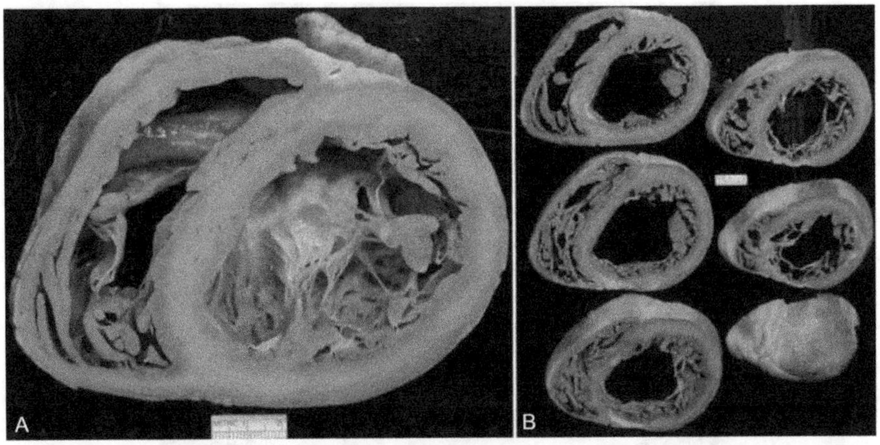

FIGURE 16. Idiopathic dilated cardiomyopathy. Heart in a 62-year-old woman who developed evidence of heart failure at age 55 years, which progressed thereafter. During the 7 months before cardiac transplant, the heart failure worsened considerably. Coronary angiography showed the major epicardial coronary arteries to be wide open. (a) Basal portion of heart exposing both tricuspid and mitral valves. Both ventricular cavities are considerably dilated. No foci of fibrosis or necrosis were noted in this portion of the ventricular walls. (b) Views of the ventricles caudal to the atrioventricular valves. In this view the posterior wall is thinned by scar tissue as is the most posterior portion of ventricular septum. The right coronary artery, as well as the others, was wide open. The focal scar may have been due to a coronary embolus many years earlier.

mononuclear myocarditis, the 4 with ARVC, and the 8 with cardiac sarcoidosis, a total of 35 patients, only 11 (31%) had the specific diagnosis made clinically. One could argue that including the single case without cardiac granulomas in the sarcoid group is improper. The type and distribution of the myocardial scarring, however, is absolutely typical of the other cases of cardiac sarcoidosis, a type of scarring not seen by us in any other condition.[43] Additionally, documented sarcoid granulomas in the lungs have been shown to disappear as the scarring increases.[59] Obviously, it is not sufficient to stop clinically with the diagnosis of non-IC cardiomyopathy. Ideally, of course, the specific subgroup needs to be sought even though therapy and outcome might not be altered by that knowledge.

The present study is not the first to compare the frequencies of discrepancies between the clinical and morphologic diagnoses in patients having CT. Bortman and colleagues[6] in 1994 examined the congruity-incongruity issue in 112 patients who underwent their first orthotopic CT at the authors' institution (University of Texas Southwestern

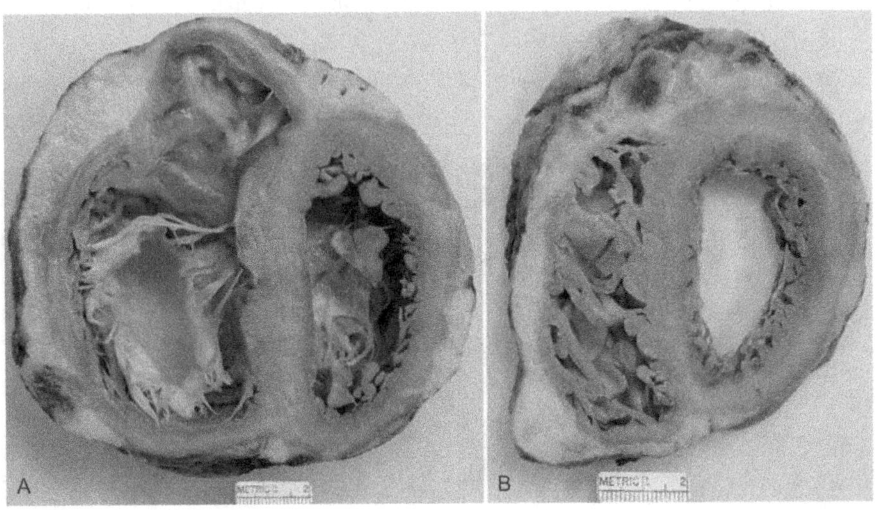

FIGURE 17. Idiopathic dilated cardiomyopathy. Heart of a 68-year-old man who was found to have heart failure at age 50 years, and, at the time, also to have severe mitral regurgitation. Coronary angiogram showed the coronary arteries to be wide open. At age 50 years, the patient underwent repair of the mitral valve including the insertion of an annular ring. The mitral regurgitation was reduced from severe to mild, but the heart failure continued and progressed. A left ventricular assist device was inserted before the cardiac transplantation. (a) View of the basal portion of the heart showing dilatation of both right and left ventricular cavities. The tricuspid annulus is quite dilated. No lesions are noted in the ventricular walls although the ventricular septum is thicker than the left ventricular free wall. (b) View more caudal showing impressive pectinate muscles within the right ventricular cavity. Again, no myocardial lesions are noted. The quantity of subepicardial adipose tissue is considerably increased.

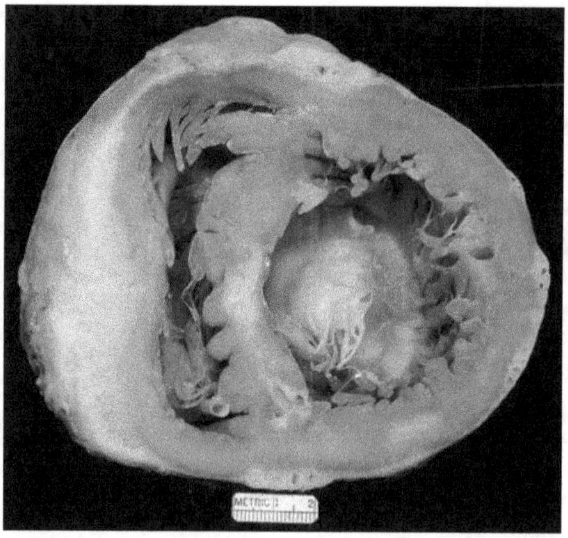

FIGURE 18. Hypertrophic cardiomyopathy. Heart in a 41-year-old man in whom hypertrophic cardiomyopathy was diagnosed when he was 6 years of age. At age 26 years, atrial fibrillation appeared and during the next 15 years he was cardioverted 98 times. He eventually developed complete heart block, and a pacemaker was inserted. At age 30 years, an intracardiac defibrillator was implanted, and at the same time an alcohol septal ablation procedure was performed. Nevertheless, evidence of heart failure persisted and a heart transplant was performed. View of the basal portion exposing both tricuspid and mitral valves. The left ventricular cavity is quite dilated. The focal scar in the ventricular septum may be the result of the alcohol septal ablation. Another small scar is present in the posterior wall of left ventricle. The thickness of the ventricular septum is greater than that of the left ventricular free wall.

Medical Center at Dallas). Among their 64 patients diagnosed with IC clinically, all had severe coronary narrowing morphologically; of their 48 patients with IDC clinically, 12 (25%) morphologically had severe coronary disease, and 3 had acute myocarditis. Thus, of their 112 patients a discrepancy between pre- and post-transplant diagnosis occurred in 15 (13%). Neither gross photographs nor definitions of the entities were provided.

In 1999, Angelini and colleagues[1] from Padua, Italy, studied the agreement or lack thereof between pre- and post-CT diagnoses in 257 patients having CT, and found a discrepancy between clinical and pathologic diagnoses in 20 patients (8%). Among their 87 patients with a clinical diagnoses of IC, 3 had IDC and 1 granulomatous myocarditis; among their 126 patients whose clinical diagnosis was non-IC, 7 morphologically had IC, 5 myocarditis, 1 ARVC, and 1 with NCLVC; among their 10 patients with a clinical diagnosis of HC, 1 had ARVC, and 1 had a cardiac fibroma.[1] No gross photographs of the heart or definitions of the conditions were provided.

In 2009, Luk and colleagues[29] from Toronto, Canada, studied the problem in 296 patients who had had CT from

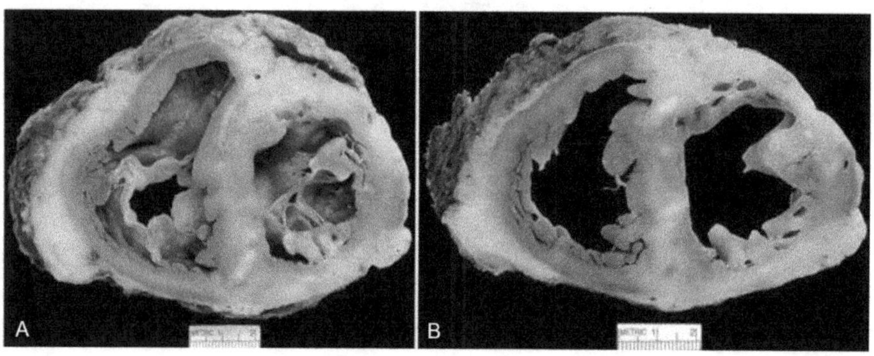

FIGURE 19. Hypertrophic cardiomyopathy. The heart in a 48-year-old man who developed heart failure at age 41 years and had an intracardiac defibrillator inserted shortly thereafter. A left ventricular assist device was inserted 2.3 years before cardiac transplantation. At age 45 years, he developed atrial fibrillation and had several cardioversion procedures performed. A parent and several cousins had heart disease of unclear type and were either asymptomatic or had died from it. (a) View of the base of the heart exposing both tricuspid and mitral valves. There is considerable scarring in the left ventricular and ventricular septal walls and in both papillary muscles. Both cavities are quite dilated. The thickness of the ventricular septum is greater than that of the left ventricular free wall. (b) Another view more caudal showing extensive scarring. The left anterior descending coronary artery is narrowed on this slice, probably the result of extensive scaring surrounding it. (Figure 19a is reprinted with permission from Elsevier.[49])

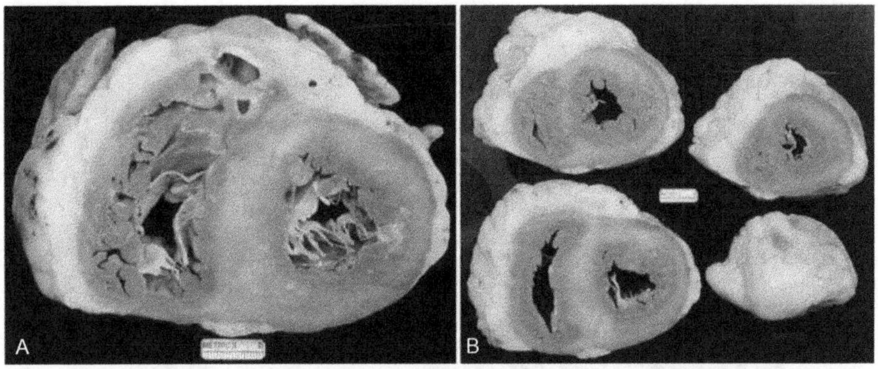

FIGURE 20. Hypertrophic cardiomyopathy. This 68-year-old man was diagnosed with hypertrophic cardiomyopathy many years earlier. His major problem was recurrent episodes of ventricular tachycardia, and he underwent an ablation procedure for that. He also had atrial fibrillation and other atrial arrhythmias. An implantable cardiac defibrillator was inserted. He also was obese, had obstructive sleep apnea, and chronic renal disease, stage 3. (a) View of the cardiac base exposing tricuspid, pulmonic, and mitral valves. The thickness of the ventricular septum is greater than that of the left ventricular free wall. The 2 ventricular cavities are only mildly dilated. Calcium was present in the mitral annular area. (b) Views of the ventricles caudal to the views shown on the left.

1987 to 2006 (Table 12). The frequency of the diagnosis made clinically and after examination of the recipient heart is shown in Table 12. It is apparent that the incongruity between the clinical and morphologic diagnoses was relatively frequent. Three gross photographs of the heart were presented. Definitions of the various conditions were not provided.

It is apparent from the present and previous studies that the largest incongruity between clinical and morphologic diagnosis in patients having CT is among the non-IC subtypes, particularly the dilated (end-stage) form of HC, mononuclear myocarditis, cardiac sarcoidosis, ARVC, and NCLVC. Would the use of additional diagnostic "instruments of precision" have allowed more precise pre-CT diagnosis among the non-IC group? Possibly so, particularly more use of magnetic resonance imaging among the patients with HC and sarcoidosis.[35] Would a more

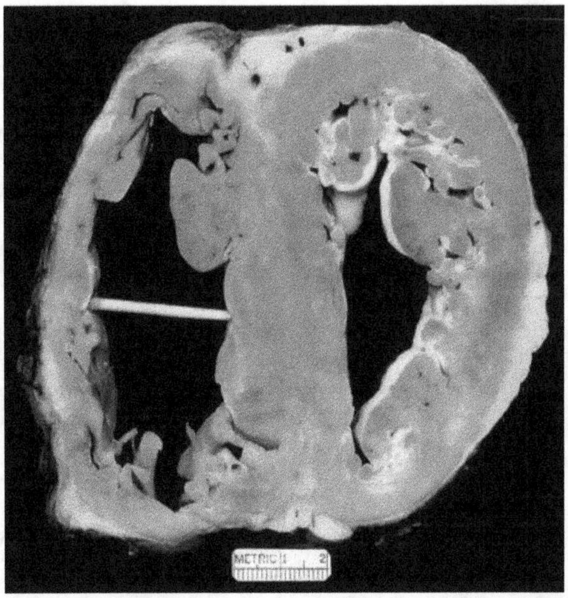

FIGURE 21. Hypertrophic cardiomyopathy. View of the heart in a 68-year-old man who was known to have some form of heart disease since age 38 years. The problem during the 30 years was various degrees of heart failure which began progressing about age 55 years. In the 2 years before cardiac transplantation he had multiple hospitalizations for decompensated heart failure. He had an intracardiac defibrillator in place for several years. Because of the severity of the heart failure, a left ventricular assist device was inserted 7 months before cardiac transplantation. The heart failure severity, however, continued, and before heart transplantation the left ventricular ejection fraction was approximately 10%. Both cardiac ventricles are dilated, the right more than the left. The ventricular septum is thicker than the left ventricular free wall. The mural endocardium of the left ventricle is thickened by white fibrous tissue. A scar is present in the posterior portion of the left ventricular free wall and also in the posterior portion of the ventricular septum.

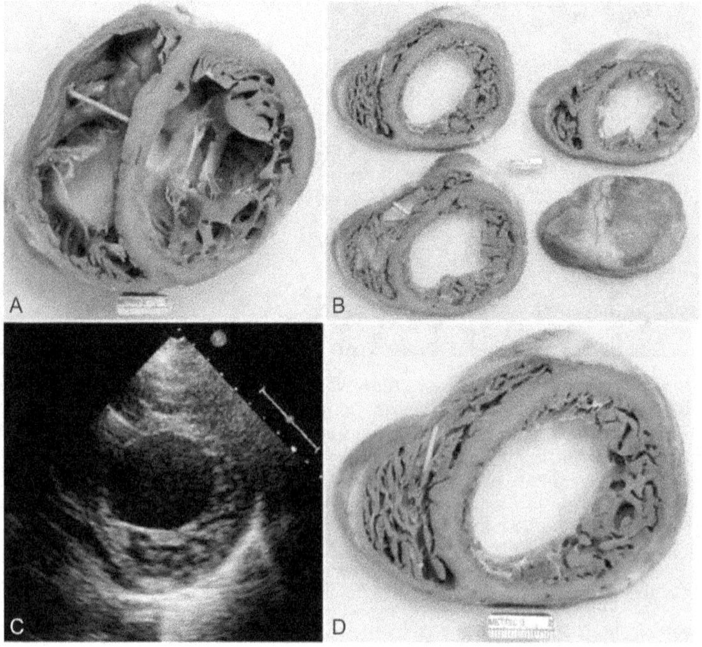

FIGURE 22. Left ventricular non-compaction cardiomyopathy. Heart in a 49-year-old man who had been well until age 33 years when symptoms of heart failure appeared. At the time, echocardiogram showed both ventricles to be dilated and the left ventricular systolic function to be severely depressed. A defibrillator was inserted at age 39 years, and cardiac resynchronization therapy at age 43 years. He underwent ablation therapy for multiple episodes of ventricular tachycardia. His left ventricular ejection fraction just before cardiac transplantation was 15%. (a) View of both ventricles just caudal to the tricuspid and mitral valves. The thickness of the ventricular septum is much greater than that of the left ventricular free wall. The compacted portion of left ventricular free wall is much thinner than the non-compacted portion. Both ventricular cavities are greatly dilated. The left ventricular free wall posteriorly is focally scarred. (a) View of the basal portion of the heart exposing the tricuspid and mitral valves. Both ventricles are greatly dilated. The posterolateral wall is focally scarred. The compacted portion of left ventricular free wall is much thinner than the trabeculated portion. (b) Views of sections of the ventricular walls caudal to the view shown in the upper left. (c) Echocardiogram showing hypertrabeculation of the left ventricular free wall. (d) Section of the left ventricular free wall corresponding to the echocardiogram. (Reprinted with permission from Elsevier.[45]).

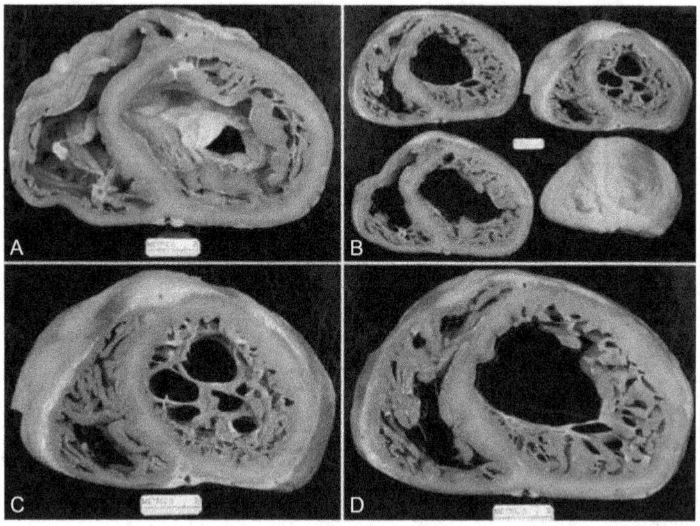

FIGURE 23. Left ventricular non-compaction cardiomyopathy. Heart of a 36-year-old woman who was well until approximately age 35 years when she developed evidence of heart failure, which slowly but gradually progressed thereafter such that when she was aged 34 years her left ventricular ejection fraction had fallen to 20% and she was in chronic atrial fibrillation. She also developed runs of ventricular tachycardia for which a defibrillator was inserted. (a) View of the heart showing both tricuspid and mitral valves. Both ventricular cavities are enormously dilated, and the ventricular walls are free of foci of fibrosis and necrosis. (b) Views of the ventricles caudal to the view shown in upper left. (c) Close-up view of 1 of the slices in upper right. (d) View showing the hypertrabeculated or non-compacted portion of the left ventricular wall to be much thicker than the compacted portion. (Reprinted with permission from Elsevier.[45]).

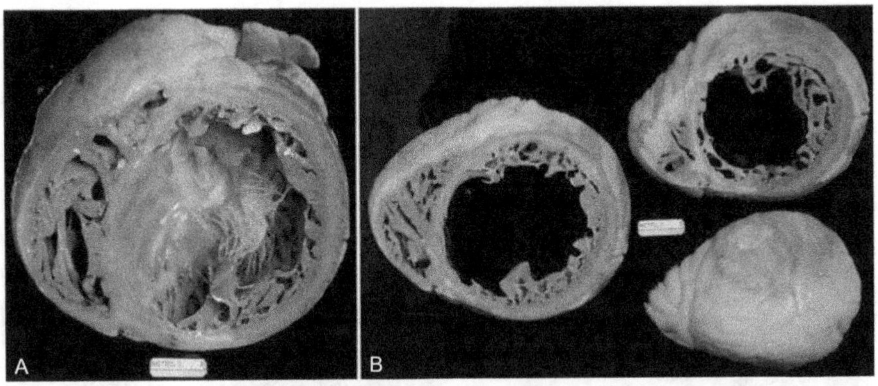

FIGURE 24. Mononuclear myocarditis. The heart in a 56-year-old man who had been well until age 48 years, when he had a cardiac event that resulted in the appearance of heart failure, which progressed thereafter. He also smoked heavily and had evidence of chronic obstructive lung disease. A defibrillator was inserted when he was 53 years old. (a) Basal portion of the heart showing severe dilatation of the left ventricular cavity with transmural scarring in the posterior and anterior left ventricular free wall and in the anterior portion of the ventricular septum. (b) Sections of the ventricular cavities caudal to the view shown on the left. The ventricular septum in 2 of the slices is completely scarred. Histologic section showed focal collections of mononuclear cells in the walls of left ventricle and ventricular septum. The coronary arteries at necropsy were wide open.

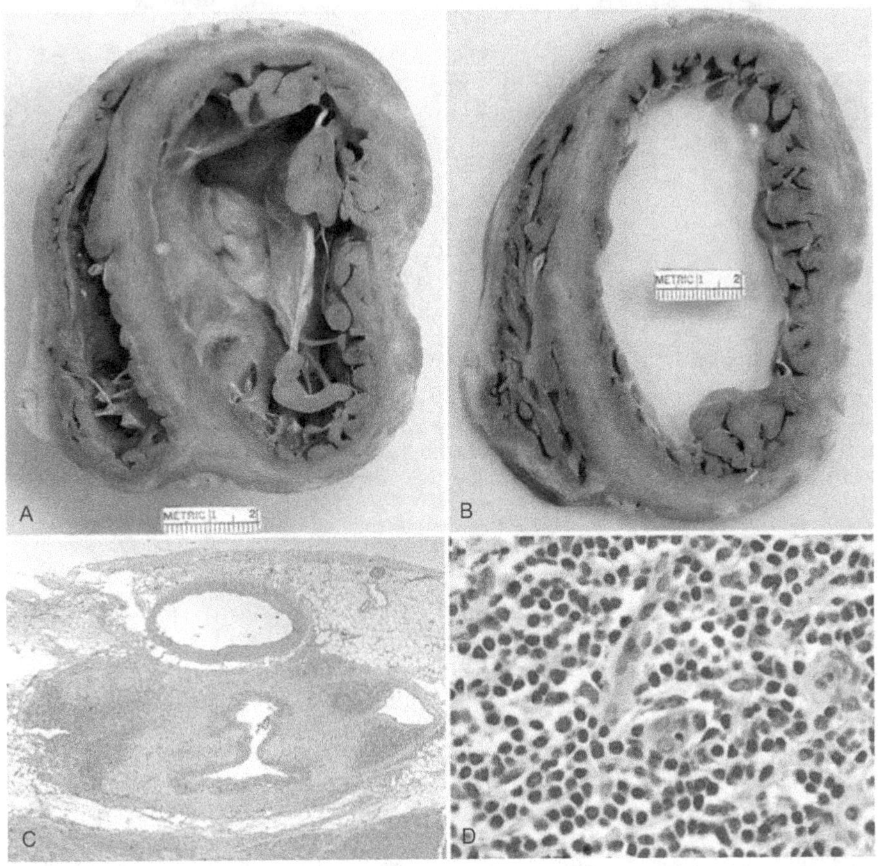

FIGURE 25. Monocytic myocarditis. Photographs and photomicrographs of the heart in a 24-year-old man who had been well until approximately 2.5 years earlier when evidence of heart failure appeared and not long thereafter his left ventricular ejection fraction was approximately 15%. A defibrillator was implanted. Progressive worsening of the heart failure prompted the CT. The echocardiogram 15 months before cardiac transplantation showed his left ventricular ejection fraction to be as low as 5%. (a) View of the cardiac base exposing the mitral valve. (b) Slice of the ventricles more caudal. The scarring and inflammatory cell infiltrates are mainly subepicardial in location. (c) Inflammatory cell collection in the subepicardial adipose tissue (Movat stain ×20). (d) Close-up of the lymphocytes (hematoxylin/eosin stain, ×100).

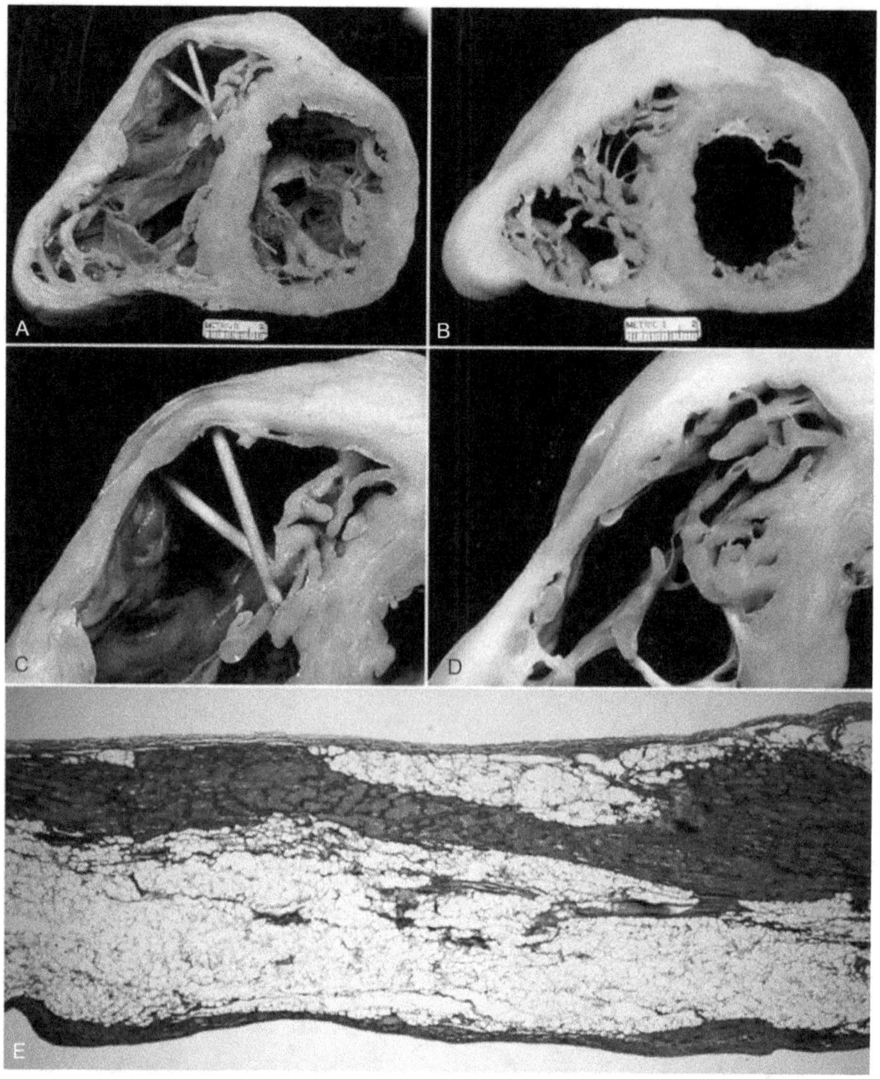

FIGURE 26. Arrhythmogenic right ventricular cardiomyopathy. The heart in a 26-year-old man who developed symptoms of heart failure at age 12 years, followed later by ventricular arrhythmias and bundle branch block. His left ventricular ejection fraction fell to 15%. (a) View of the base of the heart showing marked dilatation of both ventricles. The right ventricular wall in its outflow tract is thin (b, c, d). (e) Photomicrograph of the right ventricular wall in the right ventricular outflow tract, which consists of adipose tissue, fibrous tissue, and a few myocardial cells (Masson stain, ×20). (Reprinted with permission from Elsevier.[46]).

accurate pre-CT diagnosis among the non-IC group have led to a re-evaluation of the need for CT in the first place? Or, if clinicians had actually known the specific non-IC diagnosis, would treatment have been different and might CT have been avoided? Among the 314 patients included in this study, the morphologic and clinical diagnoses were incongruent in 42 (13%), including 7 of 17 patients with HC, 3 of 3 with NCLVC, 3 of 3 with mononuclear myocarditis, 4 of 4 with ARVC, and 8 of 8 with cardiac sarcoidosis. This incongruity certainly leaves open the possibility that, if immunosuppressive or immunomodulatory treatment had been used in certain cases, such as specific antiarrhythmic agents for ARVC or intracardiac defibrillator for non-obstructive HC with normal or near-normal left ventricular ejection fraction, this therapy might have made a difference with respect to treatment, outcome, and even potentially the need for CT.

The positive features of the present study include the fact that all hearts were examined and described and all morphologic diagnoses were provided by the same person (WCR), who has been studying cardiovascular diseases for several decades. Had many of the non-IC cases been "grossed" by a first or second year trainee, which is the modus of operation in the surgical pathology laboratory at BUMC--except for the cardiovascular cases--it is unlikely that the cases of burnt-out or end-stage HC, or ARVC, or NCLVC would have been recognized grossly, and histologic examination in these cases would unlikely have provided the proper morphologic diagnoses.

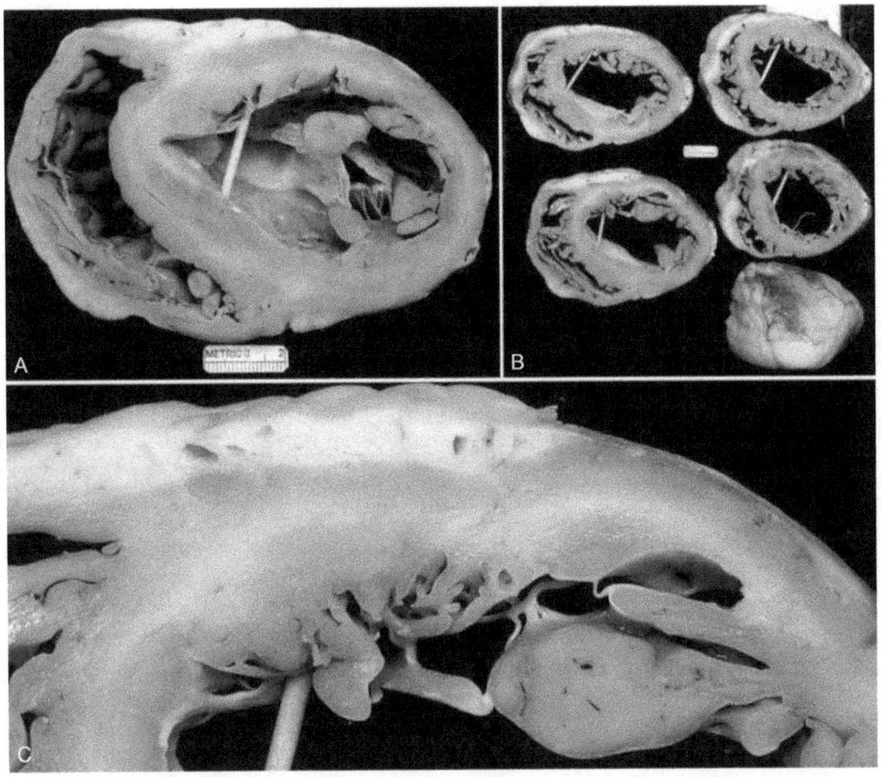

FIGURE 27. Cardiac sarcoidosis. Heart in a 52-year-old black woman who had developed evidence of heart failure beginning at age 48 years. It progressed, and an implantable cardiac defibrillator/pacemaker was placed. Runs of ventricular tachycardia occasionally were seen. Cardiac catheterization 8 months before cardiac transplantation disclosed normal coronary arteries, severe global left ventricular hypokinesis, and an estimated ejection fraction of 10%. The pressures in mm Hg were as follows: left ventricle, 115/34; right ventricle, 59/15; pulmonary artery wedge a wave 20, v wave 20, mean 18; right atrium a wave 12, v wave 10, mean 9. The cardiac index was 1.7 L/min per m2. A diagnosis of cardiac sarcoidosis was never entertained clinically. (a) Heart at the base showing the greatly dilated ventricular cavities and scarring in the ventricular septum and left ventricular free wall anteriorly. (b) Cross-section of the ventricles showing the extent of the scarring. (c) Close-up of the left ventricular free wall and ventricular septum showing the scarring. (Reprinted with permission from Elsevier.[43]).

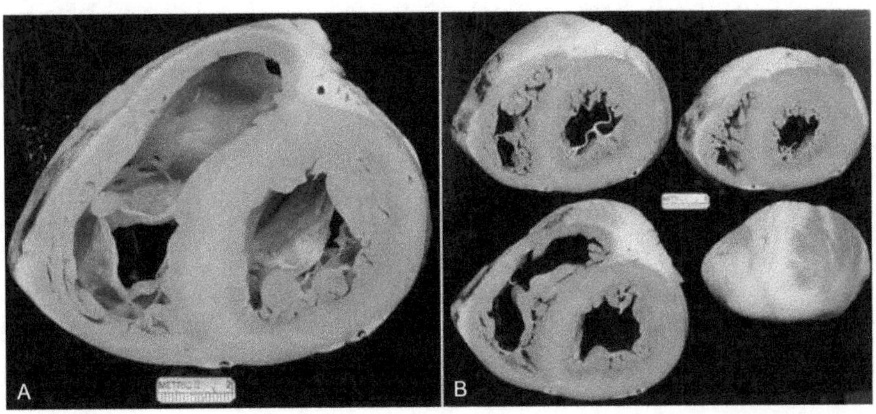

FIGURE 28. Cardiac amyloidosis. Heart in a 57-year-old man who had been well until 1 year before cardiac transplantation, when evidence of heart failure appeared. On examination 2 months later he was noted to have periorbital ecchymoses and a biopsy of an abdominal fat pad disclosed amyloidosis. During the year before CT, he lost 40 pounds, and the dyspnea and exercise intolerance progressively worsened. Echocardiogram 5 months before CT disclosed an ejection fraction of 55%, a restrictive diastolic filling pattern, and an "ineffective atrial kick." The heart weighed 420 g and amyloid deposits were extensively present in the walls of all 4 cardiac chambers. The right ventricular cavity was larger than the left ventricular cavity. The epicardial coronary arteries were wide open. Amyloid deposits were extensive in the walls of all 4 cardiac chambers. (a) View of the cardiac base. (b) Views of the more caudal portions of the heart.

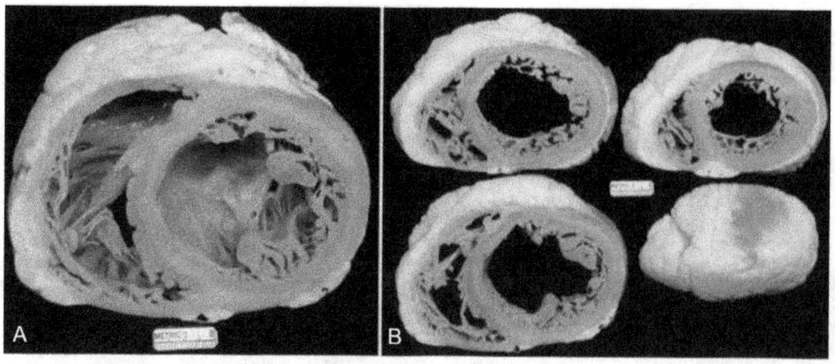

FIGURE 29. Adriamycin-induced cardiomyopathy. Heart in a 50-year-old woman who had received Adriamycin at age 38 years (12 years earlier) for cancer of the right breast with total mastectomy. She had evidence of heart failure only a couple of months before CT with rapid progression thereafter such that 1 month before CT her left ventricular ejection fraction was only 10%. The pressures in mm Hg were left ventricle 85/23; aorta 85/50. The cardiac output was 1.2 L/min, the ventricular cavities were severely dilated, and the epicardial coronary arteries were wide open. The heart weighed 405 g and the ventricles were dilated. Histologically, no specific cardiac lesions are present. (a) View of the cardiac base. (b) View of the more caudal cardiac slices.

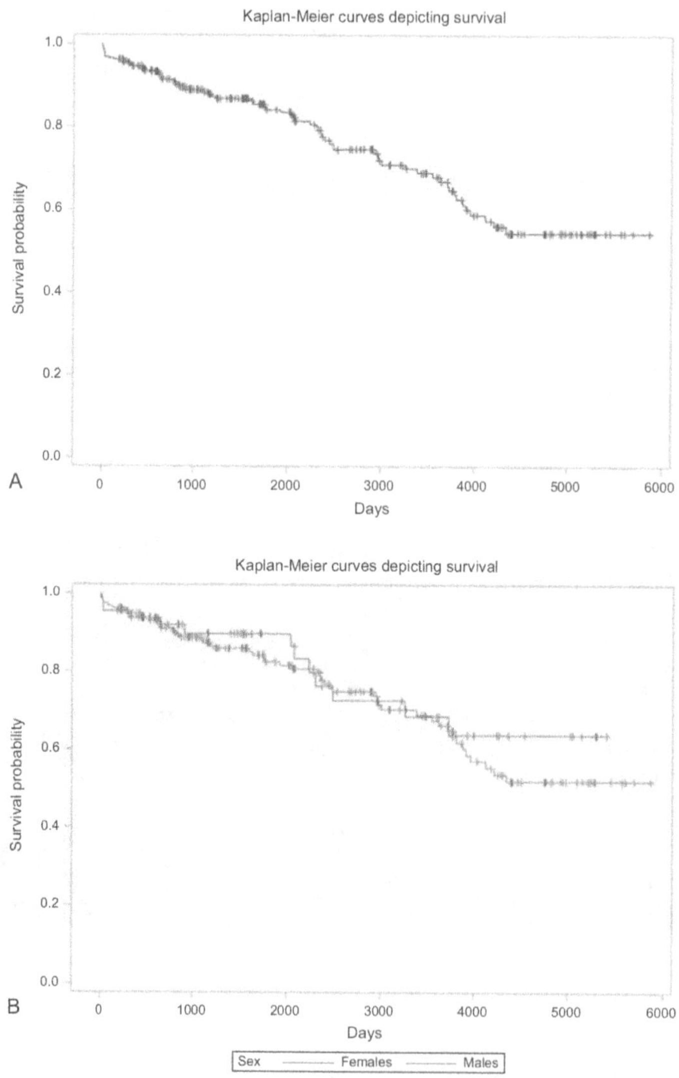

FIGURE 30. Kaplan-Meier survival curves for 257 patients whose survival data were available. (a) The unadjusted survival curve. (b) The unadjusted survival curves by sex.

REFERENCES

1. Angelini A, Boffa GM, Livi U, et al. Discordance between pre and post cardiac transplant diagnosis: implications for pre- and postoperative decision making. *Cardiovasc Pathol*. 1999; 8:17–23.
2. Avella A, d'Amati G, Zachara E, et al. Comparison between electro-anatomic and pathologic findings in a patient with arrhythmogenic right ventricular cardiomyopathy/dysplasia treated with orthotopic cardiac transplant. *Heart Rhythm*. 2010; 7:828–831.
3. Barnard CN. The Operation. A human heart transplant: an interim report of a successful operation performed at Groote Schuur Hospital, Cape Town. *S AFr Med J*. 1967; 41:1271–1274.
4. Basso C, Corrado D, Marcus FI, et al. Arrhythmogenic right ventricular cardiomyopathy. *Lancet*. 2009; 373:1289–1300.
5. Biagini E, Spirito P, Leone O, et al. Heart transplantation in hypertrophic cardiomyopathy. *Am J Cardiol*. 2008; 101:387–392.
6. Bortman G, Sellanes M, Odell DS, et al. Discrepancy between pre- and post-transplant diagnosis of end-stage dilated cardiomyopathy. *Am J Cardiol*. 1994; 74:921–924.
7. Bradshaw SH, Veinot JP. Cardiac amyloidosis: what are the indications for transplant?. *Curr Opin Cardiol*. 2012; 27:143–147.
8. Burke AP, Farb A, Tashko G, et al. Arrhythmogenic right ventricular cardiomyopathy and fatty replacement of the right ventricular myocardium: are they different diseases?. *Circulation*. 1998; 97:1571–1580.
9. Chang TI, Chi NH, Chou NK, et al. Isolated cardiac sarcoidosis in heart transplantation. *Transplant Proc*. 2012; 44:903–906.
10. Conner R, Hosenpud JD, Norman DJ, et al. Heart transplantation for cardiac amyloidosis: successful one-year outcome despite recurrence of the disease. *J Heart Transplant*. 1988; 7:165–167.
11. Conraads V, Paelinck B, Vorlat A, et al. Isolated non- compaction of the left ventricle: A rare indication for transplantation. *J Heart Lung Transplant*. 2001; 20:904–907.
12. Corrado D, Basso C, Thiene G, et al. Spectrum of clinicopathologic manifestations of arrhythmogenic right ventricular cardiomyopathy/dysplasia: a multicenter study. *J Am Coll Cardiol*. 1997; 30: 1512–1520.
13. Coutu M, Perrault LP, White M, et al. Cardiac transplantation for hypertrophic cardiomyopathy: a valid therapeutic option. *J Heart Lung Transplant*. 2004; 23:413–417.
14. Dalal D, Nasir K, Bomma C, et al. Arrhythmogenic right ventricular dysplasia: a United States experience. *Circulation*. 2005; 112:3823–3832.
15. Donsky AS, Escobar J, Capehart J, et al. Heart Transplantation for undiagnosed cardiac sarcoidosis. *Am J Cardiol*. 2002; 89:1447–1450.
16. Dubrey SW, Burke MM, Hawkins PN, et al. Cardiac transplantation for amyloid heart disease: the United Kingdom experience. *J Heart Lung Transplant*. 2004; 23:1142–1153.
17. Dubrey SW, Burke MM, Khaghani A, et al. Long term results of heart transplantation in patients with amyloid heart disease. *Heart*. 2001; 85:202–207.
18. Falk RH. Cardiac amyloidosis: a treatable disease, often overlooked. *Circulation*. 2011; 124:1079–1085.
19. Garner WL, Starling C, Kuiper JJ, et al. Lymphocytic myocarditis as a cause of fulminant fatal heart failure. *Proc (Bayl Univ Med Cent)*. 2006; 19:122–123.
20. Gungor H, Oguz E, Ayik MF, et al. Comparison of heart transplantation patients with ischemic and idiopathic dilated cardiomyopathy. *Transplant Proc*. 2011; 43:3847–3850.
21. Hamada T, Kubo T, Kitaoka H, et al. Clinical features of the dilated phase of hypertrophic cardiomyopathy in comparison with those of dilated cardiomyopathy. *Clin Cardiol*. 2010; 33:E24–E28.
22. Isner JM, Ferrans VJ, Cohen SR, et al. Clinical and morphologic cardiac findings after anthracycline chemotherapy. Analysis of 64 patients studied at necropsy. *Am J Cardiol*. 1983; 51:1167–1174.
23. Isner JM, Virmani R, Itscoitz SB, et al. Left and right ventricular myocardial infarction in idiopathic dilated cardiomyopathy. *Am Heart J*. 1980; 9:235–242.
24. Kato TS, Takayama H, Yoshizawa S, et al. Cardiac transplantation in patients with hypertrophic cardiomyopathy. *Am J Cardiol*. 2012; 110:568–574.
25. Kindermann I, Barth C, Mahfoud F, et al. Update on myocarditis. *J Am Coll Cardiol*. 2012; 59:779–792.
26. Kumar S, Marfatia R, Tannenbaum S, et al. Doxorubicin-induced cardiomyopathy 17 years after chemotherapy. *Tex Heart Inst J*. 2012; 39:424–427.
27. Lennenman AJ, Wang L, Wigger M, et al. Heart transplant survival outcomes for adriamycin-dilated cardiomyopathy. *Am J Cardiol*. 2013; 111:609–612.
28. Lobo FV, Silver MD, Butany J, et al. Left ventricular involvement in right ventricular dysplasia/cardiomyopathy. *Can J Cardiol*. 1999; 15:1239–1247.
29. Luk A, Metawee M, Ahn E, et al. Do clinical diagnoses correlate with pathological diagnoses in cardiac transplant patients? The importance of endomyocardial biopsy. *Can J Cardiol*. 2009; 25:e48–e54.
30. Mancini D, Lietz K. Selection of cardiac transplantation candidates in 2010. *Circulation*. 2010; 122:173–183.
31. Marcus FI, Zareba W, Calkins H, et al. Arrhythmogenic right ventricular cardiomyopathy/dysplasia clinical presentation and diagnostic evaluation: results from the North American Multidisciplinary Study. *Heart Rhythm*. 2009; 6:984–992.
32. Marcus GM, Glidden DV, Polonsky B, et al. Multidisciplinary Study of Right Ventricular Dysplasia Investigators. Efficacy of antiarrhythmic drugs in arrhythmogenic right ventricular cardiomyopathy: a report from the North American ARVC Registry. *J Am Coll Cardiol*. 2009; 54:609–615.
33. Maron BJ, Maron MS, Wigle ED, et al. The 50-year history, controversy, and clinical implications of left ventricular outflow tract obstruction in hypertrophic cardiomyopathy. *J Am Coll Cardiol*. 2009; 54:191–200.
34. Maron BJ, Maron MS. Hypertrophic cardiomyopathy. *Lancet*. 2013; 381:242–255.
35. Maron BJ, Wolfson JK, Epstein SE, et al. Intramural ("small vessel") coronary artery disease in hypertrophic cardiomyopathy. *J Am Coll Cardiol*. 1986; 8:545–557.
36. Maron BJ. Hypertrophic cardiomyopathy. *Lancet*. 1997; 350:127–133.
37. Maron MS, Kalsmith BM, Udelson JE, et al. Survival after cardiac transplantation in patients with hypertrophic cardiomyopathy. *Circ Heart Fail*. 2010; 3:574–579.
38. Parisi F. Heart transplantation in congenital heart disease. *Curr Cardiol Rev*. 2011; 7:50.
39. Pavie A. Heart transplantation for end-stage valvular disease: indications and results. *Curr Opin Cardiol*. 2006; 21:100–105.
40. Pelosi F, Capehart JE, Roberts WC. Effectiveness of cardiac transplantation for primary (AL) cardiac amyloidosis. *Am J Cardiol*. 1997; 79:532–535.
41. Ried M, Rupprecht L, Hirt S, et al. Sequential therapy of primary cardiac lymphoma with cardiectomy, total artificial heart support, and cardiac transplantation. *J Heart Lung Transplant*. 2010; 29: 707–709.
42. Roberts CS, Roberts WC. Morphologic features (of hypertrophic cardiomyopathy). *Progress in Cardiology 2/2*. In: Zipes DP, Rowlands DJ, editor Philadelphia: Lea & Febiger, 1989; pp. 3–32.

43. Roberts WC, Chung MS, Ko JM, et al. Morphologic features of cardiac sarcoidosis in native hearts of patients having cardiac transplantation. *Am J Cardiol*. 2014; 113:706–712.

44. Roberts WC, Glancy DL, DeVita VT. Heart in malignant lymphoma (Hodgkin's disease, lymphosarcoma, reticulum cell sarcoma and mycosis fungoides). A study of 196 autopsy cases. *Am J Cardiol*. 1968; 22:85–107.

45. Roberts WC, Karia SJ, Ko JM, et al. Examination of isolated ventricular non-compaction (hypertrabeculation) as a distinct entity in adults. *Am J Cardiol*. 2011; 108:747–752.

46. Roberts WC, Ko JM, Kuiper JJ, et al. Some previously neglected examples of arrhythmogenic right ventricular dysplasia /cardiomyopathy and frequency of its various reported manifestations. *Am J Cardiol*. 2010; 106:268–274.

47. Roberts WC, McAllister HA, Ferrans VJ. Sarcoidosis of the Heart. A clinicopathologic study of 35 necropsy patients (Group I) and review of 78 previously described necropsy patients (Group II). *Am J Med*. 1977; 63:86–108.

48. Roberts WC, Phillips SD, Escobar JM, et al. Cardiac transplantation 40 years after a stab wound to the heart. *Proc (Bayl Univ Med Cent)*. 2001; 14:241–242.

49. Roberts WC, Roberts CC, Ko JM, et al. Dramatically different phenotypic expressions of hypertrophic cardiomyopathy in male cousins undergoing cardiac transplantation with identical disease-causing gene mutation. *Am J Cardiol*. 2013; 111:1818–1822.

50. Roberts WC, Roberts CC, Ko JM, et al. Cardiac transplantation in adults with aortic valve disease with focus on the bicuspid aortic valve. *Am J Cardiol*. 2012; 109:1212–1214.

51. Roberts WC, Siegel RJ, McManus BM. Idiopathic dilated cardiomyopathy: Analysis of 152 necropsy patients. *Am J Cardiol*. 1987; 60:1340–1355.

52. Roberts WC, Vowels TJ, Ko JM, et al. Cardiac transplantation for cardiac sarcoidosis with initial diagnosis by examination of the left ventricular apical "core" excised for insertion of a left ventricular assist device for severe chronic heart failure. *Am J Cardiol*. 2009; 103:110–114.

53. Roberts WC, Waller BF. Cardiac amyloidosis causing cardiac dysfunction: analysis of 54 necropsy patients. *Am J Cardiol*. 1983; 52:137–146.

54. Roberts WC. Defining idiopathic dilated cardiomyopathy: A courtroom discussion. *Am J Cardiol*. 1989; 63:893–896.

55. Ross EM, Roberts WC. Severe atherosclerotic coronary arterial narrowing and chronic congestive heart failure without myocardial infarction; analysis of 18 patients studied at necropsy. *Am J Cardiol*. 1986; 57:51–56.

56. Ross EM, Roberts WC. Severe atherosclerotic coronary artery disease, healed myocardial infarction and chronic congestive heart failure; analysis of 81 patients studied at necropsy. *Am J Cardiol*. 1986; 57:44–50.

57. Rotela Samaniego JA, Castells E, Manito N, et al. Clinical evolution of heart transplantation in patients with previous valvular cardiomyopathy. *Transplant Proc*. 2007; 39:2355–2356.

58. Sagar S, Liu PP, Cooper LT. Myocarditis. *Lancet*. 2012; 379:738–747.

59. Scadding JG. A 'burnt-out' case of sarcoidosis. *Postgrad Med J*. 1968; 4:105–108.

60. Shirani J, Freant LJ, Roberts WC. Gross and semiquantitative histologic findings in mononuclear cell myocarditis causing sudden death, and implications for endomyocardial biopsy. *Am J Cardiol*. 1993; 72:952–957.

61. Shirani J, Maron BJ, Cannon RO, et al. Clinicopathologic features of hypertrophic cardiomyopathy managed by cardiac transplantation. *Am J Cardiol*. 1993; 72:434–440.

62. Shirani J. Subepicardial myocardial lesions. *Am Heart J*. 1993; 125:1346–1352.

63. Siân Pincott E, Burch M. Indications for heart transplantation in congenital heart disease. *Curr Cardiol Rev*. 2011; 7:51–58.

64. Tedford RJ, James C, Judge DP, et al. Cardiac transplantation in arrhythmogenic right ventricular dysplasia/cardiomyopathy. *J Am Coll Cardiol*. 2012; 9:289–290.

65. Theleman KP, Kuiper JJ, Roberts WC. Acute myocarditis (predominately lymphocytic) causing sudden death without heart failure. *Am J Cardiol*. 2001; 88:1078–1083.

66. Tops LF, Prakasa K, Tandri H, et al. Prevalence and pathophysiologic attributes of ventricular dyssynchrony in arrhythmogenic right ventricular dysplasia/cardiomyopathy. *J Am Coll Cardiol*. 2009; 54:445–451.

67. Valantine HA, Tazelaar HD, Macoviak J, et al. Cardiac sarcoidosis: response to steroids and transplantation. *J Heart Transplant*. 1987; 6:244–250.

68. Val-Bernal JF, Nistal JF, Martino M, et al. Isolated non-compaction of the left ventricular myocardium in an adult treated with heart transplantation. *Pathol Int*. 2006; 56:35–39.

69. Varr BC, Liedtke M, Arai S, et al. Heart transplantation and cardiac amyloidosis: approach to screening and novel management strategies. *J Heart Lung Transplant*. 2012; 31:325–331.

70. Waller BF, Smith ER, Blackbourne BD, et al. Congenital hypoplasia of portions of both right and left ventricular myocardial walls. Clinical and necropsy observations in two patients with parchment heart syndrome. *Am J Cardiol*. 1980; 46:885–891.

71. Waller TA, Hiser WL, Capehart JE, et al. Comparison of clinical and morphologic cardiac findings in patients having cardiac transplantation for ischemic cardiomyopathy, idiopathic dilated cardiomyopathy, and dilated hypertrophic cardiomyopathy. *Am J Cardiol*. 1998; 81:884–894.

72. Xu T, Yang Z, Vatta M, et al. Multidisciplinary Study of Right Ventricular Dysplasia Investigators. Compound and digenic heterozygosity contributes to arrhythmogenic right ventricular cardiomyopathy. *J Am Coll Cardiol*. 2010; 55:587–597.

73. Yoda M, Minami K, Fritzsche D, et al. Three cases of orthotopic heart transplantation for arrhythmogenic right ventricular cardiomyopathy. *Ann Thorac Surg*. 2005; 80:2358–2360.

The Two Extremes of Cardiac Sarcoidosis and the Effect of Prednisone Therapy

Danielle Armstrong, DO[a], Gonzalo V. Gonzalez-Stawinski, MD[b], Jong Mi Ko, BA[c], Shelley A. Hall, MD[d], and William C. Roberts, MD[a,c,d,*]

Described herein are clinical and morphologic findings in 2 patients who underwent heart transplantation because of severe heart failure resulting from cardiac sarcoidosis. Although the explanted hearts in each patient had characteristic gross changes of cardiac sarcoidosis, one patient who had been treated with prednisone, had no residual sarcoid granulomas in the myocardium, whereas the other patient, in whom diagnosis was not made until heart transplantation, had innumerable sarcoid granulomas in her heart. This report suggests that prednisone can eliminate sarcoid granulomas in the heart but that their replacement is by dense fibrous tissue, something also likely the result of the granulomas themselves, creating a situation where the treated (prednisone) and the non-treated sarcoid heart may appear similar by gross examination. **(Am J Cardiol 2015;115:150−153)**

Although it is a systemic disease, sarcoidosis uncommonly affects the heart and when it does the non-cardiac organs are usually minimally affected and they function normally.[1−6] On occasion, cardiac sarcoidosis may lead to such severe heart failure that heart transplantation (HT) is the only reasonable therapy.[3−5] In such situations, diagnosis of cardiac sarcoidosis is usually not made until HT, the usual pre-HT diagnosis being "non-ischemic cardiomyopathy".[5] Recently, 2 patients underwent HT at Baylor University Medical Center (BUMC) in the same month and examination of the explanted heart in one disclosed innumerable myocardial sarcoid granulomas (not diagnosed clinically) and, in the other patient, despite some similar gross findings in the heart, no myocardial granulomas were seen (diagnosed clinically by an earlier biopsy). This report describes findings in these 2 patients to point out the huge spectrum of myocardial changes in patients with cardiac sarcoidosis, and the potential effect of long term prednisone therapy in this condition.

Patients Studied

Pertinent findings in each of the 2 patients are detailed in Table 1. Both patients were in their 50s; both were white; both had severe (4+/4+) heart failure; both had evidence of cardiac dysfunction for approximately 4 years; both had periodic runs of non-sustained ventricular tachycardia; both had some type of heart block (complete in case #1, and right bundle branch block in case #2); neither had dysfunction of a non-cardiac body organ, and neither patient had narrowing of the epicardial coronary arteries. Diagnosis of sarcoidosis before HT was made in patient #1 by biopsy of a mediastinal lymph node 21 months before HT although 2 years earlier a cardiac biopsy had shown "granulomas". Patient #1, who had no granulomas in his explanted heart, was placed on prednisone after the granulomas were seen in the lymph node and he received this drug for 21 months, at very high doses for 10 months before dose-tapering

Table 1
Clinical and morphologic findings in the 2 patients

Variable	Case #1	Case #2
Gender	Man	Woman
Age (years)		
At heart transplantation	53	57
Onset of symptoms	49	53
Electrophysiology		
Heart block	Complete	RBBB
Ventricular tachycardia	+	+
Pacemaker	+	0
Intracardiac defibrillator	+	+
Systemic hypertension	+	0
Body mass index (Kg/m^2)	31.8	29.9
Hemodynamic data		
Lowest left ventricular EF (%)	20	15
Cardiac index (L/min/m^2)	2.01	1.36
Pressures (mm Hg)		
Blood pressure, indirect (s/d)	100/85	85/40
Right atrial mean	6	2
Right ventricle (s/d)	26/10	48/6
Pulmonary artery (s/d)	26/14	44/11
Pulmonary artery wedge mean	11	14
Prednisone therapy (months)	+ (21)	0
Heart weight (g)	535	380
Cardiac granuloma (0-4+)	0	4+
Left ventricular cavity (cm)	7.5	5.5

EF = ejection fraction; RBBB = right bundle branch block; s/d = peak systole/end diastole.

Departments of [a]Pathology, [b]Cardiothoracic Surgery, and [d]Internal Medicine (Division of Cardiology), Baylor University Medical Center, Dallas, Texas and [c]Baylor Heart and Vascular Institute, Baylor University Medical Center, Dallas, Texas. Manuscript received September 2, 2014; revised manuscript received and accepted October 5, 2014.

Support for this investigation was provided by the Baylor Health Care System Foundation.

See page 153 for disclosure information.

*Corresponding author: Tel: 214-820-7911; fax: 214-820-7533.

E-mail address: wc.roberts@baylorhealth.edu (W.C. Roberts).

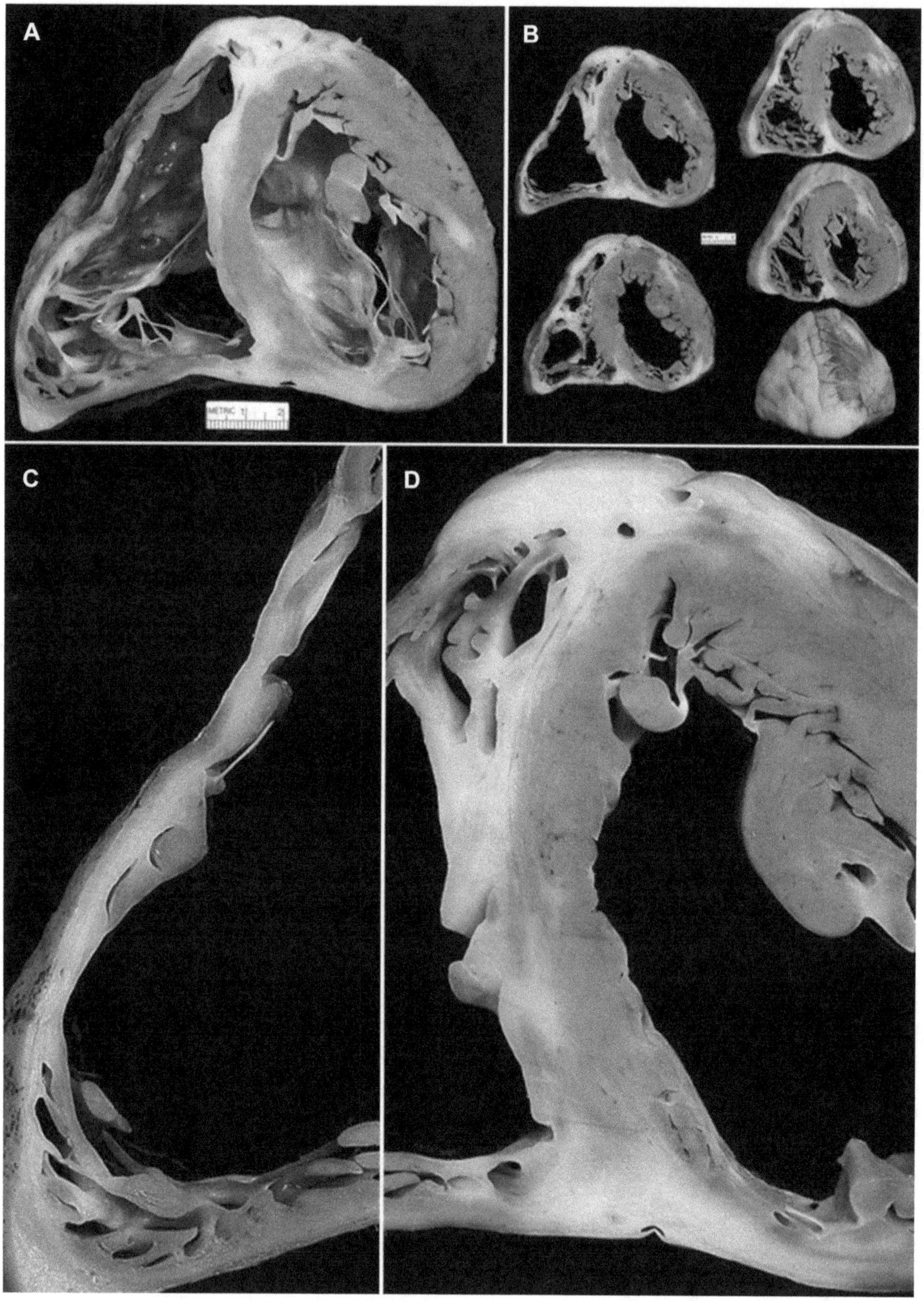

Figure 1. Heart in patient #1. *(A)* View of the base of the heart showing marked dilatation of both right and left ventricular cavities and focal scars in the left and right ventricular free walls and ventricular septum. *(B)* Transverse cuts of the cardiac ventricles caudal to the view shown in *(A)*. *(C)* Close up view of the wall of right ventricle showing extensive scarring and marked thinning of the wall (simulating arrhythmogenic right ventricular dysplasia/cardiomyopathy). *(D)* View of the ventricular septum showing the scarring primarily on the right side of the septum. Because the biotome to biopsy the heart extracts tissue from the right side of the ventricular septum that probably was the reason the biopsy was positive in this patient early in his course.

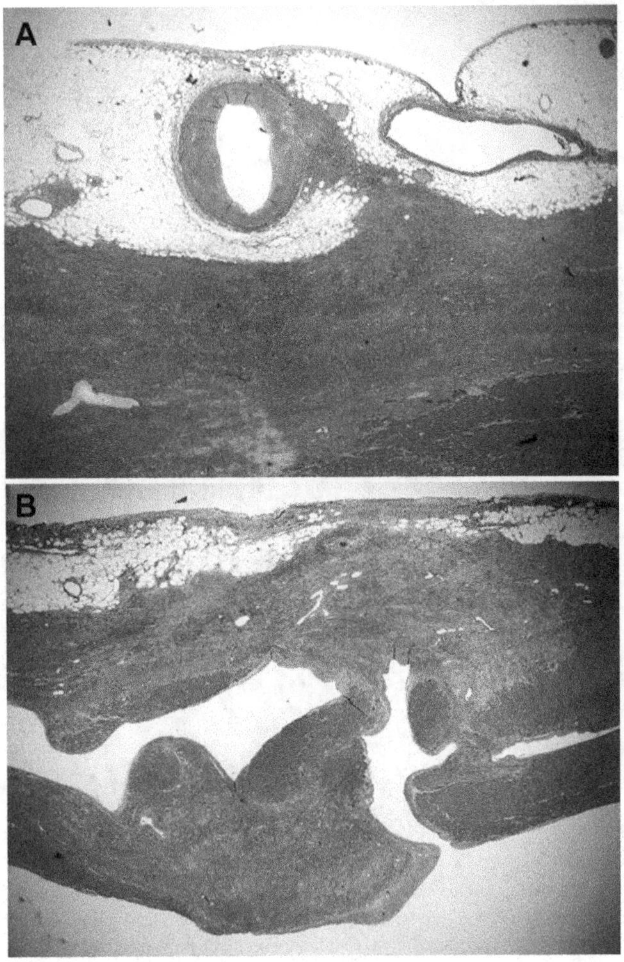

Figure 2. Photomicrographs of portions of the heart in patient #1. *(A)* View of the epicardium, subepicardium, and outer myocardial wall in the anterior portion of left ventricle. The left anterior descending coronary artery and also a coronary vein are shown. The deep blue color represents scar tissue which is located primarily in the subepicardial region rather than the sub-endocardial region. No granulomas were found in the dense fibrous tissue despite examining numerous sections of myocardium. The coronary vessels are surrounded by mainly adipose tissue. *(B)* View of the right ventricular free wall also showing extensive scarring again involving the subepicardial portion more than the subendocardial portion. Trichrome stains, each ×20.

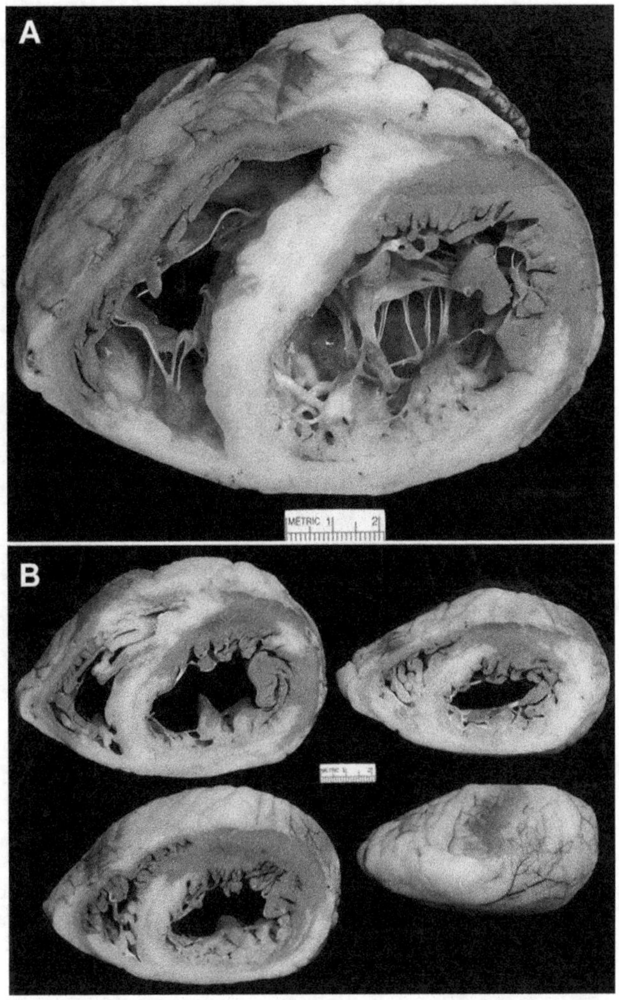

Figure 3. Views of the heart in case #2. *(A)* View of the opened basal portion of the heart showing considerable dilatation of both ventricular cavities and severe scarring of the ventricular septum, posterolateral left ventricular free wall, and posterior wall of right ventricle. Numerous sarcoid granulomas were present in the dense fibrous tissue. *(B)* One-cm thick slices of the ventricles caudal to the upper view. Much of the left ventricular free wall, ventricular septum and right ventricular free wall are replaced by sarcoid granulomas with their surrounding fibrous tissue.

began. Patient #2, whose sarcoidosis was not diagnosed until HT, never received corticosteroid therapy before HT and her explanted heart contained innumerable granulomas typical of sarcoidosis. Photographs of the heart in each patient are shown in Figures 1 to 4.

Discussion

The explanted hearts in each of the 2 hitherto described patients had gross features characteristic of cardiac sarcoidosis: involvement of the walls of both right and left ventricles and the ventricular septum; multiple lesions in each of the cardiac walls; a tendency for the gross lesions to involve the subepicardial half of the left ventricular free wall and the right ventricular half of the ventricular septum, dilation of both ventricular cavities, and absence of narrowing of the epicardial coronary arteries. Yet one patient, who previously by both cardiac and lymph node biopsies showed sarcoidosis, had no granulomas in his explanted heart; the other patient had innumerable sarcoid granulomas in her heart and diagnosis of sarcoidosis was not made until examination of the explanted heart. Patient #1 who had no granulomas in his explanted heart had received prednisone therapy for 21 months, high doses during 10 of those months. The quantity of scar tissue in both patients' hearts suggests that the sarcoid granulomas and their adjacent lymphocytes are strong fibrous-tissue stimulants, and, moreover, that prednisone therapy is a strong eliminator of sarcoid granulomas but the residue of that healing is extensive replacement fibrosis. (Sarcoidosis in the lung is also a strong fibrosis stimulator.[7]) It seems reasonable to believe that the heart in patient #1 earlier had been loaded with sarcoid granulomas as found in patient #2 but that the prednisone treatment likely played a role in eliminating the sarcoid granuloma by replacing them with dense fibrous

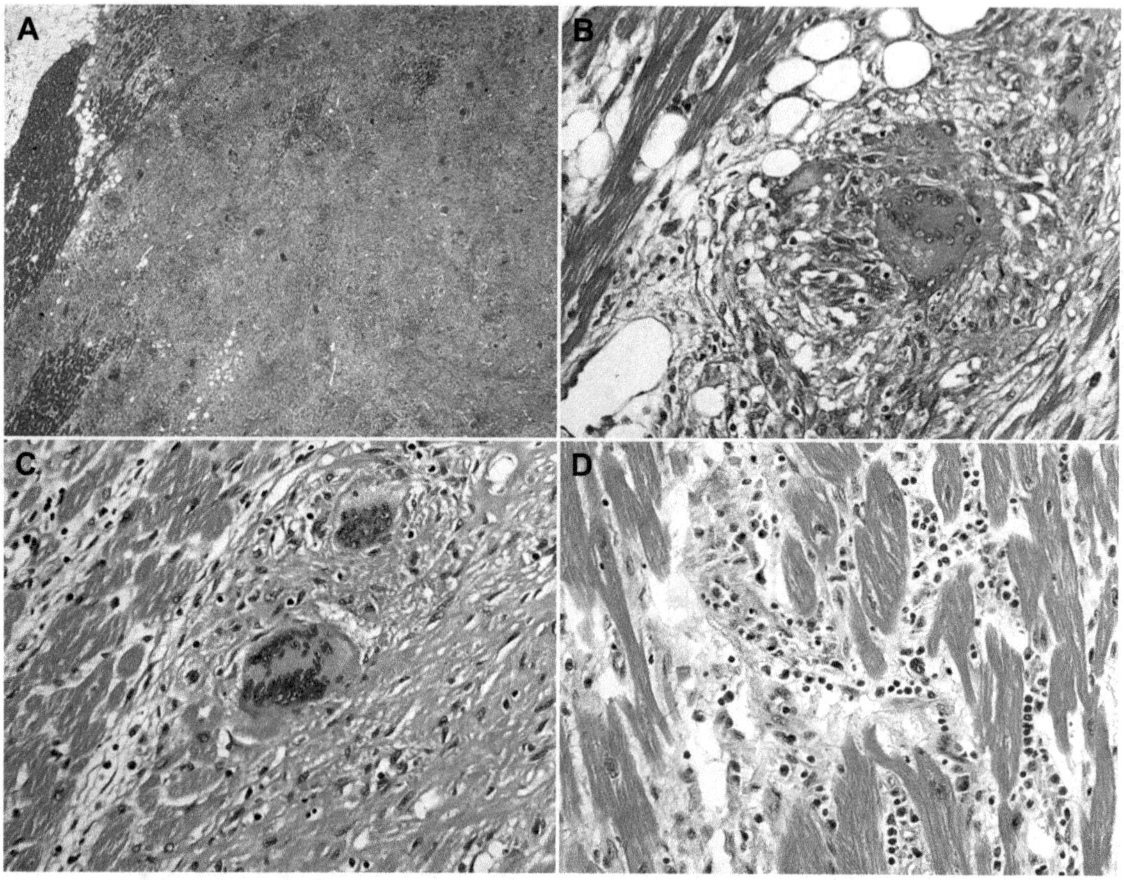

Figure 4. Photomicrographs in patient #2. *(A)* View of a portion of left ventricular free wall showing numerous granulomas surrounded by dense fibrous tissue. *(B)* Close-up view of a single sarcoid granuloma. *(C)* Another view of sarcoid granulomas showing numerous nuclei in each of the giant cells. *(D)* Infiltration between myocardial fibers of lymphocytes typical of sarcoid myocarditis. Trichrome stain, ×40 *(A)*; trichrome stain, ×400 *(B)*; hematoxylin/eosin stain, ×400 *(C)*, and hematoxylin/eosin stain, ×400 *(D)*.

tissue. Such a demonstration to our knowledge has not been provided previous to this report. Earlier we described a patient with typical gross lesions of cardiac sarcoidosis but study of numerous sections of the heart histologically failed to reveal any granulomas.[6] This earlier patient had never received corticosteroid therapy,[6] but earlier histologic examination of a portion of the left ventricular free wall excised to insert a left ventricular assist device did disclose sarcoid granulomas.

Disclosures

The authors have no conflicts of interest to disclose.

1. Roberts WC, McAllister HA Jr, Ferrans VJ. Sarcoidosis of the heart. A clinicopathologic study of 35 necropsy patients (Group I) and review of 78 previously described necropsy patients (Group II). *Am J Med* 1977;63:86–108.
2. Virmani R, Bures JC, Roberts WC. Cardiac sarcoidosis: a major cause of sudden death in young individuals. *Chest* 1980;77:423–428.
3. Donsky AS, Escobar J, Capehart J, Roberts WC. Heart Transplantation for undiagnosed cardiac sarcoidosis. *Am J Cardiol* 2002;89:1447–1450.
4. Roberts WC, Vowels TJ, Ko JM, Capehard JE, Hall SA. Cardiac transplantation for cardiac sarcoidosis with initial diagnosis by examination of the left ventricular apical "core" excised for insertion of a left ventricular assist device for severe chronic heart failure. *Am J Cardiol* 2009;103:110–114.
5. Sharma PS, Lubahn JG, Donsky AS, Yoon AD, Carry MM, Grayburn PA, Wood PB, Ko JM, Burton EC, Roberts WC. Diagnosing cardiac sarcoidosis clinically without tissue confirmation. *Proc (Bayl Univ Med Cent)* 2009;22:236–238.
6. Roberts WC, Chung MS, Ko JM, Capehart JE, Hall SA. Morphologic features of cardiac sarcoidosis in native hearts of patients having cardiac transplantation. *Am J Cardiol* 2014;113:706–712.
7. Crystal RG, Roberts WC, Hunninghake GW, Gadek JE, Fulmer JD, Line BR. Pulmonary sarcoidosis: a disease characterized and perpetuated by activated lung T-lymphocytes. *Ann Intern Med* 1981;94:73–94.

Frequency of Massive Cardiac Adiposity (Floating Heart) at Necropsy and Comparison of Clinical and Morphologic Variables With Cases With Nonmassive Cardiac Adiposity at a Single Texas Hospital, 2013 to 2014

William C. Roberts, MD[a,b,c,*], Vera S. Won, BS[a], Anupama Vasudevan, BDS, MPH, PhD[a], Jong Mi Ko, BA[a], and Joseph M. Guileyardo, MD[b]

Body weight continues to increase worldwide primarily because of the increase in body fat. This study analyzes the frequency of massive adiposity at autopsy determined by the ability of the heart to float in a container of 10% formaldehyde (because adipose tissue is lighter than myocardium) and compares certain findings in the patients with floating to those with nonfloating hearts. The hearts studied at necropsy during a 2-year period (2013 to 2014) at Baylor University Medical Center were carefully "cleaned" and weighed by the same person and tested as to their ability to float in a container of formaldehyde, an indication of severe cardiac adiposity. Of the 146 hearts studied, 76 (52%) floated in a container of formaldehyde and 70 (48%) did not. Comparison of the 76 patients with floating hearts with the 70 with nonfloating hearts showed significant differences in ages (62 ± 13 vs 58 ± 14 years). No significant differences between the 2 groups were found in gender, body mass index, frequency of systemic hypertension or diabetes mellitus, either acute or healed myocardial infarction, or whether death was due to a coronary or a noncoronary condition. A weak correlation was found between body mass index and heart weight in both men and women and in both floating and nonfloating hearts. The massive quantity of cardiac adipose tissue (floating heart) appears to have increased enormously in recent decades in the United States. **(Am J Cardiol 2016;117:1006−1013)**

Overweightness including obesity is now a worldwide problem. One commercial airline (Samoa Air) now bases ticket costs on body weight plus luggage.[1] Although the fattest major US cities seem to vary each year, Houston, San Antonio, El Paso, and Dallas rank high in virtually every annual survey.[2,3] Houston has more fast food outlets than any city in the United States.[4] We studied the frequency of massive fatty deposits in the heart at necropsy during a 2-year period (2013 to 2014) in a single hospital located in Dallas and also compared various clinical variables in the floating versus nonfloating hearts studied during the same period.

Methods

Because adipose tissue is lighter than cardiac muscle, hearts with enormous quantities of fat tend to float in containers of 10% formaldehyde and often in water.

During 2013 and 2014, Dr. Joseph M. Guileyardo, head of the autopsy service at Baylor University Medical Center, performed a total of 165 autopsies on adults. In 8, the autopsy permit did not allow examination of the heart; in 3 others, the autopsy was in patients who had previous cardiac transplantation. Of the remaining 154 autopsies in adults, WCR examined and described the hearts in 146 (95%). This study is limited to these 146 cases.

The hearts were "cleaned" of extraneous tissues, such as parietal pericardium, and then placed in a container of 10% fresh formaldehyde to determine if the heart floated to the surface after carefully removing any residual air from each chamber by compressing the heart several times when it was submerged. The heart was incised in various fashions depending on the perceived cardiac condition present (or absent) and weighed after gently "patting" all exposed surfaces by paper towels to remove extraneous water or formaldehyde. The scales used were accurate to 0.1 g (Ohaus Scott Pro Scale, Parsippany, New Jersey) or to 1.0 g (Acculab Vicon Digital Scale, Arvada, Colorado). All hearts were weighted by WCR.

The anterior surfaces of many of the 146 hearts were photographed, and, after opening, all hearts were photographed (by JMK). The clinical records were then obtained on each of the 146 patients through Baylor Health Care System's electronic medical record (Allscripts Sunrise Enterprise, Chicago, Illinois).

Statistical analysis was done using STATA 14.0.[5] The baseline characteristics of patients with floating and

[a]Baylor Heart and Vascular Institute, [b]Department of Pathology, and [c]Department of Internal Medicine, Baylor University Medical Center, Dallas, Texas. Manuscript received October 22, 2015; revised manuscript received and accepted December 16, 2015.

This study was funded by the Baylor Health Care System Foundation through the Cardiovascular Research Review Committee and in co-operation with the Baylor Heart and Vascular Institute.

See page 1012 for disclosure information.

*Corresponding author: Tel: (214) 820-7911; fax: (214) 820-7533.

E-mail address: wc.roberts@baylorhealth.edu (W.C. Roberts).

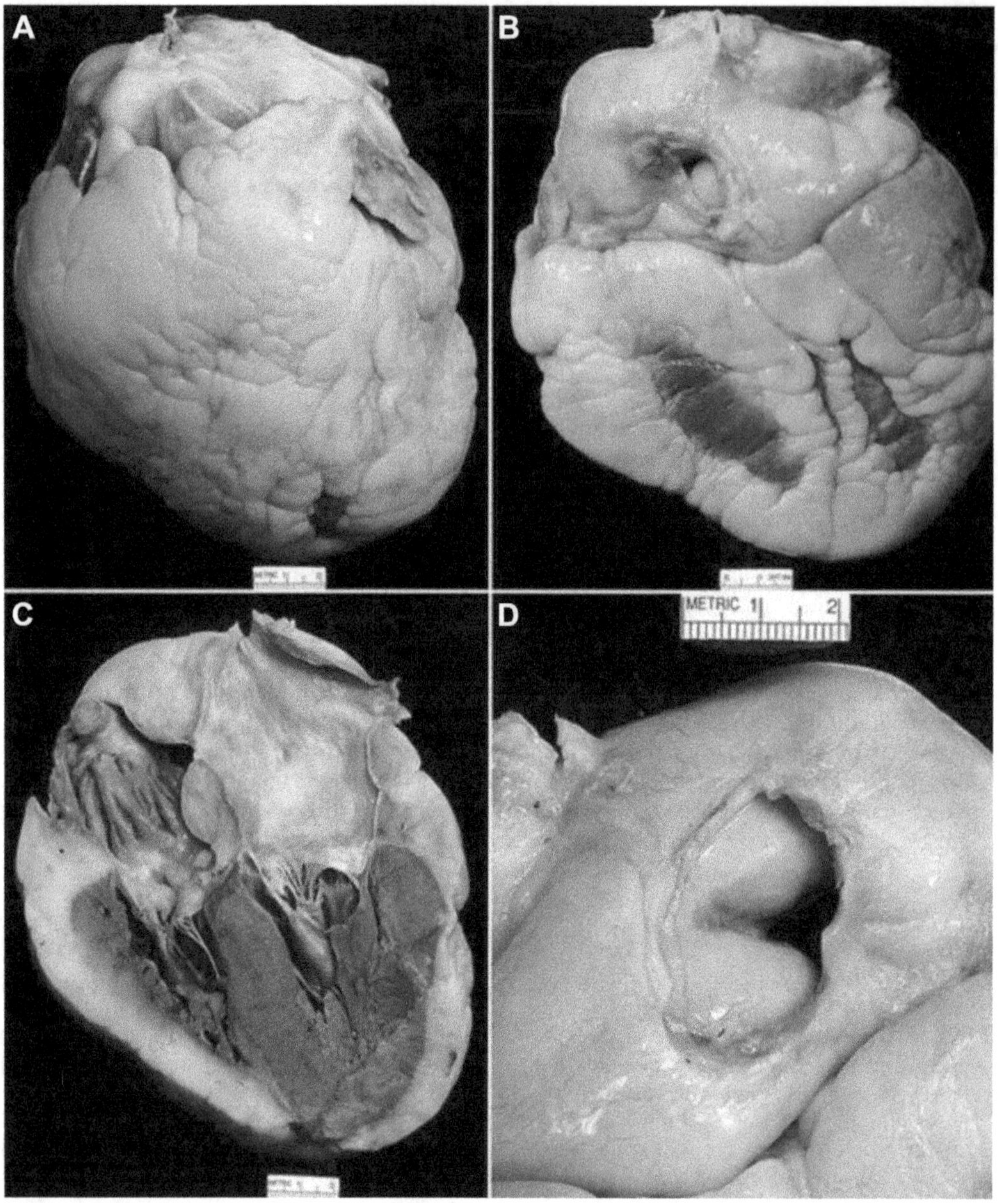

Figure 1. Shown here is a 780-g floating heart—anterior view *(A)*, posterior view *(B)*, 4-chamber view *(C)*, and view of the 2 atrial septal bulges from the orifice of the inferior vena cava *(D)* are shown. The quantity of subepicardial adipose tissue is massive and from the anterior aspect both right and left ventricles are covered by adipose tissue except for an extremely small portion of left ventricle at the apex. The photograph in *(B)* not only shows the huge quantities of fat on the posterior surface of the ventricles but also in the walls of the atria. The 4-chamber view *(C)* shows severe fatty infiltration of the atrial septum except for the fossa ovale region (lipomatous hypertrophy of the atrial septum). The coronary system in this patient was co-dominant: the lumens of the right and left circumflex coronary arteries are wide open. The adipose tissue covering the right ventricular wall is thicker than its muscular wall. Neither ventricular cavity is dilated. The 2 bulges shown in *(D)* are of the atrial septum toward the right atrium. The indentation is the area of the fossa ovale region, which is devoid of adipose tissue. This 64-year-old black woman had undergone sleeve gastrectomy 4 months before death and her BMI just before operation was >50 kg/m^2. Eighteen days after the operation, the BMI was 52 kg/m^2. The patient had diabetes mellitus, systemic hypertension, obstructive sleep apnea, chronic obstructive pulmonary disease, and rheumatoid arthritis.

nonfloating hearts were compared using the chi-square or Fisher's exact tests for proportions and *t* test/Wilcoxon's rank-sum test for continuous variables where applicable. In addition, comparisons were conducted separately for men and women. Correlations among heart weight, age, and body mass index (BMI) were evaluated using Pearson's correlation analysis. For correlation analyses, the data were rendered normal by removing any outliers.

Results

The major finding in this study was the high frequency of massive cardiac adiposity (as determined by whether the heart floated in a container of formaldehyde) at necropsy (Figures 1 to 3). Of the 146 hearts, 76 (52%) contained such large quantities of adipose tissue that they floated and 70 (48%) did not float.

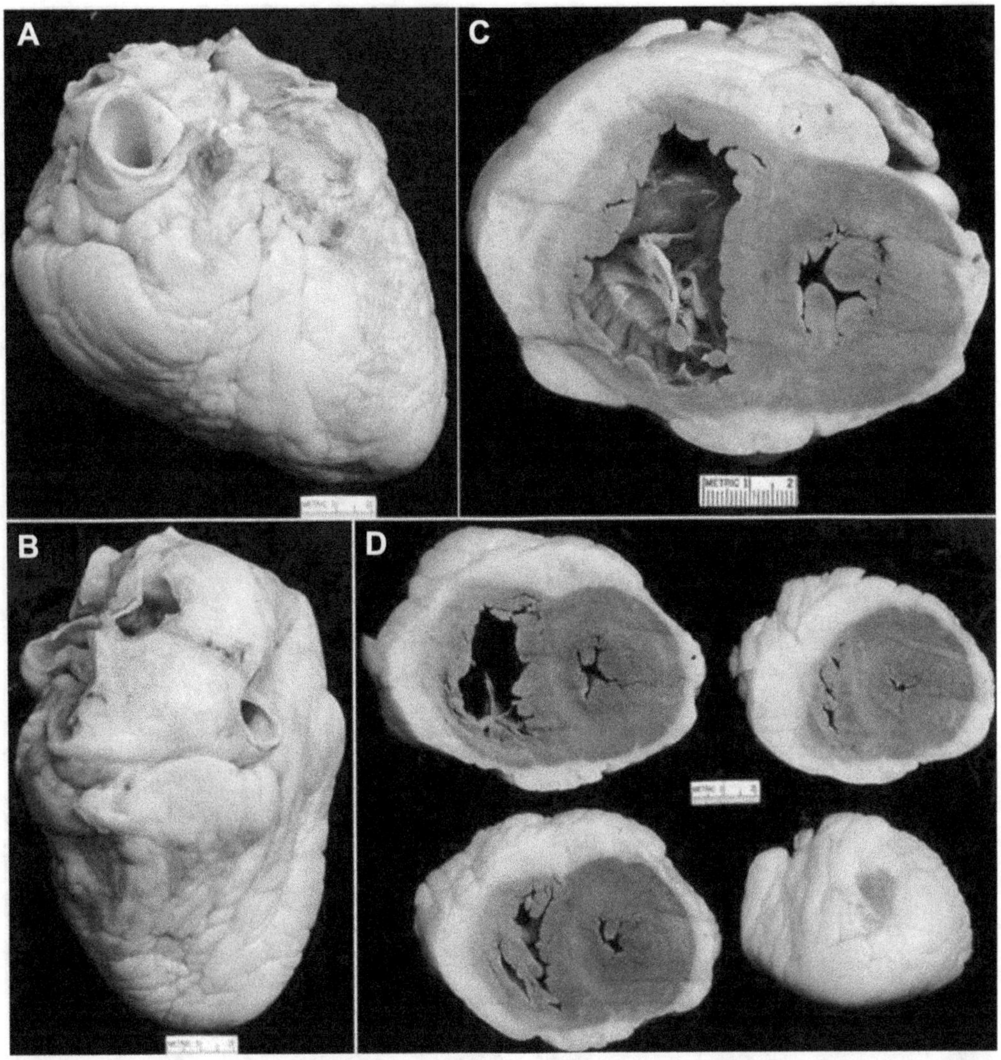

Figure 2. Shown here is the 490-g floating heart of a 55-year-old white woman who had a laparoscopic Nissen fundoplication operation 6 months before death because of a BMI >40 kg/m^2 postoperatively multiple gastrointestinal complications followed. At necropsy, the heart weighed 490 g and floated in a container of 10% formaldehyde. Shown here is the anterior view *(A)*, posterior view *(B)*, base of the heart after cutting the cardiac ventricles in several slices parallel to the posterior atrioventricular sulcus *(C)*, and 4 views of the ventricles *(D)* caudal to the view shown in *(C)*. From the anterior aspect, myocardium cannot be seen. The thickness of the adipose tissue covering the right ventricular free wall is thicker than its muscular wall. The left ventricular cavity is not dilated. The right ventricular cavity is dilated.

The second finding was comparison of various clinical and morphologic variables in the patients with floating versus nonfloating hearts (Table 1). As shown in the accompanying table, age was the only variable that was significantly different between the 76 patients with floating hearts (62 ± 13 years) and the 70 patients with nonfloating hearts (58 ± 14 years). Women with floating hearts were older (62 ± 13 years) compared with those with nonfloating hearts (52 ± 15 years), whereas no difference in age was noted among men. Comparison of the patients with floating hearts versus nonfloating hearts showed no significant differences in gender, BMI, frequency of systemic hypertension or diabetes mellitus, heart weight, either acute or healed myocardial infarcts or both at necropsy, or whether death was due to coronary or noncoronary disease (Table 1). The mean heart weights were larger in the men than in the women whether the heart floated or did not float.

Figure 4 graphically shows the relation between BMI and heart weight in both floating and nonfloating hearts in both men and women. A weak positive correlation was found. Most hearts were of increased weight (>350 g in women and >400 g in men). Figure 5 graphically shows the relation of heart weight to age in both men and women and also the relation of the 2 variations to whether the heart floated. These relations were negative.

Of the 146 patients, 37 (25%) died from consequences of coronary heart disease and 109 (75%) from noncoronary causes. There was no significant difference in the frequency of floating hearts in the 37 patients dying of coronary heart disease compared with the 109 patients dying from noncoronary cases ($p = 0.51$). Of the 146 patients, 19 had

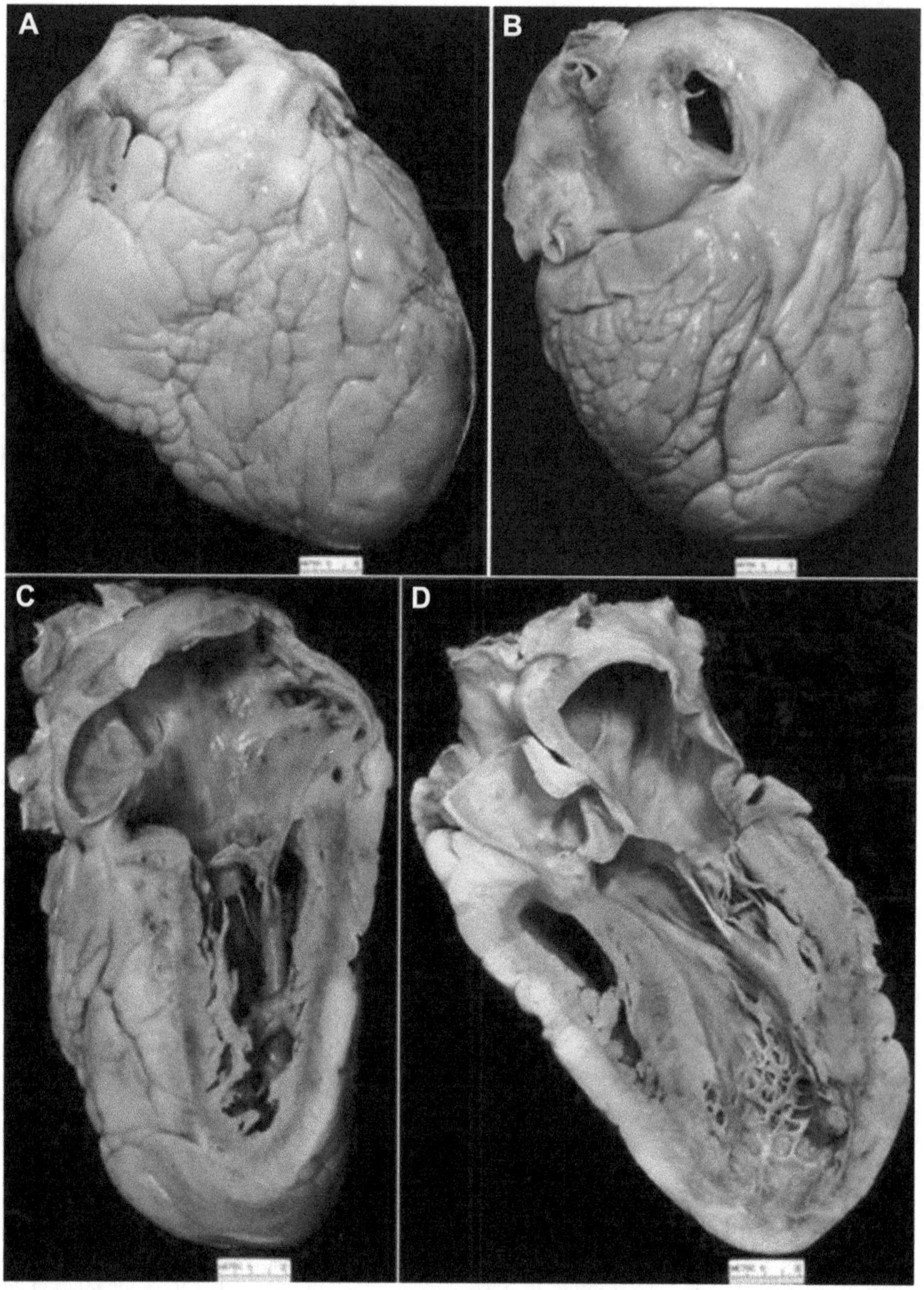

Figure 3. Shown here is the 830-g floating heart of a 64-year-old white woman whose BMI was 57 kg/m^2. This patient died of acute myocardial infarction involving the apical half of left ventricle and was in severe heart failure for some time. A thrombus developed in the apex of left ventricle. The left ventricular ejection fraction by echocardiogram was 33%. She had severe narrowing of the left anterior descending and left circumflex coronary arteries and stents were placed in both. The anterior surface of the heart *(A)*, the posterior portion of the heart *(B)*, a parasagittal view of the right side of the heart showing the right atrium, tricuspid valve, and right ventricular inflow tract *(C)*, and left parasagittal cut *(D)* showing the infarct in the apical half of the left ventricular free wall are shown. The quantity of subepicardial adipose tissue is massive. The entire walls of both right and left ventricles are covered by adipose tissue. The right coronary artery shown in *(C)* is wide open. The thickness of the subepicardial adipose tissue over the right ventricle is thicker than then the right ventricular myocardial wall.

received chronic prednisone therapy and the hearts in 10 (53%) of them floated in a container of formaldehyde; of the 127 patients who were never on chronic prednisone or other corticosteroid therapy, 66 (52%) floated in a container of formaldehyde (p = ns).

Discussion

The concept of "floating heart" was presented initially in an article by Roberts and Roberts in 1983 who described 5% frequency of floating hearts in 55 necropsy patients included in a 2.5-year period in the early 1980s.[6] The most

Table 1
Clinical and morphologic data in the 146 patients comparing various variables in those with floating and nonfloating hearts

Variable	Total (N=146)	Float (n=76)	Nonfloat (n=70)	p Value
Age (years) (Mean±SD)	60±13	62±13	58±14	0.03
Range [median]	23-90 [60]	30-87 [62]	23-90 [58]	
Men				
Mean±SD	62±13	63±14	61±12	0.39
Range [median]	30-90 [63]	30-87 [65]	42-90 [59]	
21-40	3/81 (4%)	3/3 (100%)	0/3 (0%)	
41-60	35/81 (43%)	12/35 (34%)	23/35 (66%)	
61-80	34/81 (42%)	17/34 (50%)	17/34 (50%)	
81-100	9/81 (11%)	5/9 (56%)	4/9 (44%)	0.11
Women				
Mean±SD	58±14	62±13	52±15	0.009
Range [median]	23-86 [58]	37-86 [60]	23-81 [52]	
21-40	9/65 (14%)	2/9 (22%)	7/9 (78%)	
41-60	31/65 (48%)	20/31 (65%)	11/31 (35%)	
61-80	20/65 (31%)	13/20 (65%)	7/20 (35%)	
81-100	5/65 (8%)	4/5 (80%)	1/5 (20%)	0.08
Sex				
Men	81/146 (55%)	37/81 (46%)	44/81 (54%)	0.09
Women	65/146 (45%)	39/65 (60%)	26/65 (40%)	
Body Mass Index (kg/m^2) (Mean±SD)	31±9	32±8	30±9	
Range [median]	15-72 [29]	18-55 [30]	15-72 [29]	0.19
Men				
Mean±SD	31±9	32±8	31±10	
Range [median]	16-72 [29]	21-48 [30]	16-72 [29]	0.52
≤25	19/81 (23%)	7/19 (37%)	12/19 (63%)	
>25-30	26/81 (32%)	12/26 (46%)	14/26 (54%)	
>30	36/81 (44%)	18/36 (50%)	18/36 (50%)	0.65
Women				
Mean±SD	31±9	32±8	28±7	
Range [median]	15-55 [30]	18-54 [30]	15-42 [30]	0.11
≤25	21/65 (32%)	10/21 (48%)	11/21 (52%)	
>25-30	13/65 (20%)	10/13 (77%)	3/13 (23%)	
>30	31/65 (48%)	19/31 (61%)	12/31 (39%)	0.23
Coronary Artery Disease	53 (36%)	29/53 (55%)	24/53 (45%)	0.63
Healed myocardial infarct	29 (20%)	12/29 (41%)	17/29 (59%)	0.20
Acute myocardial infarct	16 (11%)	11/16 (69%)	5/16 (31%)	0.19
Both	3 (2%)	2/3 (67%)	1/3 (33%)	1.00
Neither	13 (9%)	8/13 (62%)	5/13 (38%)	0.57
Diabetes Mellitus	54 (37%)	29/54 (54%)	25/54 (46%)	0.76
Hypertension	95 (65%)	48/95 (51%)	47/95 (49%)	0.61
Heart Weight (g) Mean±SD	490±143	469±124	512±160	0.07
Range [median]	142-1070 [475]	208-830 [455]	142-1070 [488]	
Men				
Mean±SD	548±135	519±108	572±151	0.08
Range [median]	335-1070 [515]	335-720 [505]	375-1070 [547.5]	
>400g	72/81 (89%)	32/72 (44%)	40/72 (56%)	0.53
Women				
Mean±SD	417±119	422±121	410±118	0.68
Range [median]	142-830 [410]	208-830 [395]	142-735 [410]	
>350g	45/65 (69%)	27/45 (60%)	18/45 (40%)	1.00

important finding in this study was the high frequency (52%) of massive cardiac adiposity (floating heart) at autopsy. Comparison of the patients with floating versus nonfloating hearts showed only significant differences in age and that was entirely because of a 10-year mean difference in the ages of the women (floating hearts, age 62; nonfloating, age 52 years; Table 1). There also was a significant but weak correlation between BMI and heart weight in both women and men and in both the floating and the nonfloating hearts.

The contribution of fat to heart weight can be enormous. Shirani and colleagues[7] in 1995 excised subepicardial adipose tissue and fatty atrial septa in 30 patients at necropsy and found that adipose tissue in the heart contributed up to 50% of the cardiac weight. Of the 30 cases studied by them, the heart floated in 12 and in them the adipose tissue

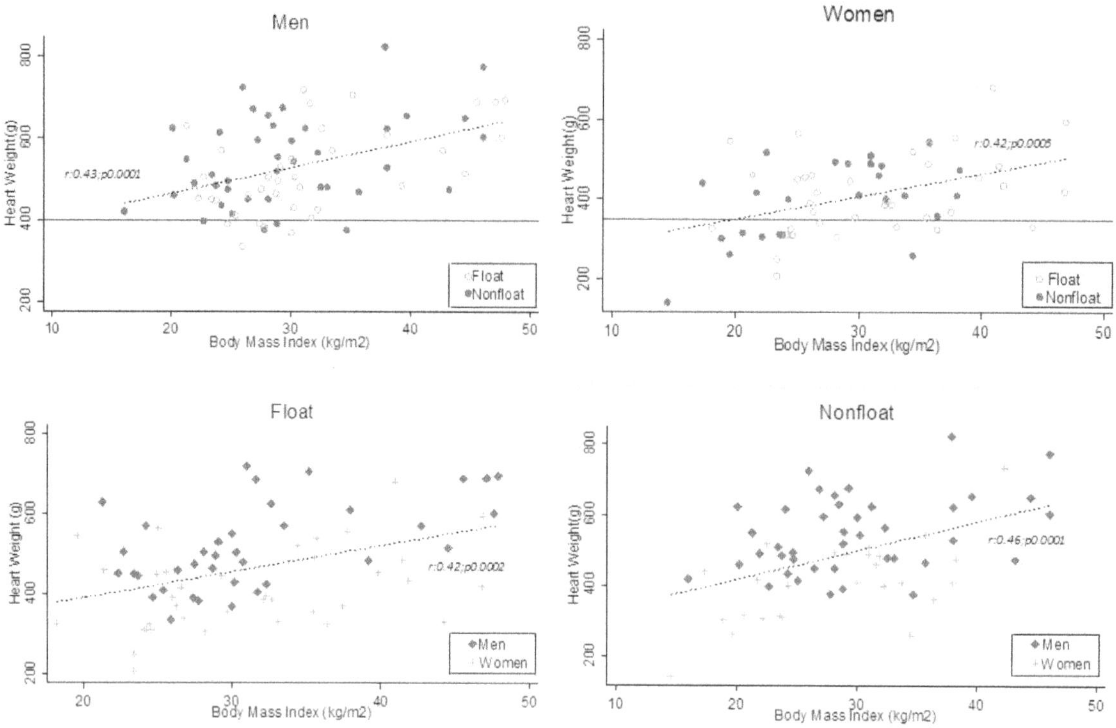

Figure 4. This graph shows the relation between BMI and heart weight in both men and women in both the hearts which floated and those which did not. There was a weak but significant correlation between BMI and heart weight in both groups. The *horizontal line* in the 2 upper graphs show the upper limits for normal heart weight in men (400 g) and women (350 g). The men are represented by *diamond* signs and the women by *plus* signs. Three men, who were outliers, were excluded from top left graph and also from the bottom right graph; 2 women, also outliers, were excluded from top right graph and 1 woman from bottom left graph.

comprised a mean of 32 ± 9% (range 21% to 52%) of the total cardiac weight at necropsy.

The occurrence of such large fatty deposits in the heart in a single Texas hospital in the second decade of the twenty-first century is astounding. It is unlikely that such huge cardiac fatty deposits were as frequent at necropsy in the United States 30, 40, or 50 years ago. Indeed, Roberts and Roberts[6] in a report in 1983 found that only 5% of hearts studied at necropsy in patients >40 years in a 2.5-year period in the early 1980s floated. Certainly, overweightness including obesity has skyrocketed in the last 30 years, and the present study did show a correlation between BMI and heart weight in both the floating and nonfloating hearts.

Osler, in his 1892, *The Principles and Practice of Medicine*[8] described "fatty overgrowth," which he defined as "...a single excess of the normal subepicardial fat, to which the term *cor adiposum* was given by older writers. In other instances, the fat infiltrates the muscular substance and, separating the strands, may reach even to the endocardium. In corpulent persons, there is always much pericardial fat. It forms part of the general obesity ...The entire heart may be enveloped in a thick sheeting of fat through which not a trace of muscle substance can be seen. On section, the fat infiltrates the muscle, separating the fibres, and in extreme cases—particularly in the right ventricle—reaches the endocardium. In some places, there may be even complete substitution of fat for the muscle substance ..." In contrast to Osler's textbook appearing 123 years ago, modern cardiologic textbooks generally fail to mention "cardiac adiposity," or "fatty heart" or "cor adiposum!".

In recent times, the quantity of subepicardial adipose tissue has received increasing attention but that attention almost entirely has been through echocardiographic,[9–16] computed tomographic,[17–25] and magnetic resonance imaging[26–28] and not from morphologic studies.[29,30] The findings in their studies, of course, were not completely uniform but most showed that the quantity (thickness of fat over the right ventricular free wall or total epicardial fat volume) correlated significantly with the quantity of visceral adipose tissue, left ventricular mass, left atrial cavity size, left ventricular diastolic function, systolic and diastolic systemic arterial pressures, the presence of and the severity of coronary atherosclerosis, the quantity of coronary arterial calcium, carotid arterial intimal-medial thickness, the level of serum triglycerides, high-density lipoprotein cholesterol, and fasting blood glucose, and the presence of the metabolic syndrome and diabetes mellitus. The cardiac adipose tissue was an independent risk factor for cardiovascular disease and even a useful predictor of recurrence of atrial fibrillation after ablation.[21]

The present study of course has strengths and limitations. The major strength is the large percent of floating hearts, namely 52%, at a single institution in a recent 2-year period. The demonstration, in 3 different views of hearts, containing enough adipose tissue to float also has not been illustrated previously. That a heart floats in formaldehyde or water indicates that the heart contains a huge quantity of adipose

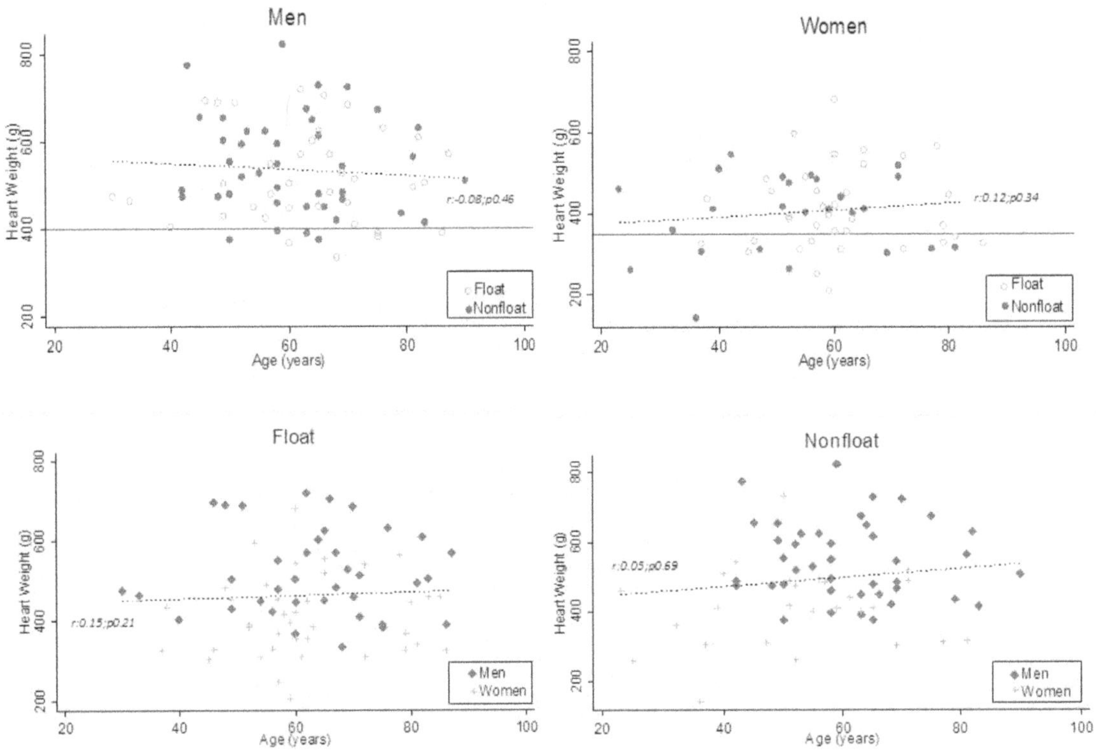

Figure 5. This diagram shows the lack of correlation of heart weight to age in hearts that floated and those that did not. In each diagram, the men and women are designated by a different symbol. The floating hearts are represented by the *"open" circles* and the nonfloating by the *"closed" circles*. The *solid line* in the women separates the hearts that weighed >350g from those that did not. The *solid line* in the men separates the hearts that weighed >400g from those that did not. Two men, who were outliers, were excluded from the top left graph and also from the bottom right graph; 2 women, who were outliers, were excluded from the top right graph and 1 woman from the bottom left graph.

tissue. If, however, the myocardial mass is considerable although the quantity of adipose is also considerable the heart may not float because the myocardial mass, by weighing more than the fatty mass, prevents the heart from floating. Although the present study focuses primarily on necropsy patients with floating hearts, indicating massive cardiac adiposity, the nonfloating hearts, with few exceptions, also had a considerably increased quantity of cardiac adipose tissue, just not quite enough to allow the heart to float. The latter fact may explain the lack of more significant clinical differences between the floating and nonfloating cases.

Disclosures

The authors have no conflicts of interest to disclose.

1. Craymer L. Weigh more, pay more: Samoa Air pegs ticket prices to passenger pounds. *Wall Street J* 2013.
2. Millado, Nate. "The fittest and fattest cities in America." Men's Fitness. Available at: *http://www.mensfitness.com/weight-loss/burn-fat-fast/the-fittest-and-fattest-cities-in-america*. Accessed on August 18, 2015.
3. Sauter MB, McIntyre DA, Weigley S. "America's fattest cities". 24/7 Wall St 2013. Available at: *http://247wallst.com/special-report/2013/04/12/americas-fattest-cities/*. Accessed on August 18, 2015.
4. Cohen J. Houston is America's fattest city. *Texas Monthly* 2013. Available at: *http://www.texasmonthly.com/articles/houston-is-americas-fattest-city/*. Accessed on August 18, 2015.
5. StataCorp. *Stata Statistical Software: Release 14*. College Station, TX: StataCorp LP, 2015.
6. Roberts WC, Roberts JD. The floating heart or the heart too fat to sink: analysis of 55 necropsy patients. *Am J Cardiol* 1983;52:1286–1289.
7. Shirani J, Berezowski K, Roberts WC. Quantitative measurement of normal and excessive (cor adiposum) subepicardial adipose tissue, its clinical significance, and its effect on electrocardiographic QRS voltage. *Am J Cardiol* 1995;76:414–418.
8. Osler W. The Principles and Practice of Medicine. Designed for the Use of Practitioners and Students of Medicine. New York: D. Appleton and Company, 1892:642–643.
9. Iacobellis G, Ribaudo MC, Leto G, Zappaterreno A, Vecci E, Di Mario U, Leonetti F. Influence of excess fat on cardiac morphology and function: study in uncomplicated obesity. *Obes Res* 2002;10: 767–773.
10. Iacobellis G, Ribaudo MC, Assael F, Vecci E, Tiberti C, Zappaterreno A, Di Mario U, Leonetti F. Echocardiographic epicardial adipose tissue is related to anthropometric and clinical parameters of metabolic syndrome: a new indicator of cardiovascular risk. *J Clin Endocrinol Metab* 2003;88:5163–5168.
11. Iacobellis G, Pond CM, Sharma AM. Different "weight" of cardiac and general adiposity in predicting left ventricle morphology. *Obesity* 2006;14:1679–1684.
12. Chaowalit N, Somers VK, Pellikka PA, Rihal CS, Lopez-Jimenez F. Subepicardial adipose tissue and the presence and severity of coronary artery disease. *Atherosclerosis* 2006;186:354–359.
13. Willens HJ, Byers P, Chirinos JA, Labrador E, Hare JM, de Marchena E. Effects of weight loss after bariatric surgery on epicardial fat measured using echocardiography. *Am J Cardiol* 2007;99: 1242–1245.
14. Willens HJ, Gómez-Marín O, Chirinos JA, Goldberg R, Lowery MH, Iacobellis G. Comparison of epicardial and pericardial fat thickness assessed by echocardiography in African American and non-hispanic white men: a pilot study. *Ethn Dis* 2008;18:311–316.
15. Iacobellis G, Willens HJ. Echocardiographic epicardial fat: a review of research and clinical applications. *J Am Soc Echocardiogr* 2009;22: 1311–1319.

16. Liu J, Fox CS, Hickson DA, May WL, Ding J, Carr JJ, Taylor HA. Pericardial fat and echocardiographic measures of cardiac abnormalities: the Jackson Heart Study. *Diabetes Care* 2011;34:341–346.
17. Gorter PM, de Vos AM, van der Graaf Y, Stella PR, Doevendans PA, Meijs MFL, Prokop M, Visseren FLJ. Relation of epicardial and pericoronary fat to coronary atherosclerosis and coronary artery calcium in patients undergoing coronary angiography. *Am J Cardiol* 2008;102:380–385.
18. Sarin S, Wenger C, Marwaha A, Qureshi A, Go BDM, Woomert CA, Clark K, Nassef LA, Shirani J. Clinical significance of epicardial fat measured using cardiac multislice computed tomography. *Am J Cardiol* 2008;102:767–771.
19. de Vos AM, Prokop M, Roos CJ, Meijs MFL, van Der Schouw YT, Rutten A, Gorter PM, Cramer MJ, Doevendans PA, Rensing BJ, Bartelink ML, Velthuis BK, Mosterd A, Bots ML. Peri-coronary epicardial adipose tissue is related to cardiovascular risk factors and coronary artery calcification in post-menopausal women. *Eur Heart J* 2008;29:777–783.
20. Djaberi R, Schuijf JD, van Werkhoven JM, Nucifora G, Jukema JW, Bax JJ. Relation of epicardial adipose tissue to coronary atherosclerosis. *Am J Cardiol* 2008;102:1602–1607.
21. Lee YJ, Wang CP, Hsu HL, Hung WC, Yu TH, Chen YH, Chiu CA, Lu LF, Chung FM, Shin SJ. Increased epicardial adipose tissue (EAT) volume in type 2 diabetes mellitus and association with metabolic syndrome and severity of coronary atherosclerosis. *Clin Endocrinol (Oxf)* 2009;70:876–882.
22. Mahabadi AA, Massaro JM, Rosito GA, Levy D, Murabito JM, Wolf PA, O'Donnell CJ, Fox CS, Hoffmann U. Association of pericardial fat, intrathoracic fat, and visceral abdominal fat with cardiovascular disease burden: the Framingham Heart Study. *Eur Heart J* 2009;30:850–856.
23. Wang TD, Lee WJ, Shih FY, Huang CH, Chang YC, Chen WJ, Lee YT, Chen MF. Relations of epicardial adipose tissue measured by multidetector computed tomography to components of the metabolic syndrome are region-specific and independent of anthropometric indexes and intraabdominal visceral fat. *J Clin Endocrinol Metab* 2009;94:662–669.
24. Ding J, Hsu FC, Harris TB, Liu Y, Kritchevsky SB, Szklo M, Ouyang P, Espeland MA, Lohman KK, Criqui MH, Allison M, Bluemke DA, Carr JJ. The association of pericardial fat with incident coronary heart disease: the multi-ethnic study of atherosclerosis (MESA). *Am J Clin Nutr* 2009;90:499–504.
25. Greif M, Becker A, Von Ziegler F, Lebherz C, Lehrke M, Broedl UC, Tittus J, Parhofer K, Becker C, Reiser M, Knez A, Leber AW. Pericardial adipose tissue determined by dual source CT is a risk factor for coronary atherosclerosis. *Arterioscler Thromb Vasc Biol* 2009;29:781–786.
26. Staten MA, Totty WG, Kohrt WM. Measurement of fat distribution by magnetic resonance imaging. *Invest Radiol* 1989;24:345–349.
27. Iacobellis G, Sharma AM. Epicardial adipose tissue as new cardio-metabolic risk marker and potential therapeutic target in the metabolic syndrome. *Curr Pharm Des* 2007;13:2180–2184.
28. Fox CS, Gona P, Hoffmann U, Porter SA, Salton CJ, Massaro JM, Levy D, Larson MG, Agostino RBD, O'onnell CJ, Manning WJ. Pericardial fat, intrathoracic fat, and measures of left ventricular structure and function. *Circulation* 2009;119:1586–1591.
29. Reiner L, Mazzoleni A, Rodriguez F. Statistical analysis of the epicardial fat weight in human hearts. *AMA Arch Pathol* 1955;60:369–373.
30. Domenico C, Roberta M, Sergio C, Paolo P, Matteo G, Tu VL, Cesare B. The ventricular epicardial fat is related to the myocardial mass in normal, ischemic and hypertrophic hearts. *Cardiovasc Pathol* 2004;13:313–316.

Characteristics of Hearts at Necropsy in Patients Treated Chronically With Prednisone (The Corticosteroid Heart)

William C. Roberts, MD[a,b,c,*], Vera S. Won, BS[a,b,c], Anupama Vasudevan, BDS, MPH, PhD[a,b,c], and Joseph M. Guileyardo, MD[a,b,c]

It is known that long-term corticosteroid therapy increases fatty deposits in several human tissues. To quantify the quantity of fatty deposits in the heart in patients on prednisone, we examined the heart at necropsy in 37 patients who had received long-term corticosteroid therapy (prednisone in 34) and compared certain findings in them to those in 194 (steroid-naïve) patients also studied at necropsy at Baylor University Medical Center, Dallas, in a 3-year period (2013, 2014, and 2015). Significant differences between the 2 groups were found in age, gender, and frequency of coronary artery disease but not in body mass index, frequency of massive cardiac adiposity, heart weight, or frequency of systemic hypertension or diabetes mellitus. Furthermore, no significant differences were observed in the patients taking ≤20 mg versus those taking >20 mg daily of prednisone. In conclusion, this study observed no significant differences in body mass index, frequency of cardiac adiposity (floating heart), heart weight, or frequencies of systemic hypertension or diabetes mellitus in the patients receiving or not receiving prednisone for a long term, but the prednisone-treated patients were younger, more often women, and had a lower frequency of severe narrowing of ≥1 major coronary arteries. **(Am J Cardiol 2016;118:1935−1940)**

Corticosteroid medicines including prednisone and its equivalents are splendid drugs for multiple different conditions, but unfortunately, they have some detrimental effects on many body organs including the heart.[1−6] The latter include an increase in blood pressure and therefore frequent left ventricular hypertrophy, an increased frequency of atrial fibrillation, and an increase in cardiac adiposity, among others. In 2015, Kitterer et al.[7] described by cardiac magnetic resonance imaging an increase in cardiac fatty deposits in corticosteroid-treated patients with rheumatic diseases compared to controls. This report describes the heart at necropsy in a group of patients treated for a long term with prednisone and compares findings in them to a control necropsy group not treated with corticosteroids.

Methods

During 3 full years (2013, 2014, and 2015), a total of 266 autopsies were performed in adults (all aged >20 years) at Baylor University Medical Center by Dr. Guileyardo: in 15 patients, the autopsy permit did not allow examination of the heart; in 11 cases, Dr. Roberts did not examine the heart, and in 9 cases, the autopsy was in subjects who previously had undergone cardiac transplantation, that is, donor heart only to examine. These 35 cases were eliminated from this study. The remaining 231 cases form the study population. Of them, 37 (16%) had received prednisone for a long term. The cardiac findings in them were compared with the other 194 autopsy cases (84%) in whom no corticosteroid drug had been administered.

Before weighing the heart, the parietal pericardium was entirely removed from the heart, the pulmonary trunk was incised about 2 cm cephalad to the level of the pulmonary valve, the ascending aorta was incised about 2 cm cephalad to the sinotubular junction, and the heart was opened in one of the following manners: The hearts were opened in both left and right parasagittal cuts (Figure 1); the ventricles were cut in "bread-loaf" fashion parallel to the posterior atrioventricular sulcus, each about 1 cm in thickness (Figure 2); or the hearts were opened in a 4-chamber cut exposing all 4 chambers in 1 view. Before weighing the heart after these cuts, each surface was gently patted with paper towels to remove any extraneous formaldehyde or water. Each of the 227 hearts was weighed by Dr. Roberts on 1 of 2 scales (Ohaus Scout Pro Scale accurate to 0.1 g or Acculab Vicon Digital Scale accurate to 1.0 g). The heart weighing was done within a week of the autopsy after fixation of the heart in formaldehyde. After describing and weighing the heart, the medical records were reviewed in each of the 231 cases.

The underlying condition prompting the prednisone therapy was lung disease in 22 patients (63%), kidney disease in 4 (11%), liver disease in 3 (9%), arthritis in 3 (9%), arteritis in 2, myasthenia gravis in 1 (3%), bone

[a]Baylor Heart and Vascular Institute, Dallas, Texas; and Departments of [b]Pathology and [c]Internal Medicine, Baylor University Medical Center, Dallas, Texas. Manuscript received July 29, 2016; revised manuscript received and accepted August 4, 2016.

Funding: This study was funded by the Baylor Health Care System Foundation through the Cardiovascular Research Review Committee and in cooperation with the Baylor Heart and Vascular Institute.

See page 1939 for disclosure information.

*Corresponding author: Tel: (214) 820-7911; fax: (214) 820-7533.

E-mail address: William.Roberts1@BSWHealth.org (W.C. Roberts).

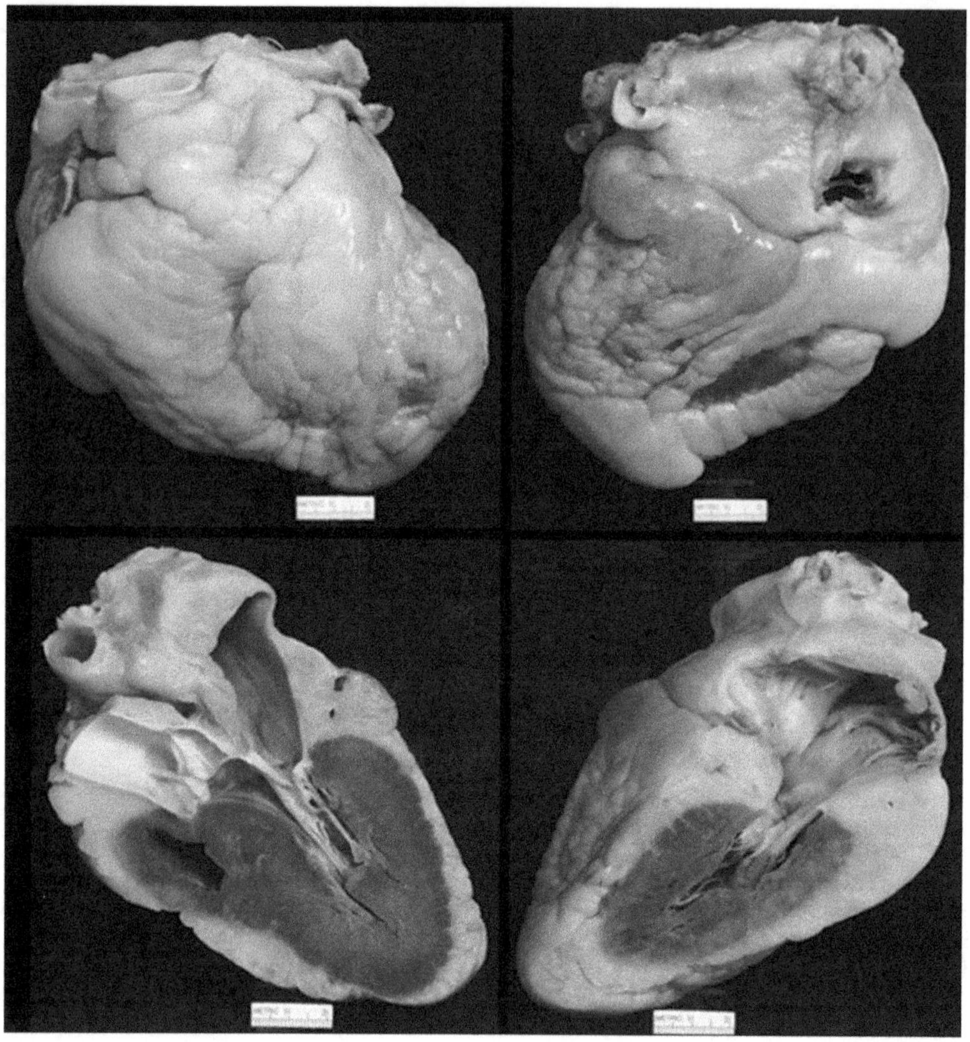

Figure 1. Heart (515 g) in a 46-year-old man (body mass index 35 kg/m^2) who had idiopathic pulmonary fibrosis and received prednisone 40 mg/day over several years. *(Upper left)* The front of the heart and adipose tissue covers most of the surface of the ventricles. *(Upper right)* The back of the heart. *(Lower left)* After a left parasagittal cut. *(Lower right)* After a right parasagittal cut. The quantity of subepicardial adipose tissue is massive, and the heart floated in a container of formaldehyde.

marrow transplant in 1 (3%), and stem-cell transplant in 1 patient (3%).

Analyses were done using STATA 14.1. Categorical variables were presented as proportions, and continuous variables were presented as mean (SD) or median (range) as applicable. We used Chi-square or Fisher's exact test to compare proportions and Student *t* test or Wilcoxon rank-sum test to compare continuous variables as appropriate. Patients treated with prednisone were gender matched with those patients not on prednisone in a ratio of 1:2. The differences in the baseline characteristics were evaluated individually by a conditional logistic regression analysis. The analysis was repeated including only the patients treated with prednisone categorizing them based on the median dose of prednisone.

The study was approved by the Baylor University Medical Center Institutional Review Board.

Results

Findings in the 37 patients and in the 194 controls are summarized in Table 1. There were significant differences in the 2 groups in gender, age, and frequency of ≥1 epicardial coronary arteries being narrowed >75% in cross-sectional area (Table 1) but not in frequency of massive cardiac adiposity (Figure 3), body mass index (BMI, Figure 4), heart weight, or frequencies of systemic hypertension or diabetes mellitus. By gender-matched analysis, we found no differences in patients with and without prednisone use (Table 2). Patients receiving ≤20 mg/day of prednisone (22 patients) compared to those receiving >20 mg/day of prednisone (15 patients) or its equivalent (3 of 37 patients) are summarized in Table 3. Findings in each of the 37 prednisone patients are detailed in Table 4.

The highest prednisone dose varied from 5 to 150 mg (mean 34 mg, median 20). The exact period the patients

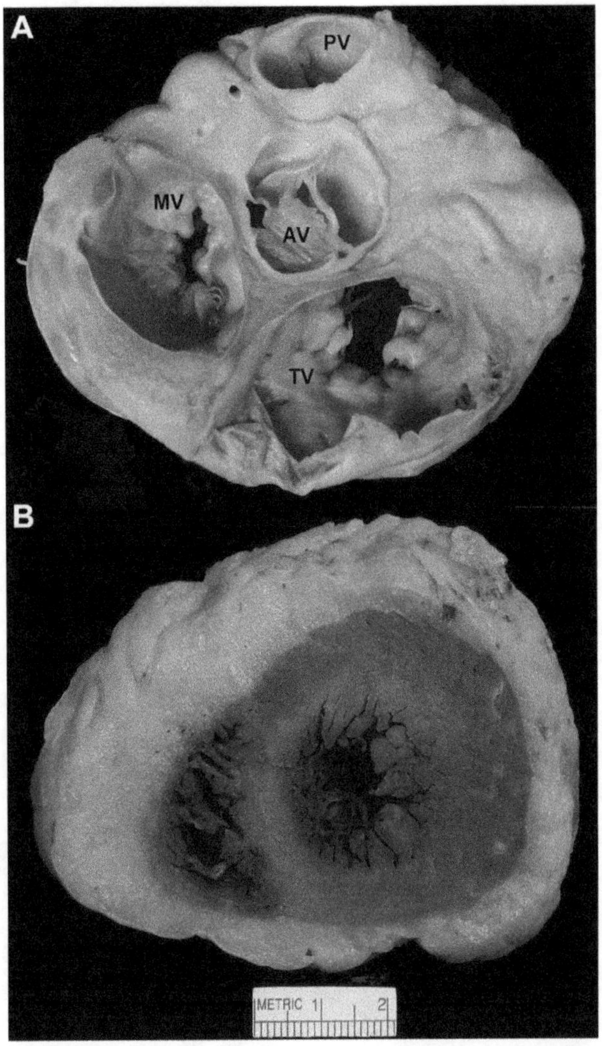

Figure 2. Heart (370 g) in a 60-year-old man who had bilateral lung transplants 17 months before death for chronic obstructive lung disease. He had been on inhaled, intravenous, and oral corticosteroids periodically for several years. The body mass index just before the lung transplant was 29 kg/m^2. *(A)* View of the 4 cardiac valves after "deroofing" the atrial walls exposing the huge amount of adipose tissue in the atrioventricular sulci. *(B)* View of both ventricles near the apex. Both ventricles are completely covered by adipose tissue. The heart floated in a container of formaldehyde. AV = aortic valve; MV = mitral valve; PV = pulmonary valve; TV = tricuspid valve.

Table 1
Findings in the 37 patients and in the 194 controls

Variable	Prednisone (n = 37)	Control (n = 194)	p Value
Age (years) (Mean±SD)	52±13	61±14	0.0007
Range [median]	23-77 [52]	24-90 [60]	
Gender			0.02
Men	13 (35%)	110 (57%)	
Women	24 (65%)	84 (43%)	
Body Mass Index (kg/m^2) (Mean±SD)	30.4±8	30.9±9	
Range [median]	18.1-51.7 [29.1]	14.6-72.3 [29.1]	0.64
Heart Weight (g) Mean±SD	455±124	487±144	
Range [median]	225-780 [455]	142-1070 [470]	0.24
Men Mean±SD	492±93	547±139	
Range [median]	360-720 [475]	265-1070 [515]	0.14
Women Mean±SD	435±135	408±110	
Range [median]	225-780 [435]	142-830 [198]	0.43
Floating Heart	24 (65%)	109 (56%)	0.33
Coronary artery disease	4 (11%)	74 (38%)	0.001
Healed myocardial infarction	3 (8%)	31 (16%)	
Acute myocardial infarction	0	19 (10%)	
Diabetes Mellitus	12 (32%)	70 (36%)	0.67
Systemic Hypertension (by history)	20 (54%)	130 (67%)	0.13

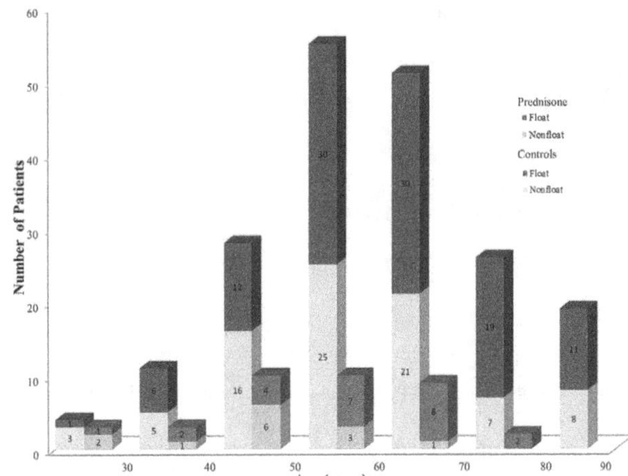

Figure 3. Bar graph shows the number of patients with floating versus nonfloating hearts in the 37 patients treated with prednisone and in the 194 patients studied at necropsy never receiving a corticosteroid drug.

received prednisone is unclear, but all were for long periods of time (at least months).

Lipoprotein results were available in 25 (68%) of the 37 patients, and in 10 of the 25 patients, the low-density lipoprotein cholesterol level was >100 mg/dl (Table 2).

Discussion

This study compares various characteristics of patients who had received prednisone for long term to those who had never received prednisone. The unexpected finding from the cardiac standpoint was the finding of few differences between those who did and did not receive prednisone. The patients who had received prednisone compared to those who had not were predominantly women (65% vs 43%); had a younger age (52 vs 61 years), and had a lower frequency of narrowing of ≥1 epicardial coronary arteries >75% in cross-sectional area by atherosclerotic plaques. There were no significant differences between the 2 groups in heart weight (both mean >450 g), BMI (both mean >30 kg/m^2), frequency of diabetes mellitus (both >30%), systemic hypertension (both >55%), or massive cardiac adiposity (both >55%). Also, comparison within the prednisone group disclosed no significant differences between the 22 patients receiving ≤20 mg/day of prednisone versus those 15 patients receiving >20 mg/day in age, gender,

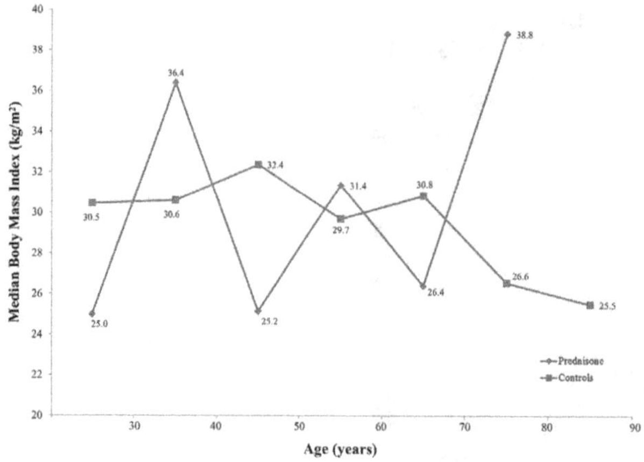

Figure 4. Diagram shows the median body mass index (kg/m^2) related to age in the 37 patients treated with prednisone *(red line)* and in the 194 patients not receiving a corticosteroid drug *(blue line)*.

Table 2
Findings in the 37 patients and in the 74 gender-matched non-prednisone controls

Variable	Prednisone (n = 37)	Matched Control (n = 74)	p Value
Age (years) (Mean±SD)	52±13	52±12	0.93
Range [median]	23-77 [52]	24-71 [52.5]	
Body Mass Index (kg/m^2) (Mean±SD)	30.4±8.3	31.6±8.4	0.49
Range [median]	18.1-51.7 [29.1]	14.6-52 [30.6]	
Heart Weight (g) Mean±SD	455±124	452±136	0.92
Range [median]	225-780 [455]	142-845 [438]	
Floating Heart	24 (65%)	44 (59%)	0.56
Coronary Artery Disease	4 (11%)	21 (28%)	0.06
Diabetes Mellitus	12 (32%)	24 (32%)	1.00
Systemic Hypertension (by history)	20 (54%)	47 (64%)	0.36

Table 3
Comparison of findings in the 37 patients receiving prednisone in doses ≤20 mg and >20 mg daily

Variable	Prednisone Dose (mg)		p-Value
	≤20 (n = 22)	>20 (n = 15)	
Age (years)	23-77 [54]	32-62 [50]	0.29
Gender			0.61
Men	7 (32%)	6 (40%)	
Women	15 (68%)	9 (60%)	
Body Mass Index (kg/m^2)	20-51.7 [31.1]	18.1-42.3 [29.2]	0.84
Systemic Hypertension (by history)	13 (59%)	7 (47%)	0.46
Diabetes Mellitus	8 (36%)	3 (20%)	0.47
Mean Heart Weight (g)	225-780 [435]	310-735 [484]	0.24
Coronary Artery Disease	3 (14%)	1 (7%)	0.63
Floating Heart	15 (68%)	9 (60%)	0.61

BMI, frequency of systemic hypertension or diabetes mellitus, mean heart weight, severe coronary arterial narrowing, or massive cardiac adiposity (floating heart[8–10]).

The only previous study comparable to the present one is the cardiac magnetic resonance imaging study by Kitterer et al.[7] which found larger quantities of "epicardial and pericardial areas of fat" in their 61 patients receiving corticosteroid therapy for "rheumatic disorders" than in their 61 control subjects who did not receive such therapy. Their investigation also found

Table 4
Findings in each of the 37 patients receiving prednisone therapy chronically

#	Sex	Age (years)	BMI (kg/m^2)	Heart Weight (g)	Heart Floated	Reason for Chronic Prednisone	Highest Prednisone Dose (mg)	CAD (Healed MI)	DM	SH	Lipids (mg/dl) TC	LDL	HDL	TG	Interval Transplant to Death (days)
1	F	23	20.4	300	0	Lung Transplant	15	0	+	+	213	142	41	169	561
2	F	23	25.0	330	+	Lung Transplant	20	0	+	0	148	90	39	208	144
3	F	23	31.6	460	0	Myasthenia gravis	20	0	0	0	-	-	-	-	-
4	F	32	36.4	360	0	Lung disease (IPF)	80	0	0	+	202	114	42	409	-
5	F	33	20.0	225	+	Lung disease (Granulomatosis)	15	0	0	0	-	-	-	-	-
6	F	37	36.4	325	+	Liver Transplant	40	0	+	0	-	-	-	-	93
7	F	44	23.3	315	0	Lung Transplant	10	0	0	+	292	126	116	278	1109
8	F	45	35.9	575	+	Arthritis (Still's disease)	40	+	0	0	-	-	-	-	-
9	F	47	23.8	310	0	Stem Cell Transplant	150*	0	0	0	-	-	-	-	40
10	F	48	41.4	485	+	Takayasu's arteritis	20	0	0	0	-	-	-	-	-
11	F	49	25.6	455	+	Kidney Transplant	50	0	0	+	163	89	61	99	6570
12	F	49	23.6	400	0	Lung disease (Sarcoidosis)	40	0	0	0	-	-	-	-	-
13	F	50	42.3	735	0	Lung disease (COPD)	40	0	0	+	171	106	38	97	-
14	F	52	26.0	390	+	Lung Transplant	50	0	0	0	171	99	44	142	94
15	F	52	42.2	420	+	Lung disease (COPD)	10	0	+	+	-	-	-	-	-
16	F	56	28.1	495	0	Kidney Transplant	10	0	0	+	160	108	34	111	5309
17	F	56	44.4	490	+	Liver Transplant	5	0	0	0	167	72	80	65	42108
18	F	57	23.4	250	+	Lung Transplant	20	0	+	0	192	96	83	80	268
19	F	57	39.8	455	+	Liver Transplant	20	0	+	+	192	140	34	84	2555
20	F	60	32.7	365	+	Arthritis (rheumatoid)	5	0	0	+	-	-	-	-	-
21	F	62	25.0	450	+	Bone Marrow Transplant	150*	0	0	0	-	-	-	-	>30
22	F	64	51.7	780	+	Arthritis (rheumatoid)	20	0	+	+	82	39	21	170	-
23	F	67	29.4	545	+	Lung Transplant	7.5	+	0	+	179	89	68	77	3265
24	F	77	46.0	515	+	Lung disease (COPD)	20	0	+	+	190	140	37	117	-
25	M	46	34.6	515	+	Lung disease (ILD)	40	0	0	0	-	-	-	-	-
26	M	48	24.7	475	0	Kidney disease (Lupus)	60	0	0	+	-	-	-	-	-
27	M	49	18.1	530	0	Lung Transplant	50	0	+	+	137	69	48	178	6570
28	M	52	30.0	595	0	Arteritis (polymyositis)	20	+(+)	0	+	154	57	67	75	-
29	M	56	33.7	540	+	Lung Transplant	70	0	0	+	151	95	41	124	6
30	M	57	22.1	455	0	Lung Transplant	10	0	0	0	225	130	80	56	38
31	M	61	21.4	475	+	Lung Transplant	30	0	0	+	185	127	39	116	1035
32	M	62	31.0	720	+	Lung Transplant	50	0	+	0	155	97	53	66	3650
33	M	65	29.1	390	+	Lung Transplant	20	0	0	0	121	71	45	84	431
34	M	65	22.3	452	+	Lung disease (COPD)	20	0	0	0	189	116	53	103	-
35	M	66	26.4	450	0	Kidney Transplant	10	0	0	+	139	80	41	61	1460
36	M	69	23.5	360	+	Lung Transplant	10	+ (+)	0	+	133	66	20	251	4015
37	M	72	31.7	435	+	Lung Transplant	10	0	+	+	291	224	37	211	792

BMI = body mass index; CAD = coronary artery disease; DM = diabetes mellitus; F = female; HDL = high-density lipoprotein; LDL = low-density lipoprotein; M = male; MI = myocardial infarction; SH = systemic hypertension; TC = total cholesterol; TG = triglycerides.
* Given a methylprednisolone as 120 mg twice daily.

larger cardiac fatty deposits in their patients receiving >7.5 mg prednisone equivalent/day than those patients receiving <7.5 mg prednisone equivalent/day. These authors also found that the quantity of "epicardial and pericardial fat" also correlated in the corticosteroid group with the BMI, a finding also at variance with the present study. Possibly, the reason the present study did not show a correlation with BMI or a difference in the frequency of massive cardiac adiposity (floating heart) between our prednisone and control groups was that the BMIs were similarly high (>30 kg/m^2) in both groups. The mean BMI in the prednisone-receiving versus steroid-naive patients studied by Kitterer et al. was lower (27 kg/m^2) although similar in both their study patients and control subjects.

The positive feature of the present study is that it is the first to examine the heart itself in patients receiving corticosteroid therapy on a long-term basis. A limitation of the present study is lack of information on the exact periods the patients received prednisone therapy.

Disclosures

The authors have no conflicts of interest to disclose.

1. Everhart JE, Lombardero M, Lake JR, Wiesner RH, Zetterman RK, Hoofnagle JH. Weight change and obesity after liver transplantation: incidence and risk factors. *Liver Transpl Surg* 1998;4:285–296.
2. Fardet L, Petersen I, Nazareth I. Suicidal behavior and severe neuropsychiatric disorders following glucocorticoid therapy in primary care. *Am J Psychiatry* 2012;169:491–497.

3. Graedon J. Prednisone side effects: Deal with the devil? *www.peoplespharmacy.com/2012/04/08/prednisone-side-effects-deal-with-the-deveil*. 2012. Available at: *www.peoplespharmacy.com/2012/04/08/prednisone-side-effects-deal-with-the-devil*. Accessed on July 1, 2016.
4. Jurgens M, Jacobs J, Geenen R, Bossema E, Bakker M. Increase of body mass index in a tight controlled methotrexate-based strategy with prednisone in early rheumatoid arthritis: side effect of the presnisone or better control of disease activity? *Arthritis Care Res* 2013;65:88–93.
5. Wei L, MacDonald TM, Walker BR. Taking glucocorticoids by prescription is associated with subsequent cardiovascular disease. *Ann Intern Med* 2004;141:764–770.
6. van der Hooft CS, Heeringa J, Brusselle GG, Hofman A, Witteman JC, Kingma JH, Sturkenboom MC, Stricker BH. Corticosteroids and the risk of atrial fibrillation. *Arch Intern Med* 2006;166:1016–1020.
7. Kitterer D, Latus J, Henes J, Birkmeier S, Backes M, Braun N, Sechtem U, Dominik Alscher M, Mahrholdt H, Greulich S. Impact of long-term steroid therapy on epicardial and pericardial fat deposition: a cardiac MRI study. *Cardiovasc Diabetol* 2015;14:130.
8. Roberts WC, Roberts JD. The floating heart or the heart too fat to sink: analysis of 55 necropsy patients. *Am J Cardiol* 1983;52:1286–1289.
9. Roberts WC, Won VS, Vasudevan A, Ko JM, Guileyardo JM. Frequency of massive cardiac adiposity (floating heart) at necropsy and comparison of clinical and morphologic variables with cases with nonmassive cardiac adiposity at a single Texas hospital, 2013 to 2014. *Am J Cardiol* 2016;117:1006–1013.
10. Roberts WC, Won VS, Vasudeven A, Ko JM, Hall SA, Gonzalez-Stawinski GV. Frequency of massive cardiac adiposity (floating heart) in the native hearts of patients having heart transplantation at a single Texas hospital (2013 to 2015) and comparison of various clinical and morphologic variables in the patients with massive versus nonmassive cardiac adiposity. *Am J Cardiol* 2016;117:1375–1380.

Usefulness of Total 12-Lead QRS Voltage as a Clue to Diagnosis of Patients With Cardiac Sarcoidosis Severe Enough to Warrant Orthotopic Heart Transplant

William C. Roberts, MD; Tiffany M. Becker, BS; Shelley A. Hall, MD

IMPORTANCE Severe heart failure caused by cardiac sarcoidosis is difficult to diagnosis without biopsy.

OBJECTIVE To assess whether total electrocardiographic 12-lead QRS voltage may be a clue to diagnosis.

DESIGN, SETTING, PARTICIPANTS Case-series study with cases collected at Baylor University Medical Center at Dallas, Dallas, Texas, from January 13, 2005, to January 24, 2017. The clinical records of 16 patients with severe heart failure caused by cardiac sarcoidosis were studied. Examination of total 12-lead electrocardiographic QRS voltage (peak of the R wave to the nadir of either the Q or S wave, whichever was deeper) was performed prior to orthotopic heart transplant (OHT). Gross and microscopic pathologic specimens of the native hearts were studied.

MAIN OUTCOMES AND MEASURES The primary outcome was to correlate the total 12-lead QRS voltage measurement with various morphologic features in the native diseased heart.

RESULTS The 16-patient study group consisted of 8 men and 8 women; 12 (75%) were white and 4 (25%) were black. At the time of OHT, patient age ranged from 50 to 67 years (mean, 57 years). Cardiac sarcoidosis was diagnosed by pre-OHT biopsy results in 2 (13%) patients and by examination of the native heart after OHT in 14 (87%) patients. Total nonpaced 12-lead QRS voltage mean was 117 mm (range, 52-155 mm) for 8 patients and total paced 12-lead QRS voltage was 90 mm (range, 67-161 mm) for 12 patients. These low mean values were similar to those of patients with carcinoid heart disease (mean [SD], 105 [40] mm), cardiac amyloidosis (104 [35] mm), and severe cardiac adiposity (120 [31] mm) studied at necropsy or after OHT. In contrast, mean (SD) values were 323 (109) mm in patients with massive cardiomegaly, 257 mm in patients with severe aortic stenosis, 272 (86) mm in patients with severe pure aortic regurgitation, 220 (67) mm in patients with severe pure mitral regurgitation, 197 (64) mm in patients with hypertrophic cardiomyopathy, and 153 (40) mm in patients with idiopathic dilated cardiomyopathy.

CONCLUSIONS AND RELEVANCE Most patients diagnosed with cardiac sarcoidosis causing severe heart failure and warranting OHT had low total 12-lead QRS voltage measurements despite having native hearts of increased weight. This finding may provide a clue to the diagnosis of this disease.

JAMA Cardiol. 2018;3(1):64-68. doi:10.1001/jamacardio.2017.4172
Published online November 15, 2017.

Author Affiliations: Baylor Heart and Vascular Institute, Baylor University Medical Center at Dallas, Dallas, Texas (Roberts, Becker, Hall); Department of Pathology, Baylor University Medical Center, Dallas, Texas (Roberts, Becker, Hall); Department of Internal Medicine, Baylor University Medical Center, Dallas, Texas (Roberts, Becker, Hall).

Corresponding Author: William C. Roberts, MD, Baylor Heart and Vascular Institute, 621 N Hall St, Ste H030, Dallas, TX 75226 (william.roberts1@bswhealth.org).

The first study of the utility of total 12-lead electrocardiographic QRS voltage was published in 1982 and reported findings for patients with aortic valve stenosis.[1] Subsequently, total 12-lead QRS voltage has been reported in a number of other conditions.[2] In each of those studies, the total 12-lead QRS voltage was compared with the weight of the native diseased heart at necropsy or after orthotopic heart transplant (OHT). The present report describes total 12-lead QRS voltage of 16 patients undergoing OHT because of severe heart failure due to cardiac sarcoidosis.

Methods

From January 13, 2005, through January 24, 2017, 16 patients at Baylor University Medical Center at Dallas (BUMC), Dallas, Texas, had OHT because of cardiac sarcoidosis. The study was approved by the Baylor Research Institute Institutional Review Board, which also waived the need for informed patient consent.

Each patient's native heart was examined by one of us (W.C.R.), and he prepared the final report. Accurate scales were used to weigh the native heart after fixation in formaldehyde for several days. The aorta and pulmonary trunk were excised about 2 cm above the sinotubular junction; all extraneous tissue was removed before weighing. Prior to weighing, the heart was opened and excessive water or formaldehyde was removed from its surfaces by gentle patting with paper towels. Clinical records and all electrocardiograms recorded at BUMC were reviewed and examined. The total 12-lead QRS voltage (defined as the distance in millimeters from the peak of the R wave to the nadir of either the Q or S wave, whichever was deeper) was measured by 2 of us (W.C.R. and T.M.B.). The statistics performed were limited to the calculation of the mean and SD. No statistical package or system was required for these calculations.

Results

The 16-patient study group consisted of 8 men and 8 women; 12 were white and 4 were black. Pertinent morphologic and electrocardiographic findings for the 16 patients are detailed in the **Table** and illustrated in **Figure 1** and **Figure 2**. At the time of OHT, the patient age ranged from 50 to 67 (mean, 57) years. Cardiac sarcoidosis was diagnosed by biopsy in 2 patients (13%) and by examination of the native heart after OHT in 14 patients (87%). The body mass index (calculated as the weight in kilograms divided by height in meters squared) ranged from 18.8 to 32.9 (mean, 27.1). Before OHT, 6 of the 16 patients (37%) had atrial fibrillation; 12 (75%) had bundle branch block (4 with left bundle branch block and 8 with right bundle branch block), and 7 (44%) had complete heart block. The low-density lipoprotein cholesterol levels before OHT ranged from 52 to 147 mg/dL (mean, 93 mg/dL) (to convert to millimoles per liter, multiply by 0.0259). Only patient 12 (Table) had greater than 75% in cross-sectional area narrowing of 1 or more major epicardial coronary arteries (defined as the right, left main, left anterior descending, and left circumflex).

Key Points

Question Is total 12-lead electrocardiographic QRS voltage a diagnostic clue for patients with cardiac sarcoidosis severe enough to warrant orthotopic heart transplant?

Findings In this case-series study, the mean total 12-lead QRS voltage in 16 patients with severe heart failure caused by extensive cardiac sarcoidosis (101 mm) was similar to that determined in patients with cardiac amyloidosis, carcinoid heart disease, and severe cardiac adiposity. In contrast, patients with fatal idiopathic dilated cardiomyopathy had a mean total 12-lead QRS voltage (153 mm).

Meaning The low total 12-lead QRS voltage measurement on electrocardiogram in patients with cardiac sarcoidosis, despite increased weight of the native heart, may be a clue to its correct diagnosis before orthotopic heart transplant.

The native heart weighed from 420 to 605 g (mean, 509 g) for the 8 men and from 370 to 600 g (mean, 442 g) for the 8 women. The quantity of cardiac adipose tissue was excessive such that the heart floated in a container of formaldehyde in 7 of the 11 hearts (64%) in which that determination was made. (Cardiac adipose tissue weighs less than myocardium.) Typical sarcoid granulomas were found in the walls of the right and left ventricles and in the ventricular spectrum in all patients. In 1 patient, however, granulomas were seen in the left ventricular wall ("button") removed for insertion of a left ventricular assist device but were not seen in the heart specimen after OHT. The number of granulomas and extent of ventricular wall scarring were subjectively quantified on a scale of 1+ (mild scarring) to 3+ (severe scarring). The distribution of sarcoid lesions is shown in the gross pathologic heart specimens for 3 of the 16 patients (Figure 2).

QRS voltage was measured using a 10-mm standard scale (10 mm = 1 mV) in all 12 leads of an electrocardiogram for all 16 patients. Mean total nonpaced 12-lead QRS voltage was 117 mm (range, 52-155 mm) for 8 patients: 3 men (mean, 137 mm [range, 121-155 mm]) and 5 women (mean, 105 mm [range, 52-144 mm]). Mean total paced 12-lead QRS voltage was 90 mm (range, 67-161 mm) for 12 patients: 6 men (mean, 81 mm [range, 47-103 mm]) and 6 women (mean, 98 mm [range, 67-161 mm]).

Discussion

Described herein are findings from measurement of total 12-lead electrocardiographic QRS voltage and findings from the examination of the native heart in 16 patients who underwent OHT because of severe heart failure due to cardiac sarcoidosis. These low total 12-lead nonpaced (mean, 117 mm) and paced (mean, 90 mm) QRS voltage values are similar to those values previously reported in patients with a variety of other conditions after OHT or necropsy.[2] The mean (SD) total 12-lead QRS voltage for several cardiac diseases is as follows: 105 (40) mm in 19 patients with carcinoid heart disease,[3] 104 (35) mm in 30 patients with cardiac amyloidosis,[4] and 120 (31) mm in 30 patients with severe cardiac adiposity.[5] In contrast, mean (SD) total 12-lead QRS voltage was 323 (109) mm in 17 patients with massive cardiomegaly (weight of native heart, >1000 g),[6] 257 mm in 50 patients with

Table. Pertinent Clinical and Morphological Findings in 16 Patients Who Underwent Heart Transplant for Cardiac Sarcoidosis

Patient No.	Age at HT, y	ECG Paced[a]	QRS Amplitude in Each ECG Lead: I	II	III	aVR	aVL	aVF	V_1	V_2	V_3	V_4	V_5	V_6	Total 12-Lead QRS Voltage, mm	Interval to ECG and HT, mo	BBB (Side)[b]	CHB[b]	LDL-C, mg/dL	SA Pressure, s/d, mm Hg	CI, $L/min/m^2$	HW, g	Location of Granulomas and Scar: RV	VS	LV	Heart Floated[c]
Men																										
1	50	0	7	11	14	5	9	12	6	14	19	7	10	7	121	31	+ (L)	0	119	130/89	1.7	605	0	1+	3+	NA
2	52	0	14	12	8	13	11	7	12	8	8	18	22	22	155	32	+ (R)	0	108	98/58 (I)	1.6	440	1+	2+	1+	NA
3	53	+	7	7	10	4	8	9	5	7	5	6	7	6	81	5	0	+	120	116/66 (I)	1.9	535	3+	3+	3+	NA
4	53	+	4	12	9	6	3	9	7	7	3	7	10	9	86	0.1	+ (R)	+	112	104/70 (I)	1.6	555	3+	3+	3+	+
5	58	+	9	9	6	4	4	6	5	3	8	8	8	7	77	1	+ (L)	0	64	88/55 (I)	1.2	420	3+	3+	3+	0
6	63	+	5	12	8	8	5	10	8	9	14	10	9	5	103	9	+ (L)	+	52	126/78	1.6	470	3+	3+	3+	+
7	63	0	8	6	3	6	6	4	9	10	13	18	22	29	134	34	+ (R)	0	86	120/84 (I)	1.7	540	3+	3+	3+	+
		+	5	8	11	5	6	11	2	4	12	17	11	3	95	2										
8	67	+	4	5	7	2	5	5	2	2	6	5	3	1	47	3	0	+	70	96/59	1.6	510	3+	3+	3+	+
Women																										
9	50	0	6	15	7	9	3	10	7	10	16	16	17	16	132	40	0	+	74	100/60 (I)	–	440	1+	3+	3+	0
		+	2	23	13	6	7	28	4	12	16	20	18	12	161	1										
10	52	+	5	5	5	5	2	8	6	7	7	5	5	7	67	3	+ (L)	0	64	115/79	2.3	440	1+	3+	2+	0
11	56	+	4	7	8	5	6	8	4	8	4	5	7	7	73	0.5	0	0	118	92/64	–	450	1+	3+	3+	+
12	57	0	5	1	6	3	6	4	5	9	5	4	2	2	52	18	+ (R)	0	94	101/58 (I)	1.4	380	3+	3+	3+	NA
13	58	0	8	8	15	3	11	12	5	7	4	4	6	6	89	49	+ (R)	0	147	102/57 (I)	2.2	560	3+	3+	3+	+
		+	3	3	4	2	3	3	3	7	3	3	4	4	69	2										
14	59	0	11	11	17	8	14	13	9	5	9	12	16	19	144	36	+ (R)	+	69	124/92	1.3	370	1+	2+	1+	NA
		+	10	12	19	8	14	15	8	9	10	13	15	14	147	35										
15	61	+	4	4	5	3	6	4	4	10	5	7	7	8	72	0.5	+ (R)	+	60	95/61 (I)	1.2	300	3+	3+	3+	+
16	62	0	10	11	10	7	7	7	10	9	7	9	10	10	107	1	+ (R)	0	129	109/68 (I)	1.5	600	1+	1+	3+	0

Abbreviations: a, augmented; BBB, bundle branch block; CHB, complete heart block; CI, cardiac index; ECG, electrocardiogram; HT, heart transplant; HW, weight of native heart; I, indirect; L, left (or left arm for ECG leads); LDL-C, low-density lipoprotein cholesterol; LV, left ventricle; NA, no information available; R, right (or right arm for ECG leads); RV, right ventricle; SA, systemic artery; s/d, systolic/diastolic; V, voltage; VS, ventricular septum.

SI conversion factor: To convert LDL-C to millimoles per liter, multiply by 0.0259.

[a] + Indicates paced; 0, nonpaced.

[b] + Indicates present; 0, not present.

[c] + Indicates present; 0, not present; and NA, no information available.

Figure 1. 12-Lead Electrocardiograms

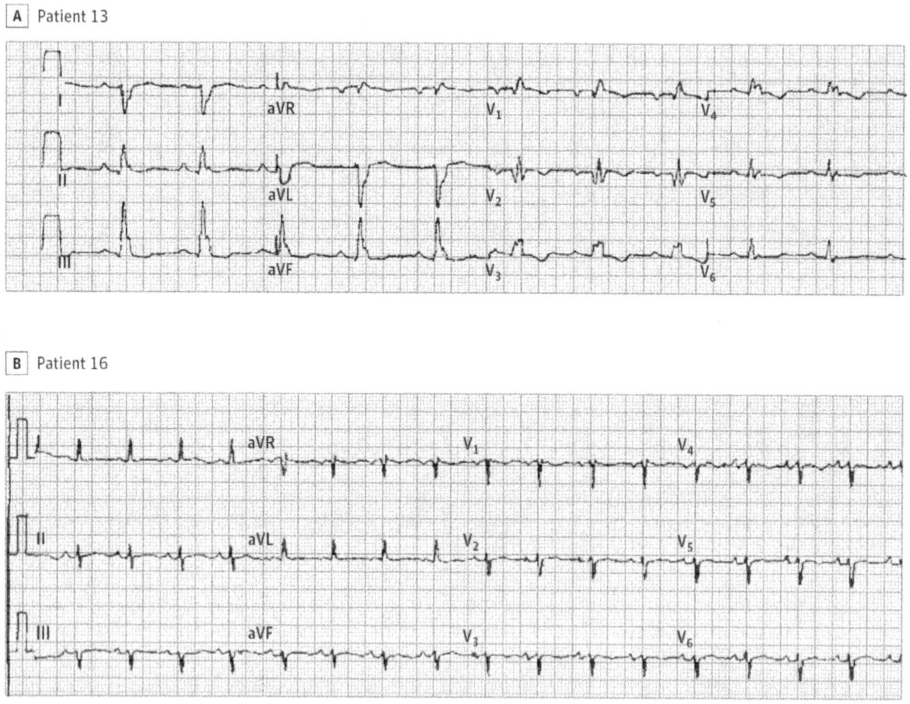

A, Patient 13: total 12-lead QRS voltage is 89 mm; weight of native heart, 560 g. B, Patient 16: total 12-lead QRS voltage is 107 mm; weight of native heart = 600 g. Leads (recording electrodes) are designated as follows: standard (bipolar) leads, I, II, and III; precordial (unipolar) leads, V_1, V_2, V_3, V_4, V_5, and V_6; and augmented limb leads/unipolar extremity leads, aVR, aVL, and aVF (a, augmented; V, voltage; R, right arm; L, left arm; and F, foot).

severe aortic stenosis,[1] 272 (86) mm in 30 patients with severe pure aortic regurgitation,[7] 220 (67) mm in 24 patients with pure mitral regurgitation,[8] 197 (64) mm in 57 patients with hypertrophic cardiomyopathy,[9,10] and 153 (40) mm in 49 patients with idiopathic dilated cardiomyopathy.[11] Thus, most of our patients (15 of 16 [94%]) with severe cardiac sarcoidosis, despite having native hearts of increased weight (>350 g in women and >400 g in men), had low total 12-lead QRS voltages.

Limitations and Strengths

A limitation of the present report is that the time interval between the recording of the electrocardiogram tracing and the OHT procedure was rather long for some patients. It is likely, however, as described previously in patients with idiopathic dilated cardiomyopathy,[12] that the total 12-lead QRS voltage would decrease as the time interval increases between initially developing cardiac sarcoidosis and OHT procedure.[12]

The strong features of the present report are that both the weight of the native heart and the extent of the cardiac sarcoid lesions were known for all 16 patients. To our knowledge, electrocardiographic QRS voltage has not been described previously in patients with cardiac sarcoidosis.[12]

Conclusions

Most patients diagnosed with cardiac sarcoidosis causing severe heart failure and warranting OHT had low total 12-lead QRS voltage measurements despite having native hearts of increased weight. This finding may provide a clue to the diagnosis of this disease.

ARTICLE INFORMATION

Accepted for Publication: September 19, 2017.

Published Online: November 15, 2017. doi:10.1001/jamacardio.2017.4172

Author Contributions: Dr Roberts and Ms Becker had full access to all of the data in the study and take responsibility for the integrity of the data and the accuracy of the data analysis.
Study concept and design: Roberts, Becker.
Acquisition, analysis, or interpretation of data: All authors.
Drafting of the manuscript: Roberts.
Critical revision of the manuscript for important intellectual content: Roberts.
Administrative, technical, or material support: Hall.
Study supervision: Roberts.

Conflict of Interest Disclosures: All authors have completed and submitted the ICMJE Form for Disclosure of Potential Conflicts of Interest and none were reported.

REFERENCES

1. Siegel RJ, Roberts WC. Electrocardiographic observations in severe aortic valve stenosis: correlative necropsy study to clinical, hemodynamic, and ECG variables demonstrating relation of 12-lead QRS amplitude to peak systolic transaortic pressure gradient. *Am Heart J*. 1982;103(2):210-221.

2. Roberts WC, Filardo G, Ko JM, et al. Comparison of total 12-lead QRS voltage in a variety of cardiac conditions and its usefulness in predicting increased cardiac mass. *Am J Cardiol*. 2013;112(6):904-909.

3. Ross EM, Roberts WC. The carcinoid syndrome: comparison of 21 necropsy subjects with carcinoid heart disease to 15 necropsy subjects without carcinoid heart disease. *Am J Med*. 1985;79(3):339-354.

Figure 2. Basal Portions of Native Heart and Photomicrograph of Myocardial Wall in Patients Who Underwent Cardiac Transplant Because of Cardiac Sarcoidosis

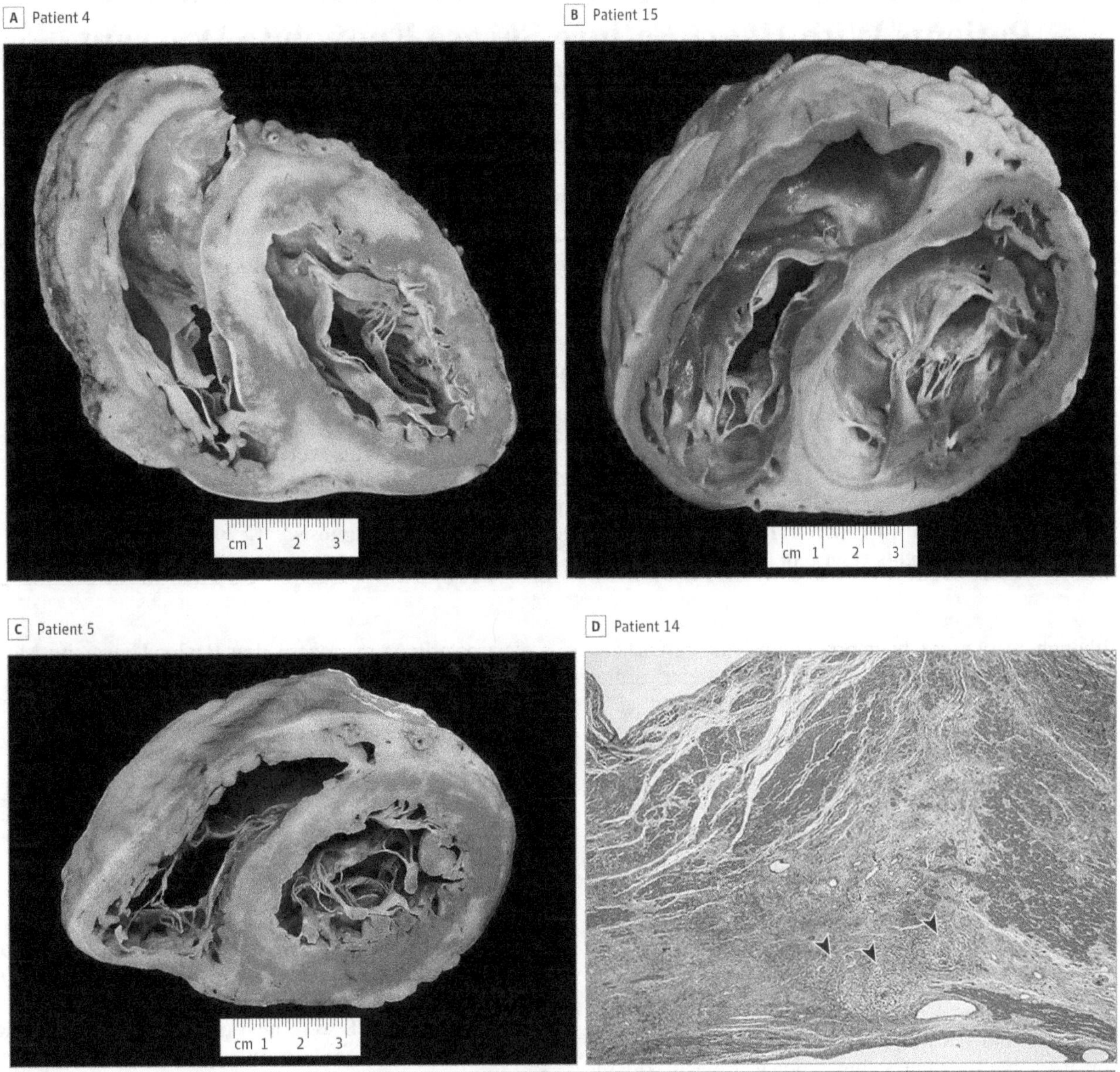

Basal portions of the heart exposing the tricuspid and mitral values. The ventricular septal and left ventricular free wall and a portion of right ventricular free wall contain white lesions; these represent scar tissue within which are sarcoid granulomas. All ventricular cavities are largely dilated. D, Photomicrograph of a portion of the left ventricular free wall of patient 14. The myocardial wall is partially, but extensively replaced by dense fibrous tissue that stains blue and contains several sarcoid granulomas (arrowheads) (trichrome stain, original magnification ×100). Scale bars in A through C are in centimeters.

4. Roberts WC, Waller BF. Cardiac amyloidosis causing cardiac dysfunction: analysis of 54 necropsy patients. *Am J Cardiol*. 1983;52(1):137-146.

5. Shirani J, Roberts WC. Clinical, electrocardiographic and morphologic features of massive fatty deposits ("lipomatous hypertrophy") in the atrial septum. *J Am Coll Cardiol*. 1993;22(1):226-238.

6. Roberts WC, Podolak MJ. The king of hearts: analysis of 23 patients with hearts weighing 1,000 grams or more. *Am J Cardiol*. 1985;55(4):485-494.

7. Roberts WC, Day PJ. Electrocardiographic observations in clinically isolated, pure, chronic, severe aortic regurgitation: analysis of 30 necropsy patients aged 19 to 65 years. *Am J Cardiol*. 1985;55(4):432-438.

8. Glick BN, Roberts WC. Usefulness of total 12-lead QRS voltage in diagnosing left ventricular hypertrophy in clinically isolated, pure, chronic, severe mitral regurgitation. *Am J Cardiol*. 1992;70(11):1088-1092.

9. Dollar AL, Roberts WC. Usefulness of total 12-lead QRS voltage compared with other criteria for determining left ventricular hypertrophy in hypertrophic cardiomyopathy: analysis of 57 patients studied at necropsy. *Am J Med*. 1989;87(4):377-381.

10. Shirani J, Maron BJ, Cannon RO III, Shahin S, Roberts WC. Clinicopathologic features of hypertrophic cardiomyopathy managed by cardiac transplantation. *Am J Cardiol*. 1993;72(5):434-440.

11. Roberts WC, Siegel RJ, McManus BM. Idiopathic dilated cardiomyopathy: analysis of 152 necropsy patients. *Am J Cardiol*. 1987;60(16):1340-1355.

12. Wilensky RL, Yudelman P, Cohen AI, et al. Serial electrocardiographic changes in idiopathic dilated cardiomyopathy confirmed at necropsy. *Am J Cardiol*. 1988;62(4):276-283.

Usefulness of Total 12-Lead QRS Voltage for Diagnosis of Arrhythmogenic Right Ventricular Cardiomyopathy in Patients With Heart Failure Severe Enough to Warrant Orthotopic Heart Transplantation and Morphologic Illustration of Its Cardiac Diversity

William C. Roberts, MD*, Nitin Kondapalli, MBBS, and Shelley A. Hall, MD

Although several electrocardiographic features of arrhythmogenic right ventricular cardiomyopathy (ARVC) (also called dysplasia) have been described, total 12-lead QRS voltage is not one of them. This report describes total 12-lead QRS voltage in 11 patients with ARVC who underwent orthotopic heart transplantation (OHT) because of progressively severe heart failure. Additionally, it illustrates the varied morphologic features of ARVC. The total 12-lead nonpaced QRS voltages before OHT ranged from 28 to 118 mm (mean 74 ± 32), and those in the paced tracings, from 33 to 129 mm (62 ± 32). The voltages are the lowest we have encountered among 12 previously reported cardiovascular conditions. The heart weights among the 11 ARVC patients ranged from 285 to 670 g (mean 448 ± 125). Very low 12-lead QRS voltage is characteristic of patients with ARVC with heart failure severe enough to warrant OHT, and thus may serve as a clue to its diagnosis. **(Am J Cardiol 2018;122:1051−1061)**

Although recognized by morphologic studies earlier,[1] the present concepts of arrhythmic right ventricular cardiomyopathy (ARVC) were introduced by Marcus et al in 1982.[2] Several reports have described various electrocardiographic features of ARVC but none have described total 12-lead QRS voltage or its potential diagnostic usefulness.[3−13] Such is one purpose of this report. Another is to illustrate several hearts of patients with ARVC to demonstrate the morphologic variability of this condition.

Methods

From 2009 to 2017, 11 adults at Baylor University Medical Center at Dallas had orthotopic heart transplantation (OHT) because of ARVC. The study was approved by the Baylor Research Institute's Institutional Review Board, which also waived the need for informed patient consent.

One of us (WCR) examined each patient's native heart and also prepared the final report. Accurate scales were used to weigh the native heart after fixation in formaldehyde for several days. The ascending aorta and pulmonary trunk were excised about 2 cm above the sinotubular junction; all extraneous tissues were removed before weighing. Before weighing, the heart was opened and excessive water or formaldehyde was removed from its surfaces by gentle patting with paper towels. Clinical records and all electrocardiograms recorded at Baylor University Medical Center were reviewed and examined. The total 12-lead QRS voltage (defined as the distance in millimeters from the peak of the R wave to the nadir of either the Q or S wave, whichever was deeper, with 10 mm standard [=1 mV]) was measured by 2 of us (WCR and NK). The statistics performed was limited to the calculation of the means and standard deviations.

Results

Pertinent clinical, morphologic, and electrocardiographic data are displayed in Tables 1 and 2. At the time of OHT, the patients' ages ranged from 21 to 70 years (mean 49 ± 17); 8 were men and 3 were women. ARVC was diagnosed before OHT in 3 patients and from examination of the operatively excised heart in the other 8 patients. All 11 patients had clinical evidence of heart failure, especially severe right-sided heart failure; by electrocardiogram, 8 had documented runs of ventricular tachycardia, 3 had epsilon waves (small amplitude distinct potentials between the end of the QRS complex and the beginning of the T wave), and 5 had inverted T waves in 1 or more precordial leads; all 11 had low QRS voltage, and 5 had right bundle branch block; by echocardiogram or computed tomography, all 11 patients had very dilated right ventricular cavities and 10 had dilated, but less so, left ventricular cavities. The body mass indexes ranged from 22 to 37 kg/m^2 (mean 29 ± 5). The progression of heart failure to class III or IV prompted the OHT.

The electrocardiographic findings before OHT are tabulated in Table 2. Six nonpaced and 7 paced electrocardiographic tracings were available for analysis. The nonpaced total 12-lead QRS voltages ranged from 28 to 118 mm (mean 74 ± 32), and those in paced tracings, from

From the Baylor Scott & White Heart and Vascular Institute, the Departments of Pathology and Internal Medicine (Division of Cardiology), Baylor University Medical Center, Part of Baylor Scott & White Health, Dallas, Texas. Manuscript received May 30, 2018; revised manuscript received and accepted June 6, 2018.

*Corresponding author: Tel: (214) 820-7911; fax: (214) 820-7533.

E-mail addresses: ajc@baylorhealth.edu, William.Roberts1@bswhealth.org (W.C. Roberts).

Table 1
Arrhythmogenic right ventricular cardiomyopathy—Clinical and morphologic features

Patient no (figure no)	Age at OHT (yrs)	Family history of SD/VT	BMI (kg/m^2)	TC (mg/dl)	LDL-C (mg/dl)	HDL-C (mg/dl)	TG (mg/dl)	LVEF (%)	CI (L/ min/m^2)	ARVC diagnosed clinically	Pressures (mm Hg) (s/d)			HW (g)	Coronary artery narrowing (>75% CSA) by plaque	Heart floated in formalin	LV involvement		Associated Condition
											SA	RV	PA				Scar	Fat	
MEN																			
1(3)	21	0	27	147	72	65	62	5	1.1	0	144/96*	21/14	17/11	490	0	0	0	0	0
2	26	0	35	204	134	56	149	10	0.8	0	180/100*	-	50/30	595	0	0	0	0	Gilbert's syndrome
3(4)	34	0	27	154	73	80	65	3	1.3	0	75/55*	48/12	20/14	515	0	0	+	0	Rheumatoid arthritis
4	44	+	22	175	112	50	87	25	1.9	0	95/60*	19/12	22/11	315	0	0	0	0	Hypothyroidism
5(5)	54	+	26	145	68	62	74	30	1.5	+	75/50*	31/4	25/10	670†	+	+	+	+	0
6(1&6)	62	0	35	173	86	82	94	20	1.4	0	100/70*	25/10	21/12	420	0	+	0	0	Guillain Barre syndrome
7(7)	66	0	29	235	107	94	184	15	1.5	0‡	80/55*	18/9	16/3	450	0	+	+	+	Hypothyroidism
8(8)	68	0	28	165	97	32	296	30	1.4	0	155/80*	26/7	24/16	460	+§	+	+	0	0
WOMEN																			
9(9)¶	44	+	37	204	149	44	119	10	1.5	0	125/85*	40/-1	42/13	420	0	+	0	0	Limb-girdle muscular dystrophy
10(10)	49	0	27	237	112	100	200	56	1.5	+	85/40*	22/12	20/13	305	0	+	0	0	0
11(2&11)	70	+	26	254	149	68	297	55	1.7	+	185/100*	17/5	17/3	285	0	+	0	0	Hypothyroidism

ARVC = arrhythmogenic right ventricular cardiomyopathy; BMI = body mass index; CABG = coronary artery bypass grafting; CI = cardiac index; CSA = cross-sectional area; g = gram(s); Hg = hydrargyrum (Mercury); HW = heart weight; ICD = Implantable Cardioverter Defibrillator; kg = kilogram(s); L = Liter(s); LDL-C = low-density lipoprotein cholesterol; LVAD = left ventricular assist device; LVEF = left ventricular ejection fraction; m = meter(s); min = minute(s); OHT = orthotopic heart transplantation; PA = pulmonary artery; RV = right ventricle; s/d = peak systole/end-diastole; SD = sudden death; SA = systemic artery; TC = total cholesterol; VT = ventricular tachycardia; Yrs = year(s).

* Indirect pressure (cuff).

† An LVAD was inserted 34 months before the OHT.

‡ The result of performed biopsy was negative for ARVC changes.

§ Patient had CABG 25 years before the OHT.

¶ Patient died 48 days after the OHT.

Table 2
Electrocardiographic features of arrhythmogenic right ventricular cardiomyopathy

Patient no. (figure no.)	Age at OHT (yrs)	ECG Paced	QRS amplitude in each electrocardiographic lead(mm)												Total 12-lead QRS voltage (mm)	ECG to OHT interval (mos)	HW (g)	ECG changes before OHT							
			I	II	III	aVR	aVL	aVF	V1	V2	V3	V4	V5	V6				AF	VPCs	VT	Epsilon wave	Inverted T waves	Right BBB	LAFB	CHB
MEN																									
1(3)	21	0	5	3	3	3	3	2	6	11	14	14	8	19	91	8.0	490	0	+	0	0	+	0	0	0
2	26	0	3	3	6	2	5	5	4	5	10	8	7	9	67	0.2	595	0	+	+	0	+	+	+	0
		+	4	3	8	2	7	5	4	5	8	8	7	7	68	3.0									
3(4)	34	+	3	4	4	3	4	5	6	6	4	7	11	8	65	0.7	515	0	+	0	0	0	0	0	+
4	44	+	1	4	4	3	2	5	2	3	6	8	9	5	52	0.5	315	+	0	+	0	0	+	0	0
5(5)	54	+	3	8	9	5	4	10	8	13	23	20	16	10	129	15.5	670*	0	+	+	0	0	0	0	0
6(1&6)	62	0	6	6	10	5	8	9	7	9	6	7	10	7	90	170.0	420	+	+	+	+	+	+	+	0
		+	3	3	5	2	4	4	2	6	2	3	3	4	41	5.0									
7(7)	66	+	3	2	3	1	3	3	1	3	3	5	4	2	33	0.3	450	+	0	+	0	0	0	0	0
8(8)	68	+	3	3	2	3	2	1	2	9	7	6	5	4	47	0.3	460	+	+	+	0	0	0	0	0
WOMEN																									
9(9)	44	0	10	10	10	10	8	9	11	12	10	10	9	9	118	23.0	420	+	+	+	0	+	+	0	0
10(10)	49	0	2	3	3	2	2	3	2	2	3	2	2	2	28	3.5	305	+	+	0	+	0	+	0	0
11(2&11)	70	0	8	3	7	4	7	3	2	5	2	2	4	5	52	1.0	285	+	+	+	+	+	0	+	0

AF = atrial fibrillation; BBB = bundle branch block; CHB = complete heart block; ECG = electrocardiogram; LAFB = left anterior fascicular block; mm = millimeter(s); OHT = orthotopic heart transplantation; VPCs = ventricular premature complexes; VT = ventricular tachycardia; Yrs = year(s).

* A left ventricular assist device was inserted 34 months before the OHT.

Table 3
Total 12-lead QRS voltage in different cardiovascular conditions*

Condition	Gender	No. of cases	Age in years (mean)	Total 12-Lead QRS voltage in mm (mean)	Patients with 12-Lead QRS voltage >175mm	Heart weight (g)	Total 12-lead QRS voltage (mm)/heart weight (g)	Year of Publication	Authors (reference Number)
Hearts weigh >1000 g	M	16	29-64 (42)	140-414 (306)	16 (94%)	1005-1360 (1102)	0.28	1985	Roberts and Podolak[14]
	F	1	20	601		1250	0.48		
Aortic valve stenosis	M	36	16-64 (48)	144-417 (249)	47 (94%)	440-880 (639)	0.39	1982	Siegel and Roberts[15]
	F	14	16-65 (47)	193-376 (277)		380-700 (521)	0.53		
Aortic regurgitation	M	22	19-59 (44)	109-428 (271)	27 (90%)	430-1100 (717)	0.38	1985	Roberts and Day[16]
	F	8	35-56 (48)	169-384 (275)		375-950 (638)	0.43		
Mitral regurgitation	M	11	24-84 (47)	111-364 (245)	17 (71%)	400-775 (629)	0.39	1992	Glick and Roberts[17]
	F	13	21-64 (37)	114-290 (199)		350-675 (472)	0.42		
Hypertrophic cardiomyopathy without cardiac transplantation	M	21	14-68 (46)	107-339 (190)	30 (53%)	325-1070 (671)	0.28	1989	Dollar and Roberts[18]
	F	36	19-87 (51)	68-327 (201)		290-1230 (547)	0.38		
Hypertrophic cardiomyopathy with cardiac transplantation	M	6	19-46 (35)	109-201 (142)	4 (40%)	310-480 (393)	0.36	1993	Shirani et al[19]
	F	4	24-45 (35)	172-378 (241)		290-650 (408)	0.59		
Idiopathic dilated cardiomyopathy	M	35	19-73 (46)	74-281 (147)	20 (41%)	400-940 (620)	0.24	1987	Roberts et al[20]
	F	14	22-75 (54)	75-243 (167)		400-860 (602)	0.28		
Lipomatous hypertrophy of the atrial septum	M	12	48-84 (67)	93-241 (140)	3 (11%)	410-795 (576)	0.24	1993	Shirani and Roberts[21]
	F	16	59-83 (74)	59-266 (124)		330-680 (502)	0.25		
Carcinoid syndrome with carcinoid heart disease	M	11	39-72 (56)	58-227 (120)	2 (11%)	220-480 (350)	0.34	1985	Ross and Roberts[22]
	F	8	28-64 (54)	58-128 (84)		200-290 (245)	0.34		
Carcinoid syndrome without carcinoid heart disease	M	10	42-75 (55)	89-129 (137)	2 (13%)	240-570 (350)	0.39		
	F	5	28-67 (50)	102-135 (121)		150-270 (230)	0.53		
Aortic syphilis	M	11	33-84 (28)	57-161 (120)	0	-	-	2015	Roberts et al[23]
	F	13	58-83 (28)	64-146 (106)		-	-		
Cardiac adiposity	M	13	51-73 (64)	73-159 (114)	1 (3%)	320-795 (485)	0.24	1995	Shirani et al[24]
	F	17	40-85 (70)	77-210 (124)		250-575 (395)	0.31		
Cardiac amyloidosis	M	15	32-69 (52)	60-197 (99)	2 (7%)	410-850 (570)	0.17	1983	Roberts and Waller[25]
	F	15	21-93 (69)	58-199 (109)		370-900 (494)	0.22		
Cardiac sarcoidosis (Nonpaced)	M	3	50,52,63 (55)	121,155,134 (137)	0	605,440,540 (528)	0.26	2018	Roberts et al[26]
	F	5	50-62 (57)	52-144 (105)		370-600 (470)	0.22		
Cardiac sarcoidosis (Paced)	M	6	53-67 (59)	47-103 (82)	0	420-555 (505)	0.16		
	F	6	50-61 (56)	67-161 (98)		300-560 (427)	0.23		
Arrhythmogenic right ventricular cardiomyopathy (Nonpaced)	M	3	21,26,62 (36)	91,67,90 (83)	0	490,595,420 (502)	0.17	2018	Roberts et al
	F	3	44,49,70 (54)	28,61,118 (69)		420,305,285 (337)	0.2		
Arrhythmogenic right ventricular cardiomyopathy (Paced)	M	7	26-68 (51)	33-129 (62)	0	315-670 (489)	0.13		
	F	0	-	-		-	-		

* Parts of this table have been published previously in the following reports: Roberts WC, Filardo G, Ko JM, Siegel RJ, Dollar AL, Ross EM, Shirani J. Comparison of total 12-lead QRS voltage in a variety of cardiac conditions and its usefulness in predicting increased cardiac mass. *Am J Cardiol* 2013; 112(6):904-909. Permission to republish this updated table is granted by the authors and the publisher, Elsevier.

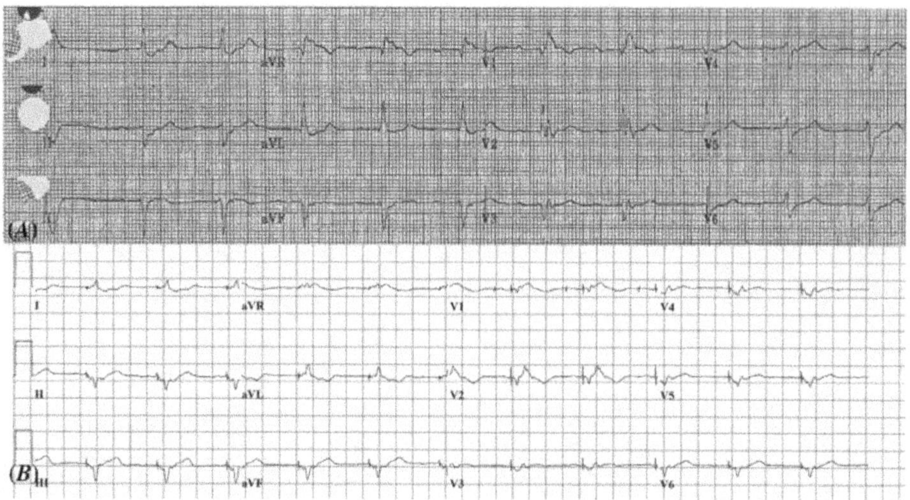

Figure 1. Case #6, Tables 1 and 2. Electrocardiograms nonpaced *(upper)* and paced *(lower)*. The total 12-lead QRS voltage in the upper tracing is 90 mm and in the lower tracing, 41 mm with 10 mm standard. Prominent epsilon waves are present in 1 or more precordial leads in the two patients.

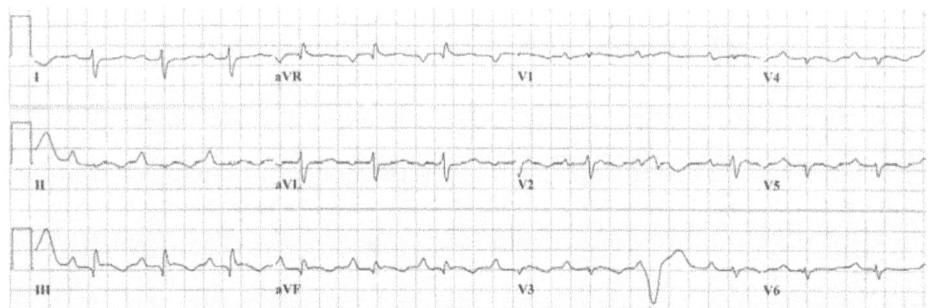

Figure 2. Case #11, Tables 1 and 2. Nonpaced electrocardiogram with total 12-lead QRS voltage of 52 mm. The PR interval is prolonged (236 ms), many T waves are inverted, and an occasional ventricular premature complex is present.

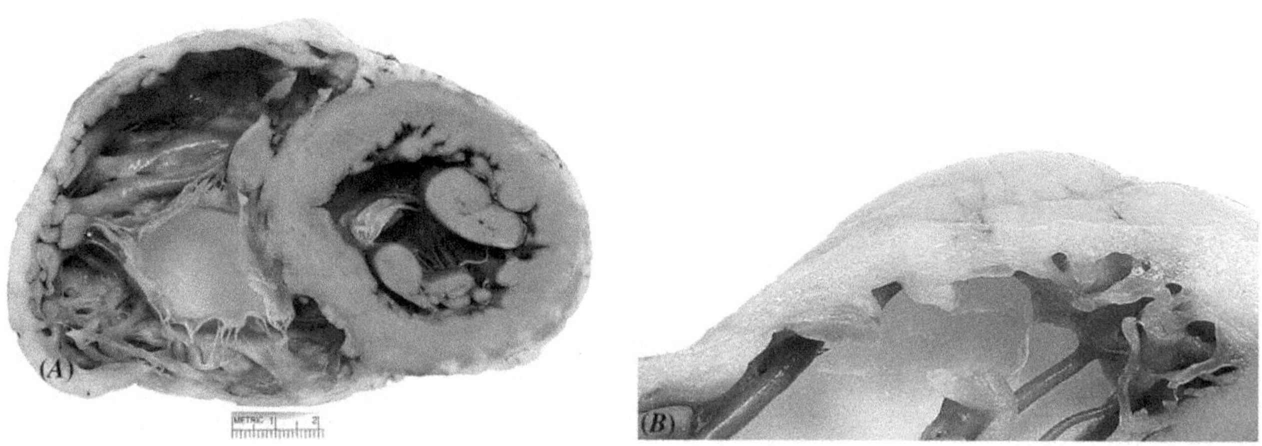

Figure 3. Case #1, Tables 1 and 2. Shown here are 2 photographs of the heart in a 21-year-old man. (*A*) Shown here is the basal portion of the heart showing marked dilatation of the right ventricular cavity and dilatation but less so of the left ventricular cavity. Most of the right ventricular wall is replaced by adipose tissue. There is some infiltration of fat in the subepicardial portion of left ventricular wall and some small scars in the subepicardial portion of left ventricular wall. (*B*) A close-up of the right ventricular outflow tract showing the right ventricular wall to be focally replaced by adipose tissue. Total nonpaced 12-lead QRS voltage in this patient was 91 mm and the heart weighed 490 g.

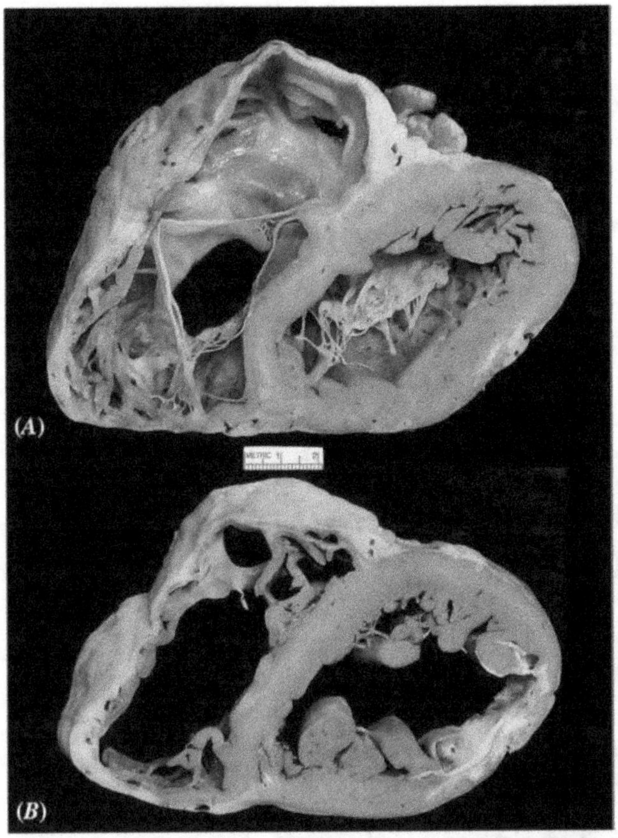

Figure 4. Case #3, Tables 1 and 2. Shown here is the basal portion of the ventricular walls in a 34-year-old man. The two ventricular cavities are dilated but the right one far more than the left. (*A*) The right ventricular free wall is replaced focally by either adipose tissue or fibrous tissue or both. (*B*) This cut of the ventricular walls not only shows the thinning of the right ventricular free wall focally but also a scar in the lateral wall of left ventricular between the two papillary muscles. The epicardial coronary arteries were wide open. Total paced 12-lead QRS voltage was 65 mm, and the heart weighed 515 g.

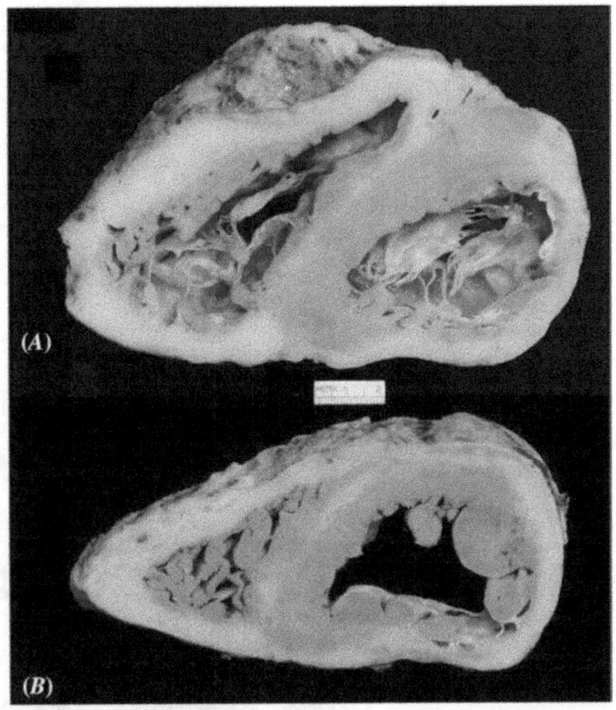

Figure 5. Case #5, Tables 1 and 2. Shown here is the basal portion of the ventricles in *A* and another portion more apically located in *B*. (*A*) The two ventricular cavities are dilated. Most of the right ventricular wall is replaced by adipose tissue. (*B*) Much of the entire left ventricular free wall, particularly the subepicardial region, is replaced by adipose tissue making the wall much thinner than the ventricular septum. The lumen of the right coronary artery was considerably narrowed by atherosclerotic plaque. Total paced 12-lead QRS voltage was 129 mm and the heart weighed 670 g. This patient had a left ventricular assist device in place for 34 months before the OHT.

33 to 129 mm (mean 62 ± 32). Before OHT, atrial fibrillation was present in 7 patients, and occasional ventricular premature complexes in 9 patients, 5 of whom also had runs of ventricular tachycardia.

The hearts of the 8 men ranged in weight from 315 to 670 g (mean 489 ± 108), and in the 3 women, from 285 to 420 g (mean 337 ± 73). The quantity of adipose tissue in the heart was huge in 7 of 11 patients causing their hearts to float in a container of formaldehyde (adipose tissue is lighter than myocardium). Two patients had narrowing of 1 or more major epicardial coronary arteries, one of whom had undergone coronary arterial bypass grafting 25 years before the OHT. All patients had dilated right ventricular cavities and all but 1 also had dilated left ventricular cavities but in all cases the right ventricular cavity was much more dilated than the left one. The right ventricular wall was focally replaced mainly by adipose tissue in which some scar tissue usually also was present. Focal scars replaced portions of the left ventricular free wall and/or ventricular septum in 4 patients, 2 of whom had narrowing >75% in cross-sectional area by plaques of 1 or more major epicardial coronary arteries. Two of 4 patients with left ventricular scars also had focal fatty replacement of these walls by adipose tissue.

Discussion

Described herein are findings from measurement of total 12-lead QRS voltage and findings from the examination of the native hearts in 11 patients who underwent OHT because of severe heart failure due to ARVC. These total 12-lead nonpaced QRS voltages (mean 74 ± 32) and paced (mean 62 ± 32) are the lowest found in any of the 12 previously reported conditions we have studied (summarized in Table 3).[14–26] The total 12-lead QRS voltage was lower in the 7 paced electrocardiograms than in the 6 nonpaced electrocardiograms.

A limitation of the present report is that the time interval between the recording of the electrocardiogram and the OHT procedure was rather long in 3 of 11 patients. It is likely, however, as described previously in patients with idiopathic dilated cardiomyopathy that the total 12-lead QRS voltage would decrease as the time interval increased

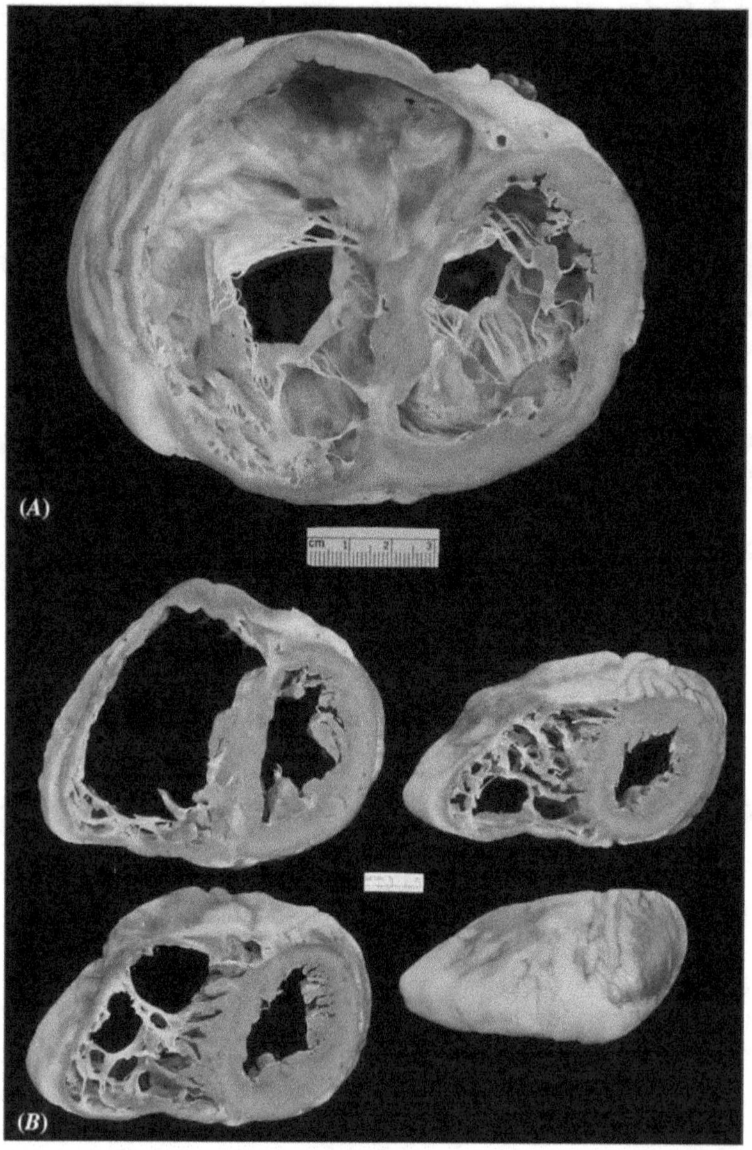

Figure 6. Case #6, Tables 1 and 2. Shown here are portions of a heart in a 63-year-old man. (*A*) The two ventricular cavities are greatly dilated, the right much more than the left. The right ventricular free wall is focally replaced, mainly by adipose tissue. Focal scars are also present in the ventricular septum. (*B*) These are transverse cuts of the ventricles caudal to the view shown in *A*. These views show scarring in the right ventricular pectinate muscles as well as focally in the ventricular septum. The right ventricular cavity is much larger than the left. Total nonpaced 12-lead QRS voltage was 90 mm and paced, 41 mm, and the heart weighed 420 g.

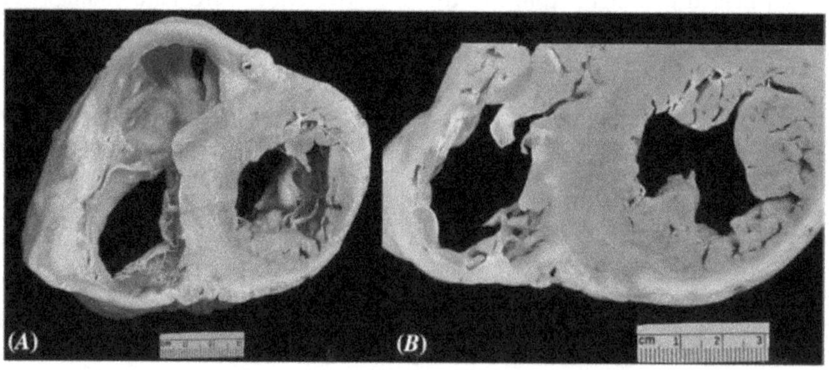

Figure 7. Case #7, Tables 1 and 2. Shown in *A* is the basal portion of the heart showing replacement of much of the walls of the two ventricles by adipose tissue. The lateral wall of the left ventricle is much thinner than the ventricular septum due to replacement of myocardium by both adipose tissue and fibrous tissue. (*B*) A closer view more apically better showing the fatty infiltration of the myocardial walls. The quantity of fat was such that the heart floated in a container of formaldehyde (adipose tissue is lighter than myocardium). The total paced 12-lead QRS voltage was only 33 mm, and the heart weighed 450 g.

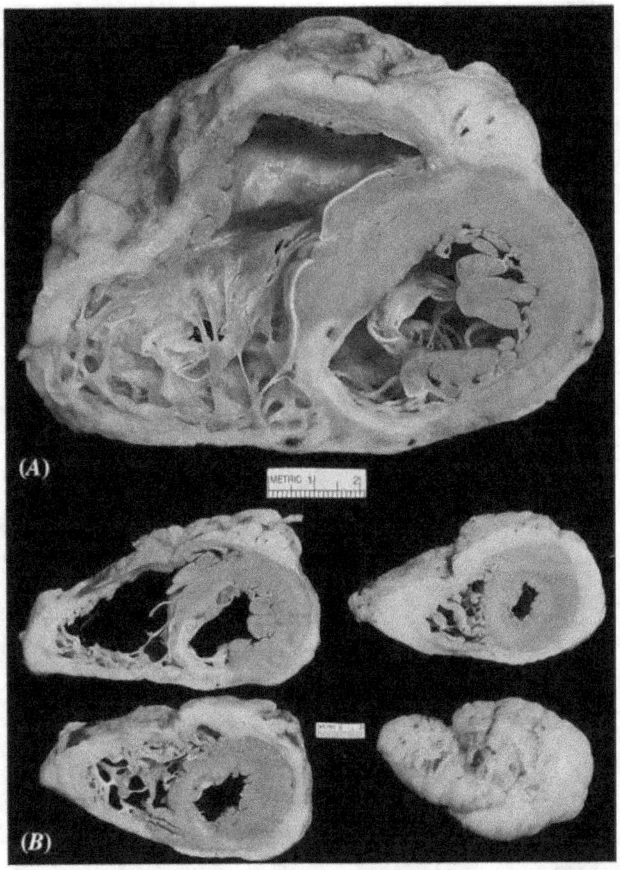

Figure 8. Case #8, Tables 1 and 2. Shown here are views of the cardiac ventricles on various levels in a 68-year-old man. The two ventricular cavities are dilated but the right far more than the left. The right ventricular cavity posteriorly and laterally is replaced by mainly adipose tissue but some scar tissue is present. The posterior portion of the ventricular septum and the posterior left ventricular free wall is replaced by scar tissue. (*B*) Photographs of the ventricular slices caudal to the view shown in *A*. The quantity of subepicardial adipose tissue is excessive such that the heart floated in a container of formaldehyde. Total paced 12-lead QRS voltage was 47 mm, and the heart weighed 460 g.

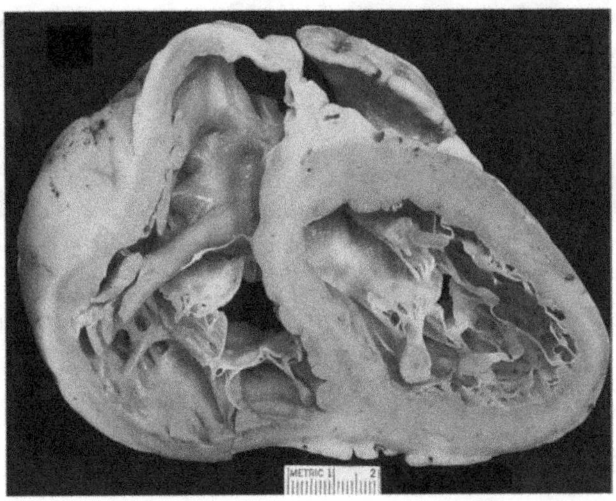

Figure 9. Case #9, Tables 1 and 2. Shown here is the basal portion of the heart in a 44-year-old woman who had limb-girdle muscular dystrophy. This photograph shows marked dilatation of the two ventricular cavities. The right ventricular free wall anteriorly adjacent to the septum is replaced by adipose tissue. The lateral wall of left ventricle between the two papillary muscles is thinner than other portions of the left ventricular free wall. Total nonpaced 12-lead QRS voltage in this patient was 118 mm, and the heart weighed 420 g.

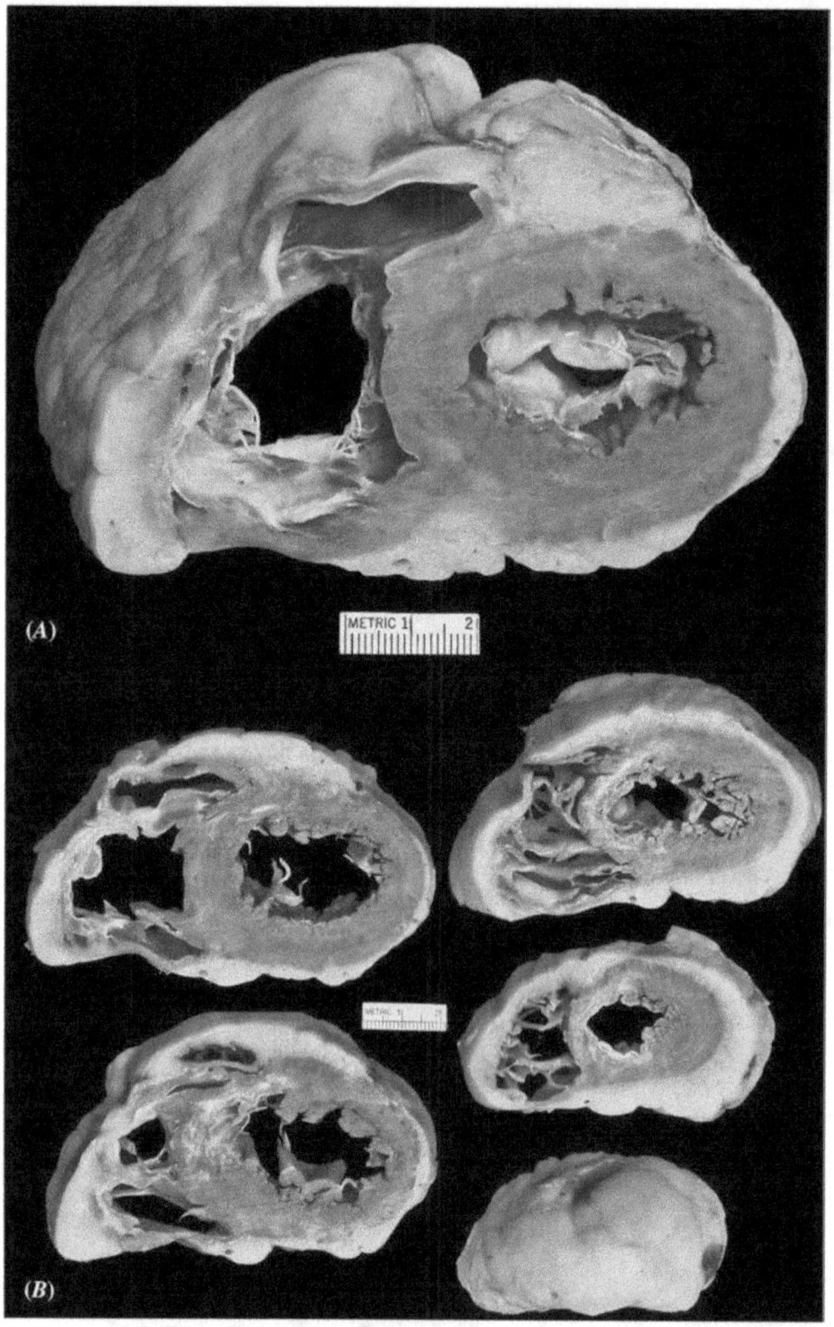

Figure 10. Case #10, Tables 1 and 2. Shown here is the heart in a 49-year-old woman. (*A*) Shown is the basal portion of the ventricles. The right ventricular cavity is considerably dilated and the left, minimally so. Portions of the endocardium of right ventricle are thickened by fibrous tissue and portions of the right ventricular free wall are replaced by fibrous tissue. No definite lesions are noted in the left ventricular free wall at the base. (*B*) Shown here are more apical cuts of the ventricular wall. The ventricular septum and the right ventricular free wall are extensively scarred. The epicardial coronary arteries were wide open. The total nonpaced 12-lead QRS voltage was 118 mm, and the heart weighed only 305 g. The heart floated in a container of formaldehyde.

between initially developing ARVC and the OHT procedure.[27] Strong features of the present report are that both the weight of the native heart and the extent of the cardiac lesions were known in all 11 patients. To our knowledge, total 12-lead electrocardiographic QRS voltage has not been described previously in patients with ARVC, and gross differing features of the hearts have not been well illustrated previously. The electrocardiographic findings may provide a clue to the diagnosis of ARVC (Figures 1–11).

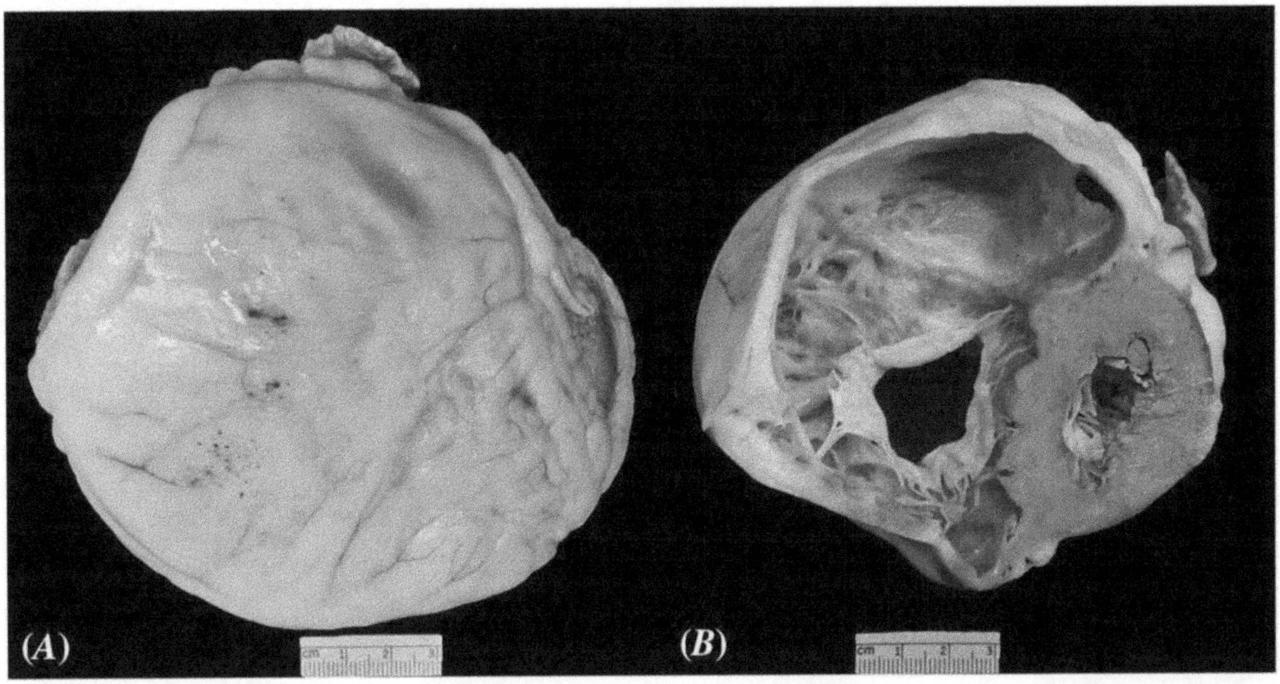

Figure 11. Case #11, Tables 1 and 2. Shown in *A* is the outside of the heart anteriorly. The right ventricular cavity is greatly dilated and totally covered by adipose tissue. (*B*) A photograph of the basal portion of the ventricles showing the enormously dilated right ventricular cavity and a normal-sized left ventricular cavity. About 90% of the right ventricular free wall is replaced by adipose tissue. The tricuspid valve annulus is greatly dilated. In contrast, no lesions are noted in the left ventricular free wall or in the ventricular septum. This patient was 70 years of age at the time of the OHT. ARVC was diagnosed clinically and the patient was found to have the nonsense mutation PKP2 c.235 C ->T (p.Arg79*), one of the mutations specific for ARVC. The same mutation was found in the patient's son and grandson, but neither had signs or symptoms of ARVC. The total nonpaced 12-lead QRS voltage was 52 mm, and the heart, which floated in formaldehyde, weighed only 285 g.

1. Roberts WC, Ko JM, Kuiper JJ, Hall SA, Meyer DM. Some previously neglected examples of arrhythmic right ventricular dysplasia/cardiomyopathy and frequency of its various reported manifestations. *Am J Cardiol* 2010;106:268–2074.
2. Marcus FI, Fontaine GH, Guiraudon G, Frank R, Laurenceau JL, Malergue C, Grosgogeat Y. Right ventricular dysplasia: a report of 24 adult cases. *Circulation* 1982;65:384–398.
3. Blomström-Lundqvist C, Sabel KG, Olsson SB. A long-term follow-up of 15 patients with arrhythmogenic right ventricular dysplasia. *Br Heart J* 1987;58:477–488.
4. Lemery R, Brugada P, Janssen J, Cheriex E, Dugernier T, Wellens HJ. Nonischemic sustained ventricular tachycardia: clinical outcome in 12 patients with arrhythmogenic right ventricular dysplasia. *J Am Coll Cardiol* 1989;14:96–105.
5. Pinamonti B, Sinagra G, Salvi A, Di Lenarda A, Morgera T, Silvestri F, Bussani R, Camerini F. Left ventricular involvement in right ventricular dysplasia. *Am Heart J* 1992;12:711–724.
6. Corrado D, Basso C, Thiene G, McKenna WJ, Davies MJ, Fontaliran F, Nava A, Silvestri F, Blomstrom-Lundqvist C, Wlodarska EK, Fontaine G, Camerini F. Spectrum of clinicopathologic manifestations of arrhythmogenic right ventricular cardiomyopathy/dysplasia: a multicenter study. *J Am Coll Cardiol* 1997;30:1512–1520.
7. Hulot JS, Jouven X, Empana JP, Frank R, Fontaine G. Natural history and risk stratification of arrhythmogenic right ventricular dysplasia/cardiomyopathy. *Circulation* 2004;110:1879–1884.
8. Dalal D, Nasir K, Bomma C, Prakasa K, Tandri H, Piccini J, Roguin A, Tichnell C, James C, Russell SD, Judge DP, Abraham T, Spevak PJ, Bluemke DA, Calkins H. Arrhythmogenic right ventricular dysplasia: a United States experience. *Circulation* 2005;112:3823–3832.
9. Marcus FI, Zareba W. The electrocardiogram in right ventricular cardiomyopathy/dysplasia. How can the electrocardiogram assist in understanding the pathologic and functional changes of the heart in this disease? *J Electrocardiol* 2009;42. 136.e1-136.e5.
10. Marcus FI, McKenna WJ, Sherrill D, Basso C, Bauce B, Bluemke DA, Calkins H, Corrado D, Cox MG, Daubert JP, Fontaine G, Gear K, Hauer R, Nava A, Picard MH, Protonotarios N, Saffitz JE, Sanborn DM, Steinberg JS, Tandri H, Thiene G, Towbin JA, Tsatsopoulou A, Wichter T, Zareba W. Diagnosis of arrhythmogenic right ventricular cardiomyopathy/dysplasia: proposed modification of the task force criteria. *Circulation* 2010;121:1533–1541.
11. Hauer RN, Cox MG, Groeneweg JA. Impact of new electrocardiographic criteria in arrhythmogenic cardiomyopathy. *Front Physiol* 2012;3:352.
12. Mast TP, James CA, Calkins H, Teske AJ, Tichnell C, Murray B, Loh P1, Russell SD, Velthuis BK, Judge DP, Dooijes D, Tedford RJ, van der Heijden JF, Tandri H, Hauer RN, Abraham TP, Doevendans PA, Te Riele AS, Cramer MJ. Evaluation of structural progression in arrhythmogenic right ventricular dysplasia/cardiomyopathy. *JAMA Cardiol* 2017;2:293–302.
13. Corrado D, Link MS, Calkins H. Arrhythmogenic right ventricular cardiomyopathy. *N Engl J Med* 2017;376:61–72.
14. Roberts WC, Podolak MJ. The king of hearts: analysis of 23 patients with hearts weighing 1000 grams or more. *Am J Cardiol* 1985;55:485–494.
15. Siegel RJ, Roberts WC. Electrocardiographic observations in severe aortic valve stenosis: correlative necropsy study to clinical, hemodynamic, and ECG variables demonstrating relation of 12-lead QRS amplitude to peak systolic transaortic pressure gradient. *Am Heart J* 1982;103:210–221.
16. Roberts WC, Day PJ. Electrocardiographic observations in clinically isolated, pure, chronic, severe aortic regurgitation: analysis of 30 necropsy patients aged 19 to 65 years. *Am J Cardiol* 1985;55:432–438.
17. Glick BN, Roberts WC. Usefulness of total 12-lead QRS voltage in diagnosing left ventricular hypertrophy in clinically isolated, pure, chronic, severe mitral regurgitation. *Am J Cardiol* 1992;70:1088–1092.
18. Dollar AL, Roberts WC. Usefulness of total 12-lead QRS voltage compared with other criteria for determining left ventricular hypertrophy in hypertrophic cardiomyopathy: analysis of 57 patients studied at necropsy. *Am J Med* 1989;87:377–381.
19. Shirani J, Maron BJ, Cannon RO III, Sheyda S, Roberts WC. Clinicopathologic features of hypertrophic cardiomyopathy managed by cardiac transplantation. *Am J Cardiol* 1993;72:434–440.

20. Roberts WC, Siegel RJ, McManus BM. Idiopathic dilated cardiomyopathy: analysis of 152 necropsy patients. *Am J Cardiol* 1987;60:1340–1355.
21. Shirani J, Roberts WC. Clinical electrocardiographic and morphologic features of massive fatty deposits ("lipomatous hypertrophy") in the atrial septum. *J Am Coll Cardiol* 1993;22:226–238.
22. Ross EM, Roberts WC. The carcinoid syndrome: comparison of 21 necropsy subjects with carcinoid heart disease to 15 necropsy subjects without carcinoid heart disease. *Am J Med* 1985;79:339–354.
23. Roberts WC, Barbin CM, Weissenborn MR, Ko JM. Electrocardiographic total 12-lead QRS voltage in patients having operative resection of syphilitic aortic aneurysm. *Am J Cardiol* 2015;116:973–976.
24. Shirani J, Berezowski K, Roberts WC. Quantitative measurement of normal and excessive (cor adiposum) subepicardial adipose tissue, its clinical significance, and its effect on electrocardiographic QRS voltage. *Am J Cardiol* 1995;76:414–418.
25. Roberts WC, Waller BF. Cardiac amyloidosis causing cardiac dysfunction: analysis of 54 necropsy patients. *Am J Cardiol* 1983;52:137–146.
26. Roberts WC, Becker TM, Hall SA. Usefulness of total 12-lead QRS voltage as a clue to diagnosis of patients with cardiac sarcoidosis severe enough to warrant orthotopic heart transplant. *JAMA Cardiol* 2018;3:64–68.
27. Wilensky RL, Yudelman P, Cohen AI, Fletcher RD, Atkinson J, Virmani R, Roberts WC. Serial electrocardiographic changes in idiopathic dilated cardiomyopathy confirmed at necropsy. *Am J Cardiol* 1988;62:276–283.

Total 12-Lead QRS Voltage in Patients Having Orthotopic Heart Transplantation for Heart Failure Caused by Adriamycin-Induced Cardiomyopathy

William C. Roberts[a, b] Sarah Haque[c] Shelley A. Hall[b]

[a]Baylor Scott and White Heart and Vascular Institute, Baylor University Medical Center, Dallas, TX, USA; [b]Division of Cardiology, Departments of Pathology and Internal Medicine, Baylor University Medical Center, Dallas, TX, USA; [c]Austin College, Sherman, TX, USA

Keywords

Adriamycin cardiomyopathy · Cardiotoxicity · Orthotopic heart transplantation

Abstract

Objective: Although several studies have described the effects of adriamycin on the heart, electrocardiographic total 12-lead QRS voltage (distance in millimeters from the peak of the R wave to the nadir of either the Q or S wave, whichever was deeper, with 10 mm [1 mV] being standard) both before and after orthotopic heart transplantation (OHT) has not been reported. This study describes the total 12-lead QRS voltage in 8 patients studied at Baylor University Medical Center at Dallas, from 1994 to June 2018, who underwent OHT for severe heart failure caused by anthracycline-induced cardiomyopathy. ***Method:*** Prior to OHT, the total 12-lead non-paced QRS voltages ranged from 86 to 189 mm (mean 125 ± 56) and for paced QRS voltages from 82 to 113 mm (mean 97 ± 15). The total 12-lead QRS voltages post-OHT ranged from 100 to 190 mm (mean 130 ± 30). Total 12-lead QRS voltages were lower in patients with a pacemaker than without. ***Results/Conclusion:*** These low voltages are like those found in patients with carcinoid syndrome, severe cardiac adiposity, cardiac amyloidosis, and cardiac sarcoidosis.

Introduction

Orthotopic heart transplantation (OHT) has proven to be a useful therapy for patients with heart failure (HF) secondary to adriamycin cardiotoxicity [1]. Little electrocardiographic data are available in patients with HF secondary to adriamycin toxicity severe enough to warrant OHT. To fill this void, we measured the total 12-lead QRS voltage in 8 patients who underwent OHT for severe HF secondary to adriamycin cardiotoxicity.

Materials and Methods

Review of all OHT cases performed at Baylor University Medical Center at Dallas from 1994 through June 2018, a 24-year period, yielded 8 patients who had received anthracycline therapy. The native hearts for all 8 patients were examined and described by one of us (W.C.R.). The clinical records and all available electrocardiograms recorded between the onset of HF and OTH for each patient were reviewed. The total 12-lead QRS voltage was measured by S.H. and confirmed by W.C.R.

Results

The pertinent clinical, electrocardiographic, and morphologic findings are summarized in Table 1. Three patients had non-Hodgkin lymphoma, 3 had breast cancer, and 2 had leukemia. At the time of cancer diagnosis and treatment, the patients ranged in age from 6 to 64 years (mean 36 ± 20),

Table 1. Pertinent clinical and morphological findings in 8 patients with adriamycin-induced cardiomyopathy

Case No.	Age at cancer Dx and Rx, years	Age at OHT, years	Year of OHT	Type of cancer	Rad Rx	Height, in	Body weight, lb	BMI	EF, %	Paced	QRS amplitude in each electrocardiographic lead												Total 12-lead QRS voltage, mm	HW, g	Floating heart	Alive in 6/2018	Intervals, days	
											I	II	III	aVR	aVL	aVF	V1	V2	V3	V4	V5	V6					P or NP ECG to OHT	OHT to PHT ECG
Men																												
1	8	26	4/2015	Leukemia	no	70	183	26	10	NP	11	7	10	7	9	9	20	36	24	15	19	22						
										PHT	12	9	13	8	11	9	6	13	14	8	9	9	121					
2	6	30	9/2008	Leukemia	no	71	185	27	15	P	2	5	5	2	5	4	11	14	18	6	5	5	82	365	no	no	109	14
										PHT	7	7	7	6	6	5	16	35	49	32	12	8	190					
3	50	55	5/2011	Lymphoma[1]	no	68	220	33	15	P	4	12	10	5	5	8	5	5	5	7	10	8	84	525	yes	yes	46	135
										PHT	11	7	5	9	8	3	9	16	15	16	15	10	124					
Women																												
4	30	37	5/2017	Lymphoma[1]	yes	62	180	33	15	NP	4	7	12	4	8	10	9	14	10	8	7	6	99	260	yes	yes	252	32
										PHT	9	1	9	5	10	5	8	23	7	8	8	7	100					
5	38	50	5/2007	Breast	yes	64	180	31	10	NP	5	3	5	2	4	4	5	9	18	12	11	8	86	405	yes	yes	16	27
										PHT	12	5	11	7	11	4	8	9	10	10	12	10	109					
6	41	64	5/2004	Breast	yes	63	135	24	10	P	7	6	7	6	6	6	5	2	28	18	11	9	111	325	no	no	47	14
										PHT	9	10	8	10	6	6	9	20	24	21	17	11	151					
7	49	65	3/2011	Lymphoma[1]	yes	61	146	28	–	P	8	10	16	8	4	16	6	6	13	5	14	7	113	560	yes	yes	74	184
										PHT	12	8	11	10	14	6	8	7	8	8	9	12	113					
8	64	68	9/2011	Breast	no	64	155	27	15	P	4	5	8	2	6	5	3	5	20	18	11	8	95	500	yes	yes	98	14
										PHT	10	5	7	7	9	3	5	14	18	23	20	14	135					

AF, atrial fibrillation; BMI, body mass index; CI, cardiac index; Dx, diagnosis; ECG, electrocardiogram; EF, ejection fraction; HW, heart weight; LV, left ventricular; NP, non-paced; OHT, orthotopic heart transplant; P, paced; PHT, post-OHT; Rad, radiation; Rx, treatment; –, no information available. [1] Non-Hodgkin lymphoma.

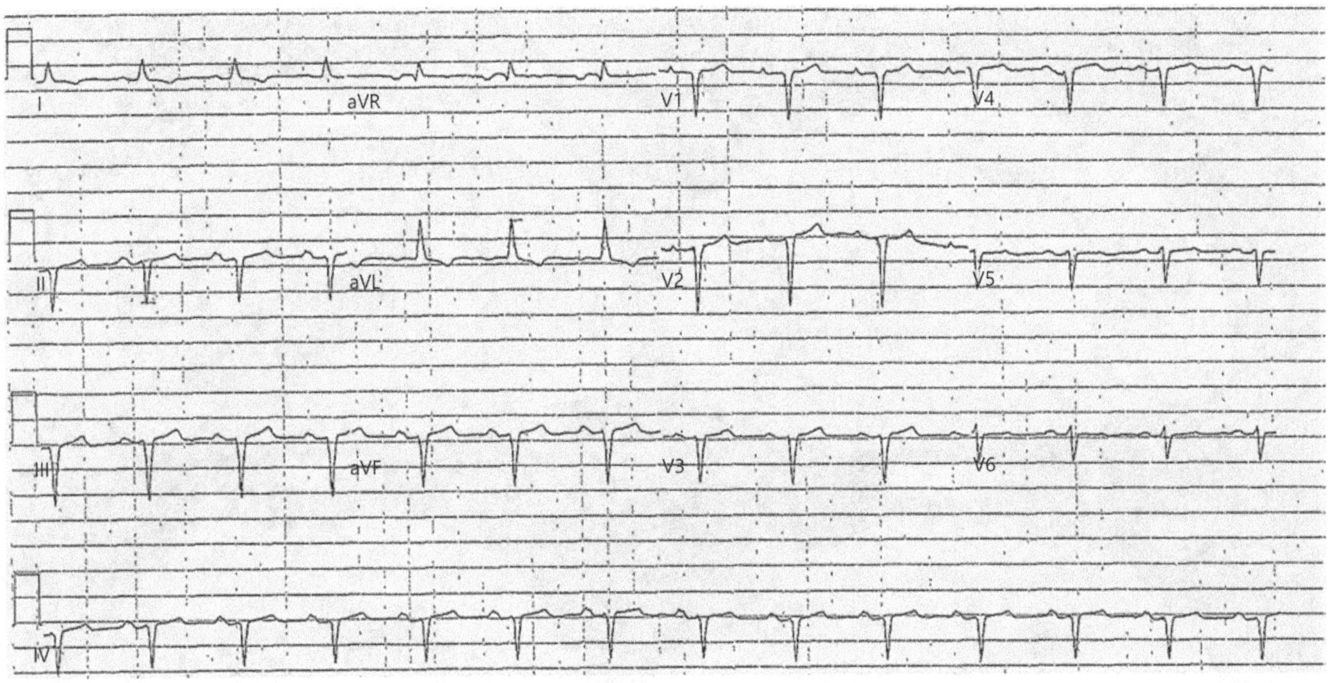

Fig. 1. Case No. 4. Pre-OHT non-paced electrocardiogram. The total 12-lead QRS voltage was 99 mm.

and at OHT from 26 to 68 years (mean 49 ± 17). The interval from the start of anthracycline treatment to OHT ranged from 4 to 24 years (mean 14 ± 8). Of the 8 patients, 3 were men and 5 were women. The body mass index ranged from 24 to 33 (mean 29 ± 3). The heart weights ranged from 260 to 558 g (mean 414 ± 105). Four patients were known to have received mediastinal irradiation at some point during chemotherapy. Adriamycin-induced cardiomyopathy was diagnosed prior to OHT in all 8 patients.

We obtained 3 non-paced and 5 paced pre-OHT electrocardiographic tracings and all 8 post-transplant tracings (Fig. 1). The total 12-lead QRS voltages prior to OHT ranged from 82 to 189 mm (mean 107 ± 49). Tracings for pre-OHT non-paced patients ranged from 86 to 189 mm (mean 125 ± 56), while pre-OHT paced voltages ranged from 82 to 113 mm (mean 97 ± 15). The total 12-lead QRS voltage post-OHT ranged from 100 to 190 mm (mean 130 ± 30). The basal portions of the cardiac ventricles in 4 of the 8 patients are shown in Figure 2.

Discussion and Conclusion

Described herein are total 12-lead electrographic QRS voltages and characteristics of the native hearts of 8 patients who underwent OHT for HF caused by adriamycin-induced cardiomyopathy. The total paced and non-paced (means 97 ± 15 and 125 ± 56 mm, respectively) 12-lead QRS voltages seen in these 8 patients are similar to those found in carcinoid syndrome (mean 117 mm), cardiac adiposity (mean 120 mm), cardiac amyloidosis (mean 104 mm), and cardiac sarcoidosis (mean 117 mm) [2]. The native hearts had no grossly visible myocardial lesions in any of the 8 patients [3, 4].

A positive feature of this report is that it is the first to describe total 12-lead electrocardiographic QRS voltages in patients with HF secondary to adriamycin-induced cardiomyopathy severe enough to warrant OHT. A limitation of the present report is the small number of patients studied and particularly the small number of electrocardiograms available before pacemaker insertion. Also, the amount of adriamycin administered years before the OHT is not known.

Acknowledgements

We thank Saba Ilyas for her excellent photographic work.

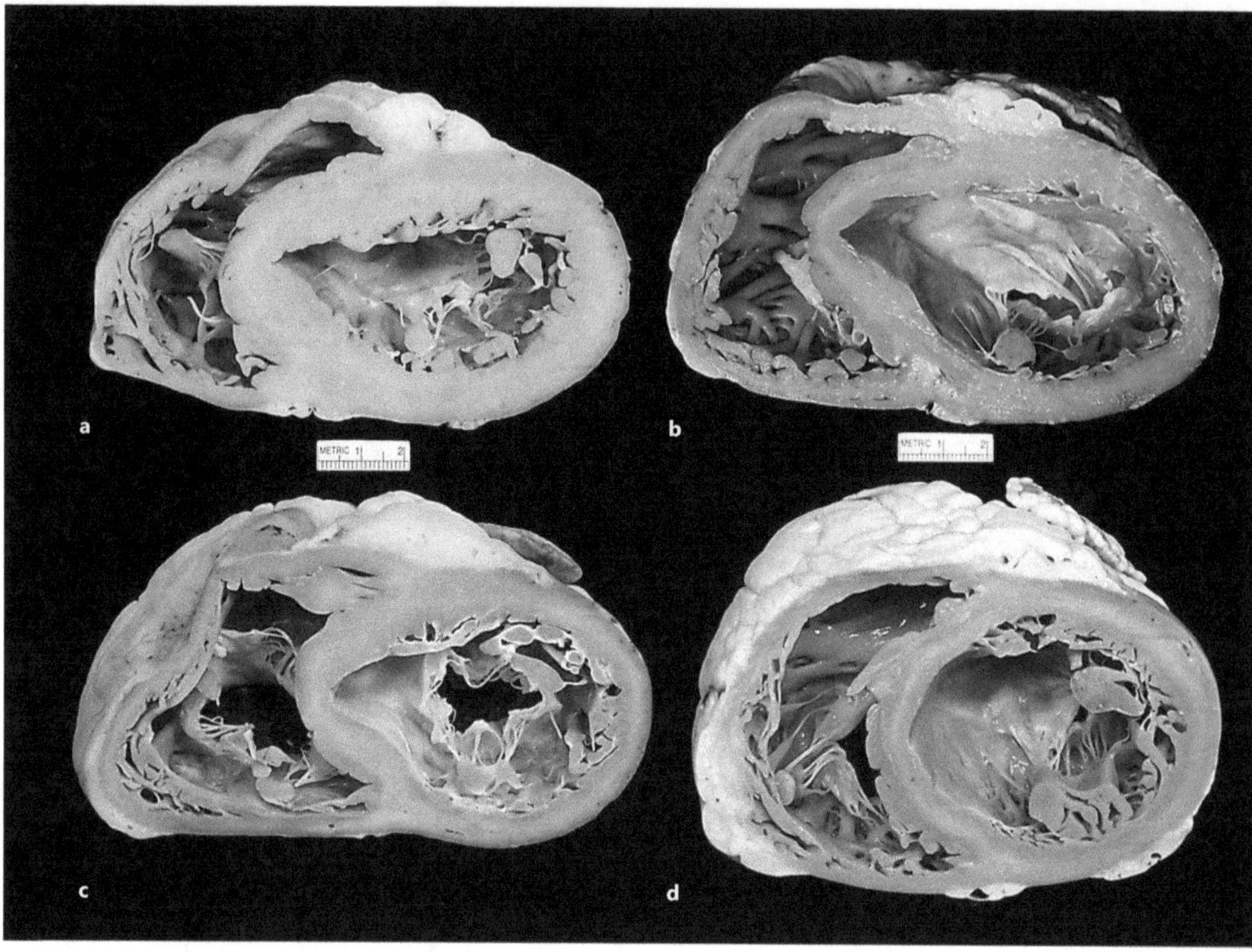

Color version available online

Fig. 2. Views of the basal portion of the ventricles in 4 patients having OHT for adriamycin cardiotoxicity. **a** Case No. 1. The total non-paced 12-lead QRS voltage prior to OHT was 189 mm and the heart weighed 370 g. **b** Case No. 2. The total non-paced 12-lead QRS voltage prior to OHT was 82 mm and the heart weighed 365 g. **c** Case No. 4. The total non-paced 12-lead QRS voltage prior to OHT was 99 mm and the heart weighed 260 g. **d** Case No. 5. The total non-paced 12-lead QRS voltage prior to OHT was 86 mm and the heart weighed 405 g.

Statement of Ethics

The authors have no ethical conflicts to disclose.

Disclosure Statement

The authors have no conflicts of interest to declare.

References

1 Lenneman AJ, Wang L, Wigger M, Frangoul H, Harrell FE, Silverstein C, et al. Heart transplant survival outcomes for adriamycin-dilated cardiomyopathy. Am J Cardiol. 2013 Feb; 111(4):609–12.

2 Roberts WC, Filardo G, Ko JM, Siegel RJ, Dollar AL, Ross EM, et al. Comparison of total 12-lead QRS voltage in a variety of cardiac conditions and its usefulness in predicting increased cardiac mass. Am J Cardiol. 2013 Sep; 112(6):904–9.

3 Lefrak EA, Pitha J, Rosenheim S, Gottlieb JA. A clinicopathologic analysis of adriamycin cardiotoxicity. Cancer. 1973 Aug;32(2):302–14.

4 Isner JM, Ferrans VJ, Cohen SR, Witkind BG, Virmani R, Gottdiener JS, et al. Clinical and morphologic cardiac findings after anthracycline chemotherapy. Analysis of 64 patients studied at necropsy. Am J Cardiol. 1983 Apr; 51(7):1167–74.

Comparison of Clinical and Morphologic Findings in Patients With Cardiac Sarcoidosis Severe Enough to Warrant Heart Transplantation in Those With -vs- Those Without Non-Caseating Granulomas in the Explanted Heart (Burnt-Out Sarcoid)

Samreen Fathima, MBBS[a,b], and William C. Roberts, MD[a,b,*]

Can cardiac sarcoidosis with heart failure severe enough to warrant orthotopic heart transplantation (OHT) be present without non-caseating granulomas in the explanted heart? The objective is to compare clinical and morphological features in patients with cardiac sarcoidosis severe enough to warrant OHT with -vs-without non-caseating granulomas in the explanted heart. The study was conducted at Baylor University Medical Center in Dallas, Texas. From a total of 671 explanted hearts examined from 1993 to 2018, twenty-five (4%) had gross morphologic features characteristic of cardiac sarcoidosis. At the time of OHT, the patients ranged in age from 50 to 69 years [mean 57]. Cardiac sarcoidosis was diagnosed before OHT in 3 (12%) patients, by percutaneous biopsy of the heart in 2 patients and by histologic examination of the "left ventricular core" in 1 patient who had a left ventricular assist device inserted, and, by examination of the native heart after OHT in the remaining 22 (88%) patients. Of the 25 patients, 16 (64%) had typical sarcoid non-caseating granulomas in the explanted heart, and 9 (36%) had no granulomas in the explanted heart. Comparison of certain clinical and morphologic features in the group with -vs- the group without cardiac granulomas showed no significant differences. In conclusion, of patients with cardiac sarcoidosis severe enough to warrant OHT, some have typical non-caseating granulomas in the explanted heart and some do not. The clinical and gross morphologic features of those with and those without cardiac granulomas are similar. **(Am J Cardiol 2019;124:599−603)**

Sarcoidosis has usually been defined by the presence of non-caseating granulomas containing multinucleated giant cells, epithelioid cells and lymphocytes in one or more body organs. When sarcoidosis attacks an organ, scar tissue develops in the areas of the granulomas and eventually it appears that the scar tissue can obliterate all evidence of previous inflammation, including the giant cells. This scenario appears to occur in cardiac sarcoidosis. Herein, we describe certain clinical and cardiac morphologic findings in 25 patients who had orthotopic heart transplant (OHT) for what proved to be cardiac sarcoidosis. We compared clinical and morphologic features of the cases with to those without non-caseating granulomas in the explanted hearts.

Methods

Since March 1993 one of us (WCR) has examined all specimens excised by cardiac surgeons at Baylor University Medical Center (BUMC) and submitted the report on each. From March 1993 through December 2018, we examined 671 native hearts excised at the time of OHT at BUMC. All hearts were opened and sections made by WCR. The weights of the hearts were all done by the same investigator after opening the chambers, removing any excess tissue (parietal pericardium for example), and incising the aorta and pulmonary trunk about 2 cm cephalad to the sino-tubular junction. The hearts were weighed within one week after their fixation in formaldehyde. Photographs were prepared on virtually all the explanted hearts, all of which have been retained. Of these 671 native hearts examined since 1993, twenty-five (4%) had gross morphologic features characteristic of cardiac sarcoidosis. Histologic sections were prepared in each heart, and stained by both hematoxylin/eosin and trichrome. At least 5 sections of myocardium were prepared in each case: 4 from the ventricles and 1 from the atria. All sections were examined by WCR. Photomicrographs were prepared from many of the cases. After examination of the heart and before submitting the final pathology report, the medical records in each case were examined.

Results

Of the 25 cases, 16 (64%) had typical sarcoid non-caseating granulomas in the explanted heart, and 9 (36%) had no granulomas in the explanted heart. Comparison of

[a]Division of Cardiology, Departments of Internal Medicine, Baylor Scott & White Heart and Vascular Institute, Baylor University Medical Center, Baylor Scott & White Health, Dallas, Texas; and [b]Department of Pathology, Baylor Scott & White Heart and Vascular Institute, Baylor University Medical Center, Baylor Scott & White Health, Dallas, Texas. Manuscript received April 19, 2019; revised manuscript received and accepted May 7, 2019.

*Corresponding author: Tel: (214) 820-7911.

E-mail address: William.Roberts1@bswhealth.org (W.C. Roberts).

certain clinical and gross morphologic features in the group with -vs- the group without cardiac granulomas showed no significant differences (Table 1). Pertinent data in each of the 25 patients is tabulated in Table 2. Three patients (cases #2, #11 and #18 Table 2) had left ventricular assist devices inserted before OHT and all 3 had granulomas in the excised "left ventricular core", including one (case #18, Table 2) who did not have granulomas in the explanted heart. Of the 9 patients without granulomas in the explanted heart, 3 previously had morphologic proof of cardiac sarcoidosis (2 by percutaneous biopsies of the heart [cases #19 and #22, Table 2] and one by examination of the portion of left ventricular free wall excised to insert a left ventricular assist device [case #18, Table 2].) Each of these 3 patients in whom cardiac sarcoidosis was proven by tissue examination before OHT were treated with corticosteroid therapy (cases #18, #19, and #22, Table 2). Additionally, two of the remaining 22 patients in whom the diagnosis of cardiac sarcoidosis was not proven before OHT also were treated with corticosteroid drugs because of biopsy proved pulmonary sarcoidosis (Cases #2 and #24, Table 2). Two patients (case #4 and #7, Table 2) had significant coronary narrowing, one (case #4, Table 2) of whom had coronary artery bypass grafting. Electrocardiographic features before OHT in each of the 25 patients are tabulated in table 3.

Table 1
Comparison in patients with clinical and morphologic findings of cardiac sarcoidosis severe enough to warrant heart transplantation in those with -vs- those without non-caseating granulomas in the explanted heart

Variable	Total (n = 25)	Cardiac granulomas		p Value
		No (n = 9)	Yes (n = 16)	
Age (years)	57 ± 6	56 ± 9	57 ± 5	0.81
Men	13 (52%)	6 (67%)	7 (44%)	0.41
Women	12 (48%)	3 (33%)	9 (56%)	
White	19 (76%)	6 (67%)	13 (81%)	0.63
Black	6 (24%)	3 (33%)	3 (19%)	
Duration (months), symptoms	72 ± 53	76 ± 65	70 ± 48	0.79
Atrial arrhythmias	7 (28%)	4 (44%)	3 (20%)	0.36
Ventricular arrhythmias	8 (32%)	1 (11%)	7 (47%)	0.18
Bundle branch block				0.28
Left	4 (16%)	1 (11%)	3 (19%)	
Right	10 (40%)	3 (33%)	7 (44%)	
Indeterminate	3 (12%)	0	3 (19%)	
Total 12-lead QRS Voltage (mm)	88 ± 36	99 ± 20	82 ± 41	0.30
Total cholesterol (mg/dl)	150 ± 42	160 ± 47	145 ± 40	0.44
LDL cholesterol (mg/dl)	90 ± 29	96 ± 27	87 ± 30	0.48
Body mass index (Kg/m^2)	28 ± 5	29 ± 7	28 ± 3	0.70
Prior LVAD	3 (12%)	2 (22%)	1 (6%)	0.60
Corticosteroid therapy	5 (24%)	4 (44%)	1 (6%)	0.097
Heart weight (g)				
Men	490 ± 58	491 ± 80	492 ± 51	0.91
Women	423 ± 86	438 ± 141	418 ± 71	0.75
Floating heart	12 (48%)	4 (44%)	8 (53%)	1.00

LDL = low density lipoprotein; LVAD =left ventricular assist device.

Discussion

The present report describes 25 patients who underwent OHT because of chronic severe heart failure resulting from cardiac sarcoidosis: 16 of the patients had classic non-caseating granulomas in the operatively-excised native hearts and 9 had no granulomas in the explanted hearts, although 3 of them had typical granulomas in percutaneous biopsies of heart or in the "left ventricular core" excised at the time of insertion of left ventricular assist device. Comparison of various clinical and gross morphologic features of the 16 patients with granulomas in the explanted hearts to the 9 patients without disclosed no significant differences.

Typical gross and histologic features of cardiac sarcoidosis severe enough to warrant OHT include focal but extensive scars in the walls of both left and right ventricles and ventricular septum.[1–8] Scars in the atrial walls are infrequent.[5] The focal scars in the right ventricular wall are usually transmural; those involving the left ventricular wall may also be transmural but often they are only subepicardial, the opposite of what occurs in hearts of patients with coronary heart disease, which is subendocardial or transmural or both but not subepicardial.[9] The ventricular walls are more often thinner than normal rather than thicker than normal. The ventricular cavities are severely dilated (unless a left ventricular assist device had been inserted earlier). Histologically, the non-caseating granulomas are typically located within the scars and numerous ones are present in some scars. In most patients some ventricular wall scars contain granulomas and others do not. The numbers of nuclei present in the giant cells may exceed 50. Lymphocytes also are present.

How can we be certain that the 9 patients without non-caseating granulomas in the explanted hearts have cardiac sarcoidosis? In 3 of these 9 patients an earlier percutaneous biopsy (in 2) or examination of the portion of left ventricular wall excised to insert a left ventricular assist device (in 1) did indeed contain non-caseating granulomas. The interval from this tissue examination to the OHT in these 3 patients was 0.1, 7, and 53 months, respectively. Another supporting factor was that many of the ventricular wall scars in the 16 patients with granulomas present in the explanted heart also had ventricular-wall scars without any granulomas. The latter observation suggests it would not be a "stretch" for all the scars to eventually be devoid of granulomas. Three of the 9 patients without granulomas in the explanted hearts were treated with cortico-steroid therapy, a known cause of converting non-caseating granulomas into scars without granulomas.[1] (Each of the 3 patients in whom the diagnosis was made by examination of cardiac tissue some time before the OHT were treated with prednisone.)

The positive features of this report are the following: (1) no previous report has emphasized that cardiac sarcoidosis may be present without non-caseating granulomas being present in the heart. (2) No previous study has compared clinical and gross morphologic findings in the patients with to those without non-caseating granulomas in the heart.

Limitations of the present study include the following: (1) perhaps not enough histologic sections of myocardium were studied. (We examined at least 4 large

Table 2
Pertinent clinical and morphological findings in 25 patients who had orthotopic heart transplantation for cardiac sarcoidosis

Case	Age (years)	Sex	Race	Duration of symptoms before OHT (months)	BMI (Kg/m^2)	TC (mg/dl)	LDL (mg/dl)	CI $(l/min/m^2)$	P-Rx	Clinical cardiac diagnosis	ICD	HW (g)	Heart floats	G	Location of granulomas		
															RV	VS	LV
1	50	F	B	132	25	124	74	–	0	IDC	+	440	0	+	1+	3+	3+
2	52	M	W	192	28	172	108	1.6	+	IDC*	0	440	0	+	1+	2+	1+
3	52	F	B	50	31	166	64	2.3	0	IDC	+	440	0	+	1+	3+	3+
4	53	M	W	12	27	188	112	1.6	0	IDC	0	555	+	+	3+	3+	3+
5	54	F	W	46	26	74	46	1.8	0	IDC	0	425	0	+	3+	3+	3+
6	54	M	W	108	30	210	134	-	0	IDC	0	511	-	+	3+	3+	3+
7	56	F	W	11	26	143	118	–	0	IDC	0	450	+	+	1+	3+	3+
8	57	F	W	46	30	138	94	1.4	0	IDC	0	380	0	+	3+	3+	3+
9	58	F	W	60	27	229	147	2.2	0	IDC	+	560	+	+	3+	3+	3+
10	58	M	W	48	25	114	64	1.2	0	IDC	0	420	0	+	3+	3+	3+
11	59	F	B	72	26	134	69	1.3	0	IDC	+	370	0	+	1+	2+	1+
12	60	F	W	36	28	130	93	1.2	0	IDC	0	401	+	+	1+	3+	3+
13	61	F	W	120	25	119	60	1.2	0	IDC	0	300	+	+	3+	3+	3+
14	63	M	W	84	33	109	52	1.6	0	IDC	+	470	+	+	3+	3+	3+
15	63	M	W	48	24	157	86	1.7	0	IDC	0	540	+	+	3+	3+	3+
16	67	M	W	48	30	116	70	1.6	0	IDC	0	510	+	+	3+	3+	3+
17	40	F	W	11	45	107	78	1.4	0	IDC	0	370	0	0	0	0	0
18	50	M	W	36	28	185	119	1.7	+	CS	+	605	0	0	0	0	0
19	53	M	W	60	31	233	120	1.9	+	CS	0	535	0	0	0	0	0
20	54	F	B	100	24	191	108	1.8	0	IDC	0	345	0	0	0	0	0
21	57	M	W	36	30	119	82	1.2	0	IDC	0	420	+	0	0	0	0
22	59	M	W	48	28	–	–	–	+	CS	+	420	+	0	0	0	0
23	62	F	B	216	19	182	129	1.5	0	IDC	+	600	0	0	0	0	0
24	65	M	B	139	29	160	82	–	+	IDC	+	475	+	0	0	0	0
25	69	M	W	36	23	101	50	1.3	0	IDC	0	475	+	0	0	0	0

AB = black; BMI = body mass index; CI = cardiac index; CS = cardiac sarcoidosis; F = female; G = granuloma; HW = heart weight; I = indirect; ICD = intracardiac defibrillator; IDC = ischemic dilated cardiomyopathy; L = left; LDL = low-density lipoprotein; LV = left ventricle; M = male; OHT = orthotopic heart transplant; P = prednisone Rx; R = right; RV = right ventricle; TC = total cholesterol; VS = ventricular septum; W = white.

* Because the patient had biopsy-proven pulmonary sarcoid, the patient clinically was considered to have cardiac sarcoid as well, but a cardiac biopsy done before the OHT was negative for sarcoid.

Table 3
Electrocardiographic findings before orthotopic heart transplantation in 25 patients with cardiac sarcoidosis

Case	Paced	QRS amplitude in each electrocardiographic lead (mm)												Total 12-lead QRS voltage (mm)	Arrhythmias		BBB (Type)	CHB	Prolonged QT Interval
		I	II	III	aVR	aVL	aVF	V1	V2	V3	V4	V5	V6		A (Type)	V (Type)			
	0	0	0	0	0	0	0	0	0	0	0	0	0	0	0	0			
1	+	2	23	13	6	7	28	4	12	16	20	18	12	161	0	0	+ (NS)	+	0
2	0	14	12	8	13	11	7	12	8	8	18	22	22	155	0	0	+ (R)	0	0
3	+	5	5	5	5	2	8	6	7	7	5	5	7	67	0	+ (VPC)	+ (L)	0	0
4	+	4	12	9	6	3	9	7	7	3	7	10	9	86	0	+ (VPC)	+ (R)	+	0
5	+	4	4	5	2	8	4	–	–	–	–	–	–	–	0	0	0	+	0
6	–	–	–	–	–	–	–	–	–	–	–	–	–	–	–	–	–	-	-
7	+	4	7	8	5	6	8	4	8	4	5	7	7	73	0	+ (VT)	0	0	0
8	0	5	1	6	3	6	4	5	9	5	4	2	2	52	+ (AT)	0	+ (R)	0	0
9	0	8	8	15	3	11	12	5	7	4	4	6	6	89	0	0			
	+	3	3	4	2	3	3	3	7	3	3	4	4	69	0	0	+ (R)	0	0
10	+	9	9	6	4	4	6	5	3	8	8	8	7	77	0	0	+ (L)	0	0
11	0	11	11	17	8	14	13	9	5	9	12	16	19	144	0	0			
	+	10	12	19	8	14	15	8	9	10	13	15	14	147	0	0	+ (R)	+	0
12	0	5	3	4	5	7	3	3	7	4	6	2	5	54	+ (AF)	+ (VPC)	0	0	0
13	+	4	4	5	3	6	4	4	10	5	7	7	8	72	0	0	+ (R)	+	+
14	+	5	12	8	8	5	10	8	9	14	10	9	5	103	0	+ (VPC)	+ (L)	+	0
15	0	8	6	3	6	6	4	9	10	13	18	22	29	134					
	+	5	8	11	5	6	11	2	4	12	17	11	3	95	+ (AF)	+ (VPC)	+ (R)	0	0
16	+	4	5	7	2	5	5	2	2	6	5	3	1	47	0	+ (VT)	+ (NS)	+	0
17	0	18	6	13	6	13	7	6	6	6	6	5	6	98	+ (APC)	+ (VPC)	0	0	0
18	0	7	11	14	5	9	12	6	14	19	7	10	7	121	+ (APC)	0	+ (L)	0	0
19	+	7	7	10	4	8	9	5	7	5	6	7	6	81	0	0	0	+	0
20	0	3	7	7	4	4	6	4	8	11	9	12	14	89	0	0	0	0	+
21	0	5	8	4	5	4	6	7	10	28	26	22	6	131	+ (APC)	0	+ (R)	0	+
22	0	4	1	5	4	3	4	–	–	–	–	–	–	–	0	0	0	0	0
23	0	10	11	10	7	7	7	10	9	7	9	10	10	107	0	0	+ (R)	0	0
24	0	5	7	5	6	4	5	5	4	5	7	10	11	74	+ (AF)	0	+ (R)	0	0
25	0	10	5	6	6	11	12	11	6	4	4	12	4	91	0	0	0	0	0

A = atrial; AF = atrial fibrillation; APC = atrial premature complexes; AT= atrial tachycardia; BBB = bundle branch block; CHB = complete heart block; L = left; NS = non-specific; R = right; V= ventricular; VPC = ventricular premature complexes; VT = ventricular tachycardia.

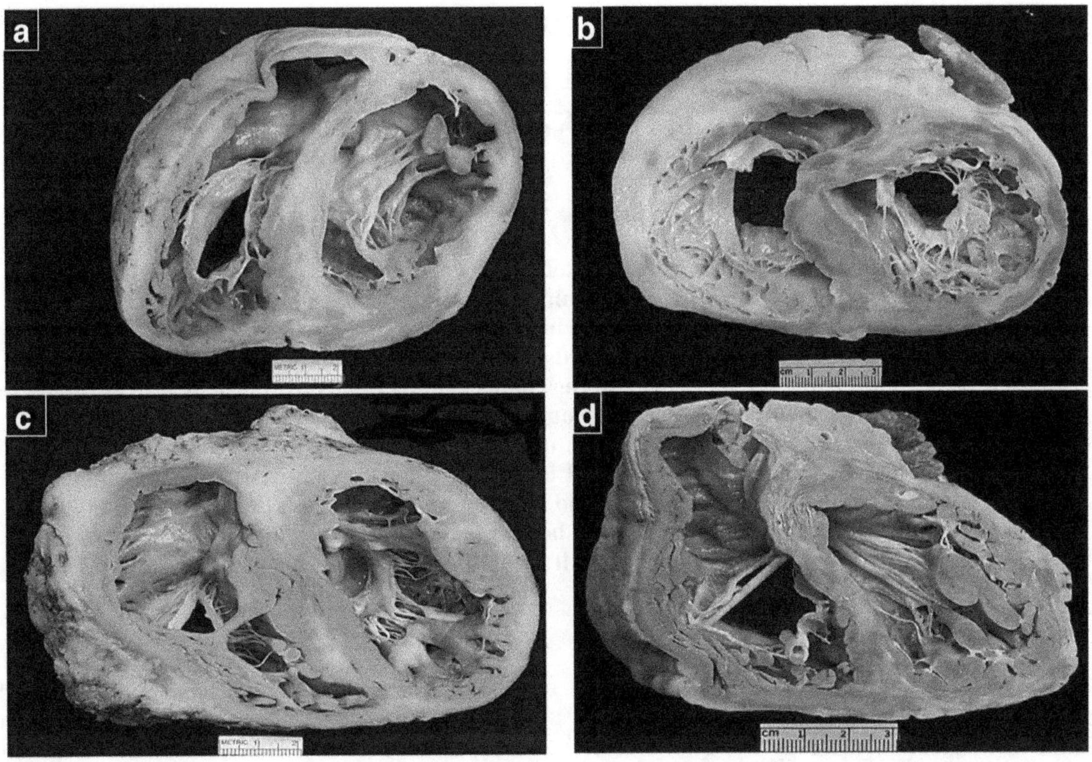

Figure 1. Shown here are basal portions of the heart in 4 patients, 2 of whom (*a* and *c*) had granulomas in the explanted heart and 2, (*b* and *d*) did not. (*a*) patient #5 (Table 2); (*b*) patient #23 (Table 2); (*c*) patient #12 (Table 2); *d*) patient #20 (Table 2). Both ventricles are dilated in each of these 4 patients. Portions of the tricuspid and mitral valves are visible in all 4 patients. The white areas of right ventricular free wall, ventricular septum and left ventricular free wall represent sites of scarring, some of which contained non-caseating granulomas and some of which did not.

[endocardium-to-epicardium] sections of the ventricular walls in all 25 patients and far more [up to 20] in a few patients.); (2) perhaps the 9 patients without tissue proof of cardiac sarcoidosis *in the explanted hearts*, namely the presence of non-caseating granulomas, did not have cardiac sarcoidosis. We believe this scenario to be highly unlikely because 3 of the 9 patients had earlier proof of cardiac sarcoidosis (biopsy or left ventricular "core" examination), and, additionally, we know of no other cardiac condition that even remotely resembles the full-blown morphologic features of cardiac sarcoidosis (Figures 1 and 2).

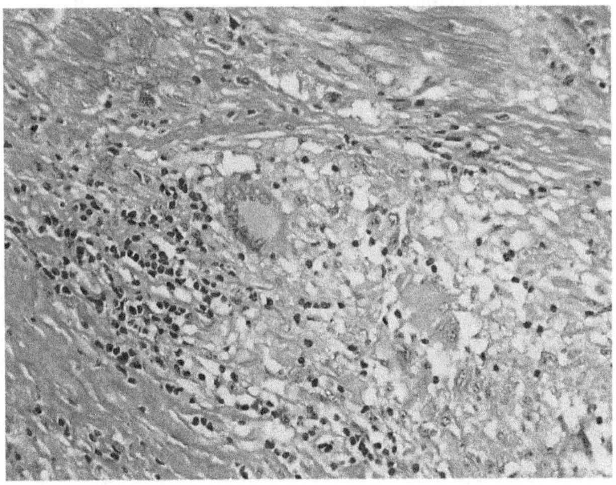

Figure 2. Photomicrograph of a portion of left ventricular free wall in patient #16 (Table 2). The myocardial wall is partially replaced by a dense fibrous tissue which stains blue within which is a sarcoid granuloma. Trichrome stain, original magnification × 40.

1. Roberts WC, McAllister HA Jr, Ferrans VJ. Sarcoidosis of the heart. A clinicopathologic study of 35 necropsy patients (Group I) and review of 78 previously described necropsy patients (Group II). *Am J Med* 1977;63:86–108.
2. Virmani R, Bures JC, Roberts WC. Cardiac sarcoidosis: a major cause of sudden death in young individuals. *Chest* 1980;77:423–428.
3. Donsky AS, Escobar J, Capehart J, Roberts WC. Heart transplantation for undiagnosed cardiac sarcoidosis. *Am J Cardiol* 2002;89:1447–1450.
4. Roberts WC, Vowels TJ, Ko JM, Capehart JE, Hall SA. Cardiac transplantation for cardiac sarcoidosis with initial diagnosis by examination of the left ventricular apical "core" excised for insertion of a left ventricular assist device for severe chronic heart failure. *Am J Cardiol* 2009;103:110–114.
5. Sharma PS, Lubahn JG, Donsky AS, Yoon ADH, Carry MM, Grayburn PA, Wood PB, Ko JM, Burton EC, Roberts WC. Diagnosing cardiac sarcoidosis clinically without tissue confirmation. *Proc (Bayl Univ Med Cent)* 2009;22:236–238.
6. Roberts WC, Chung MS, Ko JM, Capehart JE, Hall SA. Morphologic features of cardiac sarcoidosis in native hearts of patients having cardiac transplantation. *Am J Cardiol* 2014;113:706–712.
7. Armstrong D, Gonzalez-Stawinski GV, Ko JM, Hall SA, Roberts WC. The two extremes of cardiac sarcoidosis and the effect of prednisone therapy. *Am J Cardiol* 2015;115:150–153.
8. Roberts WC, Becker TM, Hall SA. Usefulness of total 12-lead QRS voltage as a clue to diagnosis of patients with cardiac sarcoidosis severe enough to warrant orthotopic heart transplant. *JAMA Cardiol* 2018;3:64–68.
9. Shirani J, Roberts WC. Subepicardial myocardial lesions. *Am Heart J* 1993;125:1346–1352.

Severe Eosinophilic Myocarditis in the Portion of Left Ventricular Wall Excised to Insert a Left Ventricular Assist Device for Severe Heart Failure

William C. Roberts, MD*, and Alexander T. Kietzman[1]

Described herein are 3 adults in whom histologic study of the left ventricular myocardium excised ("LV core") to insert a left ventricular assist device (LVAD) disclosed severe acute myocarditis and the inflammatory cells included numerous eosinophils (eosinophilic myocarditis). Examination of the clinical records disclosed elevated absolute eosinophil counts at the time of insertion of the LVAD and the counts rapidly (<30 days) returned to normal after the operation. Because of the numerous medications that each patient was taking at the time of LVAD insertion, identification of a specific initiating medication as its cause was not possible. Of the 3 patients, 2 had idiopathic-dilated cardiomyopathy and 1 had ischemic cardiomyopathy and each had had heart failure for years. The eosinophilic myocarditis in these 3 patients appears to have been transient and superimposed on the earlier cardiomyopathy. **(Am J Cardiol 2020;125:264−269)**

From 2002 to 2019 (July), a total of 425 portions of left ventricular-free wall were received in the surgical pathology unit of the department of pathology of Baylor University Medical Center after a left ventricular assist device (LVAD) had been inserted. Histologic study of the left ventricular "core" disclosed numerous inflammatory infiltrates, including numerous eosinophils in 3 (0.0072) of the 425 cases. This report describes certain clinical and morphologic findings in these 3 patients.

Case Description

Pertinent clinical and morphologic findings in the 3 patients are summarized in Table 1 and illustrated in Figures 1−8. Before insertion of the LVAD, each patient had evidence of severe heart failure for years, and it was the reason for LVAD insertion. Idiopathic-dilated cardiomyopathy had been diagnosed as its cause in 2 and ischemic cardiomyopathy in 1. The absolute eosinophil counts (2 patients) roughly 30 days before and roughly 30 days after insertion of the LVAD shown in Figures 2 and 5. The highest percent of peripheral eosinophils (2 patients) just before LVAD insertion was 6% in case #1 and 9% in case #2. Following insertion of the LVAD, the absolute eosinophil count fell to normal in both patients within 25 days. The electrocardiograms just before LVAD insertion are shown in Figures 1, 4, and 7. All 3 patients had sinus tachycardia; total 12-lead QRS voltage in all 3 cases was very low.[1]

Histologic examination of sections from the left ventricular "core" in all 3 patients showed numerous cells within the myocardium, including numerous eosinophils (Figures 3, 6, and 8). Patient #2 underwent heart transplantation 57 months after the LVAD insertion. In contrast to the findings in the LV "core," no inflammatory cells were found in the ventricular wall of the explanted native heart. The absolute

Table 1

Certain clinical data in the 2 black patients with eosinophilic myocarditis in the portion of the left ventricular free wall excised ("LV core") to insert the left ventricular assist device (LVAD)

Variable	Case #1	Case #2	Case #3
Age (years) at LVAD insertion	55	64	72
Sex	M	F	M
Underlying cardiac condition	IDC	IDC	IC
Corticosteroid Rx after LVAD	+	+	0
Orthotopic heart transplant (OHT)	0	+ (age 70)	0
Eosinophilic myocarditis diagnosis in donor heart	-	0	-
Body mass index (kg/m^2)	37	25	35
Highest eosinophil percent	6	7	9.5*
Highest absolute eosinophil count (K/μL)	1.89	1.73	0.80*
Highest absolute eosinophil count before LVAD insertion (K/μL)	1.89	0.82	0.11
Number of medications used before LVAD implanted (no known to cause eosinophilic myocarditis)	30 (9)	21 (8)	27 (3)
Interval between onset of heart failure and LVAD insertion (years)	7	7	11
Highest Troponin I (ng/mL)	0.07	0.11	0.03
Ventricular rate (bpm) before LVAD	112	131	102
Total 12-lead QRS voltage before LVAD (mm)	111	119	64
LV core weight (g)	4.22	3.44	2.19
Heart weight (g)	-	315	-

bpm = beats per minute; F = female; IDC = idiopathic dilated cardiomyopathy; IC = ischemic cardiomyopathy; M = male.

* These values were reported 1 year before the LVAD insertion. By 40 days after LVAD insertion, the percentage of eosinophils had fallen to 3, and the absolute eosinophil count had fallen to 0.35 K/μL.

Department of Internal Medicine (Cardiology) and Pathology, Baylor Scott & White Heart and Vascular Institute, Baylor University Medical Center, Baylor Scott & White Health, Dallas, Texas. Manuscript received August 9, 2019; revised manuscript received and accepted October 23, 2019.

[1]Senior, Baylor University, Waco, Texas.

*Corresponding author: Tel: (214) 820-7911; fax: (214) 820-7533

E-mail address: william.roberts1@bswhealth.org (W.C. Roberts).

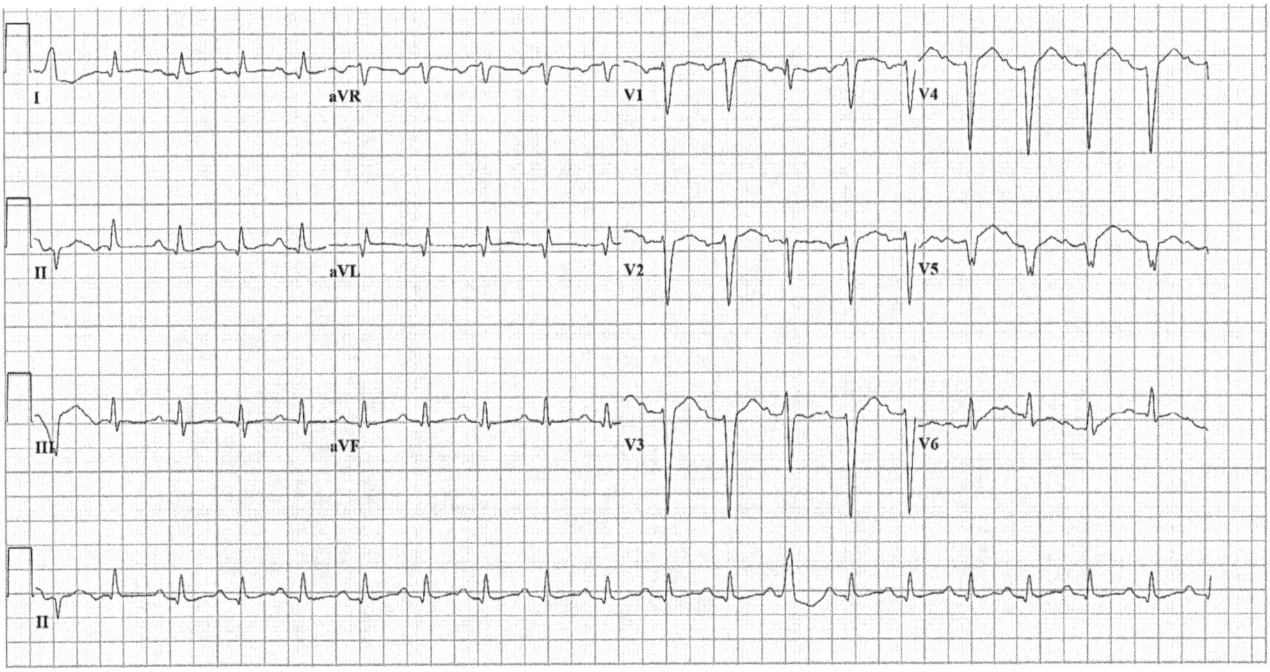

Figure 1. Case #1. Electrocardiogram recorded 6 days before insertion of the left ventricular assist device.

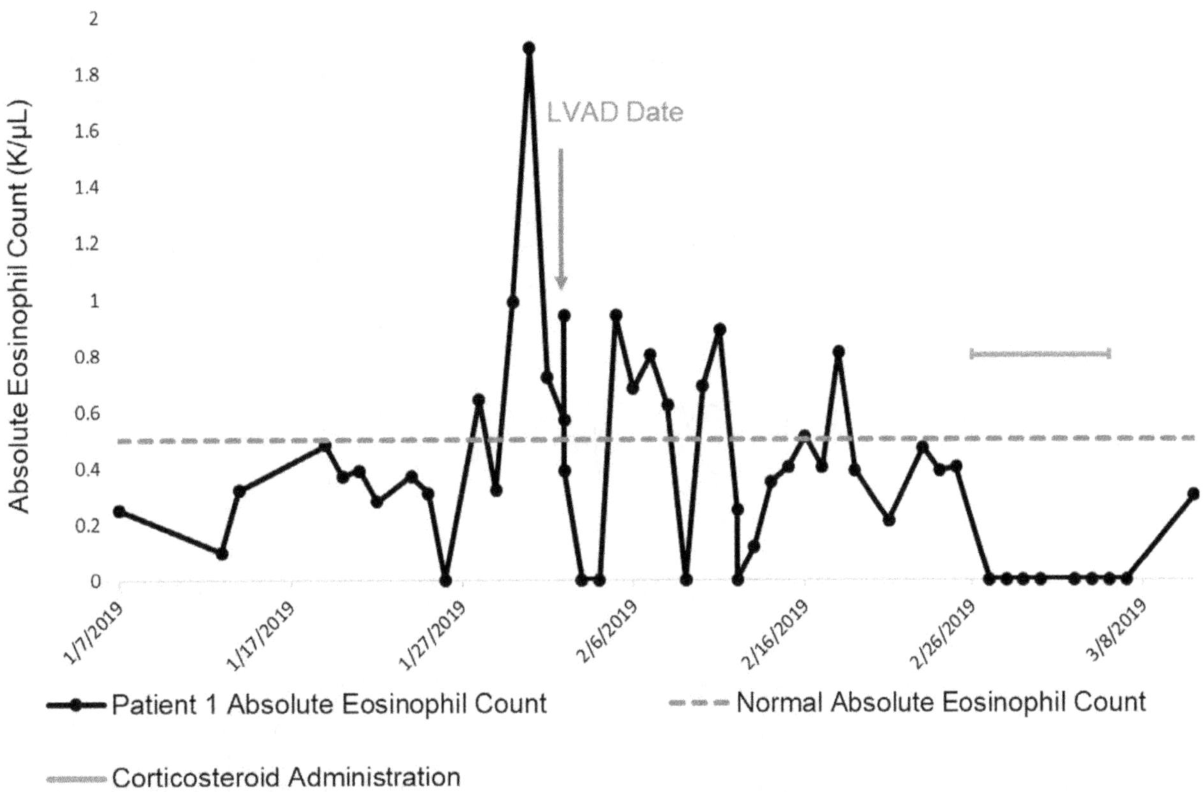

Figure 2. Case #1. Absolute eosinophil count just before and after removal of the left ventricular "core" to insert the left ventricular assist device.

eosinophil count in this patient immediately before the heart transplant was essentially normal (0.54 K/μL). The interval from the heart transplant to death in this patient was 4 months and the absolute eosinophil count just before death was 0. No eosinophils were found in the donor heart.

Discussion

Described herein are 3 patients in whom a portion of left ventricular wall was excised to insert a LVAD and histologic study of the left ventricular "core" produced

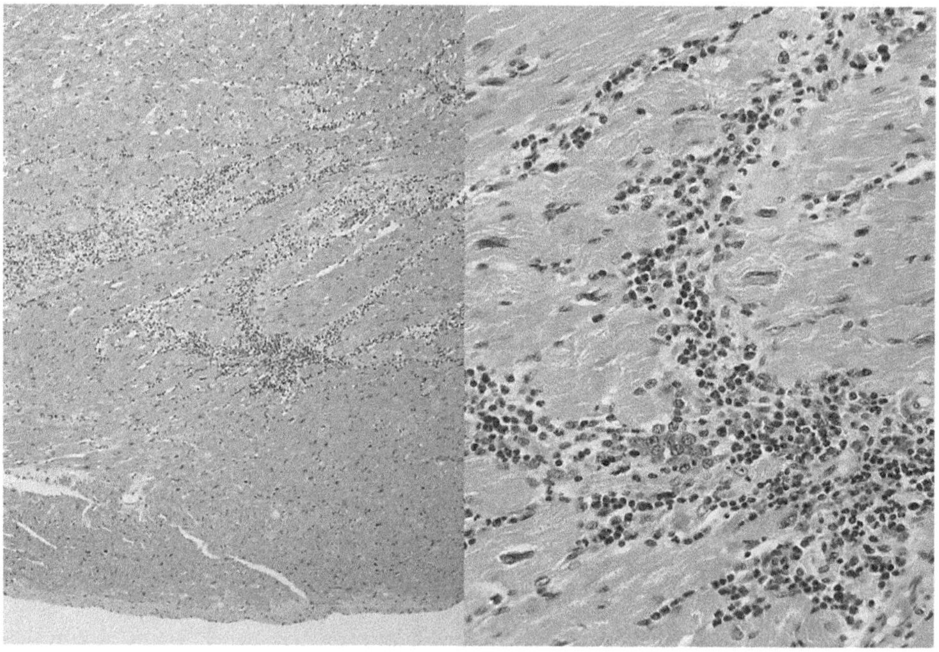

Figure 3. Case #1.Photomicrographs showing numerous collections of inflammatory cells in the myocardium (left) including numerous eosinophils (right). Hematoxylin/eosin stains ×100 (left) and ×400 (right).

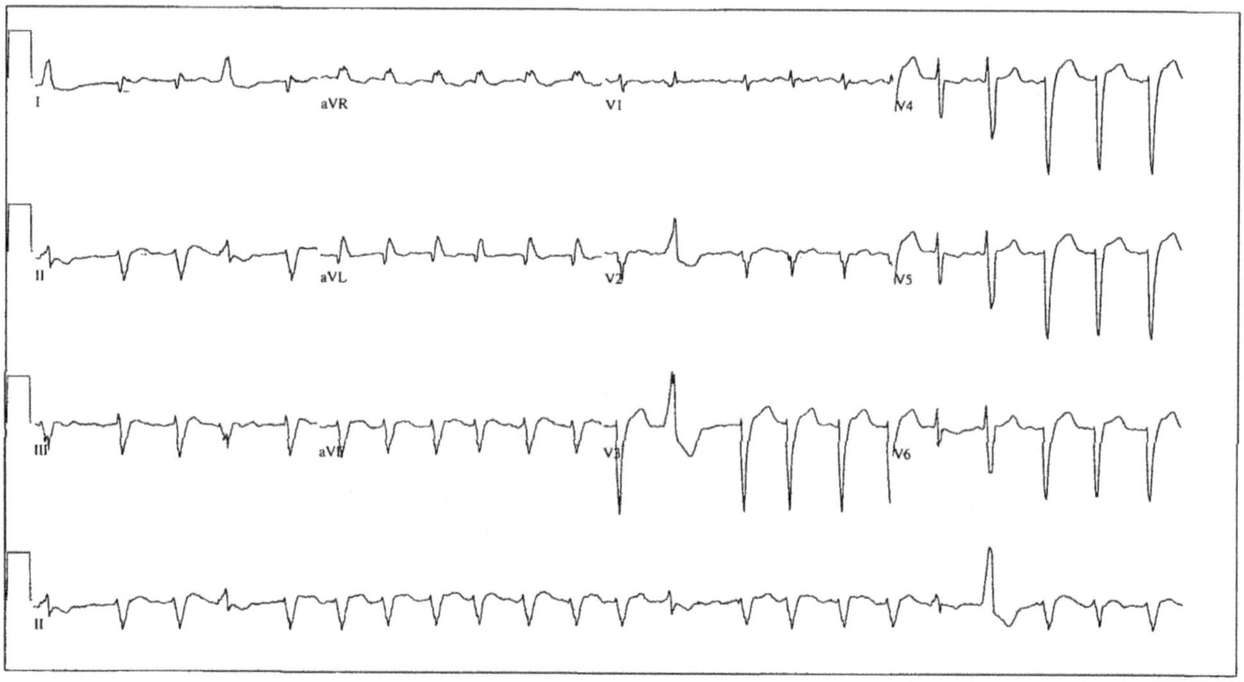

Figure 4. Case #2. Electrocardiogram recorded 1 day before LVAD insertion.

an unexpected finding, severe eosinophilic myocarditis. Idiopathic-dilated cardiomyopathy had been diagnosed clinically in 2 patients and ischemic cardiomyopathy in 1. Multiple examinations showed the percent of eosinophils and the total eosinophil counts to be elevated just before and after the LVAD was inserted in all 3 patients and their values had returned to normal by 11 days in case #1, by 18 days in case #2, and by 40 days in case #3. None of the 3 patients had received corticosteroid therapy at any time before the LVAD was inserted: case #1 received methylprednisolone (240 mg/day) for 3 days and prednisone (40 mg/day) for 7 days after the LVAD insertion; case #2 received fluticasone (usually 0.1% spray each day) for 11 days after the LVAD insertion, and case 3 did not receive any corticosteroid postoperatively.

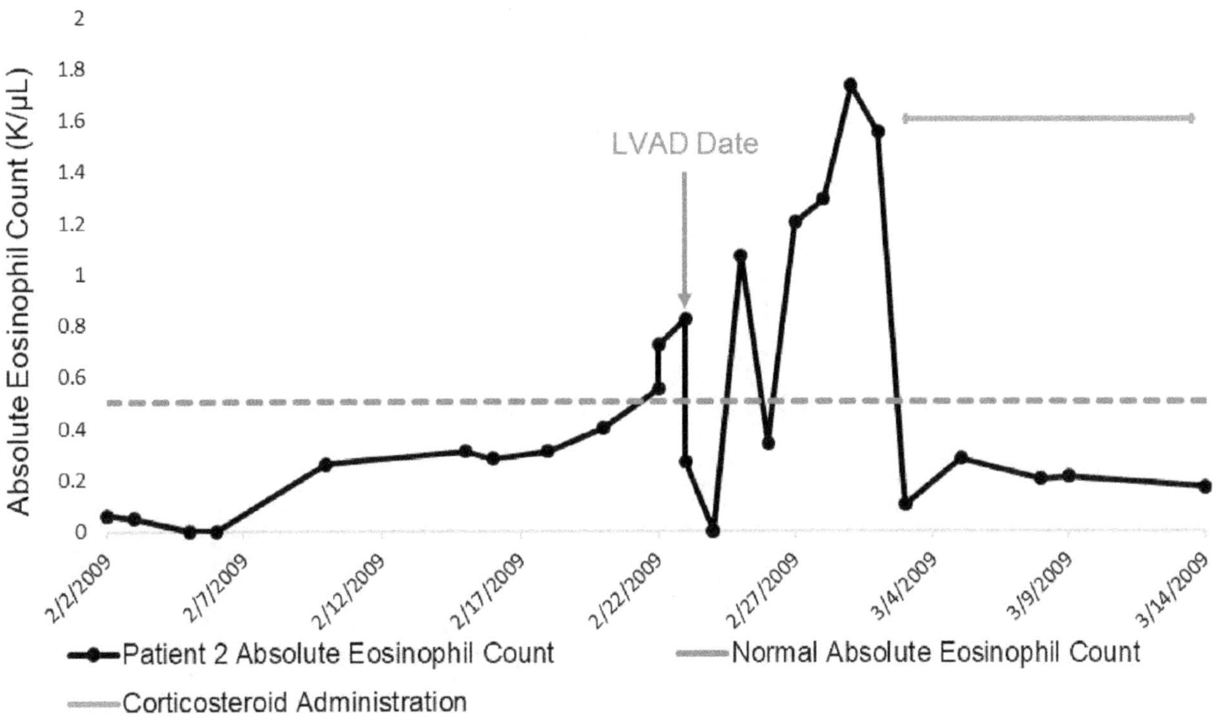

Figure 5. Case #2. Absolute eosinophil count just before and after removal of the left ventricular "core" to insert the LVAD.

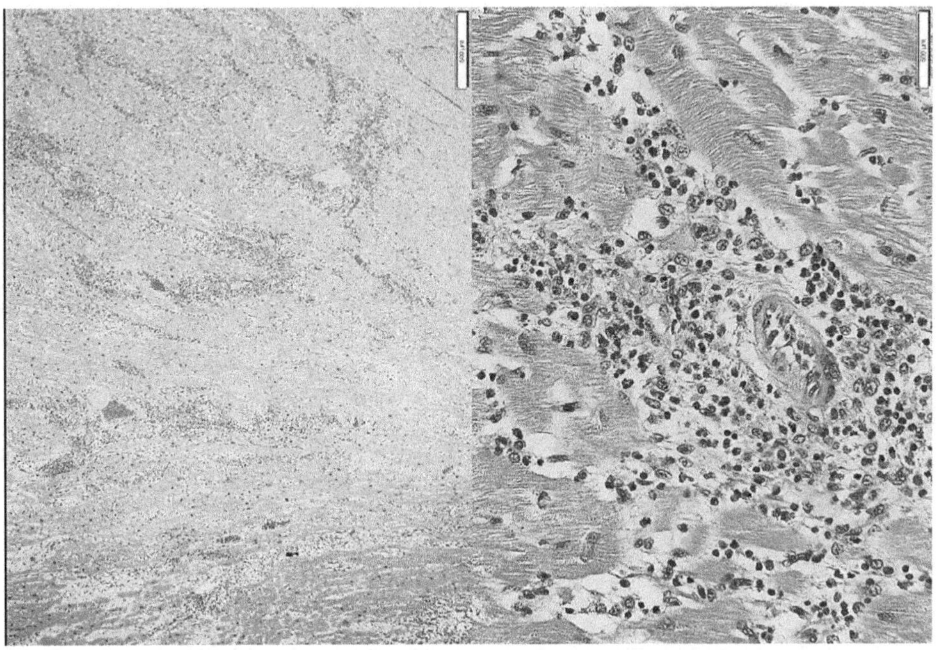

Figure 6. Case #2. Photomicrographs of the left ventricular "core" showing numerous collections of inflammatory cells including many eosinophils. Hematoxylin/eosin stains ×40 (left) and ×400 (right).

Diagnosis of eosinophilic myocarditis requires, of course, the presence of inflammatory infiltrates in the myocardial wall. Investigators have argued, however, about the extensiveness of the infiltrates and the numbers of eosinophils required for diagnosis. Some investigators require only an occasional eosinophil and no requirement that they be present on every slide.[2] We make this diagnosis only when the inflammatory infiltrates are extensive, including numerous eosinophils on every slide of myocardium.

Diagnosis of eosinophilic myocarditis has been made from myocardial samples from autopsies, from bioptome biopsies, and from left ventricular "cores" removed to insert LVADs. Previously published reports of this diagnosis made from examinations of the left ventricular "cores" are

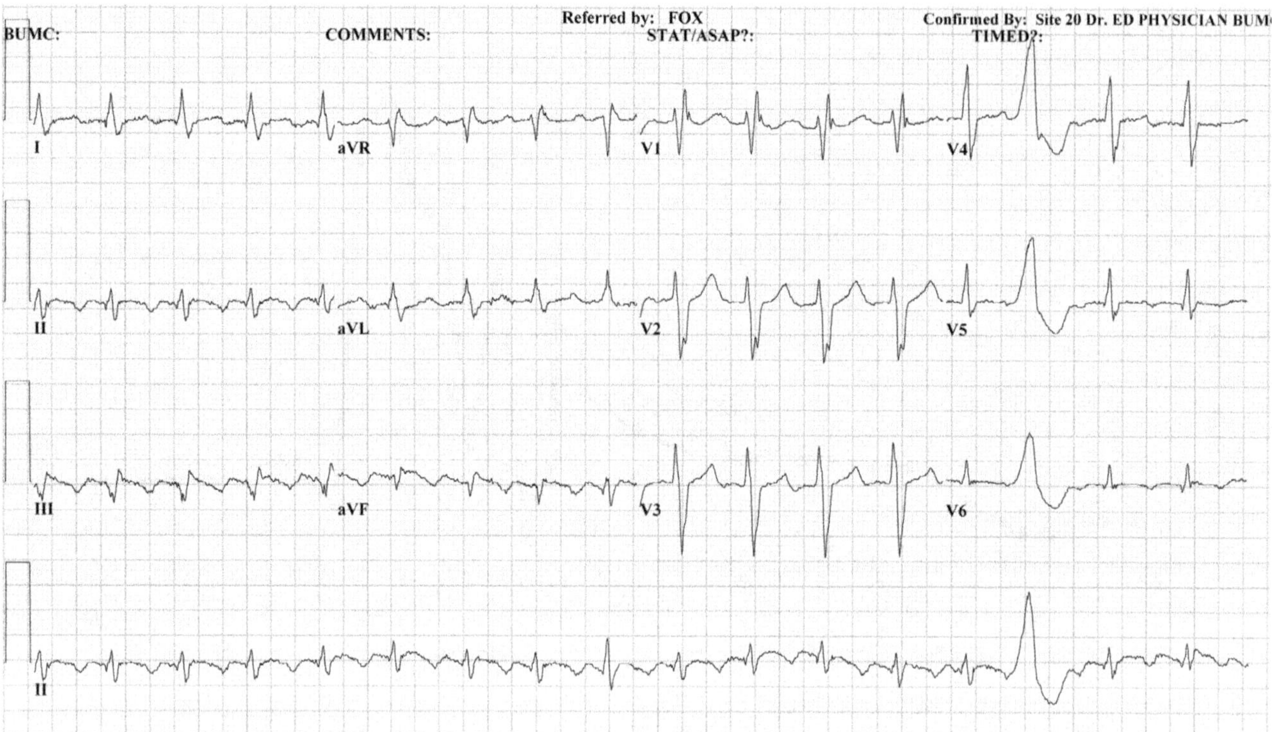

Figure 7. Case #3. Electrocardiogram recorded 7 days before the LVAD insertion. Note the standard is twice normal, so the total 12-lead QRS voltage is exceedingly low.

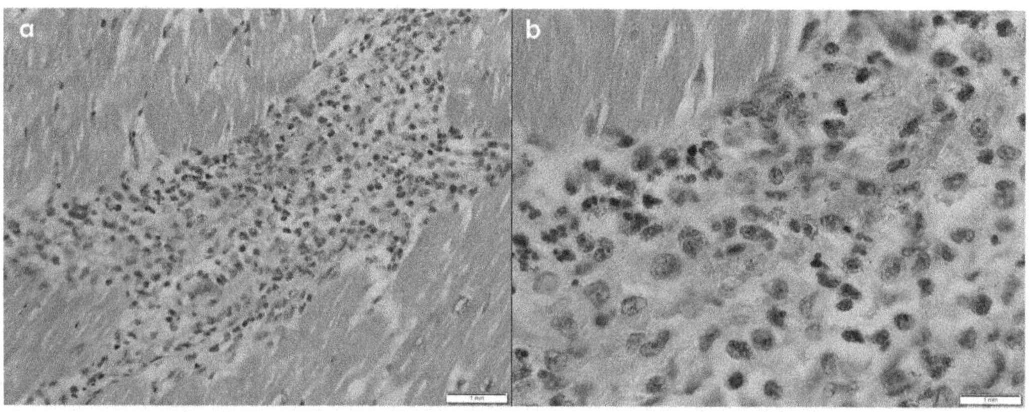

Figure 8. Case #3. Photomicrographs of the left ventricular "core" showing a collection of inflammatory cells, including numerous eosinophils. Hematoxylin/eosin stain, ×100 (left), ×400 (right).

Table 2
Findings in previously published articles where the diagnosis of eosinophilic myocarditis was made from examination of left ventricular "cores" removed at the times of left ventricular assist device insertion.

Year of publication	2002	2003	2004	2010	2014	2014	2014
First author	Maybaum	Grabellus	Takkenberg	Soon	Mody	Yoshoika	Raje
Case number	Case 1	Case 1	Case 10	Case 2	Case 7	Case 8	Case 1
Age (years)	35	52	-	28	39	55	69
Sex	M	M	-	F	M	M	M
Corticosteroid Rx before biopsy	-	-	-	+	-	-	-
Absolute eosinophil count (K/μL)	-	-	3	-	-	-	1.7
Interval (days) from histologic diagnosis to absence of any myocardial infiltrates	16	<30*	10	-	-	-	27

- = No information available
* = An estimate.

Table 3
Drugs known to have caused eosinophilic myocarditis

Acetazolamide	Isoniazid
Allopurinol	Lisinopril
Amoxicillin	Methyldopa
Ampicillin	**Milrinone**
Carvedilol	Omeprazole
Captopril	Oxyphenobutazone
Clozapine	Penicillin
Digoxin	Phenylbutazone
Dobutamine	**Spironolactone**
Enalapril	Streptomycin
Furosemide	Sulfadiazine
Hydrochlorothiazide	**Torsemide**
Imatinib	**Vancomycin**

The drugs in bold were administered to at least 1 of the 3 patients described.

summarized in Table 2.[2–8] In 4 of the 7 previously described cases listed in Table 2, subsequent myocardial biopsies performed demonstrated no evidence of residual myocarditis in <30 days in 3 patients and probably <30 in all 4 patients.

Diagnosis of eosinophilic myocarditis by "instruments of precision" other than tissue examination is not possible presently. The electrocardiogram, however, may be of potential indirect value. In all 3 patients described herein, the heart rate was >100/minute and the total 12-lead QRS voltage was low just before the LVAD was inserted.[1] Sinus tachycardia and minor T-wave and ST segment changes have been noted previously.[9–12]

The cause of the eosinophilic myocarditis in our 3 patients is unclear. Each was on multiple medications before the LVAD was inserted (Table 3), some of which have been recognized to be associated with eosinophilic myocarditis. The fact that the absolute eosinophil counts fell dramatically during the first 40 postoperative days suggests a previous allergic reaction to possibly one or more drugs. Some drugs administered immediately before LVAD insertion were eliminated immediately thereafter, a fact that may support the allergic thesis.

1. Roberts WC, Filardo G, Ko JM, Siegel RJ, Dollar AL, Ross EM, Shirani J. Comparison of total 12-lead QRS voltage in a variety of cardiac conditions and its usefulness in predicting increased cardiac mass. *Am J Cardiol* 2013;112:904–909.
2. Takkenberg JJ, Czer LS, Fishbein MC, Luthringer DJ, Quartel AW, Mirocha J, Queral CA, Blanche C, Trento A. Eosinophilic myocarditis in patients awaiting heart transplantation. *Crit Care Med* 2004;32:714–721.
3. Maybaum S, Stockwell P, Naka Y, Catanese K, Flannery M, Fisher P, Oz M, Mancini D. Assessment of myocardial recovery in a patient with acute myocarditis supported with a left ventricular assist device: a case report. *J Heart Lung Transplant* 2003;22:202–209.
4. Grabellus F, Hoffmeier A, Schmitz KJ, Kandolf R, Bültmann BD, Scheld HH, Baba HA. Resolved hypersensitivity myocarditis after ventricular circulatory assist. *Ann Thorac Surg* 2003;76:2102–2104.
5. Bourgeois GP, Cafardi JA, Groysman V, Pamboukian SV, Kirklin JK, Andea AA, Hughey LC. Fulminant myocarditis as a late sequela of DRESS: two cases. *J Am Acad Dermatol* 2011;65:889–890.
6. Mody KP, Takayama H, Landes E, Yuzefpolskaya M, Colombo PC, Naka Y, Jorde UP, Uriel N. Acute mechanical circulatory support for fulminant myocarditis complicated by cardiogenic shock. *J Cardiovasc Transl Res* 2014;7:156–164.
7. Yoshioka D, Matsumiya G, Toda K, Sakaguchi T, Yoshikawa Y, Saito S, Matsuda H, Sawa Y. Clinical results with Jarvik 2000 axial flow left ventricular assist device: Osaka University Experience. *J Artif Organs* 2014;17:308–314.
8. Raje VP, Lewis NP, Katlaps GJ, Quader MA, Shah KB, Mankad AK. Dobutamine induced eosinophilic myocarditis and right heart failure requiring emergent biventricular assist device implantation. *ASAIO J* 2015;61:213–215.
9. Cooper LT, Zehr KJ. Biventricular assist device placement and immunosuppression as therapy for necrotizing eosinophilic myocarditis. *Nat Clin Pract Cardiovasc Med* 2005;2:544–548.
10. Al Ali AM, Straatman LP, Allard MF, Ignaszewski AP. Eosinophilic myocarditis: case series and review of literature. *Can J Cardiol* 2006;22:1233–1237.
11. Li H, Dai Z, Wang B, Huang W. A case report of eosinophilic myocarditis and a review of the relevant literature. *BMC Cardiovasc Disord* 2015;15:15.
12. Brambatti M, Matassini MV, Adler ED, Klingel K, Camici PG, Ammirati E. Eosinophilic myocarditis: characteristics, treatment, and outcomes. *J Am Coll Cardiol* 2017;70:2363–2375.

Massive Cardiomegaly (>1000 g Heart) and Obesity

William C. Roberts, MD[a,b,*], and Omar S. Khan[a,b,#]

Described herein are certain clinical and morphologic findings in 9 patients who at necropsy had hearts weighing >1000 g, a weight approximately 3 times normal. With the exception of 2 patients with hypertrophic cardiomyopathy, the common finding in the remaining 7 patients was obesity. None had valvular heart disease, the previously described major cause of massive cardiomegaly. Thus, obesity needs to be added to the causes of massive cardiomegaly, a cause not previously recognized. Electrocardiograms in 4 patients disclosed high total 12-lead QRS voltage on the electrocardiogram in only one despite the massive cardiomegaly. **(Am J Cardiol 2020;125:277–281)**

Massive cardiomegaly (heart weight >1000 g) is infrequent, occurring in about 1 of every 1000 autopsies done in the USA.[1,2] In 1985, nearly 40 years ago, one of us described electrocardiographic and morphologic findings in 23 patients whose hearts weighed >1000 g[2]: 18 had primary valvular heart disease, 4 had hypertrophic cardiomyopathy, and 1 had ventricular septal defect. Since then we have collected the hearts of 9 additional patients weighing >1000 g: none had primary valvular heart disease, 2 had hypertrophic cardiomyopathy, and the remaining 7 were obese. This study seemed worthwhile because the cause of the massive cardiomegaly in most was quite different from that presented in our initial study.[3,4]

Methods

The clinical records were searched in each of the 9 patients and pertinent data recorded. The total 12-lead QRS voltage was determined in the 4 patients with available electrocardiograms (Figure 1).

All hearts were weighed by one of us (WCR) after opening the heart from 2 to 5 days after fixation in 10% formaldehyde by transverse cuts of the ventricular walls each about 1 cm in thickness and parallel to the posterior atrioventricular sulcus (Figure 2) or by left and right parasagittal cuts (Figure 3). (Previous studies have only used weights recorded in autopsy protocols.) Before weighing, all remnants of parietal pericardium were excised, and the aorta and pulmonary trunk were incised about 2 cm cephalad to their respective sinotubular junctions. Additionally, the cut surfaces before weighing were patted with paper towels to remove excess formaldehyde water. Each heart was weighed on scales accurate to 1 g. The epicardial coronary arteries including their ostia in the aorta were carefully examined by extending a probe in each and by examining their cut surface lumens after cross-sectional cuts. The myocardium was carefully examined for foci of necrosis or fibrosis or other lesions. At least 4 sections of ventricular myocardium extending from epicardium to endocardium were examined in each heart.

[a]Baylor Scott & White Heart and Vascular Institute, Dallas, Texas; and [b]Departments of Internal Medicine (Cardiology) and Pathology, Baylor University Medical Center, Baylor Scott & White Health, Dallas, Texas. Manuscript received August 17, 2019; revised manuscript received and accepted October 24, 2019.

[#]Junior, University of Texas at Dallas, Richardson, Texas.

*Corresponding author: Tel: (214) 820-7911; fax: (214) 820-7533.

E-mail address: william.roberts1@bswhealth.org (W.C. Roberts).

Results

Pertinent clinical and morphologic findings in each of the 9 patients are presented in Table 1. All were male aged 15 to 67 years (mean 44). None either clinically or at necropsy had evidence of coronary artery disease. Eight of the 9 patients had systemic hypertension and 5 had diabetes mellitus. The body weight, known in 5 patients, ranged from 242 to 434 pounds (mean 306), and their body mass indexes ranged from 32 to 65 kg/m^2 (mean 44). Two patients were known to have atrial fibrillation and 2 were known not to have this arrhythmia and all 4 of these patients were known to have complete bundle branch block, 2 left and 2 right: 4 were known to have heart block, second degree in 2 and third degree (complete) in 2. Total 12-lead QRS voltage (10 mm standard)[5] in 4 patients ranged from 133 to 249 mm (mean 172); this voltage was >175 mm (maybe the upper limit of normal[6]) in only 1 of the patients (Figure 1). Obstructive sleep apnea was recognized in 3 patients. The 4 patients recognized as having heart failure had had it from 6 to 11 years.

The causes of death are listed in the table. Four hearts are illustrated in Figures 2 and 3. Only 1 patient (#2, Table 1) died from a non-cardiovascular cause and that was opiate overdose. Two patients (#1 and #9) died from consequences of hypertrophic cardiomyopathy. Patient #6 had a 5.1 cm fusiform aneurysm involving the ascending aorta and died from extensive bleeding postoperatively after its resection. Two patients (#4 and #5) died suddenly outside the hospital. As in the other 7 patients, their coronary arteries were wide open and devoid of atherosclerotic plaques. The remaining 3 patients died from chronic heart failure of undetermined cause.

Discussion

Described herein are findings in 9 obese men whose hearts at autopsy weighed >1000 g (All were weighed by the same method by the same person [WCR].). The unusual feature is that none had evidence either clinically or

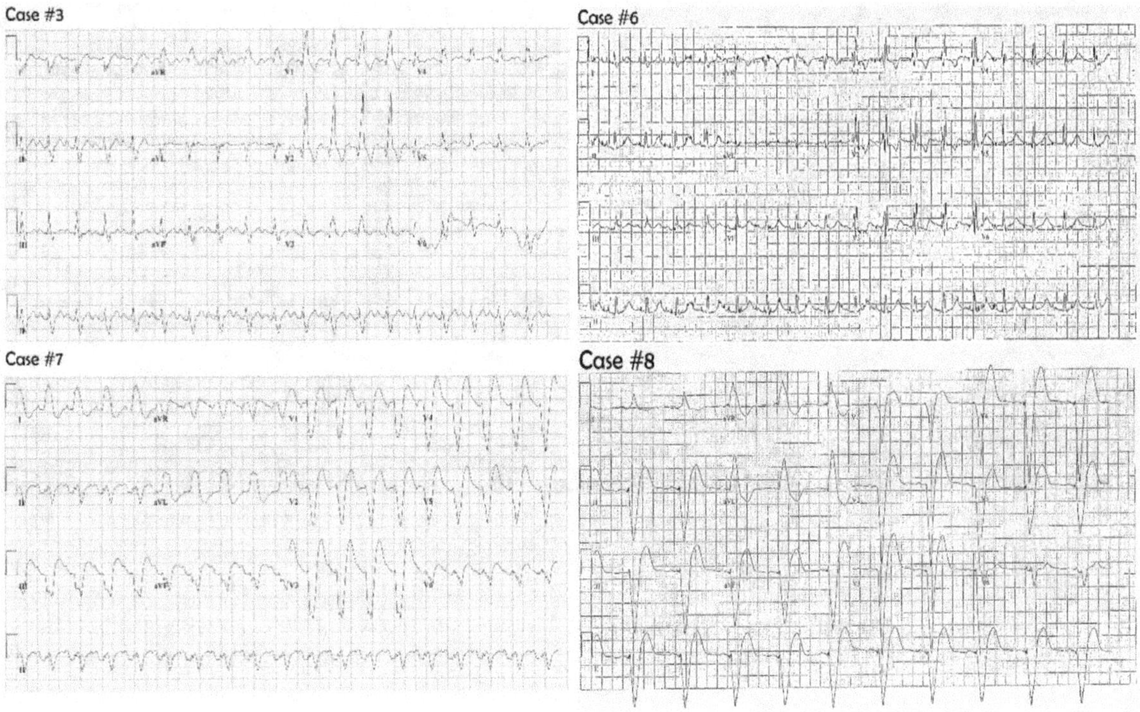

Figure 1. Electrocardiograms recorded from 1 to 10 days before death in 4 of the 9 patients: Case #3 (*top left*); case #6 (*top right*); case #7 (*bottom left*), and case #8 (*bottom right*).

morphologically of valvular heart disease, the usual cause of massive cardiomegaly. The valvular disease most commonly is pure aortic regurgitation (no element of stenosis) with or without associated mitral regurgitation or ventricular septal defect.[2] All 8 adults also had systemic hypertension; the 1 non-obese patient (#1, Table 1), who was only 15 years of age, had Danon's syndrome, a known to cause massive cardiomegaly.[7] Previously, obesity was not reported to be associated with massive cardiomegaly. Warnes and Roberts[3] in 1984, for example, reported 12 patients who weighed 310 to >510 pounds (mean 381), and their hearts ranged in weight from 380 to 990 g (mean 616): the hearts in the 7 men ranged from 410 to 990 g (mean 684). Hypertrophic cardiomyopathy has been recognized previously as a cause of massive cardiomegaly.[8]

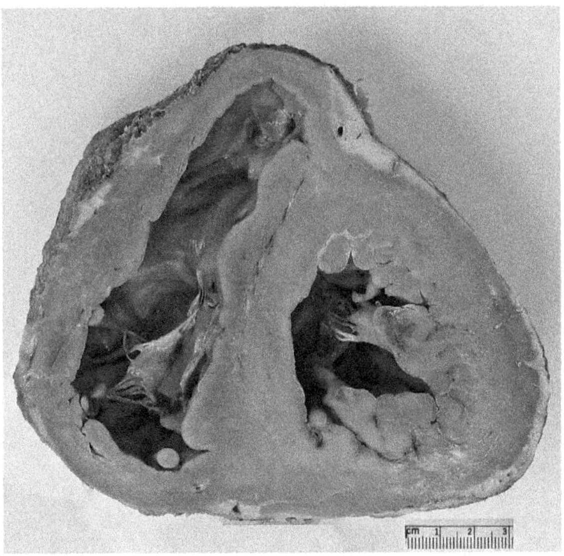

Figure 2. Case #3, Table 1. Cross section of the cardiac ventricles showing thickened walls, dilated chambers, and a small scar in the posterior wall of left ventricle. The lumens of the left anterior descending and first diagonal coronary arteries are wide open.

Several articles have been published on the relation of adiposity to heart disease. "Fatty heart" for >100 years has been considered 2 types (1) fatty infiltration, an increase in adipose tissue between myocardial fibers, primarily in the right ventricular free wall, from infiltration of the excessive subepicardial adipose, and (2) fatty degeneration, deposits of fatty droplets within myocardial cells.

In the 19th century no heart disease was regarded with more apprehension than fatty degeneration which was considered the most common form of "cardiac insufficiency," something today that would be called "heart failure".[9] George Gibson (1854-1913) in his book on "Diseases of the Heart and Aorta" published in 1898 stated that "...fatty degeneration of the heart is the most common cause of sudden death"[10] even though Osler (1849-1919) in 1892 in his first edition of "Principles and Practice of Medicine" had indicated, in his view, that coronary artery disease was its most common cause.[11]

Joseph H. Pratt (1872-1956) in 1904 reviewed the causes of "cardiac insufficiency" (i.e., heart failure) and stated "...that disease of the coronary arteries is one of the most frequent causes...".[12] Pratt also concluded "...that there is no evidence to show that fatty metamorphosis of the heart produces cardiac insufficiency."

One of the first recorded cases of fatty degeneration was reported by John Cheyne (1777-1836) in 1818 and was the

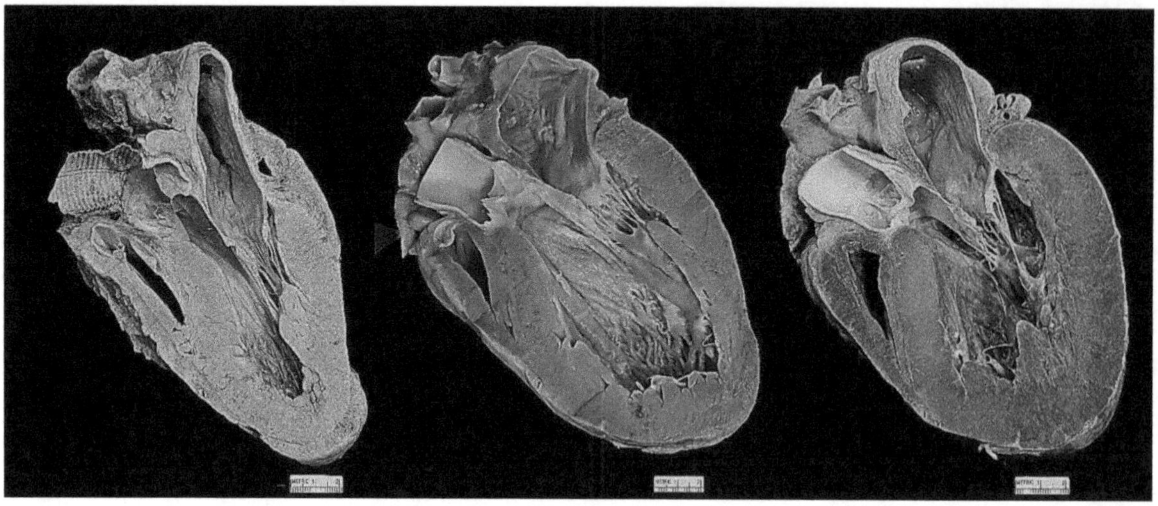

Figure 3. Left parasagittal views of the left side of the hearts in three patients: Case #6 (*left*); case #7 (*center*); and case #8 (*right*).

first case in which the peculiar modification of respiration, now known as Cheyne-Stokes Respiration, was described.[13] In 1827, Robert Adams (1791-1875) with William Stokes (1804-1878) described several cases in which a persistently slow heart rate was associated with attacks of unconsciousness, later known as the Stokes-Adams syndrome.[14] The

Table 1
Certain clinical and morphologic findings in the 9 men whose hearts at necropsy weighed >1000 g

Variable	Case numbers								
	#1	#2	#3	#4	#5	#6	#7	#8	#9
1 Age (Years)	15	28	35	36	40	51	56	65	67
2 Race	H	W	B	B	B	W	B	W	W
3 Heart weight (g)	1416	1060	1045	1190	1080	1020	1020	1070	1004
4 Body weight (lbs)	–	434	267	–	–	312	–	275	242
5 Height (inches)	–	68	70	–	–	67	–	75	72
6 Body mass index (kg/m^2)	–	65	38	–	–	50	–[††]	35	32
7 Coronary artery disease	0	0	0	0	0	0	0	0	0
8 Systemic hypertension	0	+	+	+	+	+	+	+	+
9 Diabetes mellitus	0	0	+	0	0	+	+	+	+
10 Artrial fibrillation	–	–	+	–	–	+	0	0	–
11 Bundle branch block	–	–	+(R)	–	–	+(R)	+(L)	+(L)	–
12 Total 12-lead QRS Voltage (mm)	–	–	133	–	–	142	164	249	–
13 Obstructive sleep apnea	0	0	0	0	0	+	0	+	+
14 Chronic kidney disease	0	0	+	0	0	0	0	+	0
15 Heart block (degree)	–	–	0	–	–	+ (2nd)	+ (3rd)	+ (2nd)	+ (3rd)
16 Gout	0	0	+	0	0	0	+	0	0
17 Total cholesterol (mg/dL)	–	–	67	–	–	Ó	–	205	–
18 LDL cholesterol (mg/dl)	–	–	49	–	–	–	–	125	–
19 HDL cholesterol (mg/dl)	–	–	11	–	–	–	–	23	–
20 Triglycerides (mg/dl)	–	–	158	–	–	–	–	461	–
21 Number of medications[‡‡]	–	–	9	–	–	10	17	17	–
22 Duration of HF (years)	–	–	6	–	11	–	7	7	–
23 Cause of death	DS	NC[*]	C[†]	C[‡]	C[§]	C[¶]	C[†]	C[†]	C[**]

B = black; BMI = body mass index; DS = Danon's Syndrome; H = Hispanic; HDL = high-density lipoprotein; HF = heart failure; L = left; LDL = low-density lipoprotin; NC = non-cardiac; R = right; W = white.

* Probable opiate overdose - died suddenly;

† Chronic heart failure;

‡ Sudden death while driving with chest pain. Coronary arteries wide open;

§ Sudden death (ventricular fibrillation) outside the hospital. Coronary arteries normal;

¶ A 5.1 cm aneurysm in ascending aorta was resected and he died 39 days postoperatively from bleeding. The wall of the aneurysm was histologically normal and probably was the consequence of systemic hypertension;

** Probably hypertrophic cardiomyopathy - mitral valve replacement 19 days before death;

†† Patient had a gastric bypass;

‡‡ On admission (home medications).

underlying condition in both cases was believed by the authors to be "fatty metamorphosis."

Not much happened in this arena thereafter until 1933 when Smith and Willius[15] published "Adiposity of the Heart" describing clinical and morphologic cardiac findings in 133 obese adults (body weight ranged from 13-to-170% [mean 45] above ideal). In 51 (38%) of the 133 adults the heart was normal except for the excessive adipose tissue; in 9 patients (7%) "cardiac insufficiency" (i.e., heart failure) was present without an apparent cause; 60 patients (45%) had systemic hypertension, and of the remaining 15 cases, (11%), 9 had coronary disease and 6, miscellaneous causes. The heart in the hypertensive patients, the largest of their patients, ranged in weight from 283 to 807 g, much less than in our 9 patients.

In 1965, Amad and associates[16] described "The Cardiac Pathology of Chronic Exogenous Obesity." These authors described necropsy findings in 12 "selected" adults whose body weight ranged from 99 to 225 Kg (mean 150 Kg [330 lbs.]). The heart weights in the 12 patients ranged from 400 to 1100 g (mean 575), including only one patient whose heart weighed >1000 g. Only 4 of the patients had hearts weighing >600 g. The authors concluded "...that manifestations of myocardial insufficiency do occur in very obese subjects without evidence of other heart disease..." In their study, patients whose indirect blood pressure was >150/90 mm Hg were excluded. Similarly, patients with "...clinical signs or pathologic evidences of coronary atherosclerosis, rheumatic fever, syphilis, myxedema, or other chronic diseases with possible cardiac effects..." were excluded. Only 3 of their 12 patients had evidence of heart failure.

Alexander and colleagues[17] may have been the first to examine physiologic effects of extreme obesity. These authors concluded that "...massive amounts of adipose tissue bring about an increase in systemic blood flow which is distributed largely to the fat deposits themselves, and which may be great enough to double the cardiac output at rest." This increased demand upon the heart "...leads to ventricular hypertrophy, and, on occasion, to the development of myocardial failure."

In the last 20 years a number of studies, mainly reviews, have described effects of obesity on left ventricular structure and function,[18–23] and its role in heart failure. In essence, these studies have shown that obese patients compared to those without obesity have increased left ventricular mass; an increased frequency of heart failure, systemic hypertension and diabetes mellitus, and reduced left ventricular systolic and diastolic function. There was a strong association between the degree of obesity and the frequency of these consequences. MaGavock and associates[22] have suggested that the mechanism for heart disease in obese patients is excessive lipid (triglyceride) accumulation within myocardial cells, a direct cardiotoxic effect leading to left ventricular remodeling and dilated cardiomyopathy.

An interesting paradox exists in obese patients and the quantity of adipose tissue in their hearts. In those containing a great deal of adipose tissue, the heart may float in a container of formaldehyde (fat is lighter than myocardium) but these hearts with few exceptions weigh <600 g, usually quite a bit less.[24–26] In hearts weighing >1000 g the amount of myocardium overwhelms the quantity of fat and therefore these huge hearts, despite their association with generalized obesity, are unable to come to the surface in a container of formaldehyde. Additionally, as in our 9 patients described herein, there was relatively little subepicardial adipose tissue.

1. Pena C. Massive cardiac hypertrophy. Report of 15 hearts weighing 1000 g or more. *Am J Cardiol* 1963;11:18–23.
2. Roberts WC, Podolak MJ. The king of hearts: analysis of 23 patients with hearts weighing 1000 g or more. *Am J Cardiol* 1985;55:485–494.
3. Warnes CA, Roberts WC. The heart in massive (more than 300 pounds or 136 kilograms) obesity: analysis of 12 patients studied in necropsy. *Am J Cardiol* 1984;54:1087–1091.
4. Roberts WC. The heart at necropsy in massive obesity (>300 pounds or >136 kilograms). *Am J Cardiol* 2002;89:1451.
5. Roberts WC, Filardo G, Ko JM, Siegel RJ, Dollar AL, Ross EM, Shirani J. Comparison of total 12-lead QRS voltage in a variety of cardiac conditions and its usefulness in predicting increased cardiac mass. *Am J Cardiol* 2013;112:904–909.
6. Odom H II, Davis JL, Dinh H, Baker BJ, Roberts WC, Murphy ML. QRS voltage measurements in autopsied men free of cardiopulmonary disease: a basis for evaluating total QRS voltage as an index of left ventricular hypertrophy. *Am J Cardiol* 1986;58:801–804.
7. Maron BJ, Roberts WC, Arad M, Haas TS, Spirito P, Wright GB, Almquist AK, Baffa JM, Saul JP, Ho CY, Seidman J, Seidman CE. Clinical outcome and phenotypic expression in LAMP2 cardiomyopathy. *JAMA* 2009;301:1253–1259.
8. Roberts CS, Roberts WC. Hypertrophic cardiomyopathy as a cause of massive cardiomegaly (>1000 g). *Am J Cardiol* 1989;64:1209–1210.
9. Bedford E. The story of fatty heart. A disease of Victorian times. *Br Heart J* 1972;34(1):23–28.
10. Gibson GA. *Diseases of the Heart and Aorta*. Edinburgh: Young J. Pentland; 1898:649.
11. Osler W. *The Principles and Practice of Medicine: Designed for The Use of Practitioners and Students of Medicine*. New York: D. Appleton & Co.; 1892:1079.
12. Pratt JH. On the causes of cardiac insufficiency. *Bull Johns Hopkins Hosp* 1904;15:301–309.
13. Cheyne J. A case of apoplexy in which the fleshy part of the heart was converted into fat. *Dublin Hospital Reports* 1818;2:216–223.
14. Stokes W. *The Diseases of the Heart and the Aorta*. Dublin: Hodges and Smith; 1854:689.
15. Smith HL, Willius FA. Adiposity of the heart: a clinical and pathologic study of one hundred and thirty-six obese patients. *Arch Intern Med (Chic)* 1933;52:911–931.
16. Amad KH, Brennan JC, Alexander JK. The cardiac pathology of chronic exogenous obesity. *Circulation* 1965;32:740–745.
17. Alexander JK, Dennis EW, Smith WG, Amad KH, Duncan WC, Austin RC. Blood volume, cardiac output, and distribution of systemic blood flow in extreme obesity. *Cardiovasc Res Cent Bull* 1962-1963 Winter;1:39–44.
18. Crisostomo LL, Araújo LM, Câmara E, Carvalho C, Silva FA, Vieira M, Mendes CM, Rabelo A Jr. Left ventricular mass and function in young obese women. *Int J Obes Relat Metab Disord* 2001;25:233–238.
19. Kenchaiah S, Evans JC, Levy D, Wilson PW, Benjamin EJ, Larson MG, Kannel WB, Vasan RS. Obesity and the risk of heart failure. *N Engl J Med* 2002;347:305–313.
20. Wong CY, O'Moore-Sullivan T, Leano R, Byrne N, Beller E, Marwick TH. Alterations of left ventricular myocardial characteristics associated with obesity. *Circulation* 2004;110:3081–3087.
21. Peterson LR, Waggoner AD, Schechtman KB, Meyer T, Gropler RJ, Barzilai B, Dávila-Román VG. Alterations in left ventricular structure and function in young healthy obese women: assessment by echocardiography and tissue Doppler imaging. *J Am Coll Cardiol* 2004;43:1399–1404.
22. McGavock JM, Victor RG, Unger RH, Szczepaniak LS, American College of Physicians and the American Physiological Society. Adiposity of the heart, revisited. *Ann Intern Med* 2006;144:517–524.
23. Cuspidi C, Rescaldani M, Sala C, Grassi G. Left-ventricular hypertrophy and obesity: a systematic review and meta-analysis of echocardiographic studies. *J Hypertens* 2014;32:16–25.

24. Roberts WC, Won VS, Vasudevan A, Ko JM, Guileyardo JM. Frequency of massive cardiac adiposity (floating heart) at necropsy and comparison of clinical and morphologic variables with cases with nonmassive cardiac adiposity at a single Texas hospital, 2013 to 2014. *Am J Cardiol* 2016;117:1006–1013.

25. Roberts WC, Won VS, Vasudevan A, Ko JM, Hall SA, Gonzalez-Stawinski GV. Frequency of massive cardiac adiposity (floating heart) in the native hearts of patients having heart transplantation at a single Texas hospital (2013 to 2015) and comparison of various clinical and morphologic variables in the patients with massive versus nonmassive cardiac adiposity. *Am J Cardiol* 2016;117:1375–1380.

26. Roberts WC, Won VS, Vasudevan A, Guileyardo JM. Characteristics of hearts at necropsy in patients treated chronically with prednisone (The Corticosteroid Heart). *Am J Cardiol* 2016;118:1935–1940.

www.ingramcontent.com/pod-product-compliance
Lightning Source LLC
LaVergne TN
LVHW062139200926
848484LV00007B/1834